# Pancreatic Transplantation

# Pancreatic Transplantation

Edited by

## Robert J. Corry

*Thomas E. Starzl Transplantation Institute*
*University of Pittsburgh School of Medicine*
*Pittsburgh, Pennsylvania, U.S.A.*

## Ron Shapiro

*Thomas E. Starzl Transplantation Institute*
*University of Pittsburgh School of Medicine*
*Pittsburgh, Pennsylvania, U.S.A.*

**informa**
healthcare

New York London

Informa Healthcare USA, Inc.
270 Madison Avenue
New York, NY 10016

© 2007 by Informa Healthcare USA, Inc.
Informa Healthcare is an Informa business

No claim to original U.S. Government works
Printed in the United States of America on acid-free paper
10 9 8 7 6 5 4 3 2 1

International Standard Book Number-10: 0-8247-2879-3 (Hardcover)
International Standard Book Number-13: 978-0-8247-2879-3 (Hardcover)

**Visit the Informa Web site at**
**www.informa.com**

**and the Informa Healthcare Web site at**
**www.informahealthcare.com**

# DEDICATION

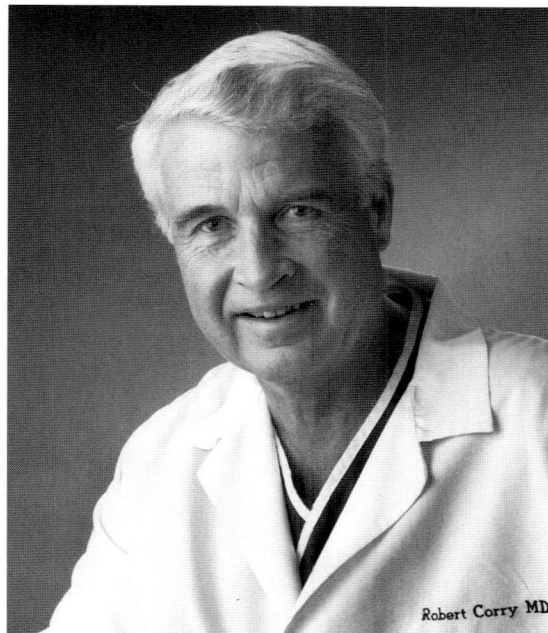

Robert Corry MD

*This book is dedicated to the memory of Robert J. Corry, M.D.,*
*pioneer transplant surgeon, gifted mentor, and warm and generous friend.*
*We miss you still—may this book be your legacy.*

# Preface

This book started out as a companion to a textbook on renal transplantation that we published in 1997. At the time that we began this project in 1998, there had not been a textbook on pancreatic transplantation since Carl Groth's book, which had been published in 1988, and the field had clearly advanced to the point where an updated text was needed. Professor Groth and his group in Stockholm, while kind enough to contribute three chapters to this book, had made it clear that they would not be writing a second edition. Thus, we began the long process of a new book on pancreatic transplantation. The path took a sad and unexpected twist with the premature passing of the lead editor, Dr. Robert J. Corry, in February 2002. At the time, the book was over 60% complete, and we elected to finish the book, keeping Dr. Corry as the senior editor and dedicating it to his memory.

The book, while not divided into specific sections, is clearly composed of many parts. The introductory chapters discuss the short-time outcomes, long-term outcomes, and the history of pancreatic transplantation. The main body of the book goes on to describe specific topics in clinical pancreas transplantation, including recipient evaluation, donor selection and organ recovery, anesthetic aspects, technical aspects, issues in patient management and immunosuppression after transplantation, pathologic and radiologic features, a number of chapters on complications after pancreatic transplantation, and additional topics on islets, pregnancy, and transplant coordination. The final part of the book comprises a number of single center chapters from many of the major programs in the United States and Europe. The result is a true multi-authored text, with a number of different points of view described. This is appropriate, for while pancreatic transplantation has matured into a worthwhile therapeutic endeavor, it is still early enough in its development that there are a number of divergent approaches regarding both the technical aspects and immunosuppressive management after transplantation. It is thus our hope that this book will serve not to define the one and only true approach to pancreatic transplantation, but to describe the ongoing variation in clinical practice today.

This book has been a long time in coming. We hope you enjoy it.

*Ron Shapiro*

# Acknowledgments

It is not possible to write a book of this nature without the support of a large number of individuals. First, we would like to recognize the critical support of Drs. Thomas E. Starzl, Director Emeritus of the Thomas E. Starzl Transplantation Institute, and Richard L. Simmons, former Chair of the Department of Surgery at the University of Pittsburgh. Dr. Corry was recruited to Pittsburgh during their respective tenures, and his arrival sparked the revival of pancreatic transplantation in Pittsburgh. Drs. John J. Fung and Amadeo Marcos, who succeeded Dr. Starzl in the running of the Transplant Institute, and Dr. Tim Billiar, current Chair of the Department of Surgery, have continued to support the work of the program. Drs. Henkie Tan, Amit Basu, Liise Kayler, and Deanna Blisard, who comprise the current kidney transplant surgical team in Pittsburgh, and Dr. Ngoc Thai, who directs the pancreas program, continue the work today. The current pancreas and kidney transplant coordinators, including Deborah Good, R.N., B.S., C.C.T.C., Janice Glidewell, R.N., B.S.N., C.C.T.C., Jareen Flohr, R.N., B.S.N., C.C.T.C., Cheryl Buzzard, R.N., B.S.N., C.C.T.C., Gerri James, R.N., C.C.T.C., Angela Barber, R.N., B.S., C.C.T.C., Corde McFeaters, R.N., B.S.N., C.P.N., C.C.T.C., Mitzi Barker, R.N., C.C.T.C., Annie Smith, R.N., Kim Meyer, R.N., Cindy Anderson, R.N., C.C.T.C., C.C.R.N., Maureen Vekasy, R.N., C.C.T.C., Amy Singh, R.N., B.S.N., Stacy Acevedo, R.N., and Nancy Eger, R.N., B.S.N., the Head Nurse on the Transplant Floor, Lisa Fox-Hawranko, R.N., M.S.N., and her team, the Case Manager, Anne Rafail, R.N., B.S.N., C.C.T.C., the Transplant Pharmacist, Kristine Schonder, Pharm. D., the Social Workers, Shirley Grube, M.S.W., B.C.D., L.C.S.W., M.P.H., Greta Coleman, M.Ed., M.S.W., L.C.S.W., and Eleanor Hershberg, M.S.W., L.C.S.W., and the Physician Assistants, Michelle Bauer, P.A.-C., and Kelly Felmet, P.A.-C., have all played incredibly important roles in the day-to-day functioning of the service. My current assistant, Judy Canelos, M.A., and her predecessors, Amanda Gregan, B.A., and Christine DiPerna, provided critical technical support in the preparation of the chapters and the figures. Judy's help was especially important during the latter half of the book's preparation, compilation, and copyediting. Finally, I would like to thank my wife, Mary K. Austin, and my daughters, Rachel and Ana, for their patience and support in putting up with the unpredictable life of a transplant surgeon.

*Ron Shapiro*

# Contents

# Contributors

**Avinash Agarwal** Department of Surgery, Indiana University School of Medicine, Indianapolis, Indiana, U.S.A.

**Rita Alloway** The Israel Penn International Transplant Tumor Registry, University of Cincinnati, Cincinnati, Ohio, U.S.A.

**Stephen T. Bartlett** Department of Surgery, University of Maryland, Baltimore, Maryland, U.S.A.

**Amit Basu** Thomas E. Starzl Transplantation Institute, University of Pittsburgh School of Medicine, Pittsburgh, Pennsylvania, U.S.A.

**Thomas M. Beebe** The Israel Penn International Transplant Tumor Registry, University of Cincinnati, Cincinnati, Ohio, U.S.A.

**W. Bennet** Karolinska Institute, Stockholm, Sweden

**Ugo Boggi** U.O. di Chirurgia nell'Uremico e nel Diabetico, University of Pisa, Pisa, Italy

**Jan Bolinder** Departments of Transplantation Surgery, Neurophysiology and Medicine, Karolinska University Hospital, Stockholm, Sweden

**Rita Bottino** Islet Isolation Core, University of Pittsburgh, Pittsburgh, Pennsylvania, U.S.A.

**Manuel Brown** Department of Radiology, Henry Ford Health System, Detroit, Michigan, U.S.A.

**Joseph F. Buell** The Israel Penn International Transplant Tumor Registry, University of Cincinnati, Cincinnati, Ohio, U.S.A.

**Ginny L. Bumgardner** Division of Transplantation, Department of Surgery, College of Medicine, The Ohio State University, Columbus, Ohio, U.S.A.

**Robert J. Corry**[‡] Thomas E. Starzl Transplantation Institute, University of Pittsburgh School of Medicine, Pittsburgh, Pennsylvania, U.S.A.

**Marco Del Chiaro** U.O. di Chirurgia nell'Uremico e nel Diabetico, University of Pisa, Pisa, Italy

**Anthony J. Demetris** Department of Pathology, University of Pittsburgh Medical Center, Pittsburgh, Pennsylvania, U.S.A.

**Alp Demirag** Division of Transplantation, Department of Surgery, College of Medicine, The Ohio State University, Columbus, Ohio, U.S.A.

**S. Forrest Dodson** Thomas E. Starzl Transplantation Institute, University of Pittsburgh School of Medicine, Pittsburgh, Pennsylvania, U.S.A.

**David L. Dunn** Department of Surgery, University of Minnesota, Minneapolis, Minnesota, U.S.A.

**M. Francesca Egidi** The University of Tennessee Health Science Center, Methodist University, Transplant Institute, Memphis, Tennessee, U.S.A.

**Benjamin H. Eidelman** Department of Neurology, Mayo Clinic, Jacksonville, Florida and Mayo Clinic College of Medicine, Rochester, Minnesota, U.S.A.

**Elmahdi A. Elkhammas** Division of Transplantation, Department of Surgery, College of Medicine, The Ohio State University, Columbus, Ohio, U.S.A.

**Michael P. Federle** Department of Radiology, University of Pittsburgh Medical Center, Pittsburgh, Pennsylvania, U.S.A.

---

[‡] Deceased.

**Ronald M. Ferguson** Division of Transplantation, Department of Surgery, College of Medicine, The Ohio State University, Columbus, Ohio, U.S.A.

**James V. Ferris** Department of Radiology, University of Pittsburgh Medical Center, Pittsburgh, Pennsylvania, U.S.A.

**M. Roy First** The Israel Penn International Transplant Tumor Registry, University of Cincinnati, Cincinnati, Ohio, U.S.A.

**Jonathan A. Fridell** Department of Surgery, Indiana University School of Medicine, Indianapolis, Indiana, U.S.A.

**A. Osama Gaber** Department of Surgery, Cornell University, and The Methodist Hospital, Houston, Texas, U.S.A.

**Lillian W. Gaber** Department of Pathology, College of Medicine, The University of Tennessee Health Science Center, Memphis, Tennessee, U.S.A.

**David A. Geller** Thomas E. Starzl Transplantation Institute, University of Pittsburgh School of Medicine, Pittsburgh, Pennsylvania, U.S.A.

**Frederick C. Goetz** Department of Medicine, University of Minnesota, Minneapolis, Minnesota, U.S.A.

**Deborah S. Good** Thomas E. Starzl Transplantation Institute, University of Pittsburgh School of Medicine, Pittsburgh, Pennsylvania, U.S.A.

**Hani P. Grewal** Mayo Clinic, Jacksonville, Florida, U.S.A.

**Thomas M. Gross** The Israel Penn International Transplant Tumor Registry, University of Cincinnati, Cincinnati, Ohio, U.S.A.

**C. G. Groth** Karolinska Institute, Stockholm, Sweden

**Angelika C. Gruessner** Department of Surgery, University of Minnesota, Minneapolis, Minnesota, U.S.A.

**Rainer W. G. Gruessner** Department of Surgery, University of Minnesota, Minneapolis, Minnesota, U.S.A.

**Michael J. Hanaway** The Israel Penn International Transplant Tumor Registry, University of Cincinnati, Cincinnati, Ohio, U.S.A.

**Donna K. Hathaway** Department of Surgery, College of Medicine, The University of Tennessee Health Science Center, Memphis, Tennessee, U.S.A.

**Mitchell L. Henry** Division of Transplantation, Department of Surgery, College of Medicine, The Ohio State University, Columbus, Ohio, U.S.A.

**Keyanoosh Hosseinzadeh** Department of Radiology, University of Pittsburgh Medical Center, Pittsburgh, Pennsylvania, U.S.A.

**Abhinav Humar** Department of Surgery, University of Minnesota, Minneapolis, Minnesota, U.S.A.

**Raja Kandaswamy** Department of Surgery, University of Minnesota, Minneapolis, Minnesota, U.S.A.

**Dixon B. Kaufman** Division of Transplantation, Department of Surgery, Feinberg School of Medicine, Northwestern University, Chicago, Illinois, U.S.A.

**Liise K. Kayler** Thomas E. Starzl Transplantation Institute, University of Pittsburgh School of Medicine, Pittsburgh, Pennsylvania, U.S.A.

**William R. Kennedy** Department of Neurology, University of Minnesota, Minneapolis, Minnesota, U.S.A.

**Akhtar S. Khan** Milton S. Hershey Medical Center, Division of Transplantation, Hershey, Pennsylvania, U.S.A.

**A. Tarik Kizilisik** Vanderbilt University Medical Center, Kidney/Pancreas Transplant Program, Nashville, Tennessee, U.S.A.

**Stuart J. Knechtle** Division of Organ Transplantation, Department of Surgery, University of Wisconsin Medical School, Madison, Wisconsin, U.S.A.

**Venkatesh Krishnamurthi** Department of Surgery, University of Maryland, Baltimore, Maryland, U.S.A.

**Shimon Kusne** Mayo Medical School, Mayo Clinic Scottsdale, Scottsdale, Arizona, U.S.A.

**Eun Jeong Kwak** Division of Infectious Diseases, Department of Medicine, Thomas E. Starzl Transplantation Institute, University of Pittsburgh School of Medicine, Pittsburgh, Pennsylvania, U.S.A.

**Amadeo Marcos** Thomas E. Starzl Transplantation Institute, University of Pittsburgh School of Medicine, Pittsburgh, Pennsylvania, U.S.A.

**Arthur J. Matas** Department of Surgery, University of Minnesota, Minneapolis, Minnesota, U.S.A.

**S. Michael Mauer** Department of Pediatrics, University of Minnesota, Minneapolis, Minnesota, U.S.A.

**Jerry McCauley** Thomas E. Starzl Transplantation Institute, University of Pittsburgh School of Medicine, Pittsburgh, Pennsylvania, U.S.A.

**Franco Mosca** U.O. di Chirurgia Generale e Trapianti, University of Pisa, Pisa, Italy

**John S. Najarian** Department of Surgery, University of Minnesota, Minneapolis, Minnesota, U.S.A.

**Joao Seda Neto** Thomas E. Starzl Transplantation Institute, University of Pittsburgh School of Medicine, Pittsburgh, Pennsylvania, U.S.A.

**Ramona Nicolau-Raducu** Department of Anesthesiology, University of Pittsburgh Medical Center, Pittsburgh, Pennsylvania, U.S.A.

**Jon S. Odorico** Division of Organ Transplantation, Department of Surgery, University of Wisconsin Medical School, Madison, Wisconsin, U.S.A.

**V. Ram Peddi** The Israel Penn International Transplant Tumor Registry, University of Cincinnati, Cincinnati, Ohio, U.S.A.

**Ronald P. Pelletier** Division of Transplantation, Department of Surgery, College of Medicine, The Ohio State University, Columbus, Ohio, U.S.A.

**Benjamin Philosophe** Division of Transplantation, Department of Surgery, University of Maryland, Baltimore, Maryland, U.S.A.

**Raymond M. Planinsic** Department of Anesthesiology, University of Pittsburgh Medical Center, Pittsburgh, Pennsylvania, U.S.A.

**John A. Powelson** Department of Surgery, Indiana University School of Medicine, Indianapolis, Indiana, U.S.A.

**Parmjeet S. Randhawa** Department of Pathology, University of Pittsburgh Medical Center, Pittsburgh, Pennsylvania, U.S.A.

**Abdul S. Rao** Tampa General Hospital and University of South Florida School of Medicine, Tampa, Florida, U.S.A.

**R. Paul Robertson** Department of Medicine, University of Minnesota, Minneapolis, Minnesota, U.S.A.

**Velma P. Scantlebury** Department of Surgery, University of South Alabama, Mobile, Alabama, U.S.A.

**Ron Shapiro** Thomas E. Starzl Transplantation Institute, University of Pittsburgh School of Medicine, Pittsburgh, Pennsylvania, U.S.A.

**M. Hosein Shokouh-Amiri** Department of Surgery, College of Medicine, The University of Tennessee Health Science Center, Memphis, Tennessee, U.S.A.

**Stefano Signori** U.O. di Chirurgia Generale e Trapianti, University of Pisa, Pisa, Italy

**Cynthia A. Smetanka** Thomas E. Starzl Transplantation Institute, University of Pittsburgh School of Medicine, Pittsburgh, Pennsylvania, U.S.A.

**Göran Solders** Departments of Transplantation Surgery, Neurophysiology and Medicine, Karolinska University Hospital, Stockholm, Sweden

**Hans W. Sollinger** Division of Organ Transplantation, Department of Surgery, University of Wisconsin Medical School, Madison, Wisconsin, U.S.A.

**Jean-Paul Squifflet** Department of Abdominal Surgery and Transplantation, University of Liege, Liege, Belgium

**Thomas E. Starzl** Thomas E. Starzl Transplantation Institute, University of Pittsburgh School of Medicine, Pittsburgh, Pennsylvania, U.S.A.

**Robert J. Stratta** Department of General Surgery, Wake Forest University School of Medicine, Winston-Salem, North Carolina, U.S.A.

**David E. R. Sutherland** Department of Surgery, University of Minnesota, Minneapolis, Minnesota, U.S.A.

**Henkie P. Tan** Thomas E. Starzl Transplantation Institute, University of Pittsburgh School of Medicine, Pittsburgh, Pennsylvania, U.S.A.

**Miguel Tan** Department of Surgery, University of Minnesota, Minneapolis, Minnesota, U.S.A.

**Seamus J. Teahan** Department of Urology and Transplantation, Beaumont Hospital, Dublin, Ireland

**Ngoc Thai** Thomas E. Starzl Transplantation Institute, University of Pittsburgh School of Medicine, Pittsburgh, Pennsylvania, U.S.A.

**Angus W. Thomson** Thomas E. Starzl Transplantation Institute, University of Pittsburgh School of Medicine, Pittsburgh, Pennsylvania, U.S.A.

**Jennifer Trofe** The Israel Penn International Transplant Tumor Registry, University of Cincinnati, Cincinnati, Ohio, U.S.A.

**Massimo Trucco** Division of Immunogenetics, Children's Hospital of Pittsburgh, Pittsburgh, Pennsylvania, U.S.A.

**Gunnar E. Tydén** Departments of Transplantation Surgery, Neurophysiology and Medicine, Karolinska University Hospital, Stockholm, Sweden

**Fabio Vistoli** U.O. di Chirurgia nell'Uremico e nel Diabetico, University of Pisa, Pisa, Italy

**E. Steve Woodle** The Israel Penn International Transplant Tumor Registry, University of Cincinnati, Cincinnati, Ohio, U.S.A.

**Holly Woods** VA Pittsburgh Healthcare System, Pittsburgh, Pennsylvania, U.S.A.

**Jennifer E. Woodward** Department of Surgery, Thomas E. Starzl Transplantation Institute, University of Pittsburgh School of Medicine, Pittsburgh, Pennsylvania, U.S.A.

**Albert Zajko** Department of Radiology, University of Pittsburgh Medical Center, Pittsburgh, Pennsylvania, U.S.A.

# 1 | Outcomes After Pancreatic Transplantation

**Ron Shapiro, Robert J. Corry,[‡] and Ngoc Thai**
*Thomas E. Starzl Transplantation Institute, University of Pittsburgh School of Medicine, Pittsburgh, Pennsylvania, U.S.A.*

## INTRODUCTION

Pancreatic transplantation has emerged as a successful therapeutic option for selected patients with type I diabetes mellitus. First performed clinically in 1966 (1), it has become increasingly common over the past 12 years, with over 1000 pancreas transplantations performed annually in the United States in 2004 (Fig. 1) and a smaller number performed outside the United States (2,3). This increase in the number of pancreas transplants is related to an improving rate of success associated with technical refinements and the development of better immunosuppression.

Pancreas transplantation generally occurs in one of three settings: in combination with a kidney transplant from the same donor (simultaneous pancreas–kidney, or SPK), after successful kidney transplantation (pancreas after kidney, or PAK), or as a solitary transplant in diabetics with normal renal function, but with other clinically significant secondary complications (pancreas transplant alone, or PTA). While SPK continues to be the most common pancreas transplant procedure, PAK and PTA make up an increasingly larger percentage of the total number of pancreas transplants. The increase in numbers of PTA and PAK is also related to better techniques and immunosuppression. The numbers of pancreas alone (PAK, PTA) transplants have increased despite an active debate as to whether pancreas transplant alone increases patient survival.

This chapter will review the early outcomes after pancreatic transplantation, focusing on patient and graft survival rates in each of the three categories, along with the causes of mortality and graft loss. It will also discuss the progress made in surgical techniques and immunosuppressive therapy, particularly the development of tacrolimus-based regimens and the utilization of antibody induction and steroid-free immunosuppression.

## SPK TRANSPLANTATION

SPK transplantation is by far the most usual context in which pancreatic transplantation has been performed, and has accounted for about 70% of the pancreases transplanted to date (Fig. 2) (2–4). SPK has been the most logical setting for the introduction of the procedure. The recipients already are in need of the kidney with concomitant immunosuppression, and monitoring the kidney for rejection is relatively straightforward, so that the kidney has been used as a marker for the pancreas. Dissynchronous rejection or drug toxicity affecting only the pancreas can also occur, but is relatively uncommon (5–7).

### Patient Survival

It is indisputable that SPK is life prolonging. The estimated survival of a diabetic on dialysis is as low as 30% to 40% at five years. Kidney transplantation in these patients increases survival to approximately 78% at five years and 45% at 10 years. The addition of a pancreas as in SPK transplantation has improved long-term patient survival compared to deceased donor (DD) kidney transplantation alone with a five-year patient survival of 82% and 10-year survival of 65% (8). Living donor kidney transplants, where the quality of the kidney is generally higher and the cold ischemia time is lower than with DD kidneys, result in similar patient survival when compared to SPK transplantation (9). Two large retrospective studies examining the United Network for Organ Sharing database from 1995 to 2003 have confirmed the significant survival advantage of an SPK for a diabetic on dialysis.

---

[‡] Deceased.

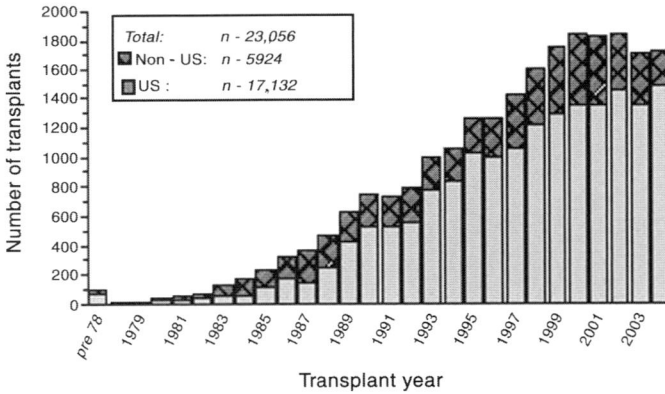

**Figure 1**  Annual number of U.S. and non-U.S. pancreas transplants reported to the IPTR, 1978–2004. *Source*: From Ref. 39.

Registry data for the period 1988–2003 have shown an improvement in the one-year actuarial patient survival rate from 90% to 95% (Fig. 3) (2–4). Individual centers have shown one- and three-year patient survival rates as high as 98% and 95% (Fig. 4) (10), and data from the Stockholm group have shown a 10-year actual patient survival rate of 80% in 14 SPK recipients who had kept their pancreases for at least two years (see Chapter 2) (11). There have also been reports of worse outcomes, with one series from the University of Minnesota demonstrating a three-year patient survival rate of 68% (12). Some of these anomalously poor outcomes may be related to patient selection issues and a willingness to offer the procedure to older, high-risk recipients. The introduction of newer and better immunosuppressive protocols and techniques (see Chapter 13) promises to improve patient survival even more.

The two important causes of death in kidney transplant recipients, cardiac and infectious complications (13), also predominate in pancreatic transplantation (12,14–16). However, it is interesting that pancreas transplantation appears to lower the rate of death related to cardiac complications of diabetics. This may be due to better glycemic control as well as improved cardiovascular function. Recent studies have shown improvements in ventricular function, cholesterol levels, and blood pressure after SPK. The recent introduction of newer and more tolerogenic immunosuppressive protocols that can minimize maintenance

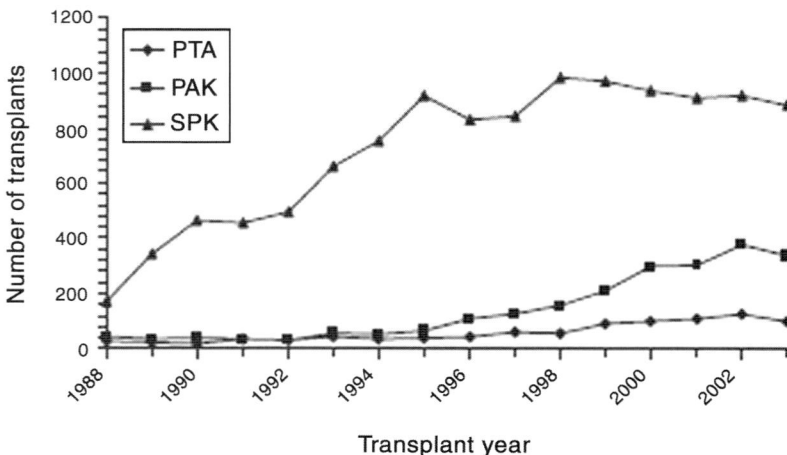

**Figure 2**  Annual number of U.S. pancreas transplants by category, 1988–2003. *Abbreviations*: PTA, pancreas transplant alone; PAK, pancreas after kidney; SPK, simultaneous pancreas kidney. *Source*: From Ref. 39.

**(A)**

**(B)**

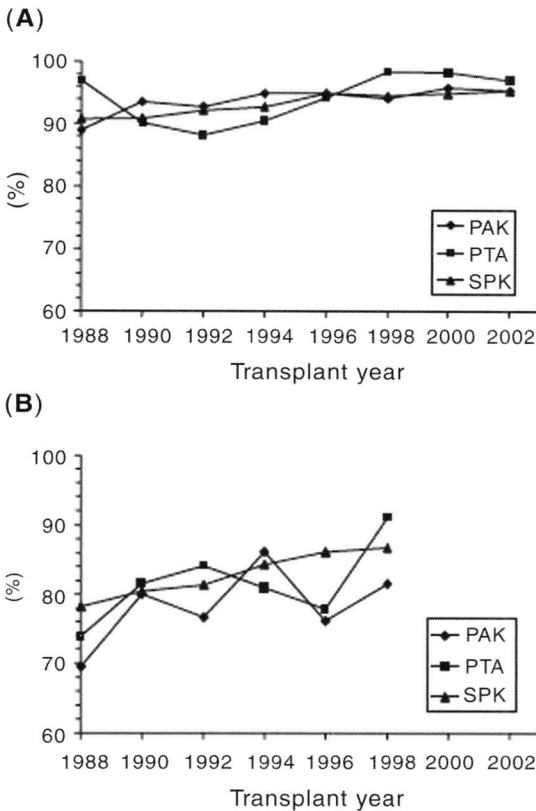

**Figure 3** Patient survival rates for U.S. deceased donor primary pancreas transplant recipients by category and era, in two-year intervals, 1988–2003: (**A**) one year, (**B**) five years. *Abbreviations*: PTA, pancreas transplant alone; PAK, pancreas after kidney; SPK, simultaneous pancreas kidney. *Source*: From Ref. 40.

immunosuppression may also reduce the number of infection-related deaths after pancreas transplantation.

## Graft Survival

Graft function after successful pancreatic transplantation is defined as euglycemia with insulin independence. Graft failure occurs when the patient returns to permanent insulin dependence. This can occur immediately after transplantation, in the setting of early allograft thrombosis; many years later, in the case of graft loss to chronic rejection; or at any intermediate time. Graft survival is conventionally defined as the time after transplantation to graft loss or patient death.

Graft survival after SPK transplantation has conventionally included both renal and pancreatic allograft survival. The kidney, being a fundamentally less fastidious organ, has been associated with persistently better short-term graft survival when compared with the pancreas. Registry data have shown a gradual improvement in one-year renal allograft survival in SPK patients, from 85% in 1988 to 92% in 1999–2003 (Fig. 5) (2–4). Corresponding one-year pancreas allograft survival rates have improved from 76% to 85% (2–4) during the same time period (Fig. 5). Individual centers have performed even better, with one-year renal and pancreatic allograft survival rates of 95% and 86% (Fig. 4) (10) [or even better (Table 1)] (17,18), respectively. Improvements in donor and recipient management, including operative techniques, nonimmunologic postoperative care, and better immunosuppression, have all contributed to this gradual improvement.

## PAK TRANSPLANTATION

PAK transplantation has increased in frequency in recent years and now accounts for 25% of the pancreatic transplantations being performed (Fig. 2) (2–4). This increase in number is largely related to the development of living donor renal transplantation. A diabetic with renal failure can now undergo a staged procedure with a living donor kidney transplant followed

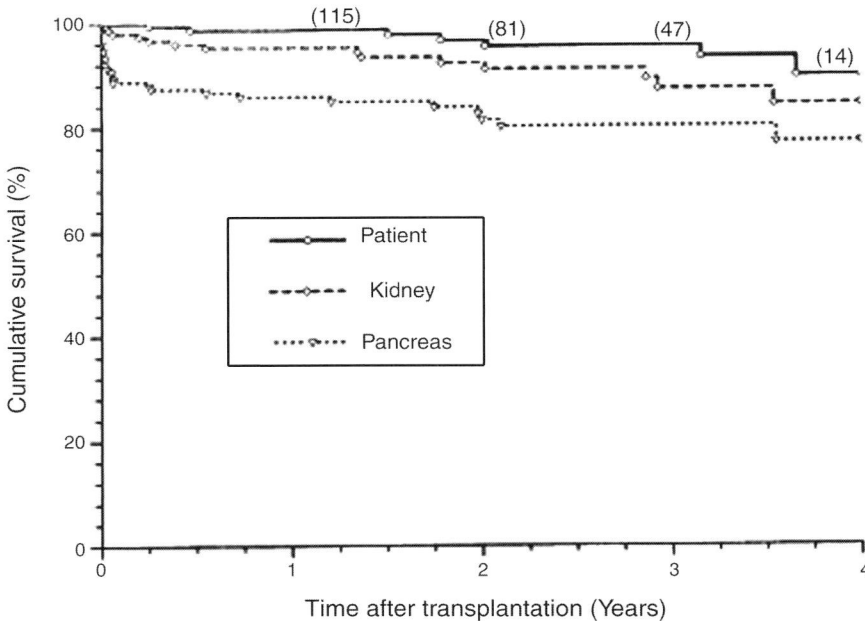

**Figure 4**  Overall patient, kidney, and pancreas allograft survival for 151 consecutive simultaneous pancreas/kidney transplants. *Source*: From Ref. 41.

by a pancreas transplant. PAKs are also performed in those who have undergone SPK transplantation and have lost the pancreatic allograft. It has been associated with comparable one-year patient survival, 95%, when compared with SPK transplantation (Fig. 3), but inferior (although improving) allograft survival, 78% (Fig. 5) (2–4). As with SPK transplantation, the causes of graft loss have been primarily technical and immunologic. Both antibody induction and tacrolimus and mycophenolate mofetil (MMF)-based immunosuppression have been associated with improved outcomes.

## PANCREATIC TRANSPLANTATION ALONE

PTA transplantation is performed in diabetics with normal renal function (CrCl > 50) who have had other secondary complications, such as significant gastropathy, retinopathy, neuropathy, fluctuating glucose levels, and lack of hypoglycemic awareness. It has accounted for 8% of the pancreatic transplantations performed in 2003 (2–4). While it has been associated with comparable one-year patient survival, as high as 97% in recent years (Fig. 3), it has had the worst graft survival, ranging from <50% to 77%, of the three forms of pancreatic transplantation (Fig. 5) (2). Here too, the advent of antibody induction and tacrolimus and MMF has led to an improvement in one-year outcomes to 77%, and a decrease in the rate of graft loss

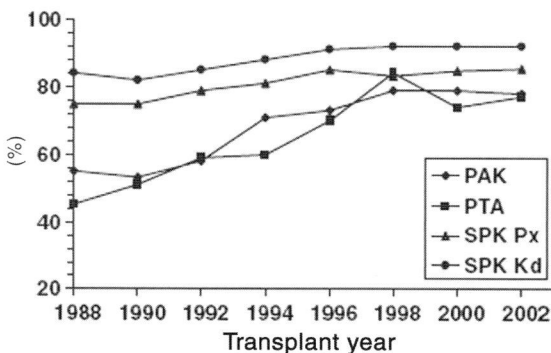

**Figure 5**  Pancreas and SPK kidney graft function for 1988–2003 U.S. deceased donor primary pancreas transplants by recipient category and era, in two-year intervals; 1988–2003, at one year. *Abbreviations*: SPK, simultaneous pancreas-kidney; PAK, pancreas after kidney; PTA, pancreas transplant alone. *Source*: From Ref. 39.

**Table 1** One- and Two-Year Actuarial Patient, and Functional Allograft Survival in 50 Simultaneous Pancreas–Kidney Recipients Receiving Mycophenolate Mofetil/Tacrolimus Primary Maintenance Immunosuppression

| Endpoint | Patient and graft survival rates (%) | |
| --- | --- | --- |
| | 1 yr | 2 yr |
| Patient survival | 97.70 | 97.70 |
| Kidney survival | 93.30 | 93.30 |
| Pancreas survival | | |
|    Including partial function | 93.70 | 90.00 |
|    Full function only | 87.70 | 83.90 |

*Source:* From Ref. 17.

to rejection from 38% to 8% (Fig. 6) (2). The technical failure rate has improved from 25% in 1988 to approximately 7% to 8% in 2003 (Fig. 7).

## IMPACT OF IMMUNOSUPPRESSION

The mid-1990s saw the introduction of the first new immunosuppressive agents in over a decade, and a number of new agents have subsequently become available (see Chapter 13). Two of these agents, tacrolimus and MMF, have been embraced rather rapidly by the pancreas transplant community, both as rescue agents and as primary immunosuppressive agents. Matched-pair control analysis has suggested that the use of tacrolimus has been associated with significant improvements in pancreatic allograft survival in the SPK setting (19). Registry data have confirmed these findings, as there has been a steady increase in pancreas graft survival in all categories (SPK, PAK, PTA) since the introduction of tacrolimus in 1994 (Fig. 5) (2–4). There has also been a corresponding decrease in the death rate of pancreas transplant recipients over the same period of time.

In general, the majority of patients undergoing pancreas transplantation (SPK, PAK, or PTA) have received anti-lymphocyte antibody induction, and registry data have suggested slightly better outcomes with antibody induction, regardless of the maintenance agent(s) being employed. However, a prospective, randomized trial involving 18 pancreas centers comparing antibody induction (including anti–T-cell antibody as well as anti–IL-2R) with no antibody induction revealed no statistically significant improvement in outcomes in SPK patients receiving antibody induction compared with no induction (20,21). Maintenance immunosuppression included tacrolimus, mycophenolate, and steroids. No difference in patient or graft survival was seen between induction and non-induction at three years, although the rate of rejection was lower in the induction group. There was also a higher rate of cytomegalovirus infection in patients who received T-cell depleting antibodies (20,22). This trial did not distinguish among the different types of antibody induction (depleting vs. non-depleting) but analyzed them all together.

For PAK and PTA recipients, induction therapy is associated with a significantly better graft survival rate. Three-year graft survival is 74% versus 64% in PAK recipients receiving or

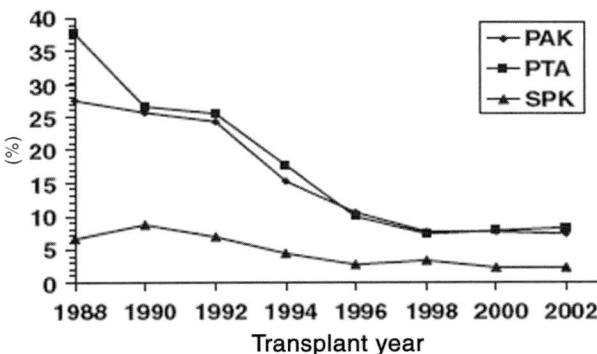

**Figure 6** Immunological graft loss rates for U.S. deceased donor primary pancreas transplants by recipient category and era, in two-year intervals; 1988–2003, at one year. *Abbreviations*: PTA, pancreas transplant alone; PAK, pancreas after kidney; SPK, simultaneous pancreas kidney. *Source*: From Ref. 39.

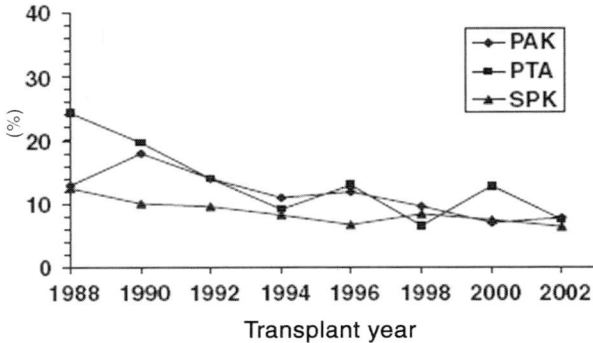

Figure 7 Early graft TFs rates for U.S. deceased donor primary pancreas transplants by recipient category and era, in two-year intervals, 1988–2003. *Abbreviations*: PTA, pancreas transplant alone; PAK, pancreas after kidney; SPK, simultaneous pancreas kidney. *Source*: From Ref. 39.

not receiving antibody induction, respectively. Antibody induction in PTA led to a one-year graft survival of 86%, compared to 74% without induction (4).

Tacrolimus has replaced cyclosporine as the maintenance immunosuppressive agent in pancreas transplantation. Tacrolimus use accounted for 89% of SPK, 93% of PAK, and 99% of PTA in 2001 (23). Most programs use tacrolimus in combination with MMF, although the combination of tacrolimus and sirolimus is gaining popularity. Maintenance protocols that include prednisone still comprise of 92% of the 820 SPK transplants performed in 2001; however, there is a trend towards a "steroid-free" immunosuppression (23,24). At the University of Minnesota, Northwestern University, and the Thomas E. Starzl Institute at the University of Pittsburgh, no steroids are used as a part of maintenance immunosuppression (25,26). At many other institutions, steroid withdrawal is rapid, usually occurring at three to six months post-pancreas transplant (22).

Recently, there has been a burgeoning interest in the use of Campath-1H antibody as an induction agent. A humanized monoclonal antibody recognizing CD52, Campath-1H, effectively depletes >99% of T- and B-cells and monocytes. As these cells do not begin to repopulate until three or more months after transplantation, the immunosuppressive effect of Campath-1H is profound and may be associated with the development of partial tolerance. It is well known in experimental models that T-cell depletion is the most effective means to promote transplant tolerance. The combination of Campath-1H induction and tacrolimus monotherapy has been shown to be highly effective in preventing renal allograft rejection (1–6%) (27). Campath-1H allows for the weaning of tacrolimus in these patients to as low as once weekly tacrolimus, suggesting partial tolerance (27). The effectiveness of Campath-1H induction and tacrolimus monotherapy has also been shown in liver transplantation (28).

The investigation into the effectiveness of Campath-1H induction in pancreas transplantation is being conducted primarily at the University of Minnesota, Northwestern University, and the Thomas E. Starzl Transplantation Institute. While the Minnesota group has eliminated calcineurin inhibitors by using MMF alone as maintenance immunosuppression, the Northwestern team has used tacrolimus combined with sirolimus.

A pilot study employing Campath-1H and tacrolimus monotherapy in pancreas transplantation has been initiated at the Thomas E. Starzl Transplant Institute. Preliminary results have been reasonable, with a patient survival rate of 98% ($N = 55$), a pancreas graft survival rate of 95%, and a rejection rate of 20% with 12 months' follow-up. The long-term follow-up of these patients is ongoing (25).

## CAUSES OF GRAFT LOSS

The main causes of pancreatic graft loss have been technical or immunologic. As the outcomes after pancreatic transplantation have improved, the incidence of these causes of graft failure has also decreased. Technical graft loss etiologies have included fistula, bleeding, thrombosis, pancreatitis, and infection. The incidence of these complications has decreased from 14% to 24% in 1987–1992 to 7% to 10% in 1999–2002 (2,3,29). The incidence of technical loss has been historically higher in enterically drained than in bladder-drained cases, although both recent registry and single center data (30) suggest that the differences are diminishing. Similarly, the immunologic pancreatic graft loss rate has decreased from 6% to 2% at one year (2,3,29).

Modifications at the Starzl Institute recently have substantially diminished technical complications and technical losses. The use of the stapler has greatly reduced both back-table and operative times, and blood loss at reperfusion. The pancreas is placed laterally, head-up and with the tail in the pelvis, allowing for a tension-free duodenojejunostomy. The thrombosis rate with this technique is <2% ($N=80$), and the anastomotic leak rate has been 0%. The re-exploration rate for bleeding has been 10%. The technical graft loss has been <2%.

## EXOCRINE DRAINAGE

The type of exocrine drainage has also evolved after SPK transplantation. The early history of pancreatic transplantation described enteric drainage, but bladder drainage became quite popular in the late 1980s and early 1990s (31,32). Recently, enteric drainage has again become increasingly popular (33–36), accounting for over half of the new cases being performed (Fig. 8) (2–4). Although earlier registry analyses showed slightly inferior outcomes in enterically drained cases, recent reports have shown equivalent pancreatic graft survival rates (Fig. 9) (2–4).

## DEBATE

While it is clear that SPK has conferred a survival advantage for the diabetic, there is still a debate whether a solitary pancreas, either as a PAK or PTA, has conferred a survival advantage for the recipient. Venstrom et al. in 2003 used the United Network for Organ Sharing database to analyze retrospectively diabetics on the transplant list between 1995 and 2000, comparing the survival of those undergoing pancreas transplantation to those listed who did not undergo transplantation over a course of four years (37). Their findings confirmed that SPK transplants conferred a significant survival advantage for the recipients, but that solitary pancreas transplantation decreased patient survival even when followed out at four years. While these conclusions are sobering to the transplant community, there are three mitigating factors: (1) the analysis of the PTA compared roughly 300 patients, so with a mortality rate in these patients of <5% comparisons of mortality may be limited by small numbers; (2) patients listed for isolated pancreas transplantation with a serum creatinine Cr >2.0 mg/dL were excluded, even those who were eventually changed and underwent SPK or PAK; (3) multiple listings of patients at different institutions were not controlled.

In 2004, Gruessner et al. analyzed the same cohort of patients between 1995 and 2003 and showed a significant survival benefit associated with solitary pancreas transplantation (38). This paper controlled for the mitigating factors listed above and included larger numbers of

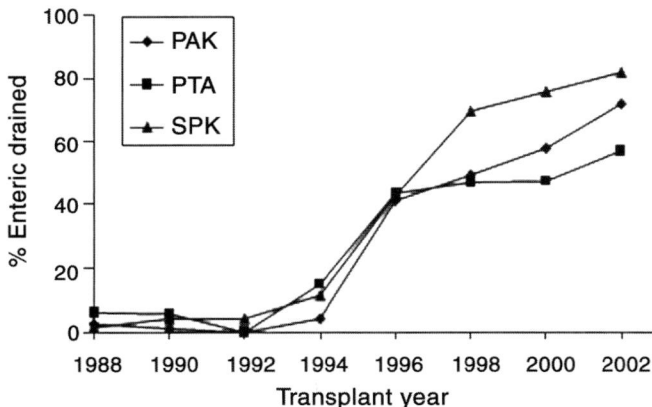

**Figure 8** Percentage of U.S. primary pancreas transplants done with ED, by recipient category and era, in two-year intervals, 1988–2003. *Abbreviations*: ED, exocrine drainage; PTA, pancreas transplant alone; PAK, pancreas after kidney; SPK, simultaneous pancreas kidney. *Source*: From Ref. 39.

(A)

(B)

(C)

(D)

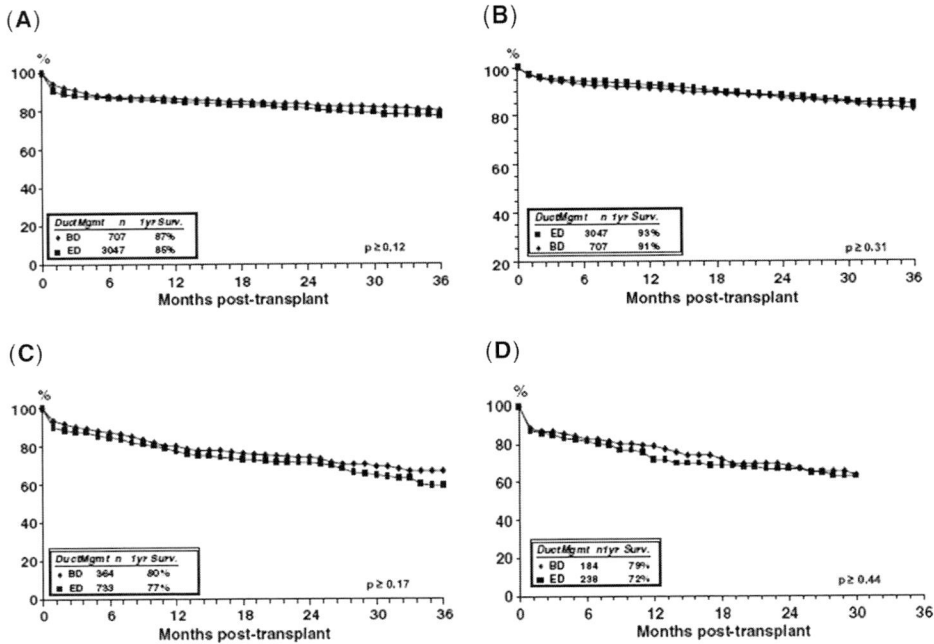

**Figure 9** Graft functional survival rates by duct management and pancreas recipient category for U.S. deceased donor primary transplants 2000–2004 cases: (**A**) SPK pancreas graft function; (**B**) SPK kidney graft function; (**C**) PAK pancreas graft function; and (**D**) PTA graft function. *Source*: From Ref. 39.

patients in each groups. Furthermore, the authors reanalyzed patients from 1995 and 2000 and also noted a survival advantage with solitary pancreas transplantation.

Finally, advances in immunosuppression and surgical techniques have led to progressively improving patient and graft survival over the past 20 years. The introduction of steroid-free immunosuppression and antibody induction over the last few years holds great promise for the future of pancreas transplantation. A reanalysis of pancreas transplants in a few years may confirm the survival advantage of solitary pancreas transplantation.

## CONCLUSION

Pancreatic transplantation has become a routinely successful procedure over the past 10 to 15 years. Technical complications have decreased, as have immunologic graft losses; newer immunosuppressive regimens have played an important role in the latter phenomenon. The next chapter will discuss the long-term outcomes of successful pancreatic transplantation, and the third chapter will focus on the history of pancreatic transplantation. The remaining chapters will describe in detail the current practices and management strategies that have brought the field its current level of development.

## REFERENCES

1. Kelly WD, Lillehei RC, Merkel FK, Idezuki Y, Goetz FC. Allotransplantation of the pancreas and duodenum along with the kidney in diabetic nephropathy. Surgery 1967; 61(6):827–837.
2. Gruessner AC, Sutherland DER. Pancreas transplant outcomes for the United States (US) and non-US cases as reported to the United Network for Organ Sharing (UNOS) and the International Pancreas Transplant Registry (IPTR) as of October 2003. In: Cecka JM, Terasaki PI, eds. Clinical Transplants 2002. Los Angeles: UCLA Tisue Typing Laboratory, 2002:41.
3. Gruessner AC, Sutherland DER. Pancreas transplants outcomes for the United States (US) and non-US cases as reported to the United Network for Organ Sharing (UNOS) and the International Pancreas Transplant Registry (IPTR) as of May 2003:21.
4. Wynn JJ, Distant DA, Pirsch JD, et al. Kidney and pancreas transplantation. Am J Trans 2004; 4(suppl 9):72.

5. Klassen DK, Weir MR, Schweitzer EJ, Bartlett ST. Isolated pancreas rejection in combined kidney–pancreas transplantation: results of percutaneous pancreas biopsy. Transplant Proc 1995; 27(1): 1333–1334.

6. Sutherland DE, Gruessner R, Moudry-Munns K, Gruessner A. Discordant graft loss from rejection of organs from the same donor in simultaneous pancreas–kidney recipients. Transplant Proc 1995; 27(1):907–908.

7. Shapiro R, Jordan ML, Scantlebury VP, et al. Renal allograft rejection with normal renal function in simultaneous kidney/pancreas recipients: does dissynchronous rejection really exist? Transplantation 2000; 69(3):440–441.

8. Reddy KS, Stablein D, Taranto S, et al. Long-term survival following simultaneous kidney–pancreas transplantation versus kidney transplantation alone in patients with type 1 diabetes mellitus and renal failure. Am J Kidney Dis 2003; 41:464–470.

9. Bunnapradist S, Cho YW, Cecka JM, et al. Kidney allograft and patient survival in type I diabetic recipients of cadaveric kidney alone versus simultaneous pancreas kidney transplant: a multivariate analysis of the UNOS database. Am Soc Nephrol 2003; 14:208–213.

10. Corry RJ, Chakrabarti PK, Shapiro R, et al. Simultaneous administration of adjuvant donor bone marrow in pancreas transplant recipients. Ann Surg 1999; 230(3):372–379.

11. Tyden G, Bolinder J, Solders G, Brattstrom C, Tibell A, Groth CG. Improved survival in patients with insulin-dependent diabetes mellitus and end-stage diabetic nephropathy 10 years after combined pancreas and kidney transplantation. Transplantation 1999; 67(5):645–648.

12. Manske CL, Wang Y, Thomas W. Mortality of cadaveric kidney transplantation versus combined kidney–pancreas transplantation in diabetic patients. Lancet 1995; 346(8991–8992):1658–1662.

13. Shapiro R. Outcome after renal transplantation. In: Shapiro R, Simmons RL, Starzl TE, eds. Renal Transplantation. Stamford, CT: Appleton and Lange, 1997:1.

14. Stratta RJ. Mortality after vascularized pancreas transplantation. Surgery 1998; 124(4):823–830.

15. Secchi A, Caldara R, DiCarlo V, Pozza G. Mortality of cadaveric kidney transplantation versus combined kidney–pancreas transplantation in diabetic patients. Lancet 1996; 347(9004):827.

16. Sutherland DE, Dunn DL, Goetz FC, et al. A 10-year experience with 290 pancreas transplants at a single institution. Ann Surg 1989; 210(3):247–285.

17. Kaufman DB, Leventhal JR, Stuart J, Abecassis MM, Fryer JP, Stuart FP. Mycophenolate mofetil and tacrolimus as primary maintenance immunosuppression in simultaneous pancreas–kidney transplantation: initial experience in 50 consecutive cases. Transplantation 1999; 67(4):586–593.

18. Odorico JS, Pirsch JD, Knechtle SJ, D'Alessandro AM, Sollinger HW. A study comparing mycophenolate mofetil to azathioprine in simultaneous pancreas–kidney transplantation. Transplantation 1998; 66(12):1751–1759.

19. Gruessner RW. Tacrolimus in pancreas transplantation: a multicenter analysis. Clin Transplant 1997; 11(4):299–312.

20. Kaufman DB, Iii GW, Bruce DS, et al. Prospective, randomized, multicenter trial of antibody induction therapy in simultaneous pancreas–kidney transplantation. Am J Transplant Jul 2003; 3(7):855–864.

21. Burke GW, Kaufman DB, Millis JM, et al. Prospective, randomized trial of the effect of antibody induction in simultaneous pancreas and kidney transplantation: three year results. Transplantation 2004; 77(8):1269.

22. Kaufman DB, Leventhal JR, Koffron AJ, et al. A prospective study of rapid corticosteroid elimination in simultaneous pancreas–kidney transplantation: comparison of two maintenance immunusuppression protocols: tacrolimus/mycophenylate mofetil versus tacrolimus. Transplantation 2002; 73:169.

23. Kaufmann DB, Shapiro R, Lucey MR, et al. Immunosuppression: practice and trends. Am J Transplant 2004; 4(suppl 9):38.

24. Jordan ML, Chakrabarti P, Luke P, et al. Results of pancreas transplantation after steroid withdrawal under tacrolimus immunosuppression. Transplantation 2000; 69:265.

25. Thai NL, Abu-Elmagd K, Khan A, et al. Pancreatic transplantation at the University of Pittsburgh. In: Cecka JM, Terasaki PI, eds. Clinical Transplants 2004. Los Angeles, CA: UCLA Immunogenetics Center, 2005:205–214.

26. Gruessner RWG, Kandaswamy R, Humar A, Gruessner AC, Sutherland DER. Transplantation 2005; 79(9):1184–1189.

27. Shapiro R, Basu A, Tan H, et al. Kidney transplantation under minimal immunosuppression after pretransplant lymphoid depletion with Thymoglobulin or Campath. J Am Coll Surg 2005; 200(4):505–515.

28. Marcos A, Eghtesad B, Fung JJ, et al. Use of alemtuzumab and tacrolimus monotherapy for cadaveric liver transplantation: with particular reference to hepatitis C virus. Transplantation 2004; 78(7): 966–971.

29. Humar A, Ramcharan T, Kandaswamy R, et al. Technical failures after pancreas transplants: why grafts fail and the risk factors—a multivariate analysis. Transplantation 2004; 78(8):1188–1192.

30. Corry RJ, Chakrabarti P, Shapiro R, Jordon ML, Scantlebury VP, Vivas CA. Comparison of enteric versus bladder drainage in pancreas transplantation. Transplant Proc 2001; 33(12):1647–1651.

31. Sollinger HW, Cook K, Kamps D, Glass NR, Belzer FO. Clinical and experimental experience with pancreaticocystomy for exocrine pancreatic drainage in pancreas transplantation. Transplant Proc 1984; 16:749–751.

32.  Nghiem DD, Corry RJ. Transplantation with urinary drainage of pancreatic secretions. Am J Surg 1987; 153:405.
33.  Kuo PC, Johnson LB, Schweitzer EJ, Bartlett ST. Simultaneous pancreas/kidney transplantation—a comparison of enteric and bladder drainage of exocrine pancreatic secretions. Transplantation 1997; 63(2):238–243.
34.  Corry RJ, Egidi MF, Shapiro R, et al. Pancreas transplantation with enteric drainage under tacrolimus induction therapy. Transplant Proc 1997; 29(1–2):642.
35.  Pirsch JD, Odorico JS, D'Alessandro AM, Knechtle SJ, Becker BN, Sollinger HW. Posttransplant infection in enteric versus bladder-drained simultaneous pancreas–kidney transplant recipients. Transplantation 1998; 66(12):1746–1750.
36.  Stratta RJ, Gaber AO, Shokouh-Amiri MH, et al. Evolution in pancreas transplantation techniques: simultaneous kidney-pancreas transplantation using portal-enteric drainage without antilymphocyte induction. Ann Surg 1999; 229(5):701–708.
37.  Venstrom JM, McBride MA, Rother KI, et al. Survival after pancreas transplantation in patients with diabetes and preserved kidney function. JAMA 2003; 290:2817.
38.  Gruessner RWG, Sutherland DER, Gruessner AC. Mortality assessment for pancreas transplantation. Am J Trans 2004; 4:2018.
39.  Gruessner AC, Sutherland DER. Pancreas outcomes for United States (US) and non-US cases as reported to the United Network for Organ Sharing (UNOS) and the International Pancreas Transplant Registry (IPTR) as of June 2004. Clin Transplant 2005; 19:435.
40.  Gruessner AC, Sutherland DER. Pancreas transplant outcomes for United States (US) and non-US cases as reported to the United Network for Organ Sharing (UNOS) and the International Pancreas Transplant Registry (IPTR) as of June 2004. Clin Transplant 2005; 19:441.
41.  Corry RJ, Chakrabarti PK, Shapiro R, Rao AS, Dvorchik I, Jordan ML, Scantlebury VP, Vivas CA, Fung JJ, Starzl TE. Simultaneous administration of adjuvant donor bone marrow in pancreas transplant recipients. An Surg 1999; 230(3):374.

# 2 | The Effect of Pancreatic Transplantation on Secondary Complications of Diabetes

**Gunnar E. Tydén, Göran Solders, and Jan Bolinder**
*Departments of Transplantation Surgery, Neurophysiology and Medicine, Karolinska University Hospital, Stockholm, Sweden*

## INTRODUCTION

After successful pancreatic transplantation, the diabetic patient will become insulin-independent and euglycemic. Although this undoubtedly improves the patient's quality of life, the patient must now start lifelong immunosuppressive therapy. One of the theoretical goals of pancreatic transplantation is to reverse or stop the progression of the secondary complications of diabetes. Whether this goal can be achieved by normalization of glycemic control has been debated for some time. One reason is that the number of patients who have had functioning pancreatic grafts for a prolonged period of time has been small. Furthermore, in the past, many transplant patients had already developed severe diabetic vascular changes by the time of transplantation, changes that could perhaps be halted in their progress, but could not be reversed. Today, however, a number of centers have cohorts of patients who have had functioning pancreatic transplants for more than 10 years.

A number of studies have examined the effect of a successful pancreatic transplantation on diabetic nephropathy, retinopathy, neuropathy, quality of life, and survival. In this chapter, these studies will be reviewed.

## NEPHROPATHY

Most pancreatic transplantations have been performed in uremic diabetic patients and thus in conjunction with a renal graft. As a consequence, the pancreatic transplantation could obviously not be expected to have an effect on the native kidneys in these patients. However, a combined kidney and pancreas transplantation creates a unique opportunity to assess whether the pancreatic transplantation can prevent the development of diabetic lesions in the renal allograft. Normal kidneys transplanted into diabetic individuals develop clear-cut morphological signs of diabetic nephropathy as early as two years after transplantation (1–3). In contrast, it has been found that, in patients who have undergone successful combined pancreatic and renal transplantation, the renal transplant is protected from recurrence of diabetic nephropathy (4). Graft biopsies obtained 1 to 6.8 years after transplantation show no light microscopic changes suggestive of diabetic nephropathy, while electron microscopic measurements reveal that the thickening of the glomerular basement membrane, which is the hallmark of early diabetic nephropathy, can also be avoided (Fig. 1) (5,6). These findings indicate that normoglycemia, as achieved by a pancreatic transplantation, prevents the development of diabetic nephropathy in humans.

The question of whether established diabetic renal lesions are reversible by pancreatic transplantation is crucial for the timing of the intervention. In one study from the University of Minnesota, renal biopsies were taken from 13 nonuremic, insulin-dependent diabetic patients with micro- and macroalbuminuria before and five years after successful pancreatic transplantation, and compared with baseline and five-year biopsy specimens from 10 nonuremic, insulin-dependent diabetic patients who did not undergo transplantation (7). The glomerular basement membrane thickness in either group did not change significantly at any time, and there was no difference between the groups. The mesangial fractional volume increased significantly in both groups and here again, there was no difference between pancreas transplant recipients and the untransplanted diabetic patients. However, the total volume of mesangium per glomerulus did not change in the pancreas recipients, while it

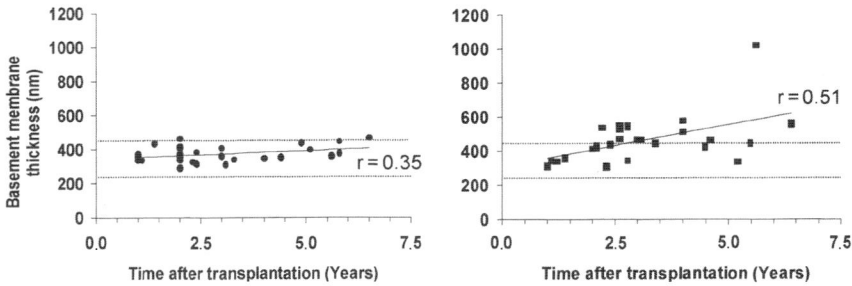

**Figure 1** Glomerular basement membrane thickness, as determined by electron microscopic morphometry, in renal allograft biopsy specimens from diabetic recipients of combined pancreatic and kidney grafts and from diabetic recipients of kidney grafts only. Area between dotted lines indicates mean ±2 standard deviation of normal human glomerular basement membrane thickness.

increased in the control patients. The creatinine clearance fell in the transplant recipients, while it remained unchanged in the control group. The fall in glomerular filtration rate occurred in the first year after transplantation and remained unchanged thereafter. Obviously, the follow-up study of the patients' native kidneys was complicated by the fact that recipients were treated with cyclosporine for immunosuppression, and it is associated with functional impairment of the native kidneys.

In a follow-up study from the same group, it was reported that normoglycemia after pancreatic transplantation not only stabilized, but also induced regression of the characteristic lesions of diabetic nephropathy in patients with functioning pancreas transplants at 10 years (8). In this cohort of patients with persistently normal glycosylated hemoglobin values and stable renal function, native kidney biopsies at 10 years demonstrated regression of glomerulosclerosis, with reduction in glomerular basement membrane width and mesangial thickness.

Thus, pancreatic transplantation can reverse the lesions of diabetic nephropathy, but this reversal requires more than five years of normoglycemia. As will be shown below, normoglycemia for at least five to six years appears to be a prerequisite for an impact not only on nephropathy, but also on any of the secondary complications of diabetes.

## NEUROPATHY

Most patients undergoing pancreatic transplantation have more or less advanced diabetic neuropathy. Signs of peripheral neuropathy include paresthesia, hypoesthesia, muscle weakness, restless legs, and cramps. Autonomic dysfunction may present as gastrointestinal, sexual, sudomotor, and/or cardiovascular disturbances. For the most part, the subjective symptoms of these disturbances improve following transplantation. However, it should be borne in mind that such improvements almost invariably follow combined renal and pancreatic transplantation and, thus, the improvement in neuropathy may be the result of an improvement in the uremic status as well as in glycemic control.

Peripheral neuropathy is usually studied by measuring nerve conduction velocity and amplitudes of sensory and motor nerves. Moderate improvements in the nerve conduction velocity have been found early after kidney/pancreas transplantation (9–11). However, when these improvements were compared with those in diabetic recipients of renal allografts alone, there was no difference. The measured improvements in nerve conduction velocity were therefore most probably attributable to the cure of uremia. When the observation time was extended to three years and more, however, a significant and lasting improvement in diabetic polyneuropathy was noted only in recipients of successful pancreas/kidney grafts, while in diabetic patients receiving kidney transplants alone a progression of diabetic neuropathy was noted (Fig. 2A) (12–14).

The effect of pancreatic transplantation on autonomic neuropathy has primarily been addressed by studies of cardiovascular disturbances. Thus, the relative beat-to-beat variation of the electrocardiogram (RR variation) during deep breathing has been used to assess the parasympathetic vagal reflex arc. Several studies have shown that, in diabetic patients,

**(A)**

**(B)**

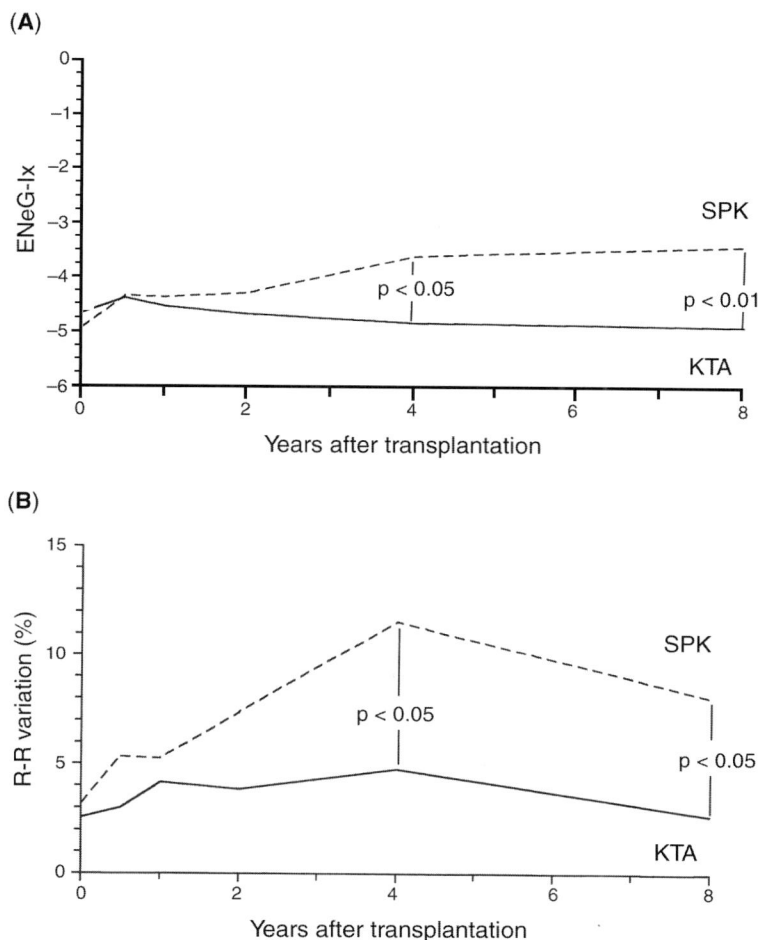

**Figure 2** (**A**) ENeG–Ix in recipients of SPK grafts and in diabetic recipients of KTA, 0.5, 2, 4, and 8 years after transplantation. (**B**) Autonomic nerve function, as asessed by the R–R variation test (%), in recipients of SPK and in diabetic recipients of KTA. *Abbreviations*: SPK, simultaneous pancreas and kidney grafts; KTA, kidney transplants alone; ENeG–Tx, electroneyrography index.

the autonomic nervous system is severely affected, and no significant improvement is achieved during the first few years following successful pancreatic transplantation. However, after four years, significantly better values in the RR variations have been found in patients with functioning pancreatic grafts compared with kidney-only transplant patients, and this difference was sustained with up to eight years' follow-up (Fig. 2B) (14). Almost identical findings have previously been reported (15), with only moderate improvement during the first year posttransplantation. At 5 and 10 years after pancreas transplantation, improvements were noted not only in cardiorespiratory reflexes, but also in sudomotor functions (sweating and evaporation).

In another study, mortality rates of groups of patients with and without autonomic neuropathy and with a functioning pancreas transplantation, a failed pancreas transplantation, or no pancreas transplantation were compared (16). The authors reported a 40% mortality rate in the cohort of patients with abnormal cardiorespiratory reflexes after seven years, compared with a 14% mortality in the patients with normal cardiorespiratory reflexes (16).

A profound difference in long-term patient survival between patients with successful pancreas/kidney transplants and diabetic patients with kidney-only transplants was recently reported (14). After 10 years, 80% of the pancreas/kidney transplant recipients, but only 20% of the patients in the kidney-only transplant group, were alive. When patients were grouped according to those who survived for 10 years and those who died during follow-up, the survivors had significantly better peripheral nerve function at four and eight years, and also better RR variations at four and eight years. This correlation between improvement in overall autonomic function and improved long-term survival may well be one of the most important effects of a successful pancreatic transplantation.

## RETINOPATHY

The vast majority of uremic diabetic patients receiving combined renal and pancreatic transplants have severe preproliferative or proliferative retinopathy and have undergone extensive laser therapy and, in many cases, vitrectomies. Assessing any effect of pancreatic transplantation on the retinal lesions in these patients has therefore been difficult. Furthermore, improvements in retinopathy posttransplantation may also be influenced by the fact that the majority of patients have been cured of their uremia.

Since the first report of a favorable effect of pancreatic transplantation on diabetic retinopathy (17), conflicting results have been published. In a study of pancreas/kidney versus kidney-only recipients 24 months after transplantation, no significant difference was found in the course of retinopathy and visual acuity (18). Despite physiological control of blood glucose for a minimum of 12 months, progression of retinopathy and deterioration of visual acuity could be observed. However, in a subsequent report, with a mean observation time of 40 months, retinopathy regressed in 9%, stabilized in 73%, and progressed in 18% of pancreas recipients, while in the control group, 34% stabilized and 46% deteriorated (19). Of interest was the observation that the patients in the study group showing a clear improvement were those in whom the degree of retinopathy was mild, indicating that amelioration can only be expected during the early stages of retinopathy. Similar observations were made in a study of retinopathy in 30 pancreas/kidney recipients, with 50 kidney recipients as controls (20). A special analysis of the few patients who had not received laser treatment prior to transplantation revealed that four eyes in the control group significantly deteriorated. In this group, glycoslated hemoglobin, which appears to be an important indicator for the development and progression of retinopathy, was clearly below 10% (mean HbA1 8.4%, normal <8%). In contrast, the mean retinopathy score remained stable in the pancreas transplant recipients.

In conclusion, it seems that the progression of diabetic retinopathy may be slowed down by a functioning pancreatic graft. However, it is also clear that established retinopathy can progress despite the restoration of normoglycemia.

## PERIPHERAL MICROCIRCULATION

To assess the effects of pancreas transplantation on microangiopathy, noninvasive methods measuring nutritional and total skin blood flow have been used. Improved skin microvascular reactivity and thermal regulation, with improvements in transcutaneous oxygen tension, reoxygenation times, skin temperature, and erythrocyte flow in pancreas recipients versus diabetic kidney-only recipients, have been reported (21). Video-photometric capillary microscopy of the nail fold capillaries of fingers measuring the superficial microcirculation has revealed an increase during both rest and reactive hyperemia posttransplant. These changes were not seen early but were noticeable at 12 months or more after pancreatic transplantation (22). In a similar study, a progressive increase in basal blood flow in the skin microcirculation was noted after successful combined kidney and pancreas transplantation, but no improvement of the impaired microvascular reactivity was seen (23).

## QUALITY OF LIFE

Although the goal of pancreatic transplantation is to prevent or halt the life-threatening secondary complications of diabetes, it is also obvious that patients enjoy the improvement in quality of life associated with normoglycemia and the avoidance of restrictions associated with the diabetic lifestyle. In recent years, it has become possible to measure quality of life in detail by structured interviews by the physician or by the use of self-administered questionnaires. There are a number of cross-sectional studies on quality of life in pancreas transplant recipients.

In one of the first studies using Spitzer's quality of life index, a benefit of a combined pancreas/kidney transplantation in comparison with kidney-only transplants was found at an evaluation two years posttransplantation (24). However, it was obvious from the study that not only the pancreas/kidney patients, but also the kidney-only transplant patients experienced a significant improvement in the quality of life after transplantation. The difference between the groups was not that impressive. However, at a follow-up five years later, that is, seven years posttransplant, a dramatic change became evident. There was an increase in most of the quality of life indices for the pancreas transplant recipients, while there was a decrease for the kidney-only transplant patients, reflecting a progression of the secondary complications (25).

In an extensive analysis of 131 pancreas recipients who were at one to 11 years posttransplantation, it was found that patients with a functioning pancreas graft described their current quality of life and rated their health significantly more favorably than did those with nonfunctioning grafts (26). It was concluded that, while a successful pancreas transplantation may not elevate all diabetic patients to the level of health and function of the general population, these patients reported a significantly better quality of life than did the patients who remained diabetic. However, in another study it was noted that, although in general all quality of life scores were higher in patients with functioning pancreas grafts, there was no significant difference between them and patients with a functioning kidney-only transplant, suggesting that the elimination of uremia and dialysis has the greatest impact on the perceived improvement in quality of life (27).

## PATIENT SURVIVAL

The ultimate goal of pancreatic transplantation must be prolongation of life. However, during the first decade of pancreatic transplantation, most papers dealing with patient survival discussed whether combined pancreas/kidney transplantation resulted in a higher mortality rate than a kidney transplant alone (28). This was indeed a relevant question in the past when the technical complication rate was high. However, as graft survival rates have improved and the morbidity associated with the procedure has decreased, increased attention has been paid to the potential beneficial effects of pancreatic transplantation on patient survival. Indeed, in a recent report (14), it was shown that by six years after transplantation, patients with functioning pancreas/kidney grafts had a significantly greater patient survival than a control group undergoing kidney transplantation alone or a group of patients in whom a simultaneous pancreas transplant had failed within the first year. This difference in patient survival became more pronounced after eight years. At 10 years, 80% of the patients with functioning pancreatic grafts were alive, while only 20% of the diabetic recipients of kidney transplants alone, or a group of patients with failed pancreatic grafts, had survived (Fig. 3). An analysis of the causes of death revealed that there was an excess mortality related to cardiovascular disease in the kidney-alone group, compared to the pancreas/kidney group.

An improvement in cardiac function has been shown as early as 12 months after a successful combined renal and pancreatic transplantation (29). Also, a favorable effect on lipid profiles in pancreas/kidney transplant recipients has been demonstrated (30,31). Furthermore,

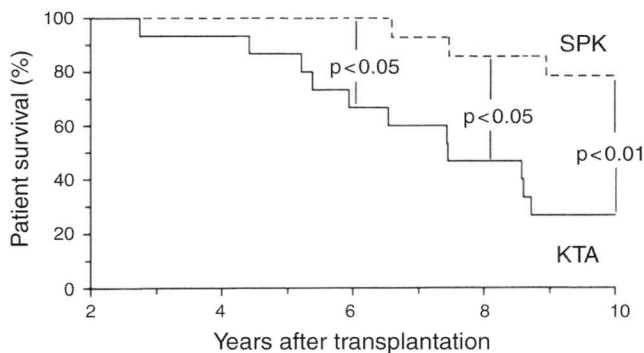

**Figure 3** Ten-year actual patient survival in recipients of SPK and in diabetic recipients of KTA. *Abbreviations*: SPK, simultaneous pancreas and kidney grafts; KTA, kidney transplants alone.

as mentioned above, a significantly better nerve conduction and RR variation was found at both four and eight years after transplantation in patients who survived 10 years when compared with patients who did not survive 10 years after transplantation. This is consistent with earlier reports of a high mortality rate associated with autonomic dysfunction in diabetics (32). It has also been shown that a neuropathy score, including cardiorespiratory and nerve conduction tests, is a better predictor of survival than are separate scores (33). In a recent report in which patient survival was analyzed in patients with type I diabetes and end-stage diabetic nephropathy, who were treated at two different centers (34), substantial differences in patient survival were noted. In one center, the primary goal was simultaneous pancreas/kidney transplantation for patients with end-stage diabetic nephropathy, whereas at the other center, kidney transplantation alone was the predominant therapeutic modality. In the first center, 73% of all patients received simultaneous pancreas/kidney transplantations, whereas at the second center, only 37% did. The 10-year patient survival rate was almost 80% at the first center; at the second center, it was 40%.

Taken together, these findings suggest that diabetic patients undergoing combined pancreas/kidney transplantation have a life expectancy superior to that of diabetic patients who undergo kidney transplantation alone.

## REFERENCES

1.  Mauer SM, Steffcs MW, Connett J, Najarian JS, Sutherland DER, Barbosa J. The development of lesions in the glomerular basement membrane and mesangium after transplantation of normal kidneys to diabetic patients. Diabetes 1983; 32:948–952.
2.  Boman SO, Wilczck H, Jaremko G, Lundgren G. Recurrence of diabetic nephropathy in human renal allografts: Preliminary report of a biopsy study. Transplant Proc 1984; 16:649–653.
3.  Mauer SM, Goetz FC, MacHugh LE, et al. Long-term study of normal kidneys transplanted into patients with type I diabetes. Diabetes 1989; 38:516–523.
4.  Boman SO, Tydén G, Wilczek H, et al. Prevention of kidney graft diabetic nephropathy by pancreas transplantation in man. Diabetes 1985; 34:306–308.
5.  Wilczek H, Jaremko G, Tydén G, Groth CG. Evolution of diabetic nephropathy in kidney grafts. Transplantation 1995; 59:51–57.
6.  Bilous RW, Mauer SM, Sutherland DER, Najarian JS, Goetz FC, Steffes MW. The effect of pancreas transplantation on the glomerular structure of renal allografts in patients with insulin dependent diabetes. N Engl J Med 1989; 321:80–85.
7.  Fioretto P, Mauer SM, Bilous RW, Goetz FC, Sutherland DER, Steffes MW. Effects of pancreas transplantation on glomerular structure in insulin dependent diabetic patients with their own kidneys. Lancet 1993; 324:1193–1196.
8.  Fioretto P, Steffes MW, Sutherland DER, Goetz FC, Mauer SM. Reversal of lesions of diabetic nephropathy after pancreas transplantation. N Engl J Mcd 1998; 339:69–75.
9.  Solders G, Tydén G, Gunnarsson R, Persson A, Wilczek H, Groth CG. Effects of combined pancreatic and renal transplantation on diabetic neuropathy: A two-year follow-up study. Lancet 1987; 2: 1232–1235.
10. Nusser J, Scheuer R, Abendroth D, Illner WD, Landgraft R. Effect of pancreatic and/or renal transplantation on diabetic autonomic neuropathy. Diabctoiogia 1991; 34:118–120.
11. Kennedy WR, Navarro X, Goetz FC, Sutherland DER, Najarian JS. Effects of pancreatic transplantation on diabetic neuropathy. N Engl J Med 1990; 332:1031–1037.
12. Solders G, Tydén G, Persson A, Groth CG. Improvement of nerve conduction in diabetic neuropathy—A follow-up study after combined pancreatic and renal transplantation. Diabetes 1992; 41:946–951.
13. Müller–Felber W, Landgraf R, Scheuer R, et al. Diabetic neuropathy three years after successful pancreas and kidney transplantation. Diabetes 1993; 42:1482–1486.
14. Tydén G, Bolinder J, Solders E, Brattström C, Tibella A, Groth CG. Improved survival in patients with insulin dependent diabetes mellitus and end-stage diabetic nephropathy 10 years after combined pancreas and kidney transplantation. Transplantation l999; 67:645–648.
15. Navarro X, Sutherland DER, Kennedy WR. Long-term effects of pancreatic transplantation on diabetic neuropathy. Ann Neurol 1997; 42:727–736.
16. Navarro X, Kennedy WR, Loewenson RB, Sutherland DER. Influence of pancreas transplantation on cardiorespiratory reflexes, nerve conduction and mortality in diabetes mellitus. Diabetes 1990; 39:802–806.
17. Uulbig M, Kampik A, Landgraf R, Land W. The influence of combined pancreatic and renal transplantation on advanced retinopathy. Transplant Proc 1987; 19:3554–3356.
18. Ramsay RC, Goetz FC, Sutherland DER, et al. Progression of diabetic retinopathy after pancreas transplantation for insulin dependent diabetes mellitus. N Engl J Med 1988; 318:208–214.

19. Königsreiner A, Miller K, Steurer W, et al. Does pancreas transplantation influence the course of diabetic retinopathy? Diabetologia 1991; 34:86–88.
20. Schneider A, Meyer-Schwickerath V, Nusser J, Land W, Landgraf R. Diabetic retinopathy and pancreas transplantation, a three-year follow up. Diabetologia 1991; 34:95–99.
21. Abendroth D, Schmand J, Landgraf R, Illner WD, Land W. Diabetic microangiopathy in type I insulin dependent diabetic patients after successful pancreatic and kidney or solitary kidney transplantation. Diabetologia 1991; 34:131–134.
22. Cheung ATW, Cox KL, Ahlfors CE, Bry WI. Reversal of microangiopathy in long-term diabetic patients after successful simultaneous pancreas/kidney transplants. Transplant Proc 1993; 25:1310–1313.
23. Jörneskog G, Tydén G, Bolinder J, Fagrell B. Does combined kidney and pancreas transplantation reverse functional diabetic microangiopathy? Transplant Int 1990; 3:167–170.
24. Nakash R, Tydén G, Groth CG. Quality of life in diabetic patients after combined pancreas/kidney or kidney transplantation. Diabetes 1989; 38:40–42.
25. Nakash R, Tydén G, Groth CG. Long-term quality of life in diabetic patients after combined pancreas/kidney transplantation or kidney transplantation. Transplant Proc 1994; 26:510–511.
26. Zehrer CL, Gross CR. Quality of life of pancreas transplant recipients. Diabetologia 1991; 34:145–149.
27. Piehlmeier W, Bullinger M, Nusser J, et al. Quality of life in type I insulin dependent diabetic patients prior to and after pancreas and kidney transplantation in relation to organ function. Diabetologia 1991; 34:150–157.
28. Manske CL, Wang Y, Thomas W. Mortality of cadaveric kidney transplantation versus combined kidney/pancreas transplantation in diabetic patients. Lancet 1995; 346:1658–1662.
29. Gaber AO, Elgebeli S, Sugathan P, et al. Early improvement in cardiac function occurs in pancreas/kidney but not diabetic kidney alone transplant recipients. Transplantation 1995; 59:1105–1107.
30. Föger B, Königsrainer A, Polos RG, et al. Effect of pancreas transplantation on lipoproteinlipase postprandial lipidemia and HDL cholesterol. Transplantation 1994; 58:899–901.
31. Larsen J, Larsson C, Hirst K, et al. Lipidstatus after combined pancreas/kidney transplantation and kidney transplantation alone in type I diabetes mellitus. Transplantation 1992; 54:992–995.
32. Page MM, Watkins PJ. Cardiorespiratory arrest and diabetic autonomic neuropathy. Lancet 1978; 1:14.
33. Navarro X, Kennedy WR, Aeppli D, Sutherland DER. Neuropathy and mortality in diabetes influence of pancreas transplantation. Muscle Nerve 1996; 19:1009–1012.
34. Smetz Y, Westendorp R, van der Pijl, et al. Effect of simultaneous pancreas/kidney transplantation on mortality of patients with type I diabetes mellitus and end stage renal failure. Lancet 1999; 353:1915–1917.

# 3 | The History of Pancreas Transplantation

## Thomas E. Starzl, Ngoc Thai, and Ron Shapiro

*Thomas E. Starzl Transplantation Institute, University of Pittsburgh School of Medicine, Pittsburgh, Pennsylvania, U.S.A.*

More than 115 years ago, it was demonstrated by Von Mering and Minkowski that pancreatectomy produced diabetes mellitus in dogs (1). Nearly four decades passed before attempts were made to restore glucose homeostasis by pancreas transplantation with surgical vascular anastomoses, but only for physiologic experiments (2,3). An additional three decades went by before preclinical studies for the potential purpose of ameliorating diabetes were undertaken in the late 1950s by Brooks and Gifford (4) and DeJode and Howard (5). After surgical technical problems were worked out in the canine model (summarized in Ref. 6), the first attempt to treat human diabetes mellitus with pancreas transplantation was carried out on December 17, 1966, by William Kelly and Richard Lillehei (7) at the University of Minnesota. The patient died after two months. The same Minneapolis team recorded the first success on June 3, 1969 (8). "Success" during this pioneer period came to be defined as patient and functional graft survival for at least one year.

Thus, the pancreas became the fourth kind of organ allograft to be successfully transplanted over a 10-year period (1959–1969) in which the feasibility of kidney (9,10), liver (11), and heart (12) already had been demonstrated (Table 1) (8–13). It was a stunning "proof of principle" development that was at first considered not credible by knowledgeable authorities who had viewed such efforts with distain. Hopes for organ transplantation had been based previously on experiments in neonatal mice (14) and in irradiated adult mice (15) in which it was shown that the development of donor-specific tolerance was associated with the donor leukocyte chimerism produced by splenic or bone marrow cell infusion. In an extrapolation of the mouse findings, the production of donor leukocyte chimerism by bone marrow infusion prior to or at the time of organ transplantation was expected to play an essential role in achieving organ engraftment. However, efforts to apply this strategy in animals were uniformly unsuccessful, in part because a good histocompatibility match was a prerequisite for avoidance of graft versus host disease. When discovery of the human leukocyte antigens made tissue matching feasible, human bone marrow transplantation was finally accomplished, but this was not until 1968 (13).

In the meanwhile, two unexplained qualities of the alloimmune response had made it feasible to forge ahead precociously with organ transplantation under drug immunosuppression (16). The first observation was that kidney allograft rejection that developed under azathioprine was regularly reversible by adding large doses of prednisone. The second finding was that organ allografts under the nonspecific immunosuppression of azathioprine and prednisone appeared to self-induce variable donor-specific tolerance. Tolerance was inferred from the rapidly declining need for immunosuppression after rejection reversal. However, because of the ostensible absence of donor leukocyte chimerism in these recipients, organ engraftment, including that of the pancreas, was attributed to different mechanisms than those of bone marrow cell engraftment. This chimerism-exclusionary dogma was not challenged until low-level (micro-) chimerism was discovered in 1992 in the blood and tissues of long-surviving organ recipients (17,18). Then it was obvious that alloengraftment was a form of partial tolerance that resulted from " . . . responses of co-existing donor and recipient cells, each to the other, causing reciprocal clonal exhaustion, followed by peripheral clonal deletion" (Fig. 1) (17,18). Successfully treated organ recipients and bone marrow recipients were mirror image versions of leukocyte chimerism, differing in the proportion of donor and recipient leukocytes (Fig. 2).

## THE DOMINANT ROLE OF DRUG IMMUNOSUPPRESSION

Without the foregoing insight into the chimerism-dependent mechanisms of organ engraftment, further progress hinged almost exclusively on the development of stronger

**Table 1**  First Successful Transplantation of Human Allografts (Survival ≥1 Year)

| Organ | City (Ref.) | Date | Physician/surgeon |
|---|---|---|---|
| Kidney | Boston (9,10) | 1/24/59 | Merrill/Murray |
| Liver | Denver (11) | 7/23/67 | Starzl/Groth |
| Heart | Cape Town (12) | 1/2/68 | Barnard |
| Bone marrow | Minneapolis (13) | 8/24/68 | Gatti/Good |
| Pancreas[a] | Minneapolis (8) | 6/3/69 | Lillehei/Kelly |

[a]Kidney and pancreas allografts in uremic patient.

immunosuppression. The combined use of azathioprine and prednisone had been a critical step in the clinical development of kidney and other kinds of organ transplantation. But because allografts were being lost to acute rejections that could not be reversed, a worldwide policy drift occurred in which large doses of prednisone were administered from the time of operation, rather than in response to rejection. The addition in 1966 of a short course of post-transplant antilymphocyte globulin (ALG) to azathioprine and prednisone (the "triple drug cocktail") substantially reduced steroid needs (19,20) and was used for the first successful non-renal organ transplantations (8,11,12). Nevertheless, the heavy mortality, and particularly the devastating morbidity caused by long-term prednisone dependence, made organ transplantation (even of kidneys) as much a disease as a treatment in the view of critics. Widespread transplantation of the nonrenal organs (including the pancreas) was forestalled until the advent of cyclosporine (21,22) and tacrolimus (23).

As the more potent drugs became available, they were simply folded into the modified formula of heavy prophylactic immunosuppression that had been inherited from the 1960s and 1970s. Used in this way, the multiple drug cocktails fueled the golden age of transplantation of the 1980s and early 1990s. The dose ceilings of the individual primary and secondary drugs were imposed by drug toxicity, while the dose floors were revealed by breakthrough rejection. For example, the upper limit of azathioprine dosage [or comparably used substitutes such as cyclosphosphamide (24) or mycophenolate mofetil (MMF) (25)] was dictated by myelotoxicity that could be monitored conveniently by serial white blood counts. The more complex limiting side effects of the calcineurin inhibitors (cyclosporine and tacrolimus) are shown in Table 2. Of specific interest in the context of pancreas transplantation, both cyclosporine and tacrolimus are diabetogenic, in addition to their nephrotoxicity and neurotoxicity (26). The other T-cell directed agent, sirolimus, has its own distinctive panoply of dose-limiting side effects (27).

By using these agents in different combinations, it was possible with the various drug cocktails to reduce acute rejection to almost a non-problem during the last two decades. The unresolved issues now became the drug-specific side effects, chronic rejection, and the

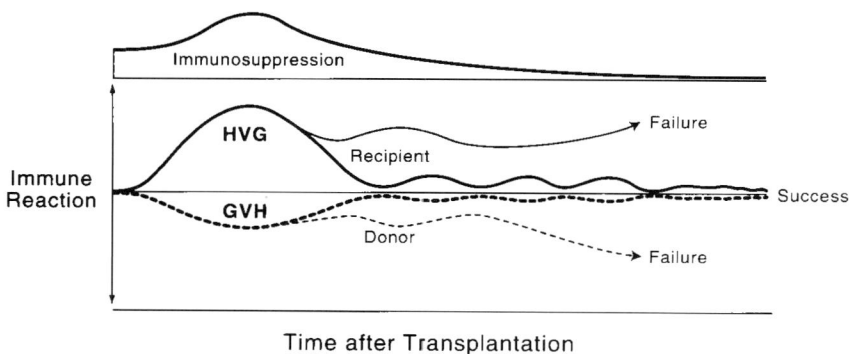

**Figure 1**  Contemporaneous host versus graft (HVG) (*upright curves*) and graft versus host (GVH) (*inverted curves*) responses after organ transplantation. If some degree of reciprocal clonal exhaustion is not induced and maintained (usually requiring protective immune suppression), one cell population will destroy the other. In contrast to the usually dominant HVG reaction of organ transplantation (shown here), the GVH reaction usually is dominant in the cytoablated bone marrow recipient. Therapeutic failure with either type of transplantation implies the inability to control one, the other, or both of the responses.

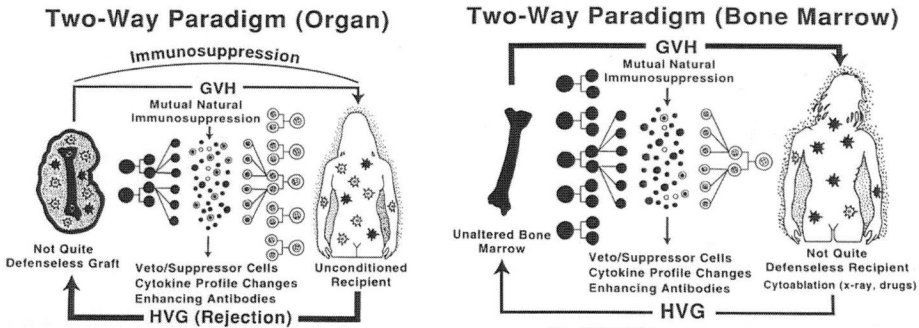

**Figure 2** Two-way paradigm in which transplantation is seen as a bidirectional and mutually canceling immune reaction that is predominantly host versus graft with whole organ grafts (*left*) and predominantly graft versus host with bone marrow grafts (*right*).

risks of long-term immunodepression. The list of complications from protracted immunodepression per se was a long one, which could be divided into two broad categories: susceptibility to infections and the development of de novo malignancies.

## PANCREAS TRANSPLANT PROCEDURES VS. IMMUNOSUPPRESSION ERA

Neither the development nor the merits of the different pancreas transplant operations could be discussed intelligently without parallel consideration of the immunosuppression that was available at the time these procedures were introduced. The point can be most easily made by perusing the 1988 textbook, *Pancreatic Transplantation*, prepared by Carl G. Groth (Huddinge Hospital, Huddinge, Sweden) (28) after it was apparent that cyclosporine had upgraded the prospects for a range of organ transplant procedures. In addition to the contributions by the Stockholm team members, Groth's book contains chapters from the seminal Minneapolis pancreas program and from programs in Cambridge (England), Iowa City, Lyon, Munich, and Pittsburgh. Because it provides a snapshot of pancreas transplantation in transition, the book is a historical treasure. In its pages, opinions about surgical technique, pancreas procurement and preservation, and other issues were discussed (circa 1987) by team leaders who continued to influence pancreas transplantation for the next dozen years and beyond.

### Azathioprine Era

The first attempts at clinical pancreas transplantation were plagued by inadequate control of rejection despite the administration of frequently myelotoxic doses of azathioprine, large

**Table 2** Nonimmunologic Profile of Calcineurin Inhibitors (Four + Worst): All Dose Related

| | Tacrolimus | Cyclosporine |
|---|---|---|
| Nephrotoxicity | ++[a] | ++ |
| Neurotoxicity | + | + |
| Diabetogenicity | + | + |
| Growth effects | | |
|   Hirsutism | 0 | +++ |
|   Gingival hyperplasia | 0 | ++ |
|   Facial brutalization | 0 | + |
|   Hepatotropic effects | ++++ | +++ |
|   Gynecomastia | 0 | + |
| Other metabolic effects | | |
|   Cholesterol increase | 0 | ++ |
|   Uric acid increase | +? | ++ |

[a]Less hypertension.
*Source*: From Ref. 26.

amounts of prednisone, and "induction" ALG. In addition to being diabetogenic, steroids were inimical to wound healing. The technical aspects of the pancreas transplant procedures developed during this period reflected efforts to work around these inadequacies of immuno-suppression. In their first human operation at the University of Minnesota (7) on December 17, 1966, Kelly and Lillehei transplanted the head and tail of a cadaveric pancreas to the left iliac fossa of a uremic recipient after removing the graft duodenum and ligating the pancreatic duct. A kidney from the same donor was placed in the right iliac fossa. The recipient immediately became insulin independent, but died at two months from a combination of rejection and sepsis.

By 1973, Lillehei and associates had implanted 13 more whole human pancreas grafts, 10 in combination with cadaver kidneys from the same donor and the final three alone (8,29). In cases 2 to 6 pancreatic secretions of the allograft were exteriorized (cutaneous graft duode-nostomy), while in cases 7 to 13 the exocrine drainage was directed via the graft duodenum into the host jejunum, using a Roux-en Y technique (8). In patient 14, a patch of graft duodenum containing the ampulla of Vater was anastomosed to recipient bowel. The only recipi-ent (the sixth) in this pioneer series of 14 cases to achieve long-lasting insulin independence beginning on the day of operation (June 3, 1969) died shortly after reaching the one-year mile-stone with a functioning pancreas after losing the kidney graft and returning to dialysis. The 13 other pancreas graft losses resulted from technical complications including vascular throm-bosis, death with a functioning graft, and, most commonly, lethal complications associated with exocrine pancreatic drainage. Similar discouraging results with pancreas transplantation during the early 1970s in Sao Paulo (Brazil), Chicago (Illinois), Irvine (California), Zurich (Switzerland), and in mostly unreported cases elsewhere caused abandonment of whole organ pancreas transplantation for more than a decade.

The grim early experience continued to influence surgical policies worldwide until the end of the 20th century. With the premise that the Achilles heel of the operation was the need for exocrine drainage, new strategies emerged to avoid entry into the host bowel, to eliminate the graft duodenum from the graft or to prevent or reduce the volume of the graft exocrine secretions. In 1973, Gliedman et al. (30) reported excision of the graft duodenum and the adjacent pancreatic head with transplantation of the rest of the pancreas; the segmen-tal pancreatic duct was anastomosed to the recipient ureter. When two of these recipients lived insulin free for two and four years (31), momentum shifted for the next dozen years to the essentially exclusive use of distal pancreas grafts. Rather than exocrine diversion into the uri-nary tract or bowel, however, most surgeons either drained exocrine secretions from the pancreatic segment into the free peritoneal cavity or blocked the segmental duct by ligation (29) or by injection of a polymer (32). Only Groth and Tydén in Stockholm systematically resisted the trend by anastomosing the duct (or the draining segmental surface) to the bowel (33).

## Cyclosporine Era

With better control of rejection and less steroid dependence made possible by cyclosporine, there was a resurgence of interest in pancreas transplantation as well as modifications of the surgical operation. Use of segmental cadaveric allografts continued until well into the 1980s, and remains an option today when live pancreas donors are used. In early 1982, we re-examined the reasons for abandonment of whole pancreas transplantation, and undertook reassessment of the procedure in dogs (34). Our conclusion was that the most logical operation of whole organ transplantation described by Lillehei and Kelly had been discontinued in favor of the inferior option of segmental pancreas transplantation. Consequently, a limited clinical trial of whole organ pancreas transplantation was begun in Pittsburgh in March 1983 (35). In a crucial modification of the original Lillehei procedure, we developed a tech-nique for draining the allograft exocrine secretions into the host jejunum through a "bubble" of graft duodenum into which the ampulla of Vater emptied. The duodenal bubble was anastomosed to the side of the host jejunum (Fig. 3) (35,36).

Although the number of cases was small, the influence of the trial was amplified by the presence in Pittsburgh at the time of fellows or visitors who had come to observe the burgeon-ing liver transplant program and who also saw how easy and successful was the whole organ pancreas transplantation. One such fellow (1981–1983), Dr. Munci Kalayoglu, subsequently joined a team at the University of Wisconsin headed by Dr. Hans Sollinger, which had

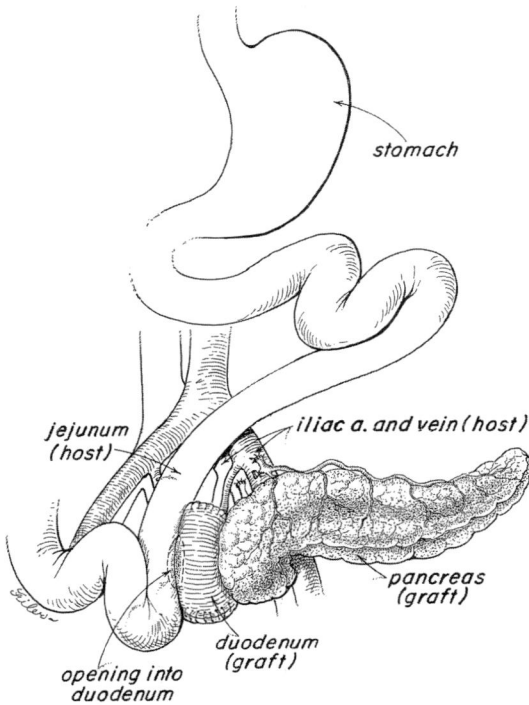

**Figure 3** Use of donor "duodenal bubble" for exocrine pancreatic drainage introduced in Pittsburgh in 1983.

previously compiled a series of segmental transplantations with exocrine drainage into the bladder. After Kalayoglu's arrival in Madison, Sollinger and Kalayoglu changed from segmental to whole organ transplantation. Similarly, Dr. Robert Corry of the University of Iowa was persuaded during a sabbatical leave in Pittsburgh in late 1983 and early 1984 to adopt the whole pancreas transplantation procedure (37).

At their home institutions, Corry and Sollinger initially drained the graft duodenal bubble into the host jejunum. However, both teams soon advocated anastomosis of the bubble to the anterolateral wall of the host bladder (Fig. 4) (38,39). Bladder drainage was adopted soon thereafter for most cases at the University of Minnesota (39). With the enthusiastic endorsement from these three centers [reflected in separate chapters in Groth's book (40–42)] the bladder drainage technique was widely accepted. Serial measurement of urine amylase concentration became a means of immune surveillance, i.e., a drop in urine amylase signaled rejection. Complications from the bladder drainage were initially viewed as acceptable. However, digestion of the urethra by activated pancreatic enzymes, less serious but common examples of cystitis, uncorrectable metabolic acidosis caused by the continuous loss of bicarbonate, and a myriad of other problems necessitating conversion to enteric drainage began to diminish enthusiasm for bladder drainage by the mid 1990s. By this time, Corry (now at the University of Pittsburgh) had switched back to enteric drainage via the duodenal bubble. After the advent of tacrolimus, this became the reconstruction of choice at almost all centers (43–45).

## Tacrolimus Era

Despite Corry's enthusiastic advocacy of tacrolimus, the drug was not widely used for pancreas transplantation until the mid 1990s because of its dose-related diabetogenicity. This view changed dramatically when a multicenter collection of cases demonstrated the ability of the new drug to rescue most of the treatment failures that were occurring under cyclosporine-based immunosuppression (46). Moreover, the superior control of rejection with minimal dependence on prednisone using tacrolimus-based immunosuppression from the outset has further eroded the arguments for exocrine diversion to the bladder. It also became possible

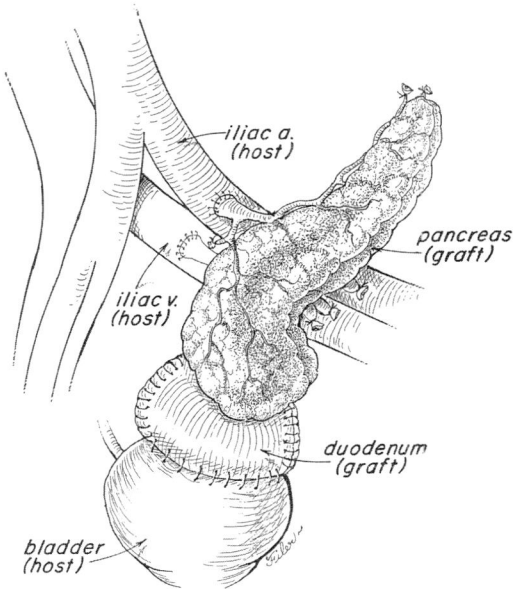

**Figure 4** Drainage of pancreas exocrine secretions into the recipient bladder. This was the most commonly used procedure from 1985 until the mid or late 1990s.

with the simplified tacrolimus-based regimens to eliminate the perioperative induction therapy with ALG that had become a standard component of cyclosporine-based immunosuppression during the mid 1980s. Since 1995, general agreement about the superiority of tacrolimus-based immunosuppression was finally reached (33,43–45,47–49).

## A New Era?

The long-term efficacy of pancreas transplantation is not yet clear. Only 16 recipients in the world are known to have functioning pancreas allografts that were transplanted before 1986 and none who were treated before 1981 (50). With the improvements that occurred since the 1980s, there have been many reports indicating that the survival of diabetic kidney transplant recipients is improved by cotransplantation of a pancreas (43–49). However, there has been at least one United Network for Organ Sharing-based analysis suggesting that the risk of death from staged kidney–pancreas transplantation has been greater, even in recent times, than in kidney-alone recipients who had been listed for a pancreas but failed to get one (51) (see also counter-arguments in Chapter 1). Apart from pancreas graft-related complications or functional failures, late recipient deaths have continued from cardiac, infectious, and peripheral vascular disease, and from de novo malignancies. Many, if not most, of these late complications can be traced to, or are aggravated by, the need for chronic immunosuppression.

The ideal solution would be to make organ recipients more tolerant and thereby less immunosuppression-dependent. This objective became realistic with the elucidation of the donor leukocyte chimerism-associated mechanisms of acquired tolerance (17,18) and the recognition that organ engraftment is a form of partial tolerance (52,53). With this insight, it was obvious that the seminal mechanism of alloengraftment and acquired tolerance (i.e., clonal exhaustion–deletion) can be subverted by the "conventional" use of heavy prophylactic immunosuppression (Fig. 5, right) (53). In 2001, it was proposed that this undesired consequence could be prevented by observance of two therapeutic principles: recipient pretreatment and the use of minimal posttransplant immunosuppression (Fig. 5, left) (53).

Between July and December 2001, the late Robb Corry carried out a pilot trial based on these principles in 10 recipients of simultaneous pancreas and kidney allografts and four recipients of pancreas transplants alone. All of the donors were human leukocyte antigen-mismatched, heart-beating cadavers with the same ABO types as the recipients. The patients

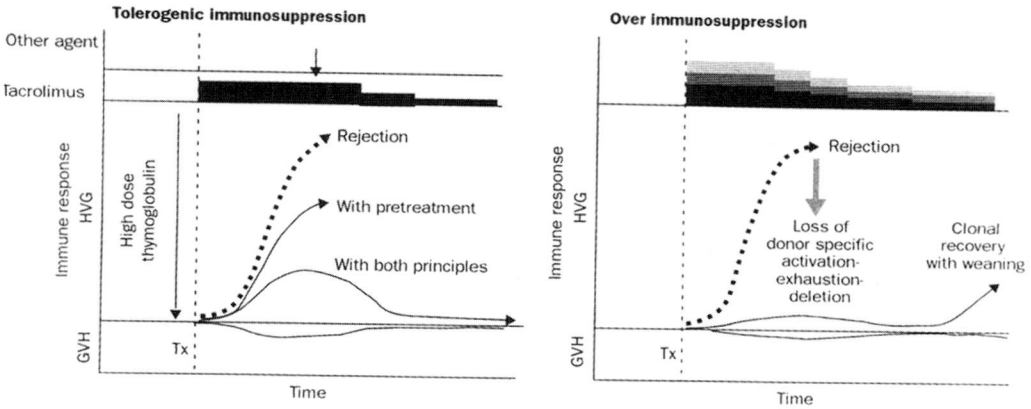

**Figure 5** Mechanisms of immunosuppression. (*Left*): Conversion of rejection (*thick dashed arrow*) to an immune response that can be exhausted and deleted by combination of pretreatment and minimalistic posttransplant immunosuppression. (*Right*): If the clonal response is eliminated by excessive posttransplant immunosuppression, exhaustion–deletion shown on the left is precluded, and subsequent graft survival is permanently dependent on immunosuppression. *Abbreviations*: GVH, graft versus host; HVG, host versus graft; Tx, transplantation.

were infused prior to organ revascularization with approximately 5 mg/kg rabbit antithymocyte globulin (Thymoglobulin[®]) and were coinfused with 1–2 g methylprednisolone to prevent cytokine reactions (54). On the first postoperative day, twice-daily tacrolimus monotherapy was begun with a target 12-hour trough level of 10 ng/mL. After four to six

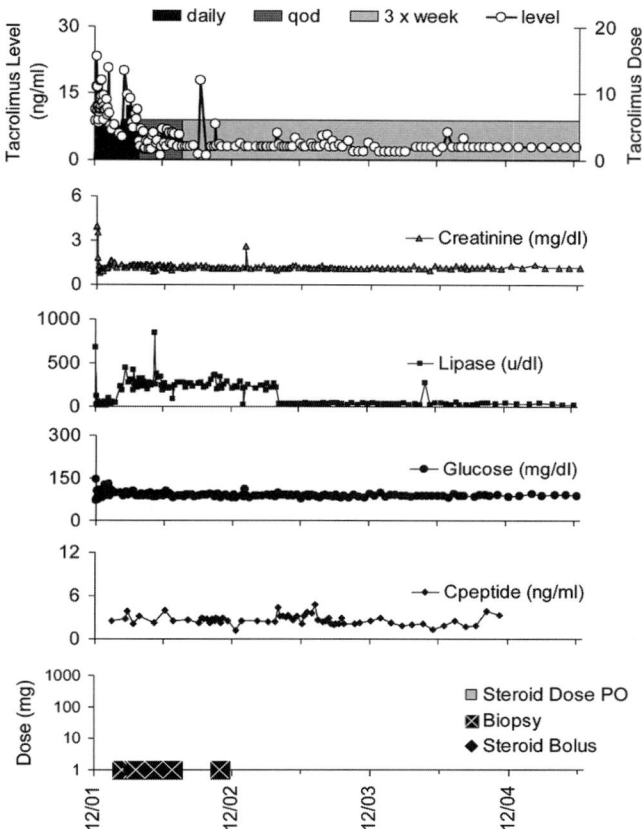

**Figure 6** The course of a simultaneous pancreas–kidney recipient pretreated with antithymocyte globulin. The dose frequency of daily monotherapy was reduced to every other day at four months and to three times a week at eight months after transplant (*top panel*). Creatinine, lipase, glucose, and C-peptide (*middle panels*), have been stable throughout. This patient did not receive any steroids or other additional treatment and was biopsied five times with no evidence of damaging acute rejection.

**Table 3**  Tolerogenic Immunosuppression for Pancreas Recipients (Corry, 2001): Results at Three Years

| Number | TX | Monotherapy (dose frequency) | Creatinine (mg/dL) | Fasting glucose (mg/dL) |
|---|---|---|---|---|
| Simultaneous pancreas–kidney | | | | |
| 1 | 7/01 | Daily | 2.0 | 80–90 |
| 2 | 8/01 | Daily | 1.3 | 80–100 |
| 3 | 8/01 | Once/wk | 1.0 | 70–80[a] |
| 4 | 9/01 | — | Failed 22 mo | Failed 5 mo |
| 5 | 9/01 | Daily | 4 | 90–100 |
| 6 | 10/01 | — | Failed 22 mo | 90–140[b] |
| 7 | 11/01 | Thrice/wk | 1.0 | 80–100 |
| 8 | 11/01 | Daily | 1.7 | 80–110 |
| 9 | 12/01 | — | Failed 13 mo | Failed 7 mo |
| 10 | 12/01 | Thrice/wk | 1.3 | 80–90 |
| Pancreas alone | | | | |
| 1 | 7/01 | Thrice/wk | 1.7[c] | 70–100 |
| 2 | 9/01 | Daily multidrug | 1.2[c] | 90–140[b] |
| 3 | 10/01 | — | 1.0[c] | Failed 5 mo |
| 4 | 12/01 | Daily | 1.6[c] | 70–90 |

Monotherapy: all tacrolimus except Case 1 (rapamycin).
—, Not applicable because of graft loss(s) and drug discontinuance.
[a]After three years, the patient developed disseminated metastases from breast cancer, and died insulin-free at 43 months.
[b]Became insulin-dependent after three years.
[c]Native kidney.
*Note*: Pancreas grafts functioning at three years: 11/14 (78.5%), currently 9/14 (64%); kidney grafts functioning at three years and now: 7/10 (70%).
*Abbreviation*: TX, transplantation.

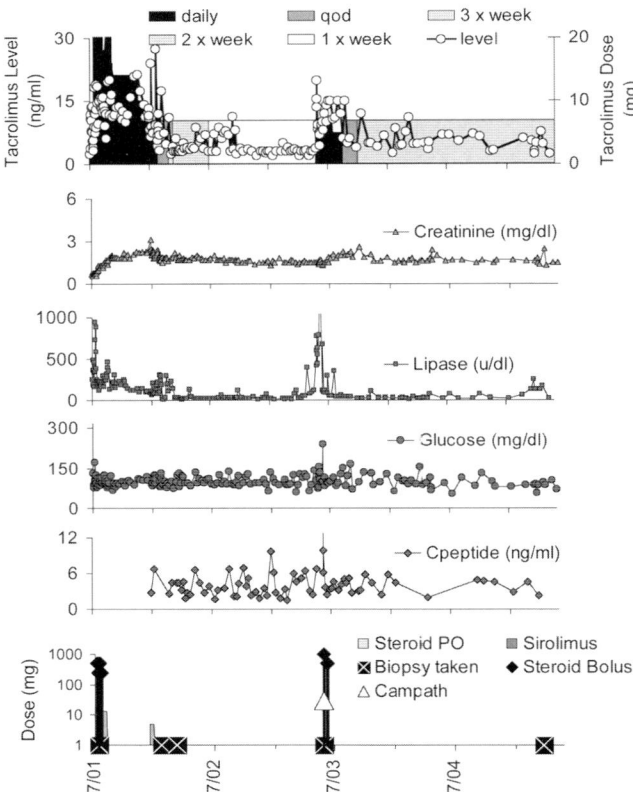

**Figure 7**  The course of the first pancreas recipient pretreated with antithymocyte globulin. The dose frequency for this pancreas-alone recipient was reduced quickly after six months reaching a minimum of one dose per week at one year. A biochemically indicated, pathology-confirmed rejection at 23 months was reversed with steroids, a dose of alemtuzumab (*lower panel*), and the temporary resumption of daily tacrolimus that subsequently was re-weaned to three times a week. The benefit of reduced exposure to tacrolimus is apparent in the creatinine levels depicted in the second panel; i.e., the patient's kidney functioned better with less treatment and worse with more treatment. Other than during the rejection episode, graft function, as reflected in the lipase, glucose, and C-peptide levels, has been stable throughout. Later patients (Fig. 6) were weaned less aggressively.

months, patients who had been on stable tacrolimus monotherapy for at least two months had extension of the interval of tacrolimus doses ("spaced weaning") to once a day, every other day, or longer if this was compatible with stable graft function (Fig. 6).

A short-term follow-up of the patients was reported in 2003 (54). The results at three years and the current results are summarized in Table 3 for each case. Eleven (78%) of the 14 recipients remained insulin free for three years, but in two of these patients, hyperglycemia recurred after 36 months. Thus, nine (64.2%) still are insulin free after 43 to 49 months. Eight of the nine insulin-free patients are on treatment with a single drug and four are on spaced doses of tacrolimus (Figs. 6 and 7). Importantly, seven of the 10 patients who also received kidneys had life-supporting renal function at three years with serum creatinine concentrations $\leq 2$ mg/dL in six. After Corry was killed in a motor vehicular accident in February 2002, the trial was placed on hold.

By the time of his death, Corry was aware that the management principles under evaluation were sound and required only fine-tuning. First, the initial step of weaning to every other day would have to be taken more cautiously. Second, weaning of monotherapy to intervals greater than every other day should be delayed until at least one year unless evidence of drug-specific side effects (e.g., nephrotoxicity, neurotoxicity, or diabetogenicity) called for earlier action. In 2003, the policy of tolerogenic immunosuppression was reinstituted with these foregoing modifications. In addition, lymphoid depletion was done with the broadly reacting antilymphoid monoclonal antibody, alemtuzumab (Campath®) rather than with Thymoglobulin. The superior early results with this management are described in Chapter 1. The chapter, along with the rest of this book, has been dedicated to Corry's memory. A Robb Corry Professorship has been established at the University of Pittsburgh, the inaugural occupant of which is Ron Shapiro.

## REFERENCES

1.  Von Mering J, Minkowski O. Diabetes mellitus nach pankreas-exstirpation. Zentralbl Klin Med 1889; 10:393–394.
2.  Gayet R, Guillaumie M. La regulation de la secretion interne pancreatique par un processus humoral, demontree par des transplantations de pancreas. Compt Rend Soc Biol 1927; 97:1613–1616.
3.  Houssay BA. Technique de la greffe pancreatico-duodenale au cou. Compt Rend Soc Biol 1929; 100:138–140.
4.  Brooks JR, Gifford GH. Pancreatic homotransplantation. Transplant Bull 1959; 23:100.
5.  DeJode LR, Howard JM. Studies in pancreaticoduodenal homotransplantation. Surg Gynecol Obstet 1962; 14:553–558.
6.  Brekke IB. Experimental background. In: Groth CG, ed. Pancreatic Transplantation. Philadelphia, PA: WB Saunders Company, 1988:21–35.
7.  Kelly WD, Lillehei RC, Merkel FK, Idezuki Y, Goetz FC. Allotransplantation of the pancreas and duodenum along with the kidney in diabetic nephropathy. Surgery 1967; 61:827–837.
8.  Lillehei RC, Simmons RL, Najarian JS, et al. Pancreaticoduodenal allotransplantation: experimental and clinical experience. Ann Surg 1970; 172:405–436.
9.  Murray JE, Merrill JP, Dammin GJ, et al. Study of transplantation immunity after total body irradiation: clinical and experimental investigation. Surgery 1960; 48:272–284.
10. Merrill JP, Murray JE, Harrison JH, Friedman EA, Dealy JB Jr., Dammin GJ. Successful homotransplantation of the kidney between non-identical twins. N Engl J Med 1960; 262:1251–1260.
11. Starzl TE, Groth CG, Brettschneider L, et al. Orthotopic homotransplantation of the human liver. Ann Surg 1968; 168:392–415.
12. Barnard CN. What we have learned about heart transplants. J Thorac Cardiovasc Surg 1968; 56:457–468.
13. Gatti RA, Meuwissen HJ, Allen HD, Hong R, Good RA. Immunological reconstitution of sex-linked lymphopenic immunological deficiency. Lancet 1968; 2:1366–1369.
14. Billingham RE, Brent L, Medawar PB. "Actively acquired tolerance" of foreign cells. Nature 1953; 172:603–606.
15. Main JM, Prehn RT. Successful skin homografts after the administration of high dosage X radiation and homologous bone marrow. J Natl Cancer Inst 1955; 15:1023–1029.
16. Starzl TE, Marchioro TL, Waddell WR. The reversal of rejection in human renal homografts with subsequent development of homograft tolerance. Surg Gynecol Obstet 1963; 117:385–395.
17. Starzl TE, Demetris AJ, Murase N, Ildstad S, Ricordi C, Trucco M. Cell migration, chimerism, and graft acceptance. Lancet 1992; 339:1579–1582.
18. Starzl TE, Demetris AJ, Trucco M, et al. Cell migration and chimerism after whole-organ transplantation: the basis of graft acceptance. Hepatology 1993; 17:1127–1152.

19.  Starzl TE, Marchioro TL, Porter KA, Iwasaki Y, Cerilli GJ. The use of heterologous antilymphoid agents in canine renal and liver homotransplantation and in human renal homotransplantation. Surg Gynecol Obstet 1967; 124:301–318.

20.  Starzl TE, Porter KA, Iwasaki Y, Marchioro TL, Kashiwagi N. The use of antilymphocyte globulin in human renal homotransplantation. In: Wolstenholme GEW, O'Connor M, eds. Antilymphocytic Serum. London: J and A Churchill Limited, 1967:4–34.

21.  Calne RY, Rolles K, White DJG, et al. Cyclosporin A initially as the only immunosuppressant in 34 recipients of cadaveric organs; 32 kidneys, 2 pancreases, and 2 livers. Lancet 1979; 2:1033–1036.

22.  Starzl TE, Klintmalm GBG, Weil R III, et al. Cyclosporin A and steroid therapy in sixty-six cadaver kidney recipients. Surg Gynecol Obstet 1981; 153:486–494.

23.  Starzl TE, Todo S, Fung J, Demetris AJ, Venkataramanan R, Jain A. FK 506 for human liver, kidney and pancreas transplantation. Lancet 1989; 2:1000–1004.

24.  Starzl TE, Putnam CW, Halgrimson CG, et al. Cyclophosphamide and whole organ transplantation in human beings. Surg Gynecol Obstet 1971; 133:981–991.

25.  Sollinger HW, for the U.S. Renal Transplant Mycophenolate Mofetil Study Group. Mycophenolate mofetil for the prevention of acute rejection in primary cadaveric renal allograft recipients. Transplantation 1995; 60:225–232.

26.  Starzl TE, Abu-Elmagd K, Tzakis A, Fung JJ, Porter KA, Todo S. Selected topics on FK 506: with special references to rescue of extrahepatic whole organ grafts, transplantation of "forbidden organs," side effects, mechanisms, and practical pharmacokinetics. Transplant Proc 1991; 23:914–919.

27.  Groth CG, Backman L, Morales JM, et al. Sirolimus (rapamycin)-based therapy in human renal transplantation: similar efficacy and different toxicity compared with cyclosporine. Sirolimus European Renal Transplant Study Group. Transplantation 1999; 67:1036–1042.

28.  Groth CG, ed. Pancreatic Transplantation. Philadelphia, PA: WB Saunders Company, 1988:1–413.

29.  Najarian J. Landmarks in clinical pancreatic transplantation. In: Groth CG, ed. Pancreatic Transplantation. Philadelphia, PA: WB Saunders Company, 1988:15–19.

30.  Gliedman ML, Gold M, Whittaker J, et al. Clinical segmental pancreatic transplantation with ureteropancreatic duct anastomosis for exocrine drainage. Surgery 1973; 74:171–180.

31.  Gliedman ML, Tellis VA, Soberman R, Rifkin H, Veith FJ. Long-term effect of pancreatic transplant function in patients with advanced juvenile-onset diabetes. Diabetes Care 1978; 1:1–9.

32.  Dubernard JM, Traeger J, Neyra P, Touraine JL, Tranchant D, Blanc-Brunat N. New method of preparation of a segmental pancreatic graft for transplantation. Trials in dogs and in man. Surgery 1978; 84:633–639.

33.  Groth CG, Tydén G. Segmental pancreatic transplantation with enteric exocrine drainage. In: Groth CG, ed. Pancreatic Transplantation. Philadelphia, PA: WB Saunders Company, 1988:99–112.

34.  Diliz-Perez HS, Hong H-Q, de Santibanes E, et al. Total pancreaticoduodenal homotransplantation in dogs immunosuppressed with cyclosporine and steroids. Am J Surg 1984; 147:677–680.

35.  Starzl TE, Iwatsuki S, Shaw BW Jr., et al. Pancreaticoduodenal transplantation in humans. Surg Gynecol Obstet 1984;159:265–272.

36.  Starzl TE, Tzakis AG. Pancreatico-duodenal transplantation with enteric exocrine drainage. In: Groth CG, ed. Pancreatic Transplantation. Philadelphia, PA: WB Saunders Company, 1988:113–129.

37.  Corry RJ, Ngheim D, Schulak J, Budtel WD, Gonwa TA. Surgical treatment of diabetic nephropathy with simultaneous pancreatic duodenal and renal transplantation. Surg Gynecol Obstet 1986; 162:547–555.

38.  Nghiem DD, Gonwa TA, Corry RJ. Metabolic effects of urinary diversion of exocrine secretions in pancreas transplantation. Transplantation 1987; 43:70–73.

39.  Sollinger HW, Kalayoglu M, Hoffman RM, Deierhoi MH, Belzer FO. Quandruple immunosuppressive therapy in whole pancreas transplantation. Transplant Proc 1987; 19:2297–2299.

40.  Sutherland DER, Goetz FC, Najarian JS. Experience with single pancreas transplantation compared with pancreas transplantation after a kidney transplantation; and with transplantation with pancreas grafts from living related compared with cadaveric donors. In: Groth CG, ed. Pancreatic Transplantation. Philadelphia, PA: WB Saunders Company, 1988:175–189.

41.  Sollinger HW, Belzer FO. Pancreas transplantation with urinary tract drainage. In: Groth, CG, eds. Pancreatic Transplantation. Philadelphia, PA: WB Saunders Company, 1988:131–146.

42.  Corry RJ. Pancreatico-duodenal transplantation with urinary tract drainage. In: Groth, CG, eds. Pancreatic Transplantation. Philadelphia, PA: WB Saunders Company, 1988:147–153.

43.  Sollinger HW, Odorico JS, Knechtle SJ, D'Alessandro AM, Kalayglu M, Pirsch JD. Experience with 500 simultaneous pancreas-kidney transplants. Ann Surg 1998; 228:284–296.

44.  Sutherland DE, Gruessner RW, Dunn DL, et al. Lessons learned from more than 1000 pancreas transplants at a single institution. Ann Surg 2001; 233:463–501.

45.  Corry RJ, Chakrabarti PK, Shapiro R, et al. Simultaneous administration of adjuvant donor bone marrow in pancreas transplant recipients. Ann Surg 1999; 230:372–379.

46.  Gruessner RW, Burke GW, Stratta R, et al. A multicenter analysis of the first experience with FK506 for induction and rescue therapy after pancreas transplantation. Transplantation 1996; 61:261–273.

47.  Tyden G, Bolinder J, Solders G, Brattstrom C, Tibell A, Groth CG. Improved survival in patients with insulin-dependent diabetes mellitus and end-stage diabetic nephropathy 10 years after combined pancreas and kidney transplantation. Transplantation 1999; 67:645–648.

48. Stratta RJ, Gaber AO, Shokouh-Amiri MH, et al. Evolution in pancreas transplantation techniques; simultaneous kidney-pancreas transplantation using portal-enteric drainage without antilymphocyte induction. Ann Surg 1999; 229:701–708.
49. Bartlett ST, Schweitzer EJ, Johnson LB, et al. Equivalent success of simultaneous pancreas kidney and solitary pancreas transplantation. A prospective trial of tacrolimus immunosuppression with percutaneous biopsy. Ann Surg 1996; 224:440–449.
50. Terasaki PI. The HLA-matching effect in different cohorts of kidney transplant recipients. In: Terasaki PI, Cecka JM, eds. Clinical Transplants 2003. Los Angeles, CA: UCLA Immunogenetics Center, 2004:466–469.
51. Venstrom JM, McBride MA, Rother KI, Hirshberg B, Orchard TJ, Harlan DM. Survival after pancreas transplantation in patients with diabetes and preserved kidney function. JAMA 2003; 290:2817–2823.
52. Starzl TE, Zinkernagel R. Antigen localization and migration in immunity and tolerance. N Engl J Med 1998; 339:1905–1913.
53. Starzl TE, Zinkernagel R. Transplantation tolerance from a historical perspective. Nat Rev Immunol 2001; 1:233–239.
54. Starzl TE, Murase N, Abu-Elmagd K, et al. Tolerogenic immunosuppression for organ transplantation. Lancet 2003; 361:1502–1510.

# 4

## Evaluation of the Pancreas Transplant Recipient

**Jerry McCauley**
*Thomas E. Starzl Transplantation Institute, University of Pittsburgh School of Medicine, Pittsburgh, Pennsylvania, U.S.A.*

## INTRODUCTION

Pancreas transplantation is the only treatment capable of reliably establishing an insulin-free, euglycemic state in patients with diabetes mellitus (1). The rate of pancreas transplantation has increased from less than 200/yr in 1987 to approximately 1000/yr in 1998 (2,3). It is no longer considered to be experimental, and both the improved quality of life and the cost-effectiveness of combined kidney–pancreas transplantation have made it the optimal therapy in type 1 diabetics with renal failure (4). The improved results of simultaneous kidney and pancreas transplantation (SPK) in the United States recently led to Medicare funding for the procedure. Further improvement in pancreas graft survival can be expected with continuing development of new immunosuppressive agents.

The evaluation of potential candidates for pancreas transplantation is critically important because many patients have preexisting cardiac disease and other complications of diabetes, and these may substantially increase the risk of death and/or graft loss. The indications for pancreas transplantation, while well established, continue to evolve, and may be highly affected by the preferences of the transplant center, improvements in allograft survival related to improved immunosuppression, and surgical technique. The contraindications to pancreas transplantation are changing as patient and graft survival continue to improve. With the advent of new immunosuppressive agents and increased funding for combined kidney and pancreas transplantation, more complicated patients will likely become potential candidates, and the preoperative evaluation of pancreas transplant recipients will become more demanding.

## GENETICS AND PATHOGENESIS OF TYPE 1 DIABETES

Evaluation of the potential pancreas transplant recipient begins with determining the type of diabetes. Conventionally, it has been generally assumed that only patients with inadequate insulin production will benefit from a second normally functioning organ. The American Diabetes Association (ADA) has recently reclassified diabetes on etiologic grounds (Table 1) (5,6). The previous classification, which was developed in 1979, was largely based upon the type of pharmacologic therapy used, and the new system has attempted to divide the types of diabetes by etiology when possible. The previous terms insulin-dependent diabetes (IDDM) and noninsulin–dependent diabetes have been eliminated. The terms type 1 and type 2 diabetes have been retained. In the revised classification primary and secondary categories of type 1 diabetes have been eliminated. Patients with low or absent insulin production (type 1 diabetics) benefit from replacement of pancreatic beta cells capable of producing insulin.

Accordingly, type 1 diabetics of the immune or idiopathic type are the most common candidates for pancreatic transplantation. Although most patients with type 1 diabetes are young (<25 years) at the time of initial diagnosis, type 1 diabetes may develop at any age, even in the geriatric population. The older description of maturity onset diabetes (MODY) was abandoned for a new classification that identifies the specific genetic defects leading to diabetes. All forms of MODY in the new classification are associated with impaired secretion of insulin but normal insulin action. Contrary to the suggestion of the term MODY, most patients with MODY develop mild hyperglycemia before the age of 25. Mutations of the gene hepatic nuclear factor 1-alpha and 4-alpha are responsible for MODY3 and 1, respectively.

**Table 1**  Etiologic Classification of Diabetes Mellitus

Type 1 diabetes (beta-cell destruction, usually leading to absolute insulin deficiency)
   Immune mediated
   Idiopathic
Type 2 diabetes (may range from predominantly insulin resistance with relative insulin deficiency to a predominantly
  secretory defect with insulin resistance)
Other specific types
   Genetic defects of beta-cell function
     Chromosome 12, HNF-1$\alpha$ (MODY3)
     Chromosome 7, glucokinase (MODY2)
     Chromosome 20, HNF-4$\alpha$ (MODY1)
     Mitochondrial DNA
     Others
   Genetic defects in insulin action
     Type A insulin resistance
     Leprechaunism
     Rabson–Mendenhall syndrome
     Lipoatrophic diabetes
     Other
   Diseases of the exocrine pancreas
     Pancreatitis
     Trauma/pancreatectomy
     Neoplasia
     Cystic fibrosis
     Hemochromatosis
     Fibrocalculous pancreatopathy
     Others
   Endocrinopathies
     Acromegaly
     Cushing's syndrome
     Glucagonoma
     Pheochromocytoma
     Hyperthyroidism
     Somatostatinoma
     Aldosteronoma
     Others
   Drug or chemical induced
   Infections
     Congenital rubella
     Cytomegalovirus
     Others
   Uncommon forms of immune-mediated diabetes
     Stiff-man syndrome
     Anti-insulin receptor antibodies
     Others
   Other genetic syndromes sometimes associated with diabetes
     Down's syndrome
     Klinefelter's syndrome
     Turner's syndrome
     Wolfram's syndrome
     Friedreich's ataxia
     Others
   (GBM)

*Abbreviations*: MODY, maturity onset diabetes; GEM, gestational diabetes.
*Source*: From Ref. 6.

A mutation of the glucokinase gene is responsible for MODY2. Mutations of mitochondrial
DNA result in ineffective conversion of proinsulin to insulin and an effective insulinopenic
state. Type 2 diabetes was retained in the new classification and represents patients with insulin resistance. Instead of insulinopenia, these patients have normal or elevated insulin levels.
There is, however, a component of defective insulin secretion even in type 2 diabetics, because
the insulin level, although elevated, is lower than would be expected for the level of hyperglycemia. A long list of other specific causes of diabetes form much of the remainder of the new

classification of diabetes, but most of these patients, such as type 2 diabetics, are conventionally not candidates for pancreatic transplantation. Finally gestational diabetes was retained in the new classification.

Autoimmune type 1 diabetes develops after immune destruction of the beta cells in the islets of Langerhans of the pancreas (7). The clinical manifestations of type 1 diabetes were once felt to result from a sudden illness, such as a viral infection, which initiated rapid destruction of beta cells and an immediate need for insulin therapy. It has now become clear that it is a chronic process of beta-cell destruction that precedes the clinical illness by many years. Hyperglycemia is an insensitive measure of pancreatic function and mass. At least 70% of the beta cells in a normal pancreas must be lost before hyperglycemia develops (8). The genetic markers of autoimmune type 1 diabetes are of course present at birth (9). These patients are felt to have a genetic predisposition, which is activated by some environmental stimulus. The major gene associated with type 1 diabetes is located on chromosome 6 in association with genes related to immune recognition (7). Both susceptibility and resistance to type 1 diabetes have been localized to HLA-DR and DQ genotypes (10). Either HLA-DR3, DQB1∗0201 or HLA-DR4, DQB1∗0302 is present in greater than 90% of type 1 diabetics. In fact, if patients have both HLA-DR3 and DR4 the lifelong risk of type 1 diabetes is even greater. Forty-five percent of the general Caucasian population in the United States have either DR3 or DR4 genotypes (10). Although this is a common antigen in the American white population, the presence of protective genotypes (DR4, DQB1∗0302/DR3, and DQB1∗0201) and others may account for the low prevalence of type 1 diabetes. Other genes are associated with susceptibility to type 1 diabetes. A recent genome-wide search based upon the human genome project has located at least 20 chromosomal regions associated with susceptibility to type 1 diabetes (11). It is now clear that the genetic predisposition and clinical expression of type 1 diabetes vary by race and geographic origin. Type 1 diabetes is most prevalent in descendants of northern Europe and less common in other ethnic groups such as those of African, Asian, or native North American descent (7,12). In Europe, the prevalence was demonstrated to have a strong North–South gradient with the highest rate in Finland and the lowest in southern Europe (7,13).

Destruction of pancreatic islet cells is mediated by autoimmune mechanisms. Genetic predisposition does not appear to be sufficient to initiate this process. Patients who are destined to develop type 1 diabetes have a genetic susceptibility but appear to require an environmental event or multiple events to initiate the autoimmune process leading to islets and ultimately leading to destruction of beta cells (7). Potential environmental factors associated with the development of diabetes include viral infection (Coxsackie, enteroviruses, and rubella), dietary factors (cow's milk in infant formula and nitrates in drinking water), and others (7). Atkinson has recently proposed two models of the pathogenesis of type 1 diabetes (Fig. 1) (7). In panel A the molecular mimicry model is illustrated. An immune response develops against a viral protein (coxsackie virus, glutamate decarboxylase, etc.) with a similar amino acid sequence between the virus and a beta-cell protein. The infected cell presents the processed to CD8 lymphocyte antigen receptors via their HLA class I molecules. Macrophages that have been infected with phagocytosed virions present the viral peptides to CD4 lymphocytes via HLA class II antigens. CD4 cells help transform CD8 cells to cytotoxic effector cells, which destroy beta cells expressing the peptide that is common to beta cells and the virus. Activated CD4 cells lead to anti-beta-cell autoantibodies. In panel B the alternative model is displayed. As in the earlier model, the process begins with beta cell viral infection. This infection leads to increased cytokine production and adhesion of lymphocytes in pancreatic islets. The virally infected beta cells are then directly attacked by cytotoxic lymphocytes. Macrophages produce additional cytokines and free radicals with the islets, which augments the cytotoxic response to beta cells. CD4 cells are also recruited to the islets by cytokines. Viral antigens are presented to CD4 cells by macrophages, and B cell activation leads to production of antibody directed against the virus and beta cells. Macrophages play the same role in both models by presenting autoantigens from virus-infected cells to activated CD4 lymphocytes, leading to the development of lymphocytes and autoantibodies that react with beta cell proteins. Beyond this initiation phase in genetically susceptible patients, other processes are recruited, such as antibody-dependent cellular cytotoxicity, delayed hypersensitivity, complement activation, and cytotoxic concentrations of interferon and interleukin-1 all of which result in continued beta cell destruction (7). The development of type 1 diabetes implies a defect in peripheral (nonthymic) tolerance.

(A)

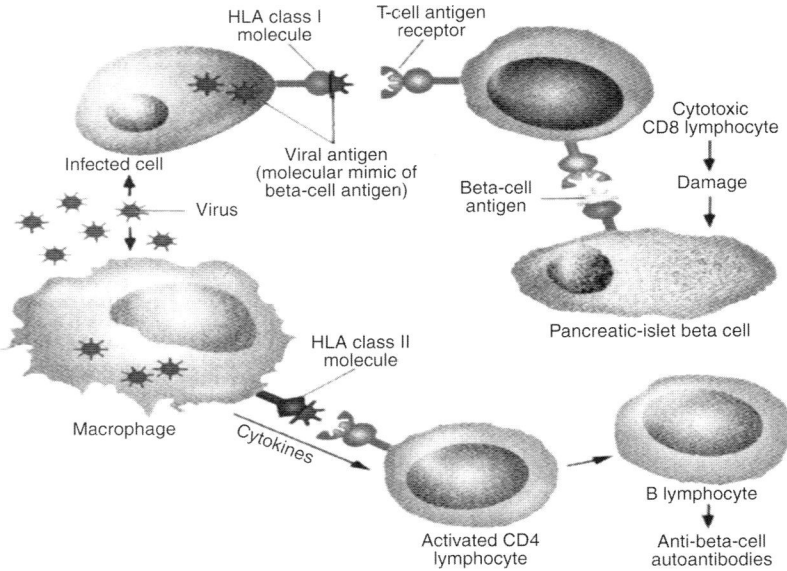

(B)

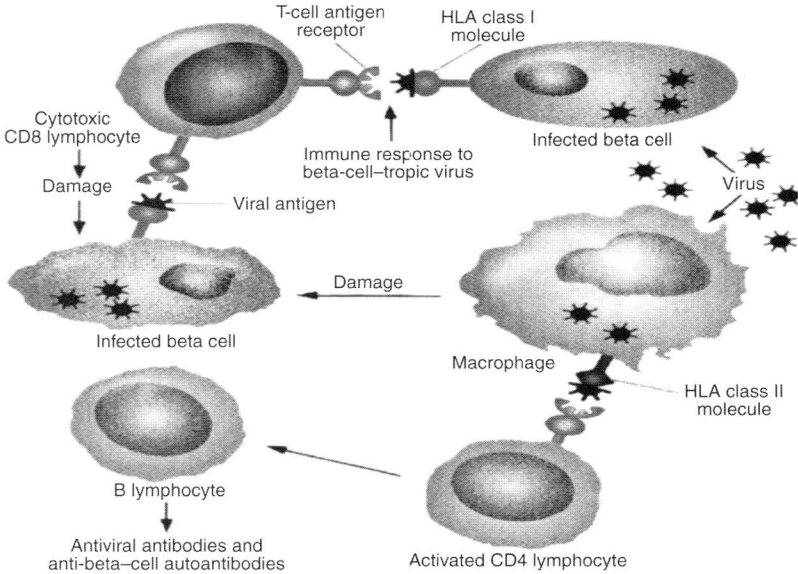

**Figure 1**  Models of the pathogenesis of IDDM. *Source*: From Atkinson MA, NEJM 1994; 331:1428.

## THE EVALUATION PROCESS
### SPK Transplantation

Until recently, approximately 88% of all pancreas transplants have been performed as SPK procedures (Fig. 2) (2). Evaluation for the potential SPK recipient is similar to the evaluation for the kidney transplant alone (KTA) recipients, with relatively small modifications (14). The protocol for recipient evaluation is detailed in Table 2. At our center, the transplant nurse coordinators obtain the initial screening medical and surgical history. Their history centers on the initial

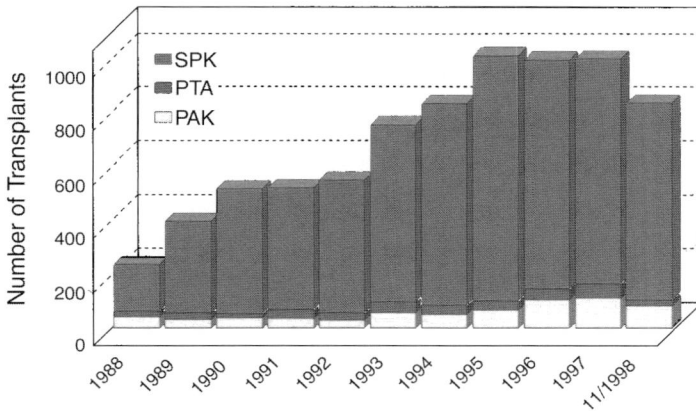

**Figure 2** Number of pancreas transplants by category and year. *Source*: From the International Pancreas Transplant Registry and United Network of Organ Sharing.

presentation of diabetes (age at diagnosis, immediate need for insulin therapy), the complications of diabetes, prior cardiovascular disease, and factors that might increase the urgency for pancreas transplantation (hypoglycemic unawareness). A history of renal failure is sought, as well as past medical and surgical history. The nurse coordinator's preliminary assessment forms the basis for the evaluation by the physician and the surgeon evaluation and helps to streamline the assessment. The nephrologist performs a complete history and physical examination and reviews medical records with the intention of identifying all previous medical conditions, paying special attention to preexisting cardiovascular disease and complications of diabetes. The surgeon's evaluations also aim to identify prior medical problems but give particular emphasis to issues that might cause surgical complications in the perioperative period. The social worker's assessment of the patient is crucial, given the burden of longstanding diabetes, which may have resulted in depression or other serious psychosocial problems. A particular concern is the ability to pay for increasingly costly immunosuppression after Medicare and state agencies stop providing support. Inability to pay for immunosuppression may become a growing cause of graft loss; identification of this often hidden risk is essential to the long-term functioning of pancreas and renal allografts.

    Laboratory studies obtained during the initial evaluation for pancreas transplant recipients are similar to those for renal transplant candidates. General laboratory studies, viral serology, and tissue typing are identical. Because pancreas transplantation is conventionally appropriate only for patients who are insulinopenic, assessment of insulin production by the patient's native pancreas is required. Absent or very low C-peptide levels are considered by most centers to be sufficient to confirm the diagnosis of type 1 diabetes. Appraisal of long-term glycemic control (hemoglobin Alc) is obtained by many centers. Other more disease-specific studies may be performed by some centers in an attempt to document the changes in diabetic complications after transplantation. These studies are usually performed

**Table 2** Pancreas and Kidney Transplant Evaluation Protocol from the University of Pittsburgh

| | |
|---|---|
| Professional evaluation | Nephrologist, surgeon, nurse coordinator, social worker, dentist |
| Laboratory Studies | *General*: Creatinine, electrolytes, calcium, phosphorus, SGOT, SGPT, GGTP, alkaline phosphatase, total cholesterol, triglyceride, LDL, HDL, amylase, lipase, total protein, albumin, CBC, platelet count, PT, PTT, RPR |
| | *Diabetes related*: C-peptide, hemoglobin Alc |
| Viral serology | CMV, Hepatitis B, Hepatitis C, Epstein Barr, Herpes Zoster, Herpes simplex, Varicella |
| Other studies | EKG, chest X ray, PPD and controls, Urine C&S |
| Immunologic evaluation | ABO type, HLA typing, DR typing, circulating antibody, quick PRA, Crossmatch |
| Urologic evaluation | Ultrasound of kidneys and right upper quadrant |
| Cancer screening | Women 35 yr or older: mammogram All women: gynecology exam and PAP smear Men $\geq$40 yr old: PSA All patients $\geq$50 yr old: sigmoidoscopy |

*Abbreviations*: CMV, cytomegalovirus; LDL, low-density lipoprotein; HDL, high-density lipoprotein.

to allow longitudinal follow-up as part of research studies, and may not be required to determine if the potential recipient is appropriate for transplantation.

As with any form of transplantation, screening for preexisting cancers is an important aspect of the medical evaluation of the pancreas recipient. Most centers follow the recommendations of major organizations for cancer prevention. We and other centers also require screening at earlier ages, given the potentially prohibitive risk of mortality from cancers in the posttransplant period. Abdominal ultrasounds screen for evidence of renal carcinoma (complex cysts) and cholelithiasis. Asymptomatic renal cell carcinoma discovered in a complex cyst usually does not require delay in listing for a pancreas transplant outside that needed for convalescence after nephrectomy. The management of asymptomatic gallstones varies from center to center. Some centers do not require pretransplant cholecystectomy but remove the gallbladder only if the usual indications are present. The mortality related to breast cancer is much higher than in nonimmunosuppressed patients. For this reason we have lowered the age for screening mammograms to 35. All sexually active women undergo gynecologic evaluations, including PAP smears. Men of age 40 years or older obtain prostate-specific antigen determinations, and all patients 50 years or older undergo a screening colonoscopy. Interestingly, patients often present for evaluation for pancreas and/or kidney transplantation without having had the routine screening studies for the general population, despite having several physicians listed as caregivers.

The indications for SPK in patients with end stage renal disease (ESRD) or near ESRD are relatively straightforward (Table 3). Once type 1 diabetes has been established, the severity of diabetic complications should be assessed. The ADA has recently released a position paper on pancreas transplantation (15). This group suggested that the potential SPK candidate should (i) already plan to have a kidney transplant, (ii) meet the medical indications and criteria for kidney transplantation, (iii) have significant clinical problems with exogenous insulin therapy, and (iv) not have excessive surgical risk for the dual procedure. Although most of these recommendations are self-explanatory, having significant clinical problems with exogenous insulin is less concrete. Patients who have frequent admissions for diabetic ketoacidosis or extreme lability of glucose control fit into this group. Similarly, those with hypoglycemic unawareness could develop significant brain damage or death, if such an event occurs while the patient is unattended. Many consider hypoglycemic unawareness to be an absolute indication for SPK. Recent animal and human studies suggest that hypoglycemic unawareness is largely, if not completely, due to recurrent or chronic hypoglycemia (16). When hypoglycemia is prevented, the awareness of hypoglycemia frequently returns. The problem of hypoglycemic unawareness can be present in any patient with IDDM, but those patients receiving intensive insulin regimes aimed at normoglycemia are two to four times more at risk than patients treated with conventional insulin protocols (17). In addition to recurrent hypoglycemia, other risk factors for hypoglycemia include duration of diabetes and presence of autonomic neuropathy.

**Table 3**  Indications for Pancreas Transplantation

| | |
|---|---|
| Simultaneous kidney–pancreas transplant | End stage renal failure with type 1 diabetes with other diabetic complications |
| | Near endstage renal failure with other diabetic complications |
| | Planned bilateral nephrectomy in diabetic with significant other diabetic complications |
| | Prior renal transplant which is failing in a type 1 diabetic |
| Pancreas after kidney transplant | Prior kidney transplant in type 1 diabetic with other diabetic complications |
| Pancreas transplant alone | Patients with a history of frequent acute severe metabolic complications requiring medical attention |
| | Clinical and emotional problems with insulin therapy that are so severe as to be incapacitating |
| | Consistent failure of other therapeutic approaches |
| | Other potential indications: |
| | Presence of diabetic complications which are progressive and unresponsive to intensive insulin therapy |
| | Early diabetic nephropathy associated with other diabetic complications |
| | Subcutaneous insulin resistance |
| | Following total pancreatectomy |
| | Insulin allergy (case report) |

*Source*: From Ref. 15.

Once patients have developed diabetic nephropathy and renal insufficiency, other diabetic complications are almost always present. The diagnosis of diabetic nephropathy, however, is seldom confirmed by renal biopsy in patients with longstanding diabetes. It is usually assumed the renal failure is secondary to diabetes. Patients without other end organ complications of diabetes and renal failure may have another underlying renal disease. Those with a short duration of diabetes (even if the C-peptide confirms type 1 diabetes) and absence of retinopathy or other complications are at high risk for having nondiabetic renal disease. Candidates without other diabetic complications but who have renal failure may not necessarily be appropriate for SPK, as the other diabetic complications may not develop in the future. In such atypical cases, a renal biopsy may be useful if the patient does not have longstanding ESRD. Patients with multiple severe diabetic complications including severe atherosclerotic disease also may not be candidates for SPK. Such patients have a very high risk of perioperative complications and may not experience a significant improvement in the quality of life apart from insulin discontinuation. The ability of pancreatic transplantation to reverse the complications of diabetes such as gastropathy, neuropathy, and retinopathy is controversial (1). This is a finding of the lack of randomized studies and limited follow-up in case series. The changes in diabetic complications are addressed in detail in Chapter 2. It is, however, generally agreed that the more severe the complication, the less likely it is to be reversible. If there is little chance of diabetic complications reversing and the cardiovascular risk is great, such patients should opt for a KTA or to continue dialysis therapy, depending upon the patient's particular clinical situation.

## Pancreas After Kidney

The evaluation of potential recipients for pancreas after kidney transplantation (PAK) is similar to that for SPK. Approximately 10% of all pancreas transplants are PAK (2). The PAK patients fall into two groups, those with a prior KTA and those with prior a SPK and a failed pancreas allograft. Because these patients have ESRD, the benefit of a functioning pancreas transplant is similar to that in the SPK group. In all potential PAK recipients, a detailed evaluation of the renal allograft must be made. Patients with poor graft function may be candidates for SPK instead. The presence significant chronic allograft nephropathy should raise the question of SPK with removal of the failing renal allograft at the time of the retransplant SPK. Patients with marginal renal function and without a recent allograft biopsy should be assumed to have chronic allograft nephropathy. Confirmation of this diagnosis by biopsy is preferred, but a clinical picture of a chronically elevated serum creatinine with or without proteinuria may be sufficient. A 24-hour urine collection for creatinine clearance and protein should be obtained to assess the level of renal impairment. No exact cutoff has been determined for creatinine clearance before replacing the prior renal allograft, but patients with creatinine clearances less than approximately 30 to 40 cc/min and significant proteinuria will likely have progressive loss of renal function and require dialysis or retransplantation in the future. The added nephrotoxicity of cyclosporine or tacrolimus after the pancreas transplant may accelerate the deterioration of renal function. The decline in glomerular filtration rate (GFR) from nephrotoxicity varies with the drug blood levels achieved and the renal function at the time of transplantation. Brennan et al. have demonstrated that the serum creatinine and creatinine clearance after a dose of cyclosporine may predict renal function in candidates for pancreas transplant alone (PTA) and by inference, PAK patients with marginal renal function (18). If it is decided that SPK may be too early (patients with creatinine clearance >30–40 cc/min), these patients must be followed with periodic assessments of their renal function if they are placed on the waiting list for PAK.

If the patient has good allograft function, the evaluation is identical to that for the SPK. For patients who were transplanted greater than one year of the time of the evaluation for PAK, all studies should be repeated. This particularly is true for the cardiovascular and immunologic evaluations.

There has been a growing interest in performing living related renal transplantation followed by PAK (KA-LD+PAK). Obtaining a planned renal transplant quickly then waiting for a pancreas transplant has been particularly attractive to some patients, and some transplant centers have offered this option as the preferred approach if a donor is available. For many patients, however, this has been a difficult decision given the superior pancreatic graft survival of the SPK. A recent cost-utility analysis has demonstrated that SPK is the optimal procedure even if a living kidney donor is available (19). In this analysis the SPK was more effective and less expensive than KA-LD+PAK. The major factor causing the KA-LD+PAK option to be less cost-effective was the inferior pancreatic graft survival compared to SPK. In order for KA-LD+PAK to be as cost-effective as SPK, the five-year PAK survival would need to exceed 86% something which has not been possible even in the large volume centers with the best graft survivals. The pretransplant evaluation of the KA-LD+PAK option is similar to the cadaveric kidney PAK scenario. It is particularly important to inform patients of the potentially inferior pancreas survival if this option is chosen.

## Solitary Pancreas

PTA has been performed in only 3% to 5% of the patients in the International Pancreas Transplantation Registry (2). As with all other pancreas transplants, PTA allograft survival has continued to improve from less than 50% at one year in the early 1990s to 76.6% in 1998 (20). The indications for PTA are listed in Table 3. As with other forms of pancreas transplantation, the ADA has proposed indications for PTA (15). Unlike SPK or PAK recipients, candidates for PTA do not otherwise require immunosuppression with their predictable side effects to prevent renal allograft rejection. There is also the additional surgical risk, which should carry a relatively small morbidity and mortality. Candidates for PTA should not have severe renal insufficiency requiring imminent renal replacement therapy. Such patients would be more appropriate candidates for preemptive SPK. It is expected that candidates for PTA should have near normal renal function, but have severe disabling nonvascular diabetic complications. The ADA has suggested that (i) patients with a history of frequent acute severe metabolic complications requiring medical attention, (ii) those with clinical and emotional problems with insulin therapy that are so severe as to be incapacitating, and (iii) those with consistent failure of other therapeutic approaches should be considered for PTA. In addition to the above recommendations, potential candidates for PTA should have diabetic complications that are progressive. Transplantation so early in the course of diabetes that few if any diabetic complications exist would pose a significant risk with little certainty of demonstrable benefit. Insulin allergy is an unusual potential indication for PTA. The evidence for this indication is in one case report only (21). A young woman with longstanding type 1 diabetes developed severe urticaria, which quickly developed into angioedema and respiratory distress after treatment with human insulin which she had taken for many years. Beef and pork insulin did not improve the symptoms. Attempts at desensitization were unsuccessful, and the fear of a life threatening anaphylactoid reaction prompted the referral for PTA. Her only diabetic complications included mild retinopathy, one episode of diabetic ketoacidosis, and rare hypoglycemic episodes. There was no evidence for renal dysfunction. She developed normoglycemia after the successful PTA without further episodes of insulin allergy. The incidence of insulin allergy has decreased from approximately 50% to 2–10% with the advent of human insulin (21). Allergy to human insulin also occurs and may be due to additives such as zinc, protamine, noninsulin proteins, and aggregates of insulin molecules and animal proteins (21,22). Pancreas transplantation for this indication should be rare, and all other measures should be exhausted if this is the only indication for PTA.

## RECIPIENT RISK FACTORS FOR PANCREAS TRANSPLANTATION

The major objective of the pretransplant recipient evaluation is to identify factors that increase the risk of death, graft loss, or major morbidity after pancreas transplantation. Many of the known risk factors are not peculiar to pancreas transplantation but must be considered during the evaluation period. As with renal transplant alone recipients, the following risk factors must be considered for potential pancreas transplant recipients: (i) increasing age, (ii) obesity, (iii) adverse psychosocial factors, (iv) preexisting cardiovascular disease, (v) chronic viral infection (hepatitis B or C, Parvovirus, HIV), (vi) gastrointestinal disorders (peptic ulcer disease, pancreatitis, diverticulosis), (vii) chronic pulmonary disease (chronic restrictive or obstructive disease), and (viii) chronic fungal disease (histoplasmosis, etc.) and previously treated malignancy. The approach to evaluation of these problems in the renal transplant setting has been examined in great detail and will not be discussed further here. The risk factors specifically affecting pancreas transplant recipients has been examined previously by

Gruessner et al. (23). This report retrospectively examined the factors predicting patient and graft survival in addition to the risks of technical complications in KTA, SPK, PAK, and PTA recipients between 1986 and 1993, with a five-year follow-up. Factors considered included (i) recipient age greater or less than 45 years, (ii) obesity, (iii) hypertension, (iv) blindness in at least one eye, (v) known cardiac disease (previous myocardial infarction, coronary bypass, or percutaneous angioplasty), (vi) peripheral vascular disease (previous cerebrovascular accident or transient ischemic attack, bypass, angioplasty, or amputation), and (vii) retransplantation (previous pancreas transplant). Patient survival was adversely affected by recipient age greater than or equal to 45 years in the SPK (relative risk 3.0) and PAK groups (relative risk 5.86). Recipients of PTA were adversely affected by recipient age. Cardiac disease increased the risk of mortality only in SPK recipients (relative risk 3.78). For PAK patients, only a previous pancreas transplant and peripheral vascular disease increased the risk of death.

Manske et al. reported a more pessimistic view of candidate factors after pancreas transplantation (24). This report summarized the patient outcomes from 1987 to 1993 in 173 consecutive IDDM patients. This center offered pancreas transplants to high-risk recipients with advanced diabetic complications and those with underlying cardiac disease, although every attempt was made to correct any anatomic lesions prior to transplantation. They also offered living related renal transplantation first followed by pancreas transplantation as the preferred option if possible. In this high-risk group of patients three-year patient survival was 68% for SPK, 86% for living related, and 90% for KTA. A Cox proportional hazard model (which included type of organ transplant in the model) identified age in five-year increments [risk ratio (RR) = 1.5, $p = 0.001$], history of congestive heart failure (RR = 2.7, $p = 0.03$), and SPK (RR = 3.1, $p = 0.02$) as predictors of increased risk of mortality. During this period the International Pancreas Transplant Registry was reporting 84% three-year patient survival for SPK, and a response to this study by Secchi et al. emphasized that excellent results were possible with SPK if patient selection differed from that described in the Manske report (25). Seechi et al. emphasized the importance of excluding patients with severe macroangiopathy (previous stokes, severe dilated cardiomyopathy, and amputations). They likewise favored SPK over living related renal transplant followed by pancreas transplantation, given the superior pancreatic graft survival with the former. Despite this careful evaluation, cardiovascular events were the major cause of death in all groups (13% KTA, 8% in kidney with segmental pancreas, and 6% in SPK). These two reports and the aggregate experience of the International Pancreas Transplant Registry suggest that excellent patient and allograft survival should be the expectation after pancreas transplantation of any type. Performing these procedures in patients with severe diabetic complications and marginally corrected cardiac disease may lead to unacceptable morbidity and mortality.

## Cardiovascular Disease

Cardiovascular disease is the leading cause of death in diabetics (26). The burden of coronary artery disease is much greater for diabetics compared to the general population, and may be present to some degree in as many as 55% of all diabetics (27,28). The purpose of the medical evaluation of potential pancreas transplant candidates is to identify risk factors that may adversely affect postoperative morbidity or mortality and to correct or minimize them prior to transplantation if possible. The potential pancreas transplant recipient is known to be at risk for accelerated atherosclerosis and thrombogenesis because of diabetes, but may also have many of the risk factors present in the general dialysis population. Table 4 lists factors responsible for the accelerated atherosclerosis in diabetics. Diabetics have been demonstrated to have higher very low-density lipoprotein, high-density lipoprotein, low-density lipoprotein, and triglyceride levels compared to nondiabetics (29). Endothelial dysfunction and impaired endothelium-dependent vasodilation have been demonstrated in diabetics with normal coronary arteries without other risk factors for coronary artery disease (30). The endothelial dysfunction has also been documented in patients with normal fasting blood glucose who later develop postprandial hyperglycemia (31). Nitric oxide is an obvious potential mediator of the impaired vasodilatation. However, administration of L-arginine did not improve the endothelial dysfunction in one study (32). Vitamin C (a free radical scavenger) and desferrioxamine (which prevents generation of hydroxyl radical) restored endothelial function in another study (33). These findings suggest that nitric oxide might play a major role in endothelial dysfunction,

**Table 4**  Causes of Accelerated Atherosclerosis in Diabetics

Dyslipidemia
Endothelial dysfuction
Platelet abnormalities
Hyperhomocysteinemia
Coagulation and fibrinolysis abnormalities
Coronary artery remodeling
Myocardial flow reserve abnormalites

but more rapid inactivation or degradation by oxygen-derived free radicals may be required to demonstrate a beneficial effect.

The evaluation can provide an opportunity to initiate preventive measures for coronary heart disease. Each of the known risk factors for atherosclerosis should be identified, and the patient should be counseled regarding all modifiable risk factors. Two major policy-setting organizations (American Heart Association and the International Task Force for Prevention of Coronary Heart Disease) have specific measures for primary prevention (34,35). Although these measures were not developed explicitly for patients with ESRD, they appear to be prudent until more specific recommendations tailored to these patients become available. The major recommendations of these two reports include (i) smoking cessation, (ii) blood pressure control, (iii) correction of hyperlipidemia, (iv) increase in physical activity, (v) weight reduction, and (vi) estrogen replacement, which is individualized. Kasiske et al. reported that approximately 25% of the dialysis patients evaluated for renal transplantation were current smokers, similar to the general population, and that hypertension was present in 70% to 85% (36). Diabetics with severe autonomic neuropathy are at risk of developing orthostatic hypotension. Once ESRD has developed and the patients are persistently hypervolemic, the orthostatic component is attenuated unless they become volume depleted after dialysis. Hyperlipidemia is also common in ESRD patients and may be a particular problem for diabetics who have recently initiated dialysis, because the nephrotic syndrome secondary to diabetic nephropathy may persist. Physical inactivity is very common in ESRD and may be particularly difficult in diabetics with labile blood glucose control. In addition, the other complications of diabetes such as neuropathy and diffuse atherosclerotic disease may make it difficult to develop a regular exercise program. Obesity is a growing problem in the dialysis population, and maintaining the appropriate body weight is even more difficult for the diabetic. Tight blood glucose control typically increases body weight, and exercise for the purpose of weight reduction is difficult. Despite the difficulties in controlling these risk factors, any evaluation of the potential candidate for pancreas transplantation should include counseling in these areas.

## The Cardiac Evaluation in the Pancreas Transplant Candidate

There is no consensus regarding the cardiovascular evaluation in the diabetic patient with ESRD. Some centers perform coronary angiography in all patients, and others attempt risk stratification, performing angiography in selected high-risk patients. The cardiac evaluation in diabetics is complicated by the high prevalence of silent ischemia and cardiomyopathy. Studies have found that exercise stress tests with or without thallium or dobutamine echocardiography are of limited predictive value in diabetics (37). Only 45% of diabetics are capable of reaching 70% to 80% of their maximum predicted heart rate. One recent study suggested that dipyridamole thallium stress tests might be predictive of perioperative cardiac events (38). In this study only 1 of 111 (0.9%) patients with a normal study developed a perioperative cardiac event, and none of those with fixed defects or reversible defects with < 50% narrowing of coronary arteries on angiography developed perioperative events. However, this optimistic impression is corroborated by others. In an attempt to stratify cardiovascular risk, Manske et al. developed an algorithm, which attempted to identify low-risk diabetic patients who could safely avoid angiography in the pretransplant evaluation (39). This group found an 88% prevalence of coronary artery disease in diabetics > 45 years of age. Given this high prevalence, they recommended angiography in all diabetics in this group. For younger patients without a smoking history or ST-T wave changes on EKG, or in those with diabetes for < 25 years, the risk of coronary disease was lower. These patients were recommended to have a pharmacologic stress test as the initial study. Any abnormality on this study would mandate angiography, even in the low-risk group. Although the sample size was small in this study, such an approach probably represents the most useful strategy for screening diabetics. Once significant coronary artery disease has been found, correction by coronary revascularization or angioplasty should be performed prior to transplantation, as it has clearly been shown to decrease the frequency of posttransplant cardiac events and mortality (40). Bypass surgery was recently shown to substantially reduce the death rate, when compared with angioplasty, in diabetics who subsequently develop Q-wave myocardial infarctions (41). Thus, if candidates for pancreas transplantation arc found to have significant coronary artery disease (CAD), bypass surgery should be recommended in most cases if the lesions are amenable to revascularization.

Many centers advocate dobutamine echocardiography as the preferred noninvasive screening study for coronary artery disease in diabetic and nondiabetic renal transplant candidates. It has the advantage of providing information on presence of ischemia, wall motion, and ejection fraction. Disadvantages of dobutamine echocardiography includes the fact that it is more difficult to perform in obese patients, and there is an increased risk of ventricular arrhythmias in patients with prior arrhythmia, severe CAD, and/or poor left ventricular function. As with dipyridamole thallium stress testing, there are limited data on the accuracy of dobutamine echocardiography in patients with ESRD. Herzog et al. have reported the only study that directly compares dobutamine stress echocardiography (DSE) with coronary angiography in renal transplant candidates (42). Fifty candidates for renal transplantation underwent dobutamine echocardiography followed by coronary angiography. Of these patients, 39 (78%) were diabetic, 10 type 1 and the remainder type 2. Twenty of the 50 dobutamine studies were positive for inducible ischemia. Three false negative dobutamine studies were found in patients with >70% stenosis, and four false negative studies were seen in patients with >75% stenosis (including the patients with >70%). The sensitivity and specificity of DSE were, respectively, 52% and 74% for 50% or greater stenosis, 75% and 71% for stenosis greater than 70%, and 75% and 76% for stenosis >75%. The positive and negative predictive values were, respectively, 70% and 57% for 50%, 45% and 90% for >70%, and 60% and 87% for >75% stenosis. The authors appropriately concluded that DSE was a useful but imperfect screening test for angiographically defined coronary artery disease.

Several algorithms have been advanced to screen for coronary artery disease in pancreas transplant candidates and other diabetic transplant candidates. They all attempt to stratify patients and perform angiography only in the high-risk group as the first diagnostic study. Williams has advocated an algorithm similar to the Manske approach but attempted to avoid any cardiac screening in low-risk patients (43). These low-risk patients would be placed directly on the waiting list without any cardiac evaluation. Our approach to cardiac evaluation (an adaptation of the Manske and Williams approaches) is displayed in Figure 3. In practice,

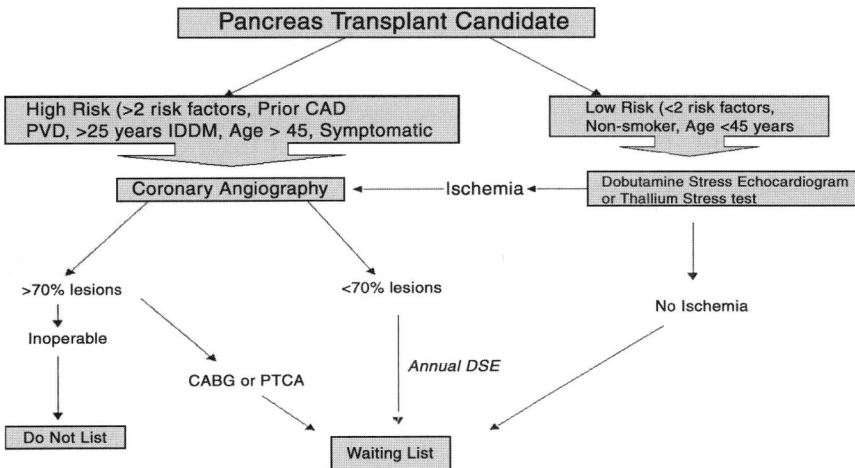

**Figure 3**  Cardiac evaluation in pancreas transplant recipients

most centers consider a pharmacologic stress test to be the minimum for all pancreas transplant candidates. A positive stress test mandates coronary angiography. In addition, because the presence of peripheral arterial disease and/or carotid artery disease increases the chances of having coronary artery disease, such patients should probably also proceed directly to angiography. Those with stenotic lesions >70% should undergo angioplasty or coronary artery bypass grafting before being placed on the waiting list. Candidates with inoperable diffuse disease should not be transplanted. Candidates with lesions <70% and no ischemia may be approved for transplantation but must be reevaluated at least annually with a pharmacologic stress test. Surveillance for ischemic heart disease should also continue after transplantation in these patients.

## CONTRAINDICATIONS TO PANCREAS TRANSPLANTATION (TABLE 5)

The contraindications to pancreas transplantation are similar to those for other types of organ transplantation, with some additional features. The presence of type 2 diabetes is the most obvious and is considered to be the major factor step in determining if patients are appropriate for pancreas transplantation. Because type 2 diabetics have insulin resistance, provision of a second functioning graft would not be thought theoretically to improve glycemic control. However, two recent studies have suggested that pancreas transplantation may be beneficial in type 2 diabetes. Elian et al. used streptozocin-treated Lewis rats to induce an insulinopenic animal with peripheral insulin resistance, and increased hepatic glucose production, similar to humans with type 2 diabetes (44). After pancreas transplantation, glycemic control and hepatic glucose production were similar to normal animals. Light et al. have recently reported the results of SPK transplants in type 2 diabetics (45). They reported excellent graft survival and glycemic control even in patients with significant pretransplant C-peptide levels. Provocative as these studies are, further study is needed before type 2 diabetics should routinely be considered for pancreas transplantation.

Cardiovascular disease that cannot be corrected is a contraindication to pancreas and other types of transplantation. Patients with severe coronary artery disease not amenable to bypass surgery or angioplasty should not be offered pancreas transplantation. Likewise severe peripheral vascular disease, which cannot be corrected sufficiently to provide adequate blood flow to the extremity and the transplanted organ, should be considered a contraindication.

Other problems that may contradict pancreas transplantation are similar to those in other types of transplantation. Recent or incompletely treated malignancies mandate a waiting period before listing. Most malignancies require two years before patients can be placed on the list ("the two year rule"). Exceptions include incidentally discovered renal cell carcinomas, which are limited to the renal parenchyma (no waiting time necessary), and those requiring more than a two-year waiting period, such as breast and colon cancer (approximately a five-year wait). Most centers will not list patients who are HIV positive, without an AIDS-defining illness, but a small number of centers are beginning to offer transplants to such patients. No centers offer transplants to patients with AIDS, active infection being an absolute contraindication.

**Table 5**  Contraindications to Pancreas Transplantation

| **Absolute contraindications** | |
| --- | --- |
| Severe cardiac disease | Coronary artery disease not amenable to anatomic correction |
| | Cardiomyopathy with low ejection fraction not corrected by surgical or medical management |
| Severe peripheral vascular disease | Aortoiliac disease without possibility of surgical correction |
| Malignancy | Recently diagnosed (requires appropriate waiting period after treatment) |
| | Metastatic and unbeatable |
| Relative contraindications (center specific) | |
| HIV infections | Acceptable at some centers if no AIDS defining illness |
| Severe diabetic complications unlikely to improve after pancreas transplantation | Only advantage to patient is cessation of insulin and relaxation of dietary restrictions. Such patients are usually high risk candidates for cardiac and other complications |

Finally, pancreas transplants probably should not be offered to patients with such severe diabetic complications that pancreas transplantation is on likely to improve their medical condition or quality of life. Elimination of insulin therapy is the most important advantage of pancreas transplantation from the patient's perspective. This benefit must be weighed against the risk of transplantation in these patients, because they will usually have severe coronary and peripheral vascular disease. If such patients are accepted for transplantation, it should be done with the realization that they will be at high risk for complications in the postoperative period and may not have significant reversal of their diabetic complications.

## ORGAN ALLOCATION SYSTEM

The United Network for Organ Sharing administers the allocation of solid organ transplants (including pancreatic organs) in the United States. This system is based upon the geographic origin of the organ, waiting time, and number of antigen mismatches (46). Pancreata are first allocated locally, regionally, and then nationally. The transplant center can chose a patient waiting for an isolated pancreas, kidney–pancreas (SPK), or solid organ-islet combination from the same donor. Zero antigen mismatched kidneys and pancreases are mandated to be shared nationally. Within each waiting list, the organs are allocated by blood type compatibility and waiting time on the transplant list. For example, blood type O organs are mandated to be transplanted into type O recipients except for O antigen mismatches.

Nationally, organs are distributed by blood type and waiting time in the following sequence: (i) isolated pancreas candidates with one A, B, or DR antigen mismatch, then (ii) isolated pancreas candidates with two A, B, or DR antigen mismatches, then (iii) isolated pancreas candidates with three A, B, or DR antigen mismatches, then (iv) combined kidney–pancreas candidates, if a kidney is available, then (v) isolated pancreas candidates with four or more A, B, or DR antigen mismatches (46).

Organs not allocated locally, regionally, or nationally can then be used for islet transplantation. The host organ procurement organization can then offer the pancreas for islet transplantation locally, regionally, and then nationally. At the regional and national levels allocation of the organ is dictated by HLA matching, medical urgency, and waiting time. Patients with zero HLA antigen mismatches receive three points, those with one mismatch two points, and those with two mismatches one point. Potential recipients with three or more antigen mismatches receive no points. Medical urgency for islet cell transplantation is based upon the presence or absence of a prior islet transplant and is divided into two groups. Status 1 patients have already received an islet cell transplant within the previous three weeks and are considered to be the most urgent. Those waiting for the first islet cell transplant are assigned to status 2. Within this classification, patients with the longest waiting time are given one point. Based upon their waiting time, a fraction of a point is assigned to subsequent patients.

## REFERENCES

1. Hricik DE. Combined kidney-pancreas transplantation. Kidney Intern 1998; 53:1091–1102.
2. 1999 Annual Report of the US Scientific Registry for Transplant Recipients and the Organ Procurement and Transplantation Network: Transplant Data: 1989–1998. US Department of Health and Human Services, Health Resources and Services Administration, Office of Special Programs, Division of Transplantation, Rockville, MD; UNOS, Richmond, VA.
3. Sutherland D. Pancreas and pancreas-kidney transplantation. Curr Opin Nephrol Hypertens 1998; 7:317–325.
4. Douzdjian V, Ferrara D, Silvestri G. Treatment strategies for insulin-dependent diabetics with ESRD: a cost-effectiveness decision analysis model. Am J Kidney Dis 1998; 31(5):794–802; ISSN: 0272–6386.
5. Anonymous. Report of the expert committee on the diagnosis and classification of diabetes mellitus. Review/Commentary/Position Statement; Special Article. 1997; 20(7):1183–1197.
6. Anonymous. Report of the expert committee on the diagnosis and classification of diabetes mellitus. Diabetes Care 1998; 21:S5–S19.
7. Atkinson MA, Maclaren NK. Mechanisms of disease: the pathogenesis of insulin-dependent diabetes mellitus. N Engl J Med 1994; 331:1428.
8. Bonner-Weir S, Trent DF, Weir GC. Partial pancreatectomy in the rat and subsequent defect in glucose-induced insulin release. J Clin Invest 1983; 71(6):1544–1553; ISSN: 0021–9738.

9.  McCulloch DK, Palmer JP. The appropriate use of B-cell function testing in the preclinical period of type 1 diabetes. Diabetes Med 1991; 8:800.
10. Todd JA, Bennett JC. A practical approach to identification of susceptibility genes for IDDM. Diabetes 1992; 41:1029–1034.
11. Davies JL, Kawaguchi Y, Bennett ST, et al. A genome-wide search for human type 1 diabetes susceptibility genes. Nature 1994; 371:130.
12. Diabetes Epidemiology Research International Mortality Study Group. Major cross-country differences in risk of dying for people with IDDM. Diabetes Care 1991; 14:49–54.
13. Green A, Gale EAM, Patterson CC. Incidence of childhood-onset insulin-dependent diabetes mellitus: the EURODIABAC study. Lancet 1992; 339:905–909.
14. McCauley J. Evaluation of the Potential Renal Allograft Recipient. Stamford, CT: Appleton & Lange, 1997:43–72.
15. Anonymous. Pancreas transplantation for patients with diabetes mellitus. Diabetes Care 1998; 21:S79.
16. Bolli GB. Counterregulatory mechanisms to insulin-induced hypoglycemia in humans: relevance to the problem of intensive treatment for IDDM. J Ped Endo Met 1998; 11(suppl 1):103–115.
17. The DCCT Research Group. Epidemiology of severe hypoglycemia in the diabetes control and complications trial. Am J Med 1991; 90:450–459.
18. Brennan DC, Stratta RJ, Lowell JA, Miller SA, Taylor RJ. Cyclosporine challenge in the decision of combined kidney-pancreas versus solitary pancreas transplantation. Transplantation 1994; 57(11):1606–1611.
19. Douzdjian V, Escobar F, Kupin W, Venkat KK, Aboujoud M. Cost-utility of living-donor kidney transplantation followed by pancreas transplantation versus simultaneous pancreas-kidney transplantation. Clin Transpl 1999; 13(1):51–58.
20. 1999 Annual Report of the US Scientific Registry for Transplant Recipients and the Organ Procurement and Transplantation Network: Transplant Data: 1989–1998. US Department of Health and Human Services, Health Resources and Services Administration, Office of Special Programs, Division of Transplantation, Rockville, MD; UNOS, Richmond, VA, 156.
21. Oh HK, Provenzano R, Hendrix J, El-Nachef MW. Insulin allergy resolution following pancreas transplantation alone. Clin Transpl 1998; 12(6):593–595.
22. Simmond JP, Russell GI, Cowley AJ, et al. Generalized allergy to porcine and bovine monocomponent insulins. Br Med J 1980; 28l(6236):355–356.
23. Gruessner RWG, Dunn DL, Gruessner AC, Matas AJ, Najarian JS, Sutherlad DER. Recipient risk factors have an impact on the technical failure and graft survival rates in bladder-drained pancreas transplants. Transplantation 1994; 57:1598–1606.
24. Manske C, Wang Y, Thomas W. Mortality of cadaveric kidney transplantation versus combined kidney-pancreas transplantation in diabetic patients. Lancet 1995; 346:1658–1662.
25. Secchi A, Caldara R, Di Carlo V, Guido P. Mortality of cadaveric kidney transplantation versus combined kidney-pancreas transplantation in diabetic patients. Lancet 1996; 347:827.
26. Grundy SM, Benjamin TJ, Burke GL, et al. Diabetes and cardiovascular disease: a statement for healthcare professionals from the American Heart Association. Circulation 1999; 100:1134.
27. Fein F, Scheuer J. Rifkin H, Porte D, eds. Heart Disease in Diabetes Mellitus: Theory and Practice. New York: Elsevier, 1990:812.
28. Nesto RW. Epidemiology of and risk factors for coronary heart disease in diabetes mellitus. Uptodate in Medicine. Vol. 8, No. 2.
29. Siegel RD, Cupples A, Schaefer EJ, Wilson PW. Lipoproteins, apolipoproteins and low density lipoprotein size among diabetics in the Framingham offspring study. Metabolism 1996; 45:1267.
30. Clarkson P, Celermajer DS, Donald AE, et al. Impaired vascular reactivity in insulin-dependent diabetes mellitus is related to disease duration and low density lipoprotein cholesterol levels. J Am Coll Cardiol 1996; 28:573.
31. Kawano H, Motoyama T, Hiroshima O, et al. Hyperglycemia rapidly suppresses flow mediated endothelium-dependent vasodilation of the brachial artery. J Am Coll Cardiol 1999; 97:736.
32. Thorne S, Mullen MJ, Clarkson P, et al. Early endothelial dysfunction in adults at risk from atherosclerosis: different responses to L-arginine. J Am Coll Cardiol 1998; 32:110.
33. Nitenberg A, Paycha F, Ledoux S, et al. Coronary artery responses to physiologic stimuli are improved by desferrioxamine but not by L-arginine in non-insulin dependent diabetic patients with angiographically normal coronary arteries and no other risk factors. Circulation 1998; 97:736.
34. Grundy SM, Balady GJ, Criqui MH, Fletcher G, et al. Guide to primary prevention of cardiovascular disease; A statement for healthcare professionals from the Task Force on Risk Reduction. Circulation 1997; 95:2329–2331.
35. Assmann G, Carmena R, Cullen P, Fruchart J, Jossa F, et al. Coronary heart disease: reducing the risk: A world wide view. International Task Force for the Prevention of Coronary Heart Disease. Circulation 1999; 100(18):1930–1938.
36. Kasiske BL et al. The adverse effects of cigarette smoking in renal transplant recipients. Presented in abstract for at the American Society of Transplantation Annual Meeting, Chicago, IL, May 1999. J Am Soc Nephrol. In press.

37. Morrow CE, Schwartz, Sutherland DER, et al. Predictive value of thallium stress testing for coronary and cardiovascular events in uremic diabetic patients before renal transplantation. Am J Surg 1983; 146:331–335.
38. Mistry BM, Bastani B, Solomon H, et al. Prognostic value of dipyridamole thallium-201 screening to minimize perioperative cardiac complications in diabetics undergoing kidney or kidney-pancreas transplantation. Clin Transpl 1998; 12(2):130–135.
39. Manske CL, Thomas W, Wang Y, Wilson R. Screening diabetic transplant candidates for coronary artery disease: identification of a low risk subgroup. Kidney Intern 1993; 44:617–621.
40. Manske CL, Wang Y, Rector T, Wilson R, et al. Coronary revascularization in insulin dependent diabetic patients with chronic renal failure. Lancet 1992; 340:998–1002.
41. Detre KM, Lombardero MS, Brooks MM, et al. The effect of previous coronary-artery bypass surgery on the prognosis of patients with diabetes who have acute myocardial infarction. Bypass Angioplasty Revascularization Investigation Investigators. N Engl J Med 2000; 342(l4):989–997.
42. Herzog CA, Marwick TH, Pheley AM, White CW, Rao VK, Dick CD. Dobutamine stress echocardiography for the detection of significant coronary artery disease in renal transplant candidates. Am J Kidney Dis 1999; 33(6):1080–1090.
43. Williams ME. Management of the diabetic transplant recipient. Kidney Int 1995; 48:1660.
44. Elian N, Bensimon C, Chapa O, Bethoux JP, Cugnene PH, Altman JJ. Pancreatic transplantation in experimental non-insulin-dependent diabetic rats. Transplantation 1996; 61(5):696–700.
45. Light JA, Sasaki TM, Currier CB, Barhyte DY. Successful long-term kidney-pancreas transplants regardless of C-peptide status or race. Transplantation 2001; 71(1):152–154.
46. 1999 Annual Report of the US Scientific Registry for Transplant Recipients and the Organ Procurement and Transplantation Network: Transplant Data: 1989–1998. US Department of Health and Human Services, Health Resources and Services Administration, Office of Special Programs, Division of Transplantation, Rockville, MD; UNOS, Richmond, VA, 418–419.

# 5 | Technical Aspects of Pancreatic Recovery

**David A. Geller, Robert J. Corry,[‡] and S. Forrest Dodson**

*Thomas E. Starzl Transplantation Institute, University of Pittsburgh School of Medicine, Pittsburgh, Pennsylvania, U.S.A.*

Over the last 15 years, there has been an evolution in the operative technique of recovering the pancreas for transplantation. The current method of choice is a rapid en bloc technique for simultaneous liver and whole organ pancreas recovery. This technique reduces operative time and is also applicable in the unstable donor, in whom a slower in situ dissection might subject the vital organs to unnecessary ischemic damage. The purpose of this chapter is to summarize the changes that have evolved in pancreatic recovery and detail the surgical technique as currently performed.

## EVOLUTION OF PANCREAS PROCUREMENT

Over the last decade, there has been great progress in the field of pancreas transplantation, including operative techniques in the donor and recipient procedures and immunosuppressive management. At the same time, there has been a steady rise in the number of patients on the United Network for Organ Sharing transplant waiting list (over 88,000 patients, United Network for Organ Sharing Registry). Unfortunately, the number of organ donors has not increased accordingly, resulting in some 6000 deaths per year on the waiting list. This disparity has led to the obvious need to maximize the number of organs retrieved from each donor. In 1984, a landmark description of a flexible procedure for multiple cadaveric organ procurement was reported by Starzl et al. (1). Noteworthy in this description were the principles of core cooling and the importance of cooperation among multiple transplant teams for the simultaneous recovery of the heart, liver, and kidneys (1). This was later modified to a rapid harvest procedure with minimal hilar dissection (2). With regard to pancreas procurement, as recently as 15 years ago, simultaneous pancreas and liver retrieval was thought to be surgically incompatible because of the shared vascular supply, and recovery of the pancreas was performed only when a suitable liver recipient was unavailable (3,4). With the growing organ shortage, the procurement technique was modified by several groups to allow recovery of both the liver and the whole pancreas from the same donor (5–10). This made sense, given that most patients who are suitable pancreas donors are also appropriate liver donors. The key technical modification was the recognition that vascular extension grafts could be used to reconstruct the pancreatic vessels, avoiding any compromise to the liver (5). Since the early reports of combined pancreas/liver procurement, others have adopted the technique, with wide acceptance (11–16). Importantly, several groups have shown no detrimental effects on either liver or pancreas transplant outcomes as a result of simultaneous retrieval (9,17,18). Recently, a technique for the procurement of intestinal, pancreatic, and hepatic grafts from the same donor has been described (19).

The initial techniques for simultaneous recovery of the pancreas and the liver generally involved extensive dissection of the vasculature of both organs prior to cross-clamping (5,8–10,20). Disadvantages of this technique included ischemic injury to the organs as a result of vasospasm related to the in situ dissection, prolonged operative time, and exclusion of unstable donors. In addition, it was commonplace even for experienced transplant teams to sacrifice one organ (usually the pancreas) when a replaced right hepatic artery was identified (8,9). However, it was shown that the superior mesenteric artery (SMA) could be divided

---

[‡] Deceased.

distal to the origin of the replaced right hepatic artery and thus retrieval of a normal pancreas for transplantation was not precluded (10,21,22).

With the increased need for and scarcity of organ donors, the technique of pancreas/ liver recovery has evolved to a rapid en bloc ("no touch") technique for liver and pancreas procurement (23–27). This technique permits utilization of the liver, pancreas, kidneys, isolated small bowel, heart, and lungs to maximize the number of potential recipients that might benefit from a single donor.

## RAPID EN BLOC TECHNIQUE FOR COMBINED PANCREAS/LIVER RECOVERY

A midline abdominal incision and a median sternotomy are performed (Even if the heart is not harvested, we prefer to include the median sternotomy to facilitate abdominal organ exposure). The round ligament is ligated and divided. The falciform ligament is divided down to the diaphragm. The left lateral segment is mobilized by taking down the triangular ligament. A nasogastric tube is passed from above through the pylorus and $200\,cm^3$ of betadine solution is instilled by the anesthesiologist. The gastrohepatic ligament is opened over the caudate lobe; this permits inspection of the pancreas in the lesser sac and also allows for detection of aberrant vascular anatomy. The upper gastrohepatic ligament is initially palpated to search for an accessory left hepatic artery originating from the left gastric artery. If it is absent, the remaining gastrohepatic ligament is divided to the diaphragm. If a left branch is present, it is helpful to make a window in the gastrohepatic ligament 1 cm cephalad to the left branch to avoid subsequent injury. Next, the presence of a replaced right hepatic artery is determined by bimanual palpation of the hepatodoudenal ligament, searching for a pulse posteriorly (as well as the main hepatic artery anteriorly). The common bile duct is ligated distally and divided. The gallbladder is then incised and flushed with saline to clear bile and prevent autolysis. Some surgeons advocate division of the gastroduodenal artery at this phase in the operation, although this is not necessary and can easily be accomplished in a bloodless field when separating the liver and pancreas after recovery. No further dissection is necessary in the porta hepatis. A generous Kocher maneuver is carried out to expose the inferior vena cava (IVC) and origins of the left and right renal veins. The duodenum and pancreatic head are freed from the retroperitoneal attachments in the avascular plane.

The infrarenal aorta is then dissected from just below the common iliac artery bifurcation to just above the take-off of the inferior mesenteric artery (IMA). Although the preceding steps in the hilum only require a few minutes of work and are useful to identify aberrant vascular anatomy, if the donor becomes at all unstable, then attention should initially focus on controlling the aorta for immediate cannulation. The IMA is ligated and divided. The aorta is encircled with umbilical tapes at its bifurcation and at the level of the IMA. It is helpful to clip the pair of lumbar arteries that usually reside between the IMA and the bifurcation that prevents back-bleeding when the aortic cannula is inserted. The donor is systemically heparinized (300 units/kg). At this time, several additional steps are useful prior to cross-clamping. One of the team members should crush ice to be ready for both the abdominal slush and the "back-table" basins. Two umbilical tapes are then passed around the pylorus and also around the proximal jejunum just beyond the ligament of Treitz. A single umbilical tape is also passed around the root of the small bowel mesentery. Pockets are made by incising the retroperitoneum lateral to Gerota's fascia to allow for adequate kidney cooling. Finally, the distal thoracic aorta is mobilized bluntly to prepare for cross-clamping in the chest. It is our experience that cross-clamping the distal thoracic aorta does not prevent the cardiac team from removing the heart easily. If the lungs are also being removed, then we place the aortic cross-clamp just below the diaphragm by dividing the crus and encircling the aorta with an umbilical tape. Some donor surgeons also perform a medial visceral rotation of the right colon in addition to the extended Kocher maneuver to allow for identification of the SMA as it arises from the aorta. Although this facilitates subsequent aortic division, there is risk of injuring the left renal vein with this maneuver. The aorta is ligated at the iliac bifurcation, and a cannula is inserted into the distal aorta and secured with umbilical tape (Fig. 1). A cannula line, pre-flushed with University of Wisconsin solution (UW) (29), is then connected. Low-volume aortic perfusion alone is used in situ, followed by portal flush ex vivo of the liver; this minimizes pancreatic flush injury and still provides adequate liver preservation (30–33). The entire dissection from the skin incision until cross-clamping usually requires 15 to 30 minutes.

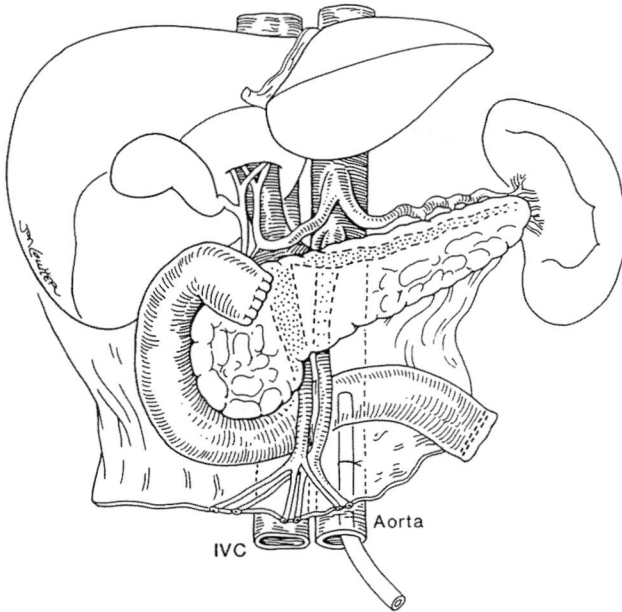

**Figure 1** En bloc procurement of liver and pancreas with duodenum and spleen. *Source*: From Ref. 28.

After coordination with the cardiac team, the aortic perfusion line is opened (Fig. 1). Ice slush is poured into the abdomen and chest, the descending thoracic aorta is cross-clamped, and the IVC is vented at the level of the right atrium. A pool-tip suction is placed in the right chest. We usually use 2–3 L of aortic flush until the effluent is rose colored. The cardiectomy is then completed concomitantly with the abdominal dissection. Care is taken to keep the abdominal organs cold with ice during the remaining dissection.

The left gastric artery is ligated along the lesser curvature at the level of the antrum and sharply dissected laterally up to the gastroesophageal junction. The proximal left gastric artery is preserved to avoid injury to an accessory left hepatic artery, if present. The nasogastric tube is aspirated and then pulled back. The duodenum is ligated at or below the pylorus with umbilical tapes and then divided (a stapler can also be used but adds cost). The greater curvature of the stomach and short gastric vessels are fully mobilized, staying close to the stomach to avoid injury to the spleen and pancreas. Next, the entire colon is sharply mobilized, beginning at the cecum and proceeding around to the distal sigmoid. The dissection line is close to the colon to avoid injury to the ureters. The terminal ileum and small bowel are then mobilized up to the root of the mesentery. The proximal jejunum is ligated and divided between the umbilical tapes. A long clamp is then applied across the root of the mesentery at the level of the previously placed umbilical tape, allowing for sufficient length of the root of the small bowel mesentery to facilitate pancreas back-table closure of the SMA, the SMV, and their branches. The small bowel mesentery is divided distal to the clamp, which then allows all of the colon and small bowel to be rotated off in a basin, leaving only the attached rectum.

Next, the spleen and tail of pancreas are carefully mobilized by dividing the retroperitoneal attachments and elevating the spleen and pancreatic tail to the midline, visualizing the left adrenal gland and left renal vein. Traumatic manipulation of the pancreas is minimized by using the spleen as a handle for elevating the pancreatic tail and body. The splenic vein is usually situated on the surface of the posterior pancreas, and great care is taken to avoid injury to the splenic vein while mobilizing the loose retroperitoneal attachments. After this maneuver and with the previously performed Kocher maneuver, the entire pancreas should be free from the retroperitoneum. The diaphragm is then split to expose the aorta while avoiding the esophagus. The descending thoracic aorta is divided, and the left anterolateral aorta is exposed by dividing the diaphragmatic crus and ganglionic tissue. This is the most difficult part of the operation and requires good exposure. It can be facilitated by inserting a finger into the open aorta, which allows palpation of the celiac and SMA orifices. The aorta is then divided distal to the SMA in a tangential fashion opposite the take-off of the SMA, to avoid injury to the renal arteries and to allow for an aortic cuff to be included with the renal arteries. After this maneuver, the retroaortic tissue and lumbar arteries are divided, which frees up the aorta with the celiac and SMA pedicles from the retroperitoneum. The IVC is divided above the renal veins. The dissection then proceeds through the right adrenal gland and right diaphragm, leaving a cuff around the suprahepatic IVC. The posterior right atrium is divided and the liver, pancreas, duodenum, and spleen are removed en bloc.

Another option is to remove the kidneys en bloc with the liver and pancreas by transecting the aorta and IVC just above the iliac vessels. The kidneys are then separated from the liver and pancreas on the back-table. Although this avoids the difficult task of dividing the aorta just below the SMA, it is cumbersome to have all organs in a single basin on the back-table and requires some experience to separate the kidneys properly when they are removed en bloc with the liver and pancreas. Donor iliac arteries and veins are then recovered in the usual fashion to allow for extension grafts, one set for the liver and the other for the pancreas. If one of the iliac arteries is injured or thrombosed, the carotid artery can be used.

## EX VIVO SEPARATION OF THE LIVER AND PANCREAS

The dissection begins in the hilum at the level of the divided common bile duct and proceeds from lateral to medial. The gastroduodenal artery is ligated and divided (leaving ties on both ends). The portal vein is dissected until the superior mesenteric vein (SMV)–splenic vein confluence is identified. Usually, the coronary vein will arise close to the confluence on the left side, and a small portal vein branch draining the pancreatic head usually comes off on the right side. The portal vein is divided 1 cm from the confluence and tagged with a vascular suture. If the portal vein is unusually long, more length can be left with the pancreas; this may avoid the need for a vein extension graft, but by no means should portal vein length compromise the donor liver just to avoid the need for a portal vein graft for the pancreas. Following portal vein division, a portal vein cannula is inserted and secured, and the liver is flushed with 1 L of UW. Usually, a small amount of hilar lymphatic and nerve tissue remains after dividing the portal vein, and requires transection. If any doubt exists as to whether a replaced right hepatic artery is present, dissection should shift to the aorta and SMA to confirm the presence of a right hepatic branch of the SMA.

The aorta is split longitudinally along the left lateral wall, exposing the orifices of the celiac and SMA. The aorta and celiac artery are dissected free of lymphatics and ganglionic tissue. The SMA is also dissected a few centimeters from the aorta to confirm the presence of a replaced right hepatic artery. The SMA is separated from the aorta leaving a Carrel patch with the celiac artery to be used with the liver. The left gastric artery is divided a few centimeters from the celiac axis, assuming that an accessory or replaced left hepatic artery is not present. The take-off of the splenic artery and the common hepatic artery are clearly identified before the splenic artery is transected at its origin from the celiac artery. The splenic artery is tagged with a vascular suture, as it can be difficult to locate later if it retracts within the pancreas. All that remains are the retroperitoneal attachments holding the liver and pancreas together along the length of the common hepatic artery; these are divided by dissecting in the plane directly along the lymph node chain accompanying the hepatic artery. The spleen and pancreas are removed together and packaged for transport.

## REPLACED RIGHT HEPATIC ARTERY

A replaced right hepatic artery originating from the SMA has been reported to occur in 10% to 20% of cadaver organ donors (34). Although once considered a contraindication for combined liver and whole pancreas procurement (8,9), it is now our practice (and that of others) to utilize the pancreas even in the presence of a replaced right hepatic artery (21,22). Once it is recognized that a replaced (or accessory) right hepatic artery exists, the SMA is dissected from the aorta to 1 cm beyond the origin of the right hepatic branch and then divided. The distal SMA on the pancreas side is also tagged with a vascular suture. The aorta, proximal SMA, and right hepatic branch then accompany the liver for subsequent reconstruction. Great care must be taken in dividing the distal SMA beyond the right branch so that the origin of the inferior pancreaticoduodenal artery is not compromised; in the transplant setting, since the gastroduodenal artery has been ligated, the inferior pancreaticoduodenal artery is the sole blood supply to the duodenum and head of the pancreas. If the distance between the right branch and the inferior pancreaticoduodenal artery is less than 2 cm, then the SMA is divided halfway in between, to allow for adequate reconstruction of both the liver and the pancreas.

## PANCREAS/KIDNEY PROCUREMENT ALONE

Occasionally, the liver is cirrhotic or grossly unsuitable, but the pancreas and kidneys are deemed acceptable for transplantation. In this setting, the procurement technique is modified. The same initial steps of dissection and aortic cannulation are performed. Once cross-clamped, the porta hepatis is clamped high in the hilum beyond the bifurcation of the left and right hepatic arteries, thereby preserving the inflow of the gastroduodenal (and superior pancreaticoduodenal) arteries to the duodenum and head of the pancreas. Venting is accomplished by dividing the portal vein high in the hilum to allow for efflux of the perfusate. The celiac axis, splenic, hepatic, and gastroduodenal arteries are preserved. Several options then exist for arterial reconstruction, and include (i) anastomosing SMA into the side of celiac, (ii) anastomosing the celiac into the side of the SMA, and (iii) using a common aortic Carrell patch.

## INTESTINE/PANCREAS/LIVER PROCUREMENT

With the increasing success and frequency of solitary intestinal organ transplantation, it has become necessary to refine the procurement procedure to permit the retrieval of the intestine, pancreas, and liver from the same cadaveric donor for transplantation into different recipients. It has been suggested, however, that this was not technically feasible. Recently, a technique for simultaneous recovery of the intestine, pancreas, and liver was described and utilized in 13 multiorgan cadaver donors during a 26-month period (19).

The most important technical consideration in this modified recovery is preservation of the inferior pancreaticoduodenal artery and vein with the pancreatic graft (19). This is accomplished by limiting the dissection of the superior mesenteric vessels to below the level of the ligated middle colic artery. In situ perfusion of UW is accomplished by aortic perfusion alone to avoid venous hypertension of the intestine and pancreas. When the in situ perfusion is completed, the intestinal graft is removed first from the surgical field by transection of the exposed segments of the SMA and SMV below the origin of the inferior pancreaticoduodenal artery from the SMA. The liver and pancreas are then removed en bloc as described above.

## BENCHWORK RECONSTRUCTION (PANCREAS BACK-TABLE)

The pancreas back-table is started by dividing the duodenum to leave an 8–10 cm remnant opposite the sphincter of Oddi (Fig. 2). This is readily identified by opening the distal common

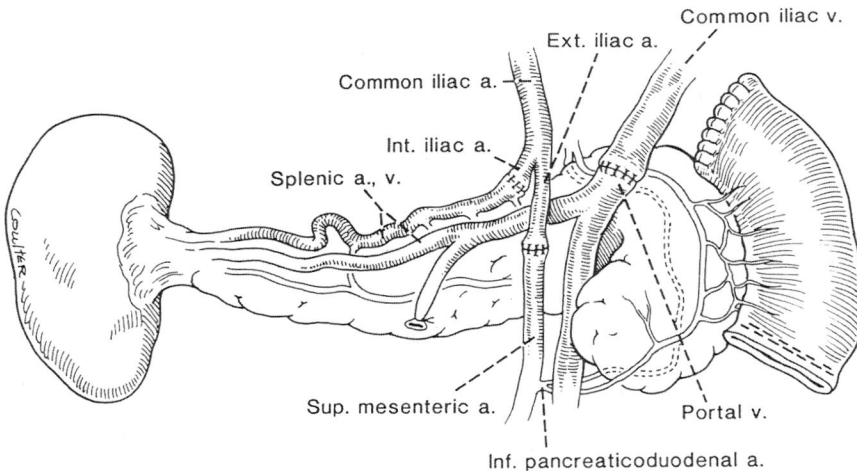

**Figure 2** Back-table reconstruction of pancreas with "Y" arterial graft and portal vein extension graft. *Source*: From Ref. 28.

bile duct and passing a pediatric feeding tube through the duct into the duodenal stump. The proximal duodenum is mobilized just enough to fire a stapler below the pylorus, and then the staple line is oversewn with Lembert sutures. The distal second portion of the duodenum is also transected with a stapler. The bile duct stump is ligated. The root of the transverse mesocolon and the root of the superior mesenteric vessels are ligated with silk ties. Any visible large arterial branches of the SMA are doubly ligated. Some surgeons favor stapling the root of the small bowel mesentery with vascular staples, followed by oversewing of the staple line. It is our belief that the SMA branches are more effectively secured with individual ties. Next, the transected inferior mesenteric vein that joins the splenic vein is ligated. The iliac extension grafts are prepared, and the common iliac vein segment is joined to the portal vein in an end–end fashion with running vascular suture. As already mentioned, occasionally the length of the portal vein left with the pancreas is sufficient, and an extension graft is not needed.

Several options have been described for the arterial reconstruction (4,14,35–37). For best size match, we usually prefer to join the external iliac artery end–end to the SMA and the internal iliac artery to the splenic artery. This leaves the end of the common iliac artery for anastomosis to the recipient external or common iliac artery. Finally, the pancreas is flushed with chilled UW and the efflux is evaluated; this usually indicates the adequacy of parenchymal flow. The spleen is left in place and excised after reperfusion in the transplant recipient.

In summary, the procedure of choice for pancreas retrieval is a rapid en bloc technique for simultaneous liver and whole organ pancreas procurement. This technique minimizes ischemic organ damage by avoiding a slower in situ dissection and is more applicable in the unstable donor. The procedure is technically straightforward and reduces operative time and costs.

## REFERENCES

1. Starzl TE, Hakala TR, Shaw BW, et al. A flexible procedure, for multiple cadaveric organ procurement. Surg Gynecol Obstet 1984; 158:223–230.
2. Starzl TE, Miller C, Broznick B, Makowka L. An improved technique, for multiple organ harvesting. Surg Gynecol Obstet 1987; 165:343–348.
3. Starzl TE, Iwatsuki S, Sahw BW, et al. Pancreaticoduodenal transplantation in humans. Surg Gynecol Obstet 1984; 159:265–272.
4. Corry RJ, Nghiem DD, Schulak JA, Beutel WD, Gonwa TA. Surgical treatment of diabetic nephropathy with simultaneous pancreatic duodenal and renal transplantation. Surg Gynecol Obstet 1986; 162:547–555.
5. Corry RJ. Pancreatico-duodenal transplantation with urinary tract drainage. In: Groth CG, ed. Pancreatic Transplantation. Philadelphia, PA: WB Saunders Co, 1988:147–153.
6. Starzl TE, Tzakis AG. Pancreatico-duodenal transplantation with enteric exocrine drainage. In: Groth CG, ed. Pancreatic Transplantation. Philadelphia, PA: WB Saunders Co, 1988:113–129.
7. Thistlethwaite JR Jr., Gaber AO, Stuart FP et al. Procurement of both liver and whole pancreas/duodenum allografts from a single donor without the use of interposition vascular grafts on transplantation. Transplant Proc 1988; 20:833–834.
8. Marsh CL, Perkins JD, Sutherland DE, Corry RJ, Sterioff S. Combined hepatic and pancreaticoduodenal procurement for transplantation. Surg Gynecol Obstet 1989; 168:254–258.
9. Sollinger HW, Vernon WB, D'Alessandro AM, Kalayoglu M, Stratta RJ, Belzer FO. Combined liver and pancreas procurement with Belzer-UW solution. Surgery 1989; 106:685–691.
10. Delmonico FL, Jenkins RL, Auchincloss H, et al. Procurement of a whole pancreas and liver from the same cadaveric donor. Surgery 1989; 105:718–723.
11. Spees EK, Orlowski JP, Temple DR, Kam I, Karrer IF. Efficacy of simultaneous cadaveric pancreas and liver recovery. Transplant Proc 1990; 22:427–428.
12. Conway MB, Saunders R, Munn SR, Perkins JD. Combined liver/pancreaticoduodenal procurement effects on allograft function. Transplant Proc 1990; 22:429–430.
13. Dunn DL, Schlumpf RB, Gressner RW, et al. Maximal use of liver and pancreas from cadaveric organ donors. Transplant Proc 1990; 22:423–424.
14. Johnson CP, Roza AM, Adams MB. Simultaneous liver pancreas procurement—a simplified method. Transplant Proc 1990; 22:425–426.
15. Stratta RJ, Taylor RJ, Spees EK, et al. Refinements in cadaveric pancreas-kidney procurement and preservation. Transplant Proc 1991; 23:2320–2322.
16. Teraoka S, Babazono T, Tomonaga O, et al. Donor criteria and technical aspects of procurement in combination pancreas and kidney transplantation from non-heart beating cadavers. Transplant Proc 1995; 27:3097–3100.

17. Schlumpf R, Morel PH, Sutherland D, et al. Combined procurement of pancreas and liver grafts does not affect transplant outcome. Transplant Proc 1990; 22:2074–2075.
18. Dunn DL, Morel P, Schlumpf R, et al. Evidence that combined procurement of pancreas and liver grafts does not affect transplant outcome. Transplantation 1991; 51:150–157.
19. Abu-Elmagd K, Fung J, Bueno J, et al. Logistics and technique for procurement of intestinal, pancreatic, and hepatic grafts from the same donor. Ann Surg 2000; 232:680–687.
20. Gruessner RW, Sutherland DE. Pancreas transplantation: Part I: the donor operation. Surg Rounds 1994; 17:311–324.
21. Ames SA, Kisthard JK, Smith JL, Piper JB, Corry RJ. Successful combined hepatic and pancreatic allograft retrieval in donors with a replaced right hepatic artery. Surg Gynecol Obstet 1991; 173:216–222.
22. Shaffer D, Lewis WD, Jenkins RL, Monaco AP. Combined liver and whole pancreas procurement in donors with a replaced right hepatic artery. Surg Gynecol Obstet 1992; 175:204–207.
23. Squifflet JP, de Hemptinne B, Gianello P, Balladur P, Otte JB, Alexandre GPJ. A new technique for en bloc liver and pancreas harvesting. Transplant Proc 1990; 22:2070–2071.
24. Dodson F, Pinna A, Jabbour N, Casavilla A, Khan F, Corry R. Advantages of the rapid en bloc technique for pancreas/liver recovery. Transplant Proc 1995; 27:3050.
25. de Ville de Goyet J, Reding R, Hausleithner V, Lerut J, Otte JB. Standardized quick en bloc technique for procurement of cadaveric liver grafts for pediatric liver transplantation. Transplant Int 1995; 8:280–285.
26. Imagawa DK, Olthoff KM, Yersiz H, et al. Rapid en bloc technique for pancreas–liver procurement. Transplantation 1996; 61:1605–1609.
27. Pinna AD, Dodson FS, Smith CV, et al. Rapid en bloc technique for liver and pancreas procurement. Transplant Proc 1997; 29:647–648.
28. Geller DA, Dodson SF, Corry RJ. Pancreas transplantation—methods of procurement. In: Sutherland D, ed. Current Opinion in Organ Transplantation. Vol. 3. Philadelphia, PA: Lippincott Williams Wilkins, 1998:242–247.
29. Kalayoglu M, Sollinger HW, Stratta RJ, et al. Extended preservation of the liver for clinical transplantation. Lancet 1988;617–618.
30. Wright FH, Wright C, Ames SA, Smith JL, Corry RJ. Pancreatic allograft thrombosis: donor and retrieval factors and early postperfusion graft function. Transplant Proc 1990; 22:439–441.
31. Ngheim DD, Cottington EM. Pancreatic flush injury in combined pancreas–liver recovery. Transplant Int 1992; 5:19–22.
32. de Ville de Goyet J, Hausleithner V, Malaise J, et al. Liver procurement without in situ portal perfusion. Transplantation 1994; 57:1328–1332.
33. Chui AK, Thompson JF, Lam D, et al. Cadaveric liver procurement using aortic perfusion only. Aust N Z J Surg 1998; 68:275–277.
34. Todo S, Makowka L, Tzakis AG, et al. Hepatic artery in liver transplantation. Transplant Proc 1987; 19:2406–2411.
35. Mayes JT, Schulak JA. Pancreas revascularization following combined liver pancreas procurement. Transplant Proc 1990; 22:588–589.
36. Corry RJ. Status report on pancreas transplantation. Transplant Proc 1991; 23:2091–2094.
37. Fernandez-Cruz L, Astudillo E, Sanfey H, et al. Combined whole pancreas and liver retrieval: comparison between y-iliac graft and splenomesenteric anastomosis. Transplant Int 1992; 5:54–56.

# 6 | Live Donor Pancreas Transplantation

**Miguel Tan, Raja Kandaswamy, David E. R. Sutherland, and Rainer W. G. Gruessner**
*Department of Surgery, University of Minnesota, Minneapolis, Minnesota, U.S.A.*

## INTRODUCTION

Although the pancreas was the first extra-renal organ to be used from living donors (LDs) (1), of the greater than 18,000 pancreas transplants performed since the 1960s less than 1% have come from LDs (2,3). Reasons for the underuse of this resource include the potential morbidity of an open distal pancreatectomy in an otherwise healthy donor, and the higher technical failure rate compared to cadaver donor transplants. In selected cases, however, LD pancreas transplantation may be an appropriate option for high panel reactive antibody (PRA) recipients who are unlikely to receive a cadaver organ or uremic diabetics on the simultaneous pancreas–kidney (SPK) waiting list. Prior to 1994, our institution only offered LD pancreas transplants as either solitary pancreas (PTA) transplants or pancreas after kidney (PAK) transplants, because of the fear that multiorgan retrieval from a LD entailed too much morbidity (4). With this approach, however, diabetic uremic recipients would have to endure two separate procedures, which many patients are reluctant to undergo. Patients will often pass up a single organ in order to receive an SPK transplant with its attendant prolonged waiting time. Furthermore, although 43% of patients with end-stage renal disease are diabetic, only 28% receive a kidney transplant (5). There are data to suggest that diabetic patients on dialysis have increased morbidity and mortality rates compared to nondiabetics on dialysis. The two- and three-year mortality rate of diabetics on dialysis is 17% and 27%, respectively, compared to 8% and 14% for nondiabetics over the same period of time (5). Consequently, we now perform LD SPK transplants to decrease morbidity and mortality while waiting for an SPK.

The donor operation is a major consideration in performing live donor pancreas transplants. The pancreas procurement can be performed using open or laparoscopic techniques. Although, open donor distal pancreatectomy can be done safely and is the more established procedure, it is associated with potentially significant postoperative morbidity associated with the bilateral subcostal incision. With the advent of laparoscopic technology, there are alternatives. This has been demonstrated most clearly with laparoscopic donor nephrectomy, which has rapidly become the procedure of choice for kidney donation because of reduced hospital stay and more rapid convalescence (6,7). Cosmetically, it is more appealing to potential donors compared to the traditional flank incision required for open nephrectomy. It is equivalent to the open procedure in terms of donor safety and quality of allograft (7). Consequently, laparoscopic techniques have rapidly been applied to other organ systems including the pancreas. Laparoscopic distal pancreatectomies have been described for treatment of a variety of pathologic states and appear to be safe with the additional benefit of reduced hospital costs, decreased pain, and accelerated postoperative recovery (8,9). In this chapter, we describe both the open technique of retrieval from a live donor, our initial experience with laparoscopic live donor pancreatectomy, the recipient operation, as well as donor and recipient outcomes of live donor pancreas transplantation.

## PREOPERATIVE DONOR EVALUATION
### Metabolic Workup

Because of the potential harm to an otherwise healthy donor, an extensive preoperative workup is essential. The goal is to ensure that the donor can safely undergo donation and the pancreatic remnant is sufficient to maintain normal metabolic function. All donors undergo an extensive multidisciplinary evaluation that includes endocrinology, nephrology, cardiology, social services, psychiatry, as well as transplant surgery.

Standard preoperative testing is performed to ensure the medical fitness of the potential donor. This includes electrocardiography, chest radiography, biochemical profiles (hemogram, electrolytes, renal function, liver function tests, coagulation profile, and lipid profile), and viral serologies (hepatitis B and C, human immunodeficiency virus, and cytomegalovirus). PRA testing, and ABO typing are also performed.

In addition, potential pancreas donors are considered only if they fit the following biochemical criteria: body mass index (BMI) $<27 \, kg/m^2$, insulin response to glucose or arginine $>300\%$ of basal insulin, $Hgb_{A1c} <6\%$, basal insulin fasting levels $<20 \, \mu mol/L$, plasma glucose $<150 \, mg/L$ during a 75 g oral glucose tolerance test, and a glucose disposal rate $>1\%$ during an intravenous glucose tolerance test (10). In related donors, no other family members other than the recipient can be diabetic. A genetically related donor should be at least 10 years older than the age of onset of diabetics in the recipient. A history of pancreatic surgery or other pancreatic disorders is also contraindicated. Furthermore, a history of gestational diabetes and high BMI are considered contraindications to donation.

## Radiologic Evaluation

Evaluation of the donor's vascular anatomy is undertaken to determine suitability for donation. At our institution, magnetic resonance angiography (MRA) is the modality of choice, although computed tomography angiogram is also acceptable. MRA appears to be as sensitive as angiography in detecting vascular abnormalities (11). It is noninvasive in nature; with it parenchymal details can be visualized and details of venous anatomy can be seen (Figs. 1 and 2) (11). Although angiography may be better at detecting small luminal abnormalities, such as fibromuscular dysplasia, it is associated with complications such as dye allergy, false aneurysms, hematomas at the puncture site, and femoral artery thrombosis (12). Although the anatomy of the splenic vessels is less variable than the renal vessels, one should try to visualize the take-off of the splenic artery and the location of the confluence of the splenic vein, inferior mesenteric vein (IMV), and superior mesenteric vein (SMV), since the IMV can sometimes join the splenic vein very close to the portal vein. MRA also allows evaluation of the location and number of renal vessels in the event that a simultaneous nephrectomy is to be done. The decision to procure the left or right kidney is taken on a case-by-case basis and determined by the number and location of accessory renal arteries. Our preference is to procure the left kidney when possible because of the longer renal vein and subsequent ease of dissection of the inferior margin of the pancreas, once the upper pole of the left kidney is dissected.

## OPERATIVE TECHNIQUE
### The Donor Operation
#### *Open Donor Distal Pancreatectomy*

The pancreas may be procured using a bilateral subcostal or midline abdominal incision. If a simultaneous nephrectomy is to be performed, the nephrectomy is done first. The technique for procuring the kidney is described in detail elsewhere (13).

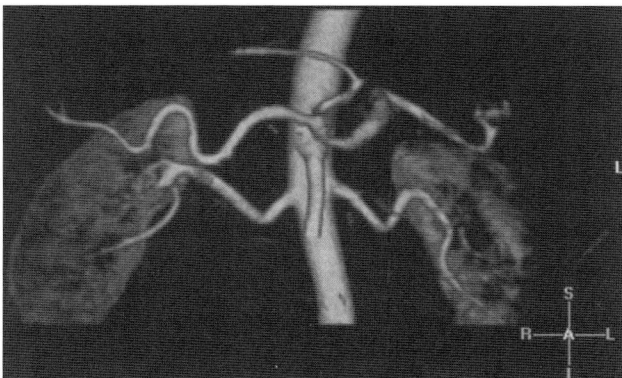

**Figure 1** Magnetic resonance angiogram showing anatomy of the splenic and renal arteries.

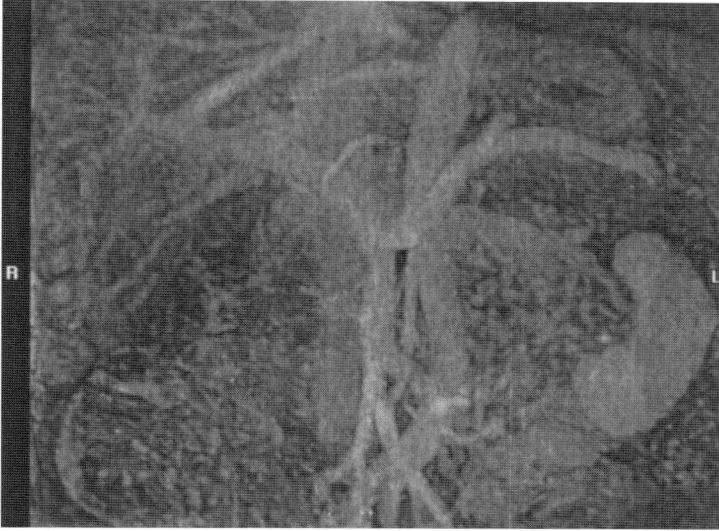

**Figure 2**  Magnetic resonance angiogram showing anatomy of splenic vein and portal confluence.

Briefly, the colon is mobilized medially. On the left side, the lienocolic ligament is preserved, if possible, as it may carry collateral vessels to the spleen. Once the kidney is ready to be procured, heparin (70 units/kg) is given prior to ligating the renal artery and vein. After the vessels are ligated, protamine (10 mg/100 units heparin) is given.

The distal pancreas is mobilized by dividing the gastrocolic ligament lateral to the inferior margin of the spleen. The right gastroepiploic and short gastric vessels are preserved to avoid devascularizing the spleen. The inferior margin of the pancreas is mobilized and a peritoneal incision is made over the tail of the pancreas where it joins the hilum of the spleen. The pancreas is dissected from the splenic surface. The splenic vessels are identified and the main trunks of the splenic artery and vein are divided proximal to the splenic branches in order to preserve the collateral vessels to the spleen.

The superior margin of the pancreas is then mobilized. As the pancreas is dissected from its retroperitoneal attachments, it is mobilized medially. The junction of the IMV with the splenic vein is visualized. The location of the junction can vary and may be close to the SMV. The IMV should be divided to allow further mobilization to the pancreatic neck. The portal vein is identified at the confluence of the SMV and splenic vein. The splenic artery is circumferentially mobilized as it takes off from the celiac axis. The pancreatic neck is divided using multiple 4–0 silk ligatures or a 45 mm ETS Flex Linear Articulating Stapler (Ethicon Endosurgery, Cincinnati, Ohio, U.S.A.). The cut edge of the pancreatic remnant can be over sewn with interrupted suture in a U-type fashion to fish mouth the edge in order to decrease the incidence of pancreatic leak.

The patient is heparinized (70 units/kg) and the splenic artery and vein are divided. The patient is then given protamine sulfate. The distal pancreatic segment is passed off to the recipient surgical team to be flushed with cold (4°C) University of Wisconsin solution prior to implantation (14).

### Laparoscopic Distal Pancreatectomy

The patient is placed in a modified right lateral decubitus position to allow the patient to be rotated from a left side up position (for a nephrectomy) to a supine position (for the distal pancreatectomy) if a nephrectomy is to be done simultaneously.

The operative table is then flexed to 45° to open up the left subcostal space to facilitate dissection of the kidney. A 6 cm midline incision is then made either supra- or periumbilically depending on the patient's body habitus. A Gelport (Applied Medical, Rancho Santa Margarita, California, U.S.A.) or HandPort device (Smith and Nephew Inc., Andover, Massachusetts, U.S.A.) is placed in the midline incision to allow for hand assistance. With standard

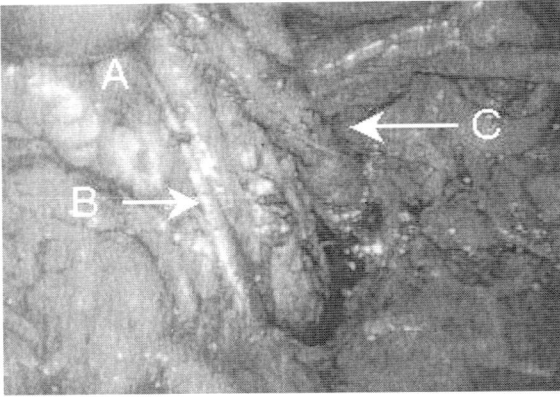

**Figure 3**  Pancreas mobilized medially to expose posterior surface of pancreas and splenic vessels. (A) Pancreas, (B) splenic vein, (C) splenic artery.

laparoscopic equipment, a 12 mm port is placed at the level of the umbilicus along the lateral edge of the left rectus for insertion of a 30° or 45° camera. A second 12 mm port is inserted in the left mid-abdomen in the plane of the anterior axillary line. This allows insertion of ultrasonic shears, laparoscopic scissors, and other instruments. Procurement of the kidney is done as per standard procedures (13). Prior to ligation of the renal vessels, the patient is given 70 units/kg of intravenous heparin, which is reversed with protamine sulfate after the vessels are ligated.

After removal of the kidney, the partially dissected inferior margin of the pancreas is mobilized using ultrasonic shears and electrocautery. The IMV is identified, ligated with staples, and divided near its insertion into the splenic vein. The posterior surface of the pancreas is then freed from its retroperitoneal attachments using electrocautery. The splenic artery and vein are identified in the hilum of the spleen and individually ligated and divided using a 35 mm vascular stapler. Care should be taken not to disturb the short gastric vessels and right gastroepiploic artery, as these constitute the main remaining blood supply to the spleen. With the pancreas retracted medially, the splenic vein is mobilized circumferentially near its junction with the SMV. The splenic artery is mobilized just as it bifurcates off the celiac axis (Fig. 3). Heparin (30 units/kg) is administered intravenously prior to ligation of the vessels. Clips are applied to the splenic artery just distal to the celiac axis and then the artery is divided with laparoscopic scissors. Two staples are applied to the splenic vein at the level of its junction with the SMV then divided. Protmaine sulfate is given as previously described. A 45 mm ETS Flex Linear Articulating Stapler is used to transect the pancreatic neck (Fig. 4). The distal pancreatic segment is then extracted by hand through the midline incision and passed off to the recipient team to be flushed immediately with cold University of Wisconsin solution. The staple line of the pancreatic remnant is over sewn with 4–0 polypropylene suture to achieve hemostasis and prevent leakage of the pancreatic duct. A drain is placed near the pancreatic remnant.

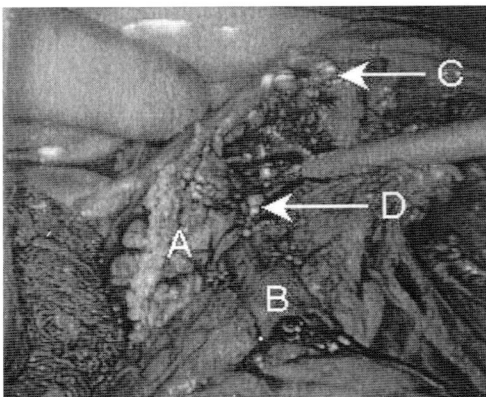

**Figure 4**  Pancreatic remnant after retrieval of distal pancreas. (A) Stapled pancreatic neck, (B) superior mesenteric vein, (C) ligated splenic arterial stump, (D) ligated splenic vein at portal confluence.

## Technical Points

In general, we try to preserve the spleen in order to prevent the potential immunologic seque-lae associated with splenectomy such as overwhelming post-splenectomy sepsis. In our five laparoscopic donors, so far, one splenectomy was performed because of a nonviable spleen that was recognized at the time of surgery. Based on the open donor pancreatectomy data, there is an 8.5% to 25% rate of splenectomy (15,16). At the current stage of evolution of this technique, we prefer the hand-assisted approach, because having tactile feedback greatly facil-itates safe dissection as well as partially overcomes the lack of three-dimensional visualization inherent in laparoscopy.

## Postoperative Care of the Donor

Postoperative care of the donor is similar to that of any patient undergoing major abdominal surgery. A nasogastric tube is left in place until return of bowel function. Hemoglobin, serum amylase, lipase, and glucose levels are followed serially. Persistently elevated amylase and lipase suggests pancreatitis, a leak, or pseudocyst formation. Persistent or severe left upper quadrant or left shoulder pain should be evaluated with CT and $^{99m}$Tc-sulfur-colloid scan of the spleen to assess splenic viability. If the spleen appears infarcted, a splenectomy should be performed.

## The Recipient Operation
### Pancreas Transplantation Using Segmental Pancreas Grafts

Segmental pancreas grafts taken from live donors may be implanted using either systemic vein and exocrine bladder drainage or systemic vein and enteric exocrine drainage. Using an intra-abdominal approach, the recipient's right side is the preferred implantation site. The cecum and ascending colon are mobilized sufficiently to provide exposure of the external and common iliac vessels on the right side. In order to achieve a tension-free venous anasto-mosis, the right internal iliac vein must often be ligated and divided. The donor splenic vein is anastomosed in an end-to-side fashion to the recipient external iliac vein using running 6-0 or 7-0 polypropylene sutures. The donor splenic artery is then positioned lateral and slightly cephalad to the venous anastomosis. It is anastomosed in an end-to-side fashion to the recipi-ent external iliac artery using 6-0 or 7-0 polypropylene sutures. Less frequently, it may be anastomosed end-to-end to the hypogastric artery (17).

### Bladder Exocrine Drainage

Pancreatic exocrine drainage into the bladder may be accomplished in two ways. Ductocystost-omy involves a direct anastomosis between the pancreatic duct and the urothelium of the bladder. The seromuscular layer of the bladder is first incised to expose 2 to 3 cm of urothelium. A posterior row of interrupted 4-0 nonabsorbable sutures is placed from the seromuscular layer of the bladder to the posterior surface of the pancreas. The urothelium is incised and an interrupted posterior row of 7-0 polydiaxanone suture is made between the urothelium and pancreatic duct. A stent is passed through the pancreatic duct and into the bladder prior to completing the anterior closure. The stent is secured to the duct using a single 5-0 absorbable suture. The stent will either be excreted spontaneously or have to be removed cytoscopically after four weeks. After the ductal anastomosis is complete, the anterior seromuscular layer is completed with interrupted 4-0 nonabsorbable sutures.

Alternatively, exocrine bladder drainage can be accomplished using an invaginated pan-creaticocystostomy. An outer posterior anastomosis is fashioned between the seromuscular layer of the bladder and the posterior surface of the pancreas. A 3 to 4 cm transverse incision is made in the bladder wall and a running 4-0 polydiaxanone suture is placed around the cir-cumference of the cut end of the pancreas and the cystostomy. Finally, the anterior outer layer is completed with 4-0 nonabsorbable sutures. A stent is placed in the pancreatic duct in the same manner as described for ductocystostomy (Fig. 5).

### Enteric Drainage

The vascular anastomosis is constructed as described above. A Roux-en-Y loop of small bowel is used for exocrine drainage. An appropriate length of jejunum is selected and divided with a GIA stapler. The stapled distal end is oversewn with 4-0 polypropelene suture. The posterior wall of the ductojejunostomy is created using 4-0 polypropylene between the posterior surface

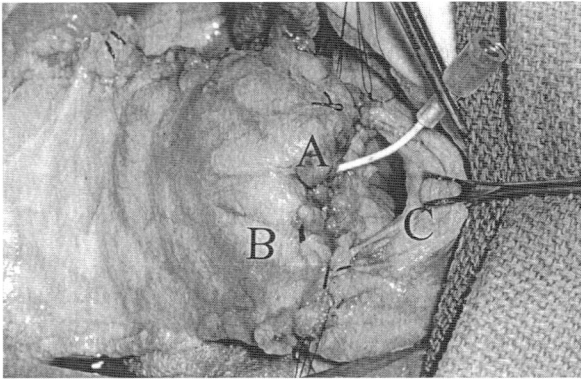

**Figure 5** Completed posterior wall of pancreati-cocystostomy using segmental pancreatic graft. (A) Cannulated pancreatic duct, (B) pancreas, (C) bladder.

of the pancreas and jejunal wall. A small incision is made on the antimesenteric side of the jejunum and a posterior row of 6-0 absorbable suture is made between the pancreatic duct and full thickness jejunum. Prior to completing the anterior inner row, stent is placed in the duct as previously described. Once the inner layer is finished, the anterior outer layer is completed with interrupted 4-0 polypropelene suture.

## DONOR OUTCOMES
### Open Donor Pancreatectomy

From January 1978 to August 2000, 115 open LD pancreas transplants were performed at our institution: 51 PTA, 32 PAK, and 32 SPK (16). There were no donor mortalities. Donor complications can include hemorrhage, splenic infarct, abscess, pancreatitis, and pseudocyst formation. Splenectomy was required in 8% of donors. Pseudocyst occurred in 10%. Percutaneous drainage was necessary in 60% of those with pseudocyst. Within the subset of SPK donors, 20% required perioperative blood transfusions. Two donors required percutaneous drainage of a noninfected peri-pancreatic fluid collection (14). The median donor age was 44 years (range 26–49). The median operative time was 6.9 hours with a median length of stay of eight days (range 6–24) (16).

Long-term follow-up was possible in 67 patients. The remaining 48 could not be located, refused to participate, lived outside of the United States, or were deceased. Ten donors had abnormal $Hgb_{A1c}$ levels. Three of them required insulin >6 years postoperatively. One of these donors had a history of gestational diabetes. The other two had pre-donation BMI >27 kg/m$^2$. One of these donors had a significant alcoholic history, which the donors did not disclose. Gestational diabetes and elevated BMI are now contraindications to donation. Since 1996, all donors have maintained normal $Hgb_{A1c}$ levels (4.9–6.2%) following these guidelines (16).

### Laparoscopic Donor Pancreatectomy

From March 1999 to August 2003, five laparoscopic pancreatectomies were performed at our center (Tan M, Kandaswamy R, Gruessner RWG. Laparoscopic donor distal pancreatectomy for LD pancreas transplantation. In press). The mean donor age was $48.4 \pm 8.7$ years with a BMI of $23.7 \pm 3.0$ kg/m$^2$. The mean length of surgery for PTA donors was $4.5 \pm 0.13$ hours, for SPK donors $7.9 \pm 0.38$ hours. Mean blood loss was $330 \pm 228$ mL. Once the learning curve has been overcome, however, the laparoscopic approach may actually have shorter operative times, as less dissection is required compared to the open technique. In two of the SPK cases, the donor surgical team had to wait 1.5 to two hours for the recipient team to receive the organs, thus prolonging the operative time. One splenectomy had to be performed at the time of the donor surgery for a nonviable spleen. No pancreatic leaks or pancreatitis was observed. The average serum glucose was $112 \pm 11.7$ mg/dL upon discharge. The amylase and lipase on discharge were $72.2 \pm 26.3$ and $67.2 \pm 34.0$ U/L, respectively. None of the donors has required oral antidiabetic medications or insulin. At three years follow-up, the mean postoperative

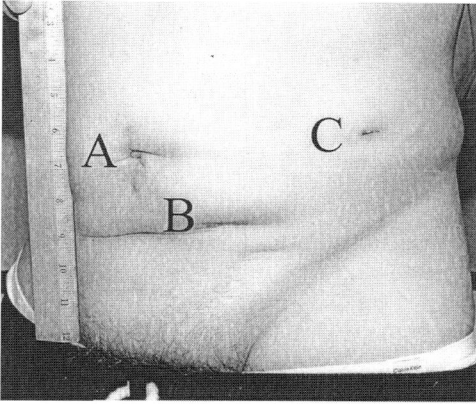

**Figure 6** Surgical incisions three weeks post laparoscopic distal pancreatectomy and left nephrectomy. (A) Gelport® site, (B) 12 mm camera port site, (C) 12 mm instrument port site.

Hgb$_{A1c}$ was $5.7 \pm 0.2\%$. One donor refused biochemical follow-up. Postoperative stay for the laparoscopic donors was $8 \pm 2$ days. No obvious statistical advantage was observed in terms of decreased hospital stay. However, based on the first handful of laparoscopic cases performed, this may be a function of over-vigilance on the part of the treating team, as tends to occur with new procedures. Certainly, in laparoscopic nephrectomy, the advantage of reduced hospital stay and earlier postoperative recovery has been demonstrated (18,19). All the donors have reported that they are back to their preoperative state of health and working. Satisfaction was high in terms of cosmetic result because the donor operation can be performed through a relatively small midline incision and only two trocar sites (Fig. 6).

## RECIPIENT OUTCOMES
### Recipient Outcomes Using Open Donor Pancreatectomy

Recipient survival rates were 93% and 90% at one and five years in those patients receiving LD segmental pancreases procured using the open technique. In the pre-tacrolimus epoch, technically successful PTA and PAK recipients had a graft survival rate of 68% and 50%, respectively. The immunologic advantage of LD pancreas transplants, at that time, was clear. Only 13% of LD pancreas recipients had graft loss secondary to rejection, whereas 41% of cadaver organ recipients lost their grafts from rejection (16). In the current immunosuppressive era, this difference hardly exists due to modern drug regimens (tacrolimus, mycophenolate mofetil), improved operative technique, and aggressive postoperative anticoagulation. Consequently, although solitary LD pancreas transplants are still performed, the focus is primarily on SPK donors in order to address the shortage of cadaver organs in this subset of pancreas transplant recipients.

Thirty-two open LD SPK transplants were done at the University of Minnesota from 1994 to 2000 (16). Patient and kidney graft survival was 100% at one year. Pancreas allograft survival was 87%. This compares favorably to current cadaver SPK transplant data that demonstrate 84% one-year survival for pancreas grafts and 90% kidney allograft survival (20). This marked improvement in patient and graft survival compared to our series of LD PTA and PAK transplants before 1994 may be attributed to improved immunosuppression, routine postoperative anticoagulation (perioperative low-dose heparin and long-term aspirin), and better infection prophylaxis (e.g., gancyclovir) (16).

### Recipient Outcomes with Laparoscopic Donor Pancreatectomy

With laparoscopically procured pancreases, patient and kidney graft survival is 100%, with 100% pancreas graft survival at three years follow-up (Tan M, Kandaswamy R, Gruessner RWG. Laparoscopic donor distal pancreatectomy for LD pancreas transplantation. In press). One patient required intermittent subcutaneous insulin postoperatively due to steroids. Once steroids were weaned, insulin requirements ceased. One of five recipients had three episodes of acute rejection that was reversed with steroids and antibody therapy. Four recipients had exocrine bladder drainage; one had enteric drainage. Two recipients had a leak at the duodenocystostomy, and three of five recipients had an intra-abdominal infection.

## SUMMARY

Although the number of available cadaver pancreata currently exceeds the number of pancreas transplants performed each year (21), the limiting factor tends to be the quality of the available pancreases, with only a disproportionately small number suitable for implantation. Consequently, the waiting list for diabetics awaiting transplantation is growing by more than 15% annually (16). In the subset of patients awaiting both a pancreas and kidney transplant, the wait time continues to be lengthy. Approximately 6% of these patients die annually while awaiting an SPK transplant (22). Compared to patients with nondiabetes-related end-stage renal disease, fewer diabetics receive kidney transplants with a two- and three-year mortality rate of dialyzed diabetics at 17% and 27%, respectively (5). The rationale, therefore, of LD pancreas transplantation, especially LD SPK transplants, is to allow for timely transplantation of high PRA recipients who are unlikely to receive a cadaver graft and to decrease the morbidity and mortality of diabetics on the waiting list.

Although the morbidity and prolonged postoperative recovery on the part of a potential pancreas donor has been a hindrance toward wider acceptance of LD pancreas transplants, use of laparoscopic techniques may make this procedure more appealing. Laparoscopic pancreatectomy appears to be safe with minimal morbidity, with recipient outcomes equivalent or better compared to open techniques of distal donor pancreatectomy. Donor satisfaction is also high in terms of postoperative cosmetic results.

### Future Trends

Currently, more institutions are performing robotic-assisted laparoscopic donor nephrectomy. The viability and safety of this modality has been demonstrated in this context (23,24). In the future, this may represent the next step in the evolution of laparoscopic donor pancreatectomy because of its advantages over traditional laparoscopic equipment, including better control of fine movements afforded by articulating instruments as well as elimination of tremor and three-dimensional visualization, which overcomes the lack of depth perception inherent in standard laparoscopic monitors.

## REFERENCES

1. Sharara AI, Dandan IS, Khalifeh M. Living-related donor transplantation other than kidney. Transplant Proc 2001; 33:2745.
2. Gruessner AC, Sutherland DER. Pancreas transplant outcomes for United States (US) and non-US cases as reported to the United Network for Organ Sharing (UNOS) and the International Pancreas Transplant Registry (IPTR) as of October 2002. Clin Transplant 2002:41.
3. Gruessner RWG, Leone JP, Sutherland DER. Combined kidney and pancreas transplants from living donors. Transplant Proc 1998; 30:282.
4. Gruessner RWG, Sutherland DER. Simultaneous kidney and segmental pancreas transplants from living related donors—the first two successful cases. Transplantation 1996; 61:1265.
5. Gruessner RWG. Should priority on the waiting list be given to patients with diabetes:pro. Transplant Proc 2002; 34:1575.
6. Schweitzer EJ, Wilson J, Jacobs S, et al. Increased rates of donation with laparoscopic donor nephrectomy. Ann Surg 2000; 232(3):392.
7. Leventhal JR, Deeik RK, Joehl RJ, et al. Laparoscopic live donor nephrectomy—is it safe? Transplantation 2000; 70(4):602.
8. Ueno T, Oka M, Nishihara K, et al. Laparoscopic distal pancreatectomy with preservation of the spleen. Surg Laparosc Endosc Percutan Tech 1999; 9(4):290.
9. Vezakis A, Davides D, Larvin M, McMahon MJ. Laparoscopic surgery combined with preservation of the spleen for distal pancreatic tumors. Surg Endosc 1999; 13(1):26.
10. Kendall DM, Sutherland DER, Najarian JS, Goetz FC, Robertson RP. Effects of hemipancreatectomy on insulin secretion and glucose tolerance in healthy humans. N Engl J Med 1990; 322:898.
11. Kandaswamy R, Stillman AE, Granger DK, Sutherland DER, Gruessner RWG. MRI is superior to angiography for evaluation of living-related simultaneous pancreas and kidney donors. Transplant Proc 1999; 31:604.

12. Gruessner RWG. Living donor pancreas transplantation. In: Gruessner RWG, Sutherland DER, eds. Transplantation of the Pancreas. Springer-Verlag, 2004:423.
13. Gruessner RWG, Kandaswamy R, Denny R. Laparoscopic simultaneous nephrectomy and distal pancreatectomy from a live donor. J Am Coll Surg 2001; 193(3):333.
14. Humar A, Gruessner RWG, Sutherland DER. Living related donor pancreas and pancreas–kidney transplantation. Br Med Bull 1997; 53(4):879.
15. Troppmann C, Grussner AC, Sutherland DE, Grussner RW. Organ donation by living donors in isolated pancreas and simultaneous pancreas–kidney transplantation. Zentralbl Chir 1999; 124(8):734.
16. Gruessner R, Sutherland D, Drangstveit M, Bland B, Gruessner A. Pancreas transplants from living donors: short- and long-term outcome. Transplant Proc 2001; (33):819.
17. Gruessner RWG. Surgical aspects of pancreas transplantation. In: Gruessner RWG, Sutherland DER, eds. Transplantation of the Pancreas. 2004:159.
18. Kercher KW, Heniford BT, Matthews BD, et al. Laparoscopic versus open nephrectomy in 210 consecutive patients: outcomes, cost, and changes in practice patterns. Surg Endosc 2003; 17(12):1889.
19. Jacobs SC, Cho E, Foster C, Liao P, Bartlett ST. Laparoscopic donor nephrectomy: the University of Maryland 6-year experience. J Urol 2004; 171(1):47.
20. International Pancreas Transplant Registry Annual Report, 2002.
21. Sutherland DER, Najarian JS, Gruessner RWG. Living versus cadaver pancreas transplants. Transplant Proc 1998; 30:2264.
22. Gruessner R, Kendall D, Drangstveit M, Gruessner A, Sutherland D. Simultaneous pancreas–kidney transplantation from live donors. Ann Surg 1997; 226(4):471.
23. Horgan S, Vanuno D, Benedetti E. Early experience with robotically assisted laparoscopic donor nephrectomy. Surg Laparosc Endosc Percutan Tech 2002; 12(1):64.
24. Horgan S, Vanuno D, Sileri P, Cicalese L, Benedetti E. Robotic-assisted laparoscopic donor nephrectomy for kidney transplantation. Transplantation 2002; 73(9):1474.

# 7 | Anesthetic Management in Kidney–Pancreas and Isolated Pancreatic Transplantation

**Raymond M. Planinsic and Ramona Nicolau-Raducu**
*Department of Anesthesiology, University of Pittsburgh Medical Center, Pittsburgh, Pennsylvania, U.S.A.*

The predominant indication for pancreatic transplantation is insulin-dependent diabetes mellitus (type I IDDM). Long-standing diabetes is often complicated by multiple end-organ dysfunction. End-organ damage is related to macroangiopathy resulting from accelerated atherosclerosis; microvascular lesions affecting the kidney, the heart, the retina, and the lower extremities; autonomic neuropathy affecting the heart, the gastrointestinal tract, and the urinary tract; and abnormal cross-linking of collagen, which is responsible for defects in connective tissue (1). The majority of pancreatic transplants ( >80%) are performed in combination with kidney transplantation. The combined procedure increases the length of the operation, thus making anesthetic management especially important.

## EVALUATION OF THE PATIENT

Preoperative assessment of end-organ pathology is one of the most important factors, and can contribute to a decrease in morbidity and mortality in diabetic patients (1).

The main cardiovascular problem observed in the diabetic patient is accelerated atherosclerosis, which leads to peripheral vascular disease and coronary artery disease (CAD). Long-standing hypertension also contributes to CAD as well as left ventricular hypertrophy.

Evaluation of cardiac risk is especially important in this patient population. A careful history and physical examination are required to ascertain cardiac risk factors and functional status. An electrocardiogram is not sufficient to screen for CAD in these patients, as they may have clinically silent ischemia. Perioperative Holter monitoring has been recommended to improve the value of preoperative electrocardiogram (2). Exercise stress testing may not be adequate if the patient is not capable of completing the study. Either a dobutamine stress echocardiogram or an adenosine thallium stress test is preferable to screen for ischemia and cardiac reserve. In Rabbat et al.'s study (3), a negative test result with nuclear scintigraphy or dobutamine stress echocardiogram was associated with a low risk of myocardial infarction and cardiac death. Conversely, patients with abnormal myocardial perfusion studies were at higher long-term risk for myocardial infarction or cardiac death. If either test shows signs of ischemia or poor cardiac performance, then coronary angiography is mandatory, and right heart catheterization may be useful to determine the cardiac output and to measure cardiac filling pressures (4).

Autonomic neuropathy associated with diabetes can make intraoperative blood pressure control difficult. In addition, there is a higher incidence of sudden death during the postoperative period in these patients (1). To evaluate autonomic dysfunction, Ewing and Winney (5) developed two tests: the cardiovascular responses to the Valsalva maneuver and to sustained handgrip. In their study, there was a reduction in the beat-to-beat variation in heart rate at rest in those patients who had abnormal Valsalva maneuvers, independent of age or the resting heart rate.

Besides cardiac dysfunction, autonomic neuropathy may cause anesthetic complications because of diabetic gastroparesis. There is often an associated alteration in esophageal motility and a decrease in lower esophageal sphincter tone, both of which may lead to delayed gastric emptying and an increase risk of aspiration during induction of anesthesia (1). The patient should be questioned for a history of gastric reflux as well as NPO status.

Chronic renal failure is characterized by a low hemoglobin level (6–8 g%), which reduces oxygen-carrying capacity of the blood and is associated with a compensatory high cardiac output. A hemoglobin concentration greater than 8 g% is necessary for adequate oxygen delivery to the heart and the transplanted organ. Blood transfusion to relieve anemia-related symptoms was the only treatment prior to the availability of erythropoietin. Patients receiving erythropoietin can have relatively normal hemoglobin levels, although they may be at increased risk of vascular access site thrombosis (6).

In patients with end-stage renal disease receiving hemodialysis or peritoneal dialysis, it is important to evaluate their acid–base, electrolyte, and volume status. In patients on dialysis, fluid and electrolyte imbalances can be optimized prior to surgery to a normal or near-normal state. Coagulation defects caused by abnormal platelet function can also be partially reversed by dialysis (7). Patients who have not received dialysis for several days may be volume overloaded, in addition to having acid–base and electrolyte disturbances.

Airway evaluation is very important for patients with type I IDDM. These patients often manifest the stiff joint syndrome, characterized by a fixation of the atlantooccipital joint along with limitation of head extension, making endotracheal intubation difficult or impossible (8). Stiff joint syndrome also affects the first small joints of the fingers and hands. Failure to oppose palms due to stiffness of the interphalangeal joints ("prayer sign") and the reduced palm print may be sensitive predictive factors of difficult laryngoscopy and intubation in diabetics (9). A lateral cervical radiograph is essential for an accurate diagnosis.

Impairment of respiratory function is another problem that must be considered in the preoperative evaluation of patients with diabetes (10). Pulmonary function abnormalities are related to a loss of lung elastic proprieties and are characterized by a decrease in cough reactivity, a significant restriction of lung volumes with a reduced tidal volume and forced expired ventilation, and a reduced resting diffusing capacity for carbon monoxide (11).

In addition to routine laboratory studies prior to the transplantation, a blood sample should be submitted to the blood bank to type and cross an appropriate number of units of red blood cells.

## INTRAOPERATIVE AND IMMEDIATE POSTOPERATIVE MANAGEMENT

All patients about to undergo isolated pancreatic or combined kidney–pancreas transplantation should have central venous pressure (CVP) monitoring capabilities and good peripheral intravenous access. The internal jugular vein is usually cannulated with a double or triple lumen catheter to allow CVP monitoring, blood sampling, and, if necessary, vasopressor drug use. If the patient has significant cardiac disease and careful measurement of pulmonary artery pressure, pulmonary capillary wedge pressure, and cardiac output are needed, a pulmonary artery catheter introducer should be inserted. Direct arterial catheterization of the radial or other artery is routinely performed, as it will allow for direct blood pressure, assessment and serial electrolyte, glucose, and hematocrit measurements both intraoperatively and during the early postoperative period.

There is an increased risk of surgical wound infection in diabetic patients, especially in patients with poor glycemic control. This leads to defects in the inflammatory phase of healing, resulting in a reduction of fibroblast growth and collagen synthesis (12). Staphylococci and gram-negative aerobic bacilli cause the majority of wound infections after pancreas or pancreas–kidney transplantation. The recommended antibiotic regimen for these patients is cefotetan 1–2 g IV at the induction of anesthesia (13).

The technique of induction of anesthesia is not as important as the maintenance of hemodynamic stability. Avoidance of hypertension, hypotension, and tachycardia are important in this patient population who may suffer from CAD. In Menigaux's study, an attenuated hemodynamic and somatic response to laryngoscopy and orotracheal intubation was obtained using esmolol (0.5–1 mg/kg) before induction (14). Induction can be achieved safely with reduced dose of sodium thiopental (2–3 mg/kg), etomidate (0.1 mg/kg), or propofol (1.5–2 mg/kg), and these can be combined with narcotics (1–2 µg/kg fentanyl) and/or benzodiazepines (2–5 µg/kg midazolam). The choice of muscle relaxant adequate for endotracheal intubation will depend on the potassium level. If potassium is not a concern, then the use of a depolarizing agent (succinylcholine 1–1.5 mg/kg) is safe; otherwise the administration of an intubating dose of a nondepolarizing agent such as cisatracurium (0.1 mg/kg) or mivacurium (0.15–0.2 mg/kg) is preferable, since these will not be affected by renal dysfunction (15).

If diabetic gastroparesis is a concern, then use of a non-particulate antacid (sodium citrate and citric acid oral solution 30 mL) immediately prior to the induction of anesthesia will decrease the acid content of the stomach. Use of metoclopramide (30 mg PO) may increase gastric emptying and lower esophageal sphincter tone. If time allows, the use of an $H_2$ blocker 6 to 12 hours prior to induction will decrease gastric acid production (16).

Diabetic neuropathy affects peripheral sensory and motor nerves. The risk of nerve compression related to improper patient positioning and padding of pressure points is increased during anesthesia (16). Pre-existing asymptomatic neuropathy may present postoperatively, and for this reason it is preferable to avoid plexus and truncal blocks in patients with pre-existing motor or sensory abnormalities (16).

The use of an epidural catheter should be considered for postoperative pain as well as intraoperative anesthetic management. Continuous infusions of low-dose local anesthetics and narcotics (bupivacaine 0.125% and hydromorphone 0.01 mg/mL) can be administered if there are no contraindications, and can decrease intraoperative systemic narcotic use as well as inhalational anesthetic concentrations. This will allow for a more rapid emergence from anesthesia and a more comfortable patient postoperatively.

Maintenance of anesthesia can be achieved with a combination of inhalational agents, narcotics, benzodiazepines, and muscle relaxants. During maintenance, a reduction in the narcotic and benzodiazepine doses should be considered, to avoid excessive respiratory depression and sedation, which may delay recovery of adequate spontaneous ventilation at the end of surgery (17). Muscle relaxant drugs such as cisatracurium (0.025 mg/kg) or mivacurium (0.05–0.1 mg/kg) are required for adequate surgical conditions, with close monitoring of the neuromuscular blockade. Use of a bispectral index monitor (BIS, Aspect Medical Systems, Inc. Natick, MA) is advocated to maintain an adequate depth of anesthesia. Beta-adrenergic blockers and antihypertensive drugs, as well as vasopressors, should be readily available for administration during the perioperative period.

Careful management of intraoperative fluid, electrolytes, and glucose is required, especially in the combined kidney–pancreas transplant recipient. Intravenous fluids should be administered to maintain CVP of 10–12 cmH$_2$O. Prior to reperfusion of the donor kidney, to enhance graft function, intravenous furosemide (1 mg/kg) and mannitol (1 g/kg) are often given. An additional dose of intravenous furosemide (1 mg/kg) may also be given over 30 minutes after reperfusion of the kidney. Finally, maintenance of good systolic pressure (120–140 mmHg) may require titration of the anesthetic or the use of vasopressors. Low-dose dopamine (1–5 µg/kg/min) is used because of its ability to enhance renal blood by flow stimulating the dopamine-1 renal receptor. Dopamine-2 renal, alpha-, and beta-adrenergic receptors, however, are also stimulated at low-dose dopamine rates. A new selective dopamine-1 agonist, fenoldopam, is now available (18). At low doses it exhibits many desirable renal effects, including decreases in renal vascular resistance accompanied by increases in renal blood flow and glomerular filtration rate, and increases in sodium excretion and urine volume. Even at high doses of fenoldopam, dopamine-2 renal, alpha-, or beta-adrenergic receptors are not stimulated, and undesirable side effects such as arrhythmias can be avoided (18). All of these maneuvers are aimed at having the newly grafted kidney produce urine immediately. With regard to the pancreas, it is preferable to avoid both glucose-containing solutions and insulin, if at all possible, to allow assessment of the pancreas after reperfusion.

Reperfusion of both kidney and pancreas grafts may be associated with hypotension. This can be related to bleeding or to a reduction in the preload as a consequence of unclamping the iliac artery. This may be treated with intravenous fluids or colloids, but may require low-dose vasopressors. If hyperkalemia results from prolonged ischemia of the donor graft or residual preservation solution, tall peaked T-waves on the electrocardiogram and ventricular arrhythmias may be observed. This can be treated with $CaCl_2$ (0.5–1 g) intravenously; hyperkalemia related to metabolic acidosis can also be treated with intravenous sodium bicarbonate.

After the procedure is completed, the patient is routinely kept intubated and taken to the intensive care unit, where extubation can be performed several hours later. As with induction of anesthesia, hemodynamic stability is essential during emergence. Hypertension can lead to increased myocardial oxygen demand, and may lead to myocardial ischemia in the patient with coexisting CAD. In addition, vascular anastomoses are susceptible to disruption and leakage under the stress of hypertension. Short-acting antihypertensive drugs such as nitroglycerin, nicardipine, or esmolol may be considered. Finally, as stated above, the use of an epidural catheter for postoperative pain and intraoperative anesthetic management, while by no means mandatory, may allow for a hemodynamically stable emergence from anesthesia.

## CONCLUSION

The patient presenting for combined kidney–pancreas or isolated pancreatic transplantation presents a number of challenges to the anesthesia team. A variety of coexisting diseases, the consequence of long-standing IDDM, makes these patients more prone to potential intraoperative and postoperative complications. Precise control of hemodynamics, electrolytes, glucose, and acid–base status are required for good outcomes. Invasive monitoring and frequent laboratory evaluations are essential for maintaining a stable physiologic state. Vigilance and anticipation of potential intraoperative and postoperative problems will protect the patient and help to ensure a smooth early posttransplant course.

## REFERENCES

1. Scherpereel PA, Tavernier B. Perioperative care of diabetic patients. Eur J Anaesthesiol 2001; 18(5):277–294.
2. Cashion AK, Hathaway DK, Milstead EJ, Reed L, Gaber AO. Changes in patterns of 24-hr heart rate variability after kidney and kidney–pancreas transplant. Transplantation 1999; 68(12): 1846–1850.
3. Rabbat CG, Treleaven DJ, Russell JD, Ludwin DC, Deborah J. Prognostic value of myocardial perfusion studies in patients with end-stage renal disease assessed for kidney or kidney-pancreas transplantation: a meta-analysis. J Am Soc Nephrol 2003; 14(2):431–439.
4. Schweitzer EJ, Anderson L, Kuo PC, et al. Safe pancreas transplantation in patients with coronary artery disease. Transplantation 1997; 63(9):1294–1299.
5. Ewing DJ, Winney R. Autonomic function in patients with chronic renal failure on intermittent haemodialysis. Nephron 1975; 15:424–429.
6. Murphy ST, Parfrey PS. Erythropoietin therapy in chronic uremia: the impact of normalization of hematocrit. Curr Opin Nephrol Hypertens 1999; 8(5):573–578.
7. Burke JF, Francos GC. Surgery in the patient with acute or chronic renal failure. Med Clin North Am 1987; 71:489.
8. Salzarulo HH, Taylor LA. Diabetic 'stiff joint syndrome' as a cause of difficult endotracheal intubation. Anesthesiology 1986; 64:366–368.
9. Nadal JL, Fernandez BJ, Escobar IC, Black M, Rosenblatt WH. The palm print as sensitive predictor of difficult laryngoscopy in diabetics. Acta Anaesth Scand 1998; 42:199–203.
10. Ramirez LC, Dal Nogare DA, Hsia C, et al. Relationship between diabetes control and pulmonary in insulin dependent diabetes mellitus. Am J Med 1991; 91:371–376.
11. Niranjan VIS, McBrayer DG, Ramirez LC, Raskin PH, Connie CW. Glycemic control and cardiopulmonary function in patients with insulin-dependent diabetes mellitus. Am J Med 1997; 103(6):504–513.
12. Leaper DJ. Blood vessels. In: Bucknall TE, Ellis H, eds. Wound Healing for Surgeons. Eastbourne: Balliere-Tindall, 1984:221–241.
13. ASHP therapeutic guidelines on antimicrobial prophylaxis in surgery. Am J Health Syst Pharm 1999; 56(18):1839–1888.
14. Menigaux CG, Adam B, Sessler F, Joly DI, Chauvin VM. Esmolol prevents movement and attenuates the BIS response to orotracheal intubation. Br J Anaesth 2002; 89(6):857–862.
15. Dierdorf SF. Anesthesia for patients with diabetes mellitus. Curr Opin Anaesthesiol 2002; 15(3): 351–357.
16. Stoelting RK. Considerations in the anesthetic management of patients with diabetes mellitus. Curr Opin Anaesthesiol 1996; 9:245–246.

17. Koehntop DE, Rodman JH. Fentanyl pharmacokinetics in patients undergoing renal transplantation. Pharmacotherapy 1997; 17:746–752.
18. Singer I, Epstein M. Potential of dopamine A-1 agonist in the management of acute renal failure. Am J Kidney Dis 1998; 31:743–755.

# 8 | Technical Aspects of Pancreas Transplantation

**Ron Shapiro, Robert J. Corry,[‡] and Ngoc Thai**
*Thomas E. Starzl Transplantation Institute, University of Pittsburgh School of Medicine, Pittsburgh, Pennsylvania, U.S.A.*

The success of pancreas transplantation is critically dependent both on sound judgment in donor selection (discussed in Chapter 4) and on technical perfection in all phases of organ recovery (Chapter 5), preparation, and implantation. It is, in many ways, perhaps the most fastidious transplantable organ, in that it has almost no tolerance for even minor irregularities in any of the above steps. This chapter will address the technical issues involved in pancreas transplantation. It will focus first on back table preparation and then go on to discuss implantation, including most of the potential variations.

## BACK-TABLE PREPARATION

The deceased donor pancreatic bloc includes the pancreas, at least the first, second, and third portion of the duodenum, and the spleen (discussion of the separation of the pancreas and liver is covered in Chapter 5) (Fig. 1) (1–4). Inspection of the pancreas is important to determine its suitability for transplantation. Fatty infiltration, fibrosis, and parenchymal injury need to be evaluated, since their presence might preclude transplantation. The arterial blood supply includes the splenic artery and the superior mesenteric artery (SMA), the former supplying the body and tail of the pancreas and the latter supplying the head of the pancreas and duodenum, via the inferior pancreaticoduodenal artery (5). The gastroduodenal artery has usually been ligated at its origin. The venous drainage includes a short segment of portal vein just beyond the confluence of the splenic and superior mesenteric veins (SMV). The tasks involved in the back table preparation of the pancreas involve visual inspection of the organ, trimming of the excess duodenum, ligating the distal superior mesenteric artery and vein and their branches and the short gastric vessels, and reconstructing, if necessary, the arterial and venous blood supply.

The first portion of the duodenum is divided a few centimeters below the pylorus proximally and the ampulla of Vater distally. It is possible to dissect the third portion of the duodenum sharply off the pancreas; as the distal aspect of the second portion is neared, it is important to ligate and divide small branches coming from the pancreas (Fig. 2). The dissection of the first portion of the duodenum should be performed with ligation and division of the small peripancreatic branches just below the pylorus. Prior to stapling and dividing the excess duodenum, the tie around the distal common bile duct should be cut, and a 5-French feeding tube should be passed through the duct into the duodenum. This maneuver ensures that the duodenum is not divided too close to the ampulla of Vater. It is important to remember to ligate the common bile duct after removing the feeding tube. Approximately 7–8 cm of duodenum is left with the pancreas (Fig. 3A). The proximal staple line should be inverted with interrupted 4–0 silk Lembert seromuscular sutures (3,4). The distal staple line may either be inverted or not, depending on whether enteric drainage using the distal end of the duodenum is to be used (Fig. 3B).

Ligation of the distal superior mesenteric vessels exiting the head of the pancreas is performed next (Fig. 4). Our personal preference is double ligation of individual vessels, although stapling with the endo-GIA stapler and reinforcing with locking 4–0 polypropylene work equally well and may save some time. The inferior mesenteric vein is identified and ligated.

[‡] Deceased.

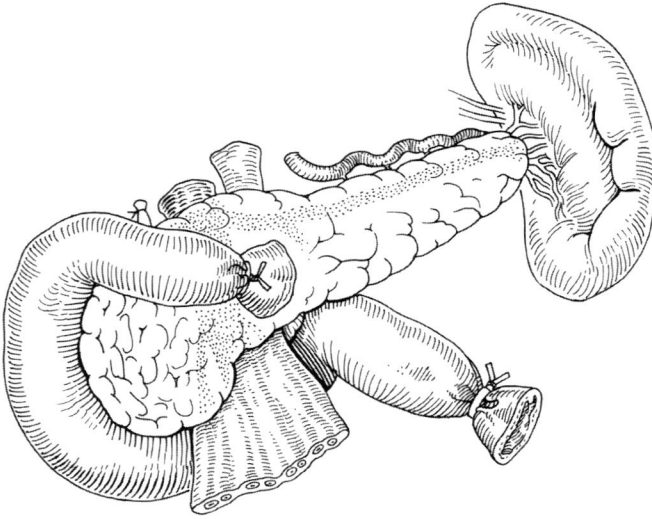

**Figure 1** The deceased donor pancreatic bloc: the pancreas, spleen, and duodenum.

Dissection then proceeds distally to ligate small incidental branches and short gastric vessels. Splenectomy can be performed at the back table or after implantation. Double ligation of splenic vessels or stapling with 4–0 prolene reinforcement works equally well. Care must be ensured that the tail of the pancreas is not damaged during the splenectomy, especially if stapling is used.

Attention is then turned to the splenic and SMA and portal vein. Lymphatic tissue on the posterior surface of the pancreas is ligated. The arteries are usually reconstructed with an iliac arterial Y-graft (Fig. 5A) (6,7). The internal iliac artery is joined end-to-end to the splenic artery, and the external iliac artery to the SMA. The common iliac is used for anastomosis to the recipient artery. Occasionally, a small caliber external iliac artery will mandate joining the common iliac artery to the SMA, leaving the external iliac for recipient anastomosis.

Variations of arterial reconstruction include end-to-side anastomosis of the splenic artery to the SMA. Usually, a graft using donor external iliac artery is required with this method if the

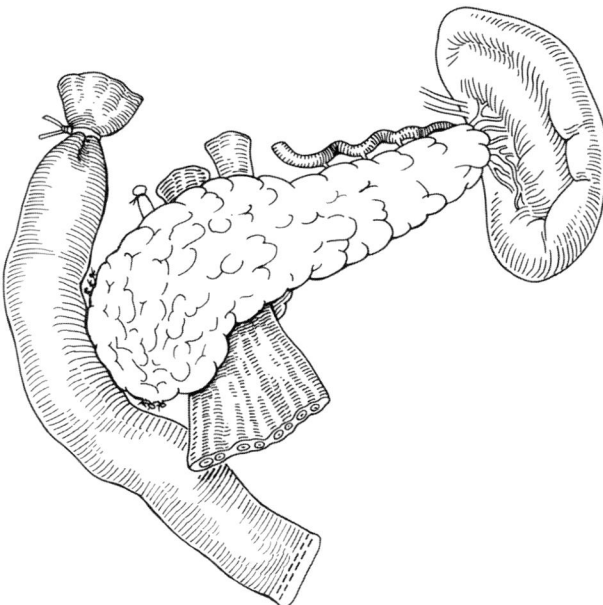

**Figure 2** Dissecting off the first and third portions of the duodenum.

**(A)**

**(B)**

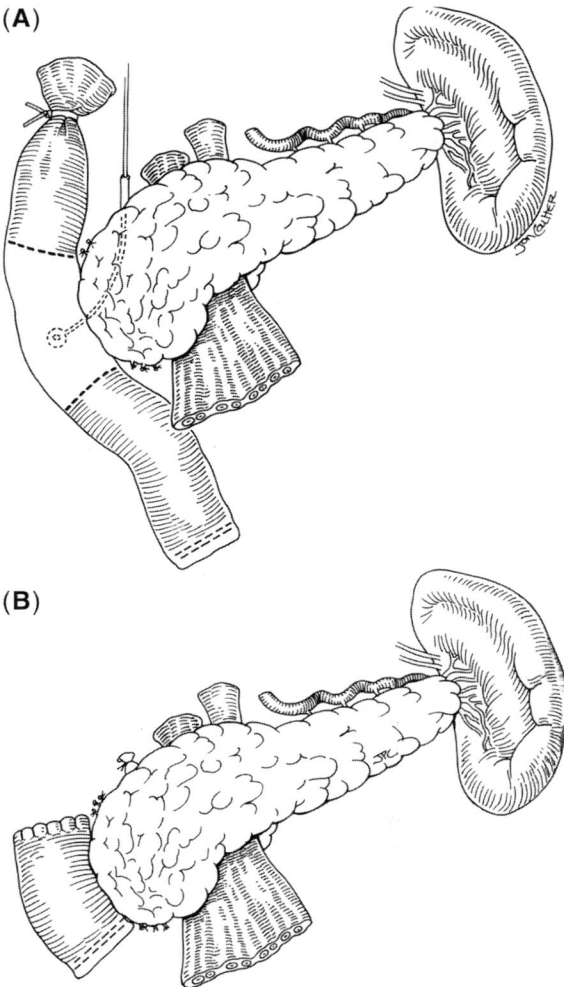

**Figure 3** (**A**) The remaining second portion of the duodenum attached to the pancreas; note the catheter identifying the ampulla. (**B**) The duodenum after division of the first and third portions.

splenic artery is not redundant (Fig. 5B). Alternatively, if a Y-graft is not available, a common orifice between the SMA and splenic artery in a "pants" configuration can be made, and a single artery extension can be placed onto this common channel. We have recently described the reperfusion of the GDA in addition to the Y-graft to augment arterial flow to the head of the pancreas. In a few cases, no reconstruction at all may be needed if a cuff of aorta with both the celiac artery and the SMA is available (Fig. 5C); this is unusual because most pancreas donors are also liver donors.

Depending on the available length of portal vein, a short common iliac vein graft anastomosed end-to-end to the portal vein may be needed (Fig. 5A). If it is used, it is important to perform the portal anastomosis to the distal end of the donor vein graft, so that no obstruction from a valve occurs.

Once the back table preparation has been completed, the pancreas is removed for a brief period from the basin, and the artery is flushed with chilled University of Wisconsin solution. It is of critical importance not to use the solution in the basin for flushing or testing of the arterial suture lines, but rather to use a new bottle of chilled University of Wisconsin solution. Small particles of tissue or fat in the basin solution will destroy the pancreas if flushed into the organ. Flushing allows the surgeon both to look at how well the pancreas perfuses and to check for unligated vessels that can be clamped and tied. If there is any doubt about a portion of the pancreas being inadequately perfused, methylene blue or indigo carmine can be added to the flush to see how well the parenchyma is perfused. Assessment of the rate of efflux is also important. Once this is accomplished, the organ is ready to be implanted.

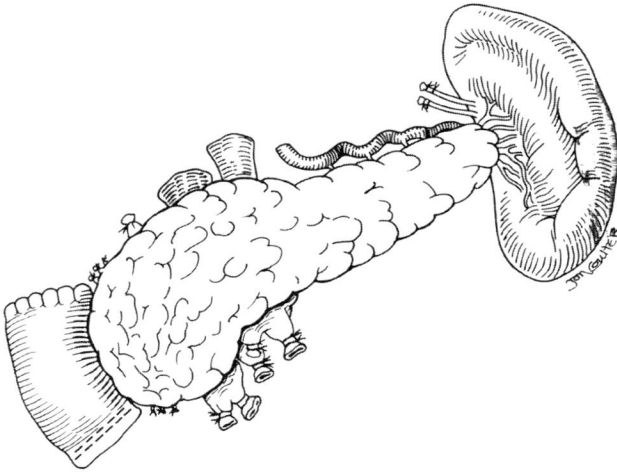

**Figure 4** Ligation of the distal superior mesenteric vessels and short gastric vessel.

## IMPLANTATION

While the details of the back table preparation are fairly uniform and straightforward, there are a number of alternatives concerning techniques of implantation of the pancreas. These variations begin with the type of incision, continue with the question of systemic venous or

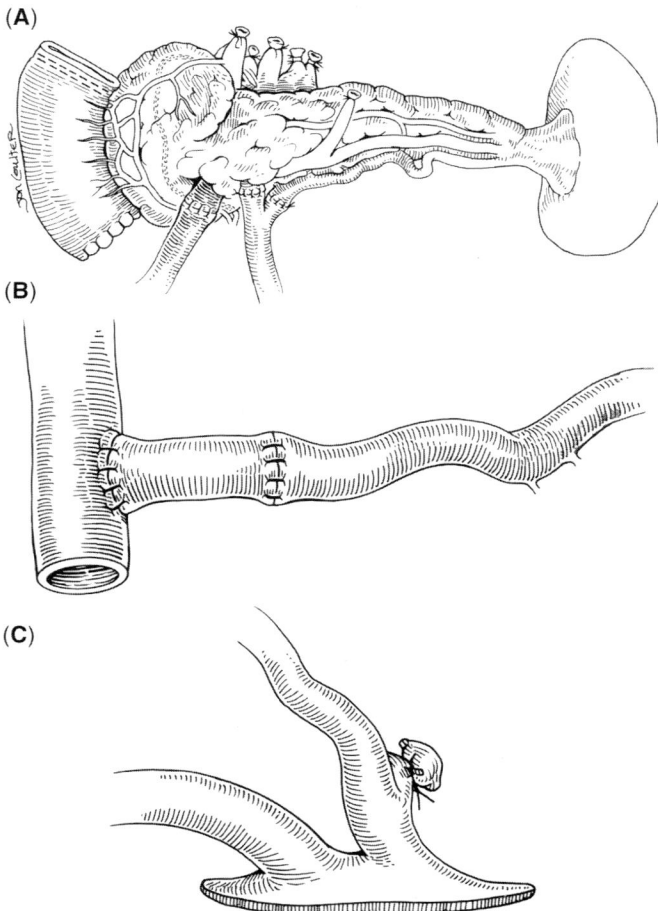

(**A**)

(**B**)

(**C**)

**Figure 5** Arterial reconstruction: (**A**) Y-graft for artery; note vein graft for portal vein. (**B**) End-to-side arterial graft anastomosing the splenic artery to the SMA. (**C**) Cuff of celiac and SMA (rare).

portal venous drainage, and conclude with the issue of bladder or enteric drainage for the exocrine secretions of the pancreas. There are advantages and disadvantages associated with all of these different technical approaches.

## The Incision

The first decision to be made concerns the use of a midline or a right (or left) lower quadrant oblique incision. Advocates of the midline incision prefer it for the advantages of a single incision, in the case of a combined pancreas/kidney transplant, and/or for access to the recipient's SMV, in the case of portal venous drainage of the transplanted pancreas. Advocates of the separate right lower quadrant (or left lower quadrant, in the case of the pancreas after kidney transplant, where the kidney was previously placed on the right side) incision argue that it allows for improved exposure of the iliac vessels, and separates the kidney, which remains retroperitoneal, from the pancreas, which is intraperitoneal. This protects the kidney in the case of a subsequent pancreas-associated infection. There is no question that a second incision, in the case of the combined procedure, adds at least an extra hour to an already lengthy procedure. Our personal preference has been to use two separate incisions, but the single midline incision is quite popular.

## Exposure of the Vessels

If the iliac vein is to be used for the venous anastomosis, the distal external iliac vein is mobilized, although the circumflex vein does not usually need to be divided. The corresponding proximal external iliac artery is mobilized just beyond its origin (3,4). Alternatively, if it is in good condition, the internal iliac artery may be used for end-to-end arterial anastomosis. This has the advantage of avoiding any risk to the lower extremity blood supply.

If the SMV is to be used for the venous anastomosis (8–11), it is exposed below the root of the mesentery in a similar fashion as in a mesocaval shunt procedure. Anastomosis is performed at a comfortable location to the main SMV. A venous extension is frequently needed for this procedure also. The corresponding arterial exposure is at the level of common iliac artery.

## Vascular Anastomosis

It is usual to perform the venous anastomosis first, followed by the arterial anastomosis. When systemic venous drainage is used, the pancreas is essentially transplanted "upside down," so that the superior aspect of the pancreas is lying posteriorly, with the still-attached spleen pointing cephalad and the duodenum caudad (Fig. 6). The portal vein, with or without an iliac vein extension, is anastomosed end-to-side to the distal external iliac vein. The distal placement relaxes the 90° angle at the portal vein–splenic vein junction (4). If bladder drainage is used, the vein should be placed a bit more proximally so that it is not compressed by the duodenum. The artery is anastomosed either end-to-side to the proximal external iliac artery, or end-to-end to the internal iliac artery. Again, if bladder drainage is used, the artery may need to be placed just proximal to the vein so that the duodenum can reach the bladder. When drained into the portal system, the donor portal vein, with the iliac venous extension, is anastomosed end-to-side to the SMV (Fig. 7A). The artery is usually anastomosed to the right common iliac artery (Fig. 7B). Standard vascular anastomotic techniques are used; our personal approaches are to use either a simple two-stitch technique or a four-stitch technique, utilizing running 5–0 polypropylene. Topical cooling of the pancreas is performed as the vessels are being anastomosed; alternatively, one can use an ice blanket. No special agents are given during the vascular anastomosis; it is important that the use of intraoperative insulin be minimized or even avoided, if possible, to allow early assessment of the function of the transplanted pancreas.

In those systemically vascularized, enterically drained cases, recently, we have been utilizing a head-up approach to minimize the tension to the duodenoenterostomy. A 30° rotation of the portal vein anastomosis allows the tail of the pancreas to be placed in the pelvis and the head laterally. This orientation also allows the portal vein to be anastomosed onto the external iliac vein. The arterial Y-graft can also be anastomosed to the external iliac artery. Results with this technique appear to be very satisfactory.

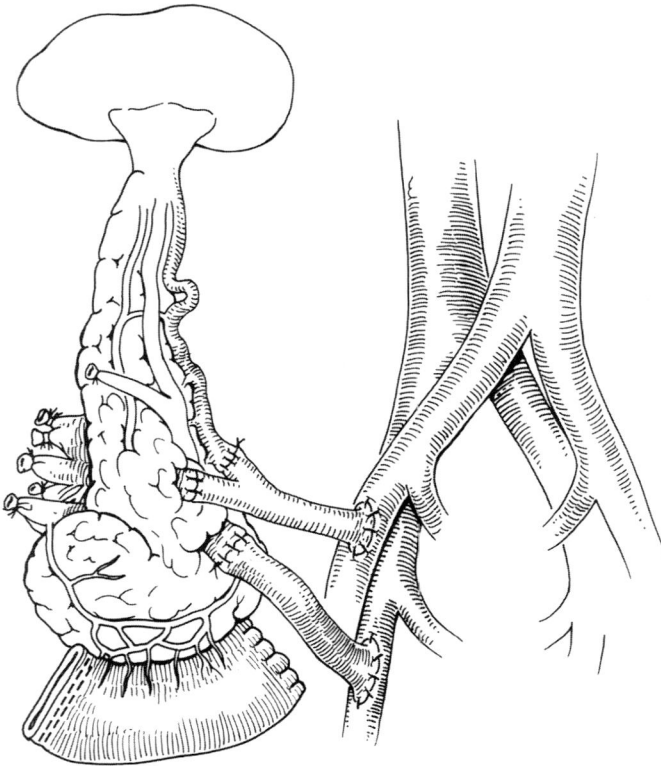

**Figure 6** Implantation of the pancreas using systemic venous drainge.

## Reperfusion

After completion of the vascular anastomoses and release of the cross clamps, perfusion of the pancreas can be assessed. A normal pancreas allograft will perfuse uniformly and turn tan-pink, and the duodenum will be pink and will soon begin to fill with mucus. Bleeders can be clamped and ligated with silk ties. After adequate reperfusion has been established, the distal splenic artery and vein are clamped, the spleen is amputated if not done on the back table, and the vessels are doubly ligated or stapled (Fig. 8). The pancreas is then placed in an appropriate position, with the body and tail resting on top of or lateral to the cecum in the right paracolic gutter, taking special care to ensure that adequate inflow and outflow are present. The splenic vein is evaluated for excessive pressure by palpation. The portal vein is inspected and palpated, to ensure a stable position and rule out the presence of a clot. If a clot exists in the portal vein, it should be removed; in addition, the pancreas will need to be repositioned to allow for better venous outflow.

## Drainage of the Exocrine Pancreas

Although the pancreas is transplanted because of its endocrine function, one of the main issues that has plagued the successful development of pancreatic transplantation has been the exocrine drainage. The two options are bladder drainage (4,12–14) or enteric drainage (3,10,15–21); duct injection with polymer (22–25) or pancreaticoureterostomy (26,27) has generally passed from serious consideration.

### Bladder Drainage

Bladder drainage involves suturing the side of the duodenum to the dome of the bladder, as described by Nghiem et al. and Sollinger et al. (Fig. 9) (4,12–14). A 4–5 cm opening is made in both the duodenum and the bladder, and the anastomosis is performed in two layers, with an

(A)

(B)

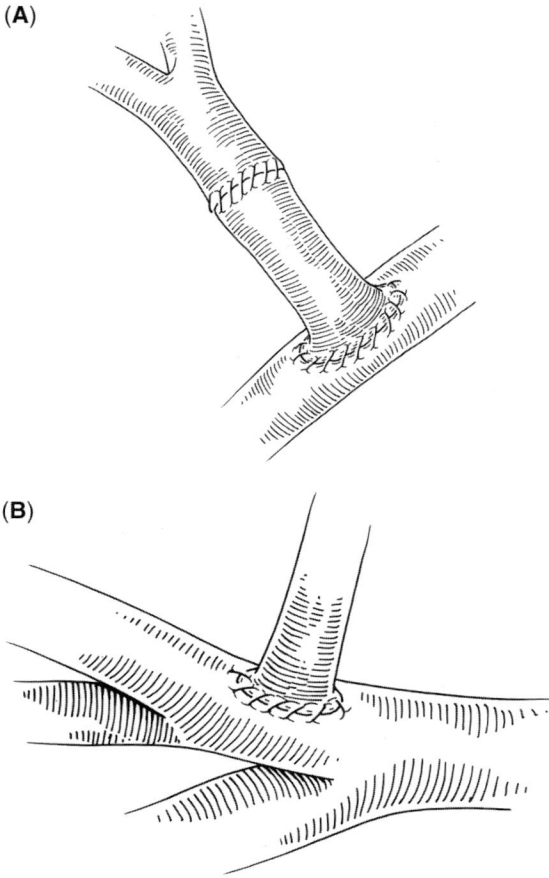

**Figure 7** Portal venous drainage: (**A**) Venous anastomosis to the SMV. (**B**) Arterial anastomosis to the right common iliac artery.

outer seromuscular layer of interrupted 4–0 silk and an inner, full-thickness layer of running 3–0 monofilament absorbable suture.

Although an unusual physiological arrangement, the bladder drainage technique allows measurement of the urinary amylase, which has been an important marker for rejection in many centers, particularly when the pancreas is transplanted alone (without the kidney). In addition, it avoids potential septic complications attendant with the enterotomy required for the enteric drainage procedure.

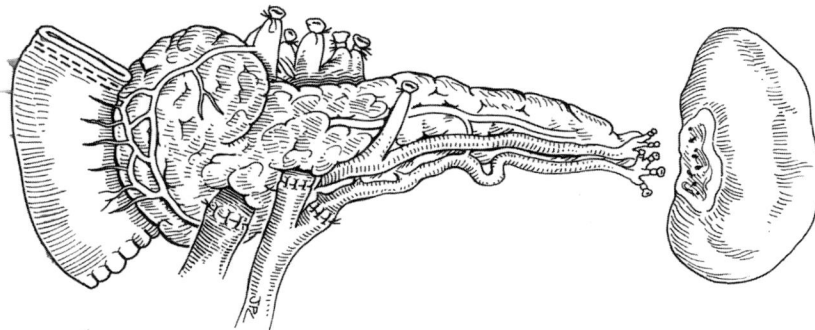

**Figure 8** Removal of the spleen.

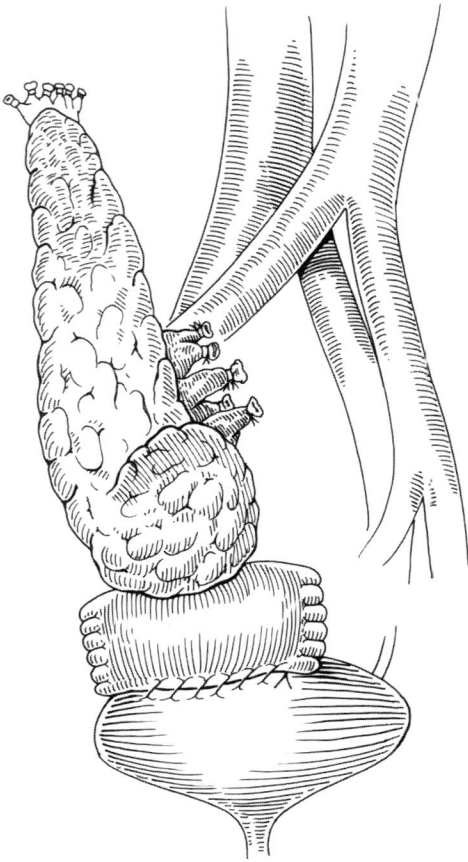

**Figure 9**   Duodenocystostomy: Bladder drainage.

### Enteric Drainage

Enteric drainage has become more popular again, after being out of favor for many years (10,20,21). The anastomosis can be constructed from the distal end (Fig. 10A) or the side (Fig. 10B) of the donor duodenum to the side of the recipient jejunum. There are a number of possible variations; all involve a standard two-layer anastomosis with an outer nonabsorbable seromuscular layer (usually interrupted 4–0 silk) and an inner absorbable full-thickness layer. Recently, the use of a circular stapler to perform a side-to-side duodenoenterostomy has also gained popularity. We recommend a layer of 4–0 silk Lemberts to reinforce the circular staple line. We have not had a single enteric leak in the last 50 pancreas transplants performed using the combined stapling with silk Lembert reinforcement. Alternatively, a roux-en-y limb of recipient jejunum can be created for the anastomosis; this has the advantage of minimizing leakage of enteric contents in the event of anastomotic breakdown, but subjects the recipient to additional surgery.

Some authors, notably the Stockholm group, have, in the past, advocated placement of a fine feeding tube to drain the pancreatic duct; this tube can even be brought out through the recipient's small bowel and the skin to permit examination of the pancreatic fluid for amylase content and cytology (6,15–19). Unfortunately, the tube also obstruct the pancreatic duct and cause pancreatitis.

After completion of the drainage procedure, the pancreas is examined carefully to make sure that it is in a good position regarding its blood supply. If possible, the omentum is draped over the duodenocystostomy or duodenojejunostomy and the intestines for further protection. The pancreas is not covered, to permit possible subsequent fine needle or small core biopsy without passing the needle through the highly vascularized omentum (Fig. 11).

Throughout the operation, topical antibiotic irrigation is used; our personal preference consists of a solution of 1000 mg of cefotetan and 5 mg of amphotericin B per liter of saline.

**(A)**

**(B)**

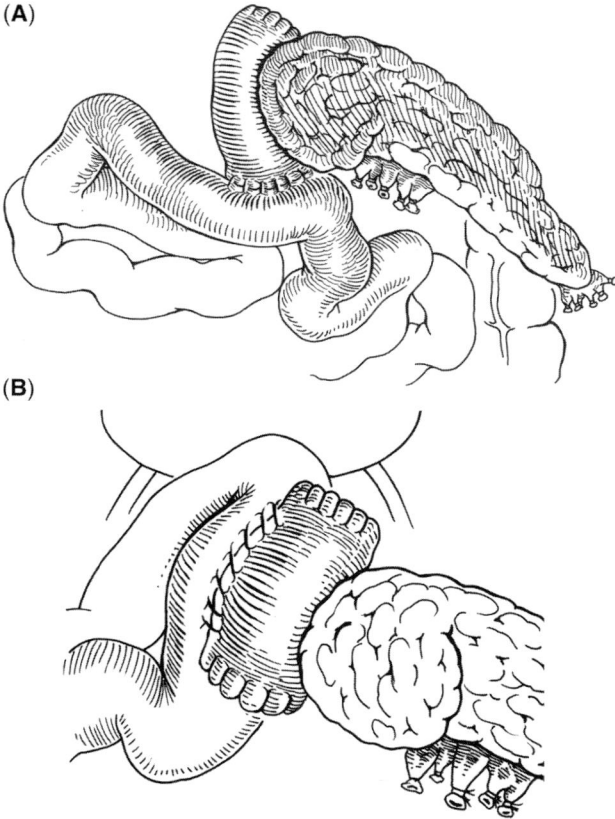

**Figure 10** Duodenojejunostomy: Enteric drainage.

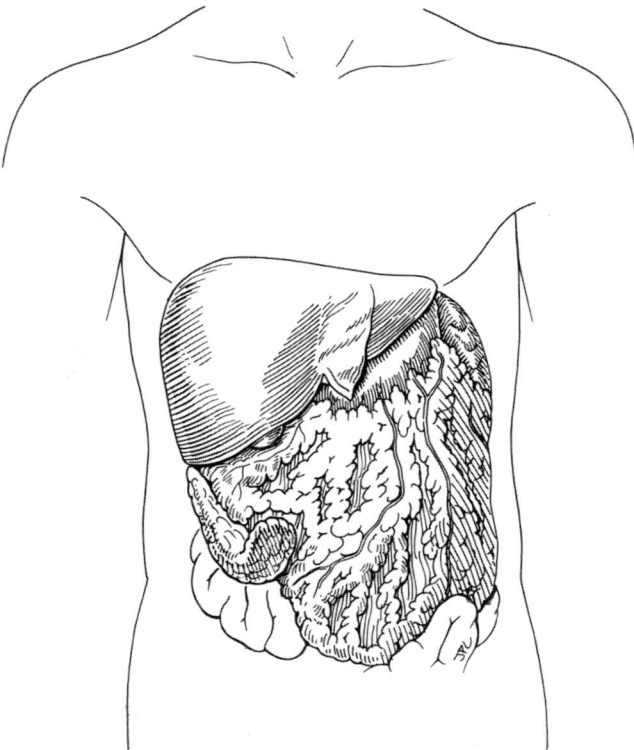

**Figure 11** Draping the omentum over the duodenojejunostomy.

Prior to closure, and after meticulous hemostasis is achieved, special care regarding final positioning of the graft is essential to avoid kinking or unnecessary pressure on the portal vein. Both artery and vein should be short, to avoid thrombosis in this low-flow organ. If there is any doubt, and one of the vessels appears to be twisted or kinked, the pancreas should be removed, cooled and flushed, and reimplanted.

Wound closure is routine; a personal preference is to close the peritoneum separately with a running absorbable suture, and then to close the fascia in two layers with a running nonabsorbable suture. Subcutaneous and skin layers are closed according to the surgeon's preference.

## REFERENCES

1.  Kelly WD, Lillehel RC, Merkel FK, Idezuki Y, Goetz FC. Allotransplantation of the pancreas and duodenum along with the kidney in diabetic nephropathy. Surgery 1967; 61(6):827–837.
2.  Lillehei RC, Simmons RL, Najarian JS, et al. Pancreatico-duodenal allotransplantation experimental and clinical experience. Ann Surg 1970; 172:405–436.
3.  Starzl TE, Iwatsuki S, Shaw BW Jr, et al. Pancreatico-duodenal transplantation in humans. Surg Gynecol Obstet 1984; 72:159–265.
4.  Corry RJ, Nghiem DD, Schulak JA, Buetel W, Gonwa TA. Surgical treatment of diabetic nephropathy with simultaneous pancreatic duodenal and renal transplantation. Surg Gynecol Obstet 1986; 162:547–555.
5.  Gray H. The organs of digestion. In: Pick TP, Howden R, eds. Gray's Anatomy. New York: Bounty Books—Crown Publishers, Inc., 1977:498.
6.  Tyden G, Groth CG. Pancreas transplantation. In: Starzl TE, Shapiro R, Simmons RL, eds. Atlas of Organ Transplantation. New York, NY: Gower Medical Publishing, 1992:8.4–8.21.
7.  Tibell A, Groth CG. Renal and pancreatic transplantation. In: Shapiro R, Simmons RL, Starzl TE, eds. Renal Transplantation. Stamford, CT: Appleton & Lange, 1997:483–494.
8.  Tyden G, Wilczek H, Lundgren G, et al. Experience with 21 intraperitoneal segmental pancreatic transplants with enteric or gastric exocrine diversion in humans. Transplant Proc 1985; 17:331–335.
9.  Sutherland DER, Goetz FC, Moudry KC, Abouna GM, Najarian JS. Use of recipient mesenteric vessels for revascularization of segmental pancreas grafts: technical and metabolic considerations. Transplant Proc 1987; 19(1):2300–2304.
10. Nymann T, Elmer DS, Shokouh-Amiri MH, Gaber AO. Improved outcome of patients with portal-enteric pancreas transplantation. Transplant Proc 1997; 29(1–2):637–638.
11. Nymann T, Hathaway DK, Soukouh-Amiri MH, Gaber LW, Abu-el-Ella K, Gaber AO. Incidence of kidney and pancreas rejection following portal-enteric versus systemic-bladder pancreas–kidney transplantation. Transplant Proc 1997; 29(1–2):640–641.
12. Sollinger HW, D'Alessandro AM, Stratta RJ, Pirsch JD, Kalayouglu M, Belzer FO. Combined kidney–pancreas transplantation with pancreaticocystostomy. Transplant Proc 1989; 21(1):2837–2838.
13. Sollinger HW, Ploeg RJ, Eckhoff DE, Stegall MD, Isaacs R, Pirsch JD. Two hundred consecutive simultaneous pancreas–kidney transplants with bladder drainage. Surgery 1993; 114:736–744.
14. Nghiem DD, Corry RJ. Technique of simultaneous renal pancreatoduodenal transplantation with urinary drainage of pancreatic secretion. Am J Surg 1987; 153(4):405–406.
15. Groth CG, Lundgren G, Klintmalm G, et al. Successful outcome of segmental human pancreatic transplantation with enteric exocrine diversion after modifications in technique. Lancet 1982; 2:522–524.
16. Groth CG, Lundgren G, Wilczek H, et al. Segmental pancreatic transplantation with duct ligature or enteric diversion: technical aspects. Transplant Proc 1984; 16(3):724–728.
17. Tyden G, Bolinder G. Surgical techniques and results in pancreatic transplantation. Bailliere's Clin Gastroenterol 1989; 3(4):835–849.
18. Tyden G, Tibell A, Groth CG. Pancreatico-duodenal transplantation with enteric exocrine drainage: technical aspects. Clin Transplant 1991: 5:36–39.
19. Tibell A, Brattstrom C, Wadstrom J, Tyden G, Groth CG. Improved results using whole organ pancreatico-duodenal transplants with enteric exocrine drainage. Transplant Proc 1994; 26(2):412–413.
20. Corry RJ, Egidi MF, Shapiro R, et al. Enteric drainage of pancreas transplants revisited. Transplant Proc 1995; 27(6):3048–3049.
21. Corry RJ, Egidi MF, Shapiro R, et al. Pancreas transplantation with enteric drainage under tacrolimus induction therapy. Transplant Proc 1997; 29(1–2):642.
22. Dubernard JM, Traeger J, Neyra P, Touraine L, Tranchang D, Blanc-Brunat N. A new method of preparation of segmental pancreatic grafts for transplantation: trials in dogs and in man. Surgery 1978; 84:633–640.
23. Dubernard JM, Traeger J, Martin X, Faure JL, Devonec M. Pancreatic transplantation in man: surgical technique and complications. Transplant Proc 1980; 12(4 suppl 2):40–43.

24. Dubernard JM, Sanseverino R, Martinenghi S, et al. Duct obstruction of segmental grafts in pancreas transplantation. Trans Proc 1989; 21(1):2799–2800.
25. Hohnke C, Illner WD, Abendroth D, Schleibner S, Landgraf R, Land W. Seven-year experience in clinical pancreatic transplantation using duct occlusion technique. Trans Proc 1989; 21(1):2862–2863.
26. Gliedman ML, Gold M, Whittaker J, et al. Clinical segmental pancreatic transplantation with ureter–pancreatic duct anastomosis for exocrine drainage. Surgery 1973; 74(2):171–180.
27. Toledo-Pereyra LH, Castellanos J, Lampe EW, Lillehei RC, Najarian JS. Comparative evaluation of pancreas transplantation techniques. Ann Surg 1975; 182(5):567–571.

# 9 | Medical Management After Pancreas Transplantation

**M. Francesca Egidi**
*The University of Tennessee Health Science Center, Methodist University, Transplant Institute, Memphis, Tennessee, U.S.A.*

## INTRODUCTION

It is well known that diabetes mellitus is characterized by systemic complications that cause recurrent morbidity and premature mortality (1). Because of this underlying pathophysiological background, pancreas transplant recipients must be considered to be at high risk to develop postoperative complications. Intensive medical follow-up care is necessary, both in the immediate posttransplant period and in the long-term management of the patient (2–5). This chapter will discuss guidelines for the management of diabetic patients who have undergone pancreatic transplantation (6–8).

## IMMEDIATE POSTOPERATIVE PERIOD: GENERAL ASPECTS

The postoperative management of pancreas transplant recipients follows the general principles followed after other transplant procedures. The routine postsurgical care includes monitoring of vital signs, central venous pressure (CVP), daily laboratory values, incentive spirometry, nasogastric tube (NG) suction, Foley catheter irrigation, bed rest for at least 48 hours (this is peculiar to pancreas transplantation, and reflects the need to prevent early shifting of the organ and possible vessel kinking when the patient stands), daily weight, pain control, and deep venous thrombosis prophylaxis with pneumatic compression stockings. However, the management of the pancreas transplant patient is complicated by specific anatomic and physiologic differences related to bladder (BD) or enteric drainage (ED) (9–12). NG tube removal and diet reinstatement will require a longer period of time for patients with ED. In order to avoid abdominal distension, possible small bowel obstruction, or anastomotic leak, the patient must be kept NPO until the patient has recovered completely from postoperative ileus. Many diabetics also suffer from gastroparesis, which affects gastrointestinal motility and the absorption of medication. During this phase, medications should be administered intravenously, if possible. The Foley catheter can be removed by postoperative day 3 or 4 in ED recipients, but should be kept longer (7–10 days) in BD recipients, because of the increased risk of urologic complications (13). In order to prevent reflux of urine into the kidney and/or the pancreas graft (reflux pancreatitis in BD), post-void residual (PVR) volumes should be checked at least three to four times after the Foley catheter has been removed. In cases of patients who have diabetic neurogenic bladders and significant PVR ($>250$ mL), the Foley catheter should remain longer. In order to minimize the risk of infection, intermittent catheterization should be limited to untreatable cases of urinary retention. In elderly men, benign prostatic hyperplasia may also be responsible for an elevated PVR, and alpha-adrenergic receptor inhibitors may be helpful.

## ANTICOAGULATION

Pancreas allografts, particularly those from older donors or with prolonged ischemia times, may be at increased risk of early thrombosis, although this is currently a less common complication (14–16). Besides technical reasons, the main cause of this devastating event is related to the low microcirculatory blood flow in the pancreas (17,18). In most transplant centers, aspirin is utilized immediately after transplantation and continued long term because of the risk of systemic thrombotic events; additional antiplatelet aggregation agents are also indicated in those patients affected by previous cerebrovascular accidents. It is important to remember that if a renal and/or pancreatic biopsy, or other surgical procedures, is required it may be useful to stop these medications two to three days in advance.

Solitary pancreas recipients are at an increased risk for graft thrombosis because of the lack of uremia. In this patient group, 3000 to 5000 units of heparin are administered as an intravenous bolus prior to implantation of the pancreas. Different heparin regimens have been proposed for the first three to five days posttransplantation, such as 5000 units subcutaneously twice daily or a continuous infusion [5–107 U/kg/hr intravenous (IV)]. Low-molecular-weight dextran, infused at 10 to 20 mL/hour, has also been used. The role of low-molecular-weight heparin (LMWH) has not yet been established. The main concern with LMWH relates to the difficulty of monitoring its efficacy only with factor Xa, which requires a special laboratory assay. A possible indication for LMWH would be in patients with hypercoagulable syndrome, a not infrequent situation in diabetics (19). After discharge, these patients may require a longer period of anticoagulation, as they may be at increased risk for late thrombosis.

## FLUID AND ELECTROLYTE BALANCE

During the first 48 hours after surgery, the patients are in the surgical intensive (or intermediate intensive) care unit, with continuous monitoring of vital signs, CVP, EKG, and laboratory tests. Once stabilized, patients are transferred to the transplant unit and spend approximately six to 10 days in the hospital. Because of the increased risk of cardiovascular complications in diabetic patients, a careful history prior to surgery will be useful in postoperative fluid management. In "high cardiac risk" patients, a Swan-Ganz catheter may be necessary in order to better assess the cardiac filling pressures. In order to avoid pulmonary edema and congestive heart failure, fluid challenges must be administered with caution in patients with ischemic heart disease or with left ventricular noncompliance. Hypertensive crises are dangerous not only because of the cardiac consequences but also because of the risk of bleeding. On the other hand, hypotension and hypovolemia should obviously be avoided as they might cause inadequate left ventricular filling pressure, decreased cardiac output, and suboptimal graft perfusion, with a risk of pancreatic thrombosis. Intravenous fluids are usually administered according to the hourly urine output (UOP), while monitoring the blood pressure (BP) and CVP. In general, the intravenous fluid replacement consists of one-half normal saline: 100% for 50–300 mL UOP and 80% for UOP >300 mL. A drop in the UOP secondary to inadequate filling pressures can be treated with a 500 mL bolus of normal saline and or 50 mL of 25% albumin. In case of oliguria or anuria, with appropriate filling pressure and no response to 80–100 mg of IV furosemide, surgical complications such as ureteral obstruction or leak, or vascular anastomotic problems must be ruled out. Losses from the NG tube must also be carefully considered in the overall fluid balance. During surgery and the immediate postoperative period, the total protein levels are reduced, not only because of large amounts of IV fluid but also because of real albumin losses (approximately 1.07 g/kg body weight). In order to mobilize "third space fluids," small amounts of intravenous albumin and furosemide can be administered cautiously. Calcium gluconate infusions (1–2 amp IV) are indicated in case of hypocalcemia, with the understanding that the serum calcium values must be adjusted as a function of the serum albumin levels. In general, transplant centers have standardized posttransplant orders for potassium (K+), sodium bicarbonate, and magnesium replacement. The K+ management is very important, not only for preventing cardiac arrhythmias but also for avoiding prolonged ileus. BD recipients can suffer massive losses of sodium bicarbonate (1–27 L/day) from pancreatic exocrine and duodenal mucosal secretions. Adequate amounts of PO and IV sodium bicarbonate are administered to prevent hyperchloremic metabolic acidosis, dehydration, and orthostatic hypotension. Blood transfusions are indicated in cases of hemorrhage and low hematocrit values (less than 30%).

## BLOOD SUGARS AND ENDOCRINE FUNCTION
### Immediate Posttransplant Period

In the case of a well-functioning pancreas, when the patient leaves the operating room, the blood sugars (BS) will normalize and insulin is not required. In the first two to three days posttransplant, BS should be monitored every one to two hours, whereas for the following seven to

10 days, accuchecks should be performed every four hours. Doppler ultrasonography and BS monitoring are the best markers for following the pancreatic function in the immediate post-transplant period (20–22). BS values between 80 and 150 mg/dL reflect stable pancreatic function; however, because of impaired glucose metabolism related to steroids and calcineurin inhibitors, slightly elevated BS (150–200 mg/dL) may also be observed. Sudden hyperglycemic episodes (BS > 280 mg/dL) in the early posttransplant phase may indicate a thrombotic event. Despite the fact that most pancreatic thrombosis leads to irreversible graft loss, early diagnosis and surgical re-exploration may occasionally lead to salvage of the allograft (23). Although infrequent, hypoglycemia secondary to massive release of insulin may require small amounts of IV dextrose (24–27). In recent years, the concept of maintaining the pancreas "at rest," with the goal of better long-term islet function, has been abandoned. Very few transplant units are still using protocols with insulin drips and total parenteral nutrition for one to two weeks posttransplantation. The use of total parenteral nutrition should be limited to cases of prolonged ileus or surgical complications.

## Intermediate and Late Posttransplant Period

From a practical point of view, fasting BS values, C-peptide levels, and glycosylated hemoglobin levels are the key components for monitoring the pancreatic endocrine function (28–31). The development of insulin resistance is not uncommon in the weeks following the transplant and, in general, is responsive to steroid and/or calcineurin inhibitor dosage reduction and agents able to increase insulin sensitivity (32,33). The pathogenesis of insulin resistance is not entirely understood. Clinical and experimental data have shown an interaction of different mechanisms. In pancreatic transplantation, hyperinsulinemia induced by the systemic release of insulin might play a larger role in the development of insulin resistance than steroids and calcineurin inhibitors. The latter have also been shown to have direct toxic effects on beta cells (34). Portal venous drainage of the pancreas has the physiologic advantage of eliminating hyperinsulinemia and perhaps insulin resistance (12,35–37). Recent data have suggested better glucose control in portally drained transplant recipients treated with nondiabetogenic agents such as sirolimus (39). Interestingly, the noninnervated state of the transplanted pancreas might play a role in the insulin pathways (39–41).

An unsolved question is why, despite the development of insulin resistance, long-term glucose control and insulin independence are achieved in most pancreatic transplant recipients (42,43). The progressive loss of pancreatic function with return to insulin dependence is perhaps related to a fibrotic process with islet exhaustion. These findings are likely similar to the development of chronic allograft nephropathy in kidney transplant recipients, where interstitial fibrosis is the predominant pathological finding. As immunological and nonimmunological factors are implicated in the development of chronic allograft nephropathy, one may speculate that pancreatic fibrosis is a consequence of chronic rejection and fibrogenic events. In addition, despite the administration of immunosuppression after transplantation, there are data that suggest the possibility of recurrent autoimmune type I insulin-dependent diabetes (44–47).

Promising results have been achieved in pancreas recipients with type II diabetes already affected by insulin resistance and severe atherosclerosis. In this patient category, the impact of hyperinsulinemia on metabolic and atherosclerotic processes should be investigated.

## EXOCRINE FUNCTION

Whereas BS are the most important marker of pancreatic endocrine function, serum amylase (AMY) and lipase (LIP) reflect the exocrine function and have an important role in assessing the inflammatory status of the allograft. Abnormalities in AMY and LIP can be detected in different situations. In the immediate posttransplant period, elevated AMY and LIP are related to ischemia-reperfusion injury. Generally, this situation is self-limited and reverses in a few days. A sudden increase in AMY and LIP values might indicate infection, toxicity, reflux pancreatitis, a surgical problem (leak, abscess, obstruction), or possible rejection (48,49). The subcutaneous or IV administration of somatostatin (octreotide acetate) might be useful (early pancreatitis immediately after transplantation may also respond to a short course of somatostatin) (50). Noninvasive procedures (Doppler ultrasonography, radionuclide blood flow, computer-assisted tomography scan, abdominal films) can be useful to help determine the etiology (51). Elevated AMY and LIP levels in the fluid from the intra-abdominal drains may raise the suspicion of surgical complications. In case of BD pancreas transplants, urinary AMY should be checked routinely, a decrease being an important marker of pancreatic dysfunction (52). Although a fall in urinary AMY excretion rate in BD pancreas is considered a reliable sign for rejection, controversy still exists about the specificity of increased serum AMY and LIP values as a marker for rejection (53) either in BD and ED pancreases. A pancreas biopsy or a fine needle aspiration biopsy should be performed if rejection is suspected (34,49,54,55). Efforts have been made to identify noninvasive markers of rejection, such as the measurement of anodal trypsinogen and pancreatic specific protein (56). Although sensitive to pancreatic dysfunction, these markers have not shown adequate specificity for rejection and can only be used as a "red flag" for further histologic evaluation (49).

## RENAL FUNCTION
### Immediate Posttransplant Period

Assessment of renal function after pancreas transplantation varies according to the type of procedure: simultaneous pancreas–kidney (SPK), pancreas after kidney (PAK) or kidney after pancreas (KAP), and pancreas alone (PTA). Whereas PAK and PTA candidates have stable (and hopefully close to normal) renal function (32,57,58), SPK and KAP recipients (if the surgery is not pre-emptive) may require dialysis before surgery. In order to reduce the cold ischemia time, hemodynamic changes, and risk of bleeding, preoperative dialysis should be considered only in cases of real need, such as hyperkalemia and volume overload. If the patient is on peritoneal dialysis, it is unlikely that there will need to be much of a delay preoperatively. Before the surgery, the peritoneal fluid must be drained and cultured even if the catheter will be removed during the surgical procedure. Delayed graft function (DGF) is an infrequent complication, but may occur because of unexpected donor factors or recipient hemodynamic instability. Situations of nonoliguric DGF can be managed with careful fluid, potassium, and acidosis control. Oliguric DGF is generally an indication for hemodialysis. Dialysis with rapid and excessive fluid removal is contraindicated and can put the pancreas at risk. Immediate renal function requires adequate fluid replacement, daily weight, and careful monitoring of calcineurin inhibitor levels or other nephrotoxic agents. The doses of medications used in the posttransplant period must be adjusted according to renal function. Nephrotoxicity or an early rejection must always be considered in the case of an unexplained rise in serum creatinine, once anastomotic leak, obstruction, and other nonimmunologic causes have been ruled out by ultrasonography and/or renal scan. In PAK, the pre-existing kidney graft can be affected either by hemodynamic events or exposure to higher levels of calcineurin inhibitors, and can develop some degree of renal dysfunction. The rejection of the pre-existing graft (PAK or KAP) is extremely unlikely, as the initial immunosuppression will exceed maintenance dosages for the previously transplanted organ. The native kidneys of PTA recipients may be already compromised by some degree of diabetic glomerulosclerosis and suffer some degree of renal dysfunction, mostly related to hemodynamic events and/or calcineurin inhibitor nephrotoxicity (59,60). In general, perioperative renal dysfunction in PAK and PTA is mild and reversible within a few days posttransplantation.

### Late Posttransplant Period

The causes of renal allograft loss (rejection, chronic allograft nephropathy, pyelonephritis, de novo glomerulonephritis) in SPK recipients resemble the causes affecting renal transplant patients, with the exception of diabetic nephropathy that can recur in diabetics not receiving a pancreas (61,62). Recent studies have shown that the SPK recipients may have an increased incidence of thrombotic microangiopathy as a possible consequence of calcineurin inhibitor toxicity or may develop polyoma virus nephropathy related to over-immunosuppression (63–65). The role of calcineurin-inhibitor sparing regimens for reversing these lesions or minimizing chronic nephrotoxicity is still being evaluated (38).

## MEDICATIONS

Different immunosuppressive regimens for induction, maintenance, and the treatment for rejection are described in Chapters 13 and 14.

The prevention of early and late infections requires effective prophylaxis against bacterial, fungal, protozoal, and viral pathogens (66,67). This is also described in Chapters 13 and 14. Perioperative treatment consists of a three-day course of a broad-spectrum non-nephrotoxic antibiotic (cefotetan is a reasonable choice). In most transplant centers, oral nystatin (or fluconazole), gancyclovir and trimethoprim–sulfamethoxazole are initiated after transplantation. Prophylaxis for cytomegalovirus (CMV) is perhaps less standardized; however, in case of a CMV seropositive donor and CMV seronegative recipient or in case of anti–T-cell therapy, clinical studies have shown the benefit of prolonged antiviral prophylaxis with either gancyclovir or valgancyclovir and (possibly) CMV immune globulin (68,69). Routine CMV antigenemia studies are performed not only for diagnosis but also for monitoring the response to treatment in the case of CMV reactivation or disease (70,71). Because of their impaired immunity, occasional insulin-dependent diabetes mellitus patients are both CMV and EBV seronegative (54). Recent reports have shown an increased incidence of post-transplant lymphoproliferative disorders with possible EBV reactivation related not only to the amount of immunosuppression but also to the lack of immunity (72,73). The prevention and the treatment of PTLD are still controversial; however, there is reasonable consensus that prolonged antiviral prophylaxis and CMV immune globulin (which has significant anti-EBV titers) should be considered in EBV seronegative recipients of EBV seropositive organs. Treatment of PTLD is discussed in Chapter 20 (74).

BP management requires a careful approach in the setting of diabetic autonomic neuropathy and possible cardiac abnormalities in these patients (75,76). In general, hypertension improves with a functioning kidney, to the point that many patients can discontinue antihypertensive medications. It is mandatory to obtain BP values in the sitting and standing position, since autonomic neuropathy in the now euvolemic recipient may lead to orthostatic hypotension. If, however, hypertension remains a problem and requires therapy, calcium channel blocking agents are particularly useful, not only for cardiovascular purposes but also for balancing the calcineurin inhibitor-induced vasoconstriction of the glomerular afferent arterioles. Angiotensin I converting enzyme inhibitors (ACE-I) and angiotensin II receptor antagonists should also be strongly considered because of their other benefits independent of reducing the BP. Treatment with ACE-I helps to prevent the expression of cytokines (TGF-β, PAI) involved in fibrogenesis. As a result, the ACE-I's and angiotensin II receptor antagonists' antiproteinuric and antifibrotic effects may protect the transplanted kidney (77–79). Clonidine and beta-blockers may be combined successfully with other agents but must be discontinued with caution because of rebound tachycardia and hypertension. In case of hypertensive emergencies, direct IV vasodilating agents such as hydralazine, nitroglycerine, or sodium nitroprusside should be considered, and are used in an intensive care unit setting.

Volume depletion (or even euvolemia) in the setting of diabetic autonomic dysfunction can induce orthostatic hypotension. In addition to oral supplementation of fluids, sodium chloride, sodium bicarbonate, PO fludrocortisone, small doses of the alpha agonist midodrine hydrochloride (80), blood transfusions (for hematrocrit < 28%), and periodic IV fluids can all be useful and may be administered via semipermanent vascular access in cases of severe dehydration and metabolic acidosis.

Pancreas transplant recipients with BD are more susceptible to metabolic acidosis and volume depletion because of massive losses of sodium and bicarbonate into the urinary tract. In these patients, enteric conversion should be considered in cases of unresolvable fluid and electrolyte imbalances.

Neurogenic bladders in diabetic patients can complicate the posttransplant follow-up and lead to recurrent infections, reflux pancreatitis, and renal dysfunction. Bethanechol chloride has limited use because of its cholinergic side effects.

Antisecretory compounds (omeprazole, pantoprazole) may be needed chronically in patients with esophagitis and other gastrointestinal tract pathologies.

Gastroparesis constitutes a serious problem that can resolve after successful kidney and pancreas transplantation, but may take some time (81–83). Patients may complain of nausea, vomiting, "failure to thrive," and severe abdominal pain and can require intensive medical treatment. Metoclopramide, either PO or IV, accelerates gastric emptying and intestinal transit time, and has antiemetic properties related to its blocking of central and peripheral dopamine receptors (84,85). As metoclopramide is often used in combination with phenothiazines, which are also dopamine antagonists, patients can present with extra-pyramidal reactions that require dose reduction or discontinuation. Cisapride is no longer available because of cardiac toxicity. Domperidone, a selective antagonist of peripheral dopamine D2 receptors, has been shown in Canadian and European trials to be associated with excellent antiemetic properties and promotion of gastric mobility (86). So far, it has not been approved in the United States. Erythromycin may provide substantial symptomatic improvement in gastropathy refractory to other agents. As with all the macrolide antibiotics, erythromycin, even in low doses, may increase calcineurin inhibitor levels; azithromycin is the exception and has been useful anecdotally to treat gastroparesis without affecting calcineurin inhibitor levels.

Hyperlipidemia is not necessarily present in insulin-dependent diabetes mellitus patients, but subtle lipoprotein abnormalities can be detected and altered posttransplantation. These changes may be significant in the management of pancreas recipients and can be related to the different vascular anastomotic techniques (87–89). Although systemic delivery of insulin does not appear to impair carbohydrate metabolism significantly, avoiding hyperinsulinemia may be relevant to lipid metabolism and the development of atherosclerosis. Portal venous drainage of the pancreas has proven to be more physiologic and beneficial for lipoprotein composition and insulin resistance minimization (90,91), although it has not impacted patient or graft survival. The combination of steroids, cyclosporine, and/or sirolimus may alter the lipid metabolism, and HMG-CoA reductase inhibitors (lipitor, zocor), fibric acid derivatives (tricor, lopid), and possibly fish oil tablets may be required, particularly in the presence of coronary artery disease (92).

Pain control related to neuropathy represents one of the most difficult aspects in the management of pancreas recipients. Although, many patients experience relatively rapid improvement after transplantation with the correction of uremia, many will continue to complain of pain and require narcotics. Several studies have shown that the resolution or improvement of the secondary diabetic complications may take several months, if not years. Unfortunately, narcotic addiction constitutes one of the biggest neglected problems in diabetics, and requires a multidisciplinary approach. Antidepressants and gabapentin have been routinely employed, with mixed results.

## CONCLUSIONS

Pancreatic transplantation represents the treatment of choice for patients affected by insulin-dependent diabetes and suffering from secondary complications, with or without end-stage renal disease (93). Improved surgical techniques and careful medical management have enormously impacted not only patient and graft survival rates but also the quality of life and the overall morbidity related to pre-existing diabetic complications (94–96).

## REFERENCES

1.  Nathan DM. Long-term complications of diabetes mellitus. N Engl J Med 1993; 328:1676–1685.
2.  Tydén G, Bolinder J, Solders G, Brattström C, Tibell A, Groth C. Improved survival in patients with insulin-dependent diabetes mellitus and end-stage diabetic nephropathy 10 years after combined pancreas and kidney transplantation. Transplantation 1999; 67:645–648.
3.  Landgraf R. Impact of pancreas transplantation on diabetic secondary complications and quality of life. Diabetologia 1996; 39:1415–1424.
4.  Gaber AO, el-Gebely S, Sugathan P, Elmer DS, Hathaway DK, McCully RB. Early improvement in cardiac function occurs in pancreas–kidney but not diabetic kidney alone recipients. Transplantation 1995; 59:1105–1124.
5.  Langone A, Helderman JH. The effect of pancreas transplantation on cardiovascular mortality. Kidney Int 2001; 60:2035–2036.
6.  Stratta RJ, Taylor R, Wahl TO, et al. Recipient selection and evaluation for vascularized pancreas transplantation. Transplantation 1993; 55:1090–1096.
7.  Pirsh JD. Medical evaluation for pancreas transplantation: evolving concepts. Transplant Proc 2001; 33:3489–3491.
8.  Lin K, Stewart D, Cooper S, Davis CL. Pre-transplant cardiac testing for kidney–pancreas transplant candidates and association with cardiac outcome. Clin Transpl 2001:269–275.
9.  Prieto M, Sutherland DER, Goetz FC, Rosemberg ME, Najarian JS. Pancreas transplant results according to the technique of duct management: bladder versus enteric drainage. Surgery 1987; 102:680–691.

10. Corry RJ, Egidi MF, Shapiro R, et al. Enteric drainage of the pancreas transplants revisited. Transplant Proc 1996; 27:3048–3049.
11. Krishnamurthi V, Philosophe B, Bartlett ST. Pancreas transplantation: contemporary surgical techniques. Urol Clin North Am 2001; 28:833–838.
12. Gaber AO, Shokouh-Amiri MH, Hathaway DK, et al. Results of pancreas transplantation with portal venous and enteric drainage. Ann Surg 1995; 221:613–622.
13. Sollinger HW, Messing EM, Eckhoff DE, et al. Urological complications in 210 consecutive simultaneous pancreas-kidney transplants with bladder drainage. Ann Surg 1993; 218:561–568.
14. Troppman C, Gruessner AC, Benedetti E, et al. Vascular graft thrombosis after pancreatic transplantation: univariate and multivariate operative and nonoperative risk factor analysis. J Am Coll Surg 1996; 182:285–316.
15. Ciancio G, Cespedes M, Olson L, Miller J, Burke GW. Partial venous thrombosis of the allografts after simultaneous pancreas–kidney transplantation. Clin Transplant 2000; 14:464–471.
16. Humar A, Johnson E, Gillingham KJ, et al. Venous thromboembolic complications after kidney and kidney–pancreas transplantation: a multivariate analysis. Transplantation 1998; 65:229–234.
17. Hotter G, Leon OS, Rosello-Catafau J, et al. Tissutal prostanoid release, phospholipase $A_2$ activity and lipid peroxidation in pancreas transplantation. Transplantation 1991; 51:987–990.
18. Kessler L, Wiesel ML, Boudjema K, et al. Possible involvement of Von Willebrand factor in pancreatic graft thrombosis after kidney-pancreas transplantation: a retrospective study. Clin Transplant 1998; 12:35–42.
19. Mellinghoff AC, Reininger AJ, Wurzinger LJ, Landgraf R, Hepp KD. Impact of pancreas and kidney transplantation on determinants of blood and plasma viscosity. Clin Hemorheol Microcirculation 1998; 18:175–184.
20. Martinez-Noguera A, Montserrat E, Torrubia S, Monill JM, Estrada P. Ultrasound of the pancreas: update and controversies. Eur Radiol 2001; 11:1594–1606.
21. Boeve WK, Kok T, Tegzess AM, van Son WJ, Ploeg R, Slutier WJ, Kamman RL. Comparison of contrast enhanced MR–angiography–MRI and digital subtraction angiography in the evaluation of pancreas and/or kidney transplant patients: initial experience. Magn Resonance Imaging 2001:19,595–19,607.
22. Eubank WB, Schmiedl UP, Levy AE, Marsh CL. Venous thrombosis and occlusion after pancreas transplantation: evaluation with breath-hold gadolinium-enhanced three-dimensional MR imaging. AJR Am J Roentgenol 2000 Aug; 175(2):387–385.
23. Ciancio G, Julian JF, Fernandez L, Miller J, Burke GW. Successful surgical salvage of pancreas allografts after complete venous thrombosis. Venous thrombosis and occlusion after pancreas transplantation: evaluation with breath-hold gadolinium-enhanced three-dimensional MR imaging. 2000 Aug; 175(2):387–385.
24. Osei K. Post-transplantation hypoglycaemia in type 1 diabetic pancreas allograft recipients. Acta Diabet 1998; 35:1716–1782.
25. Larsen J, Fellman S, Stratta R. Anti-insulin antibodies may cause hypoglycaemia following pancreas transplantation. Acta Diabetol 1998; 35:172–175.
26. Battezzati A, Bonfatti D, Benedini S, et al. Spontaneous hypoglycaemia after pancreas transplantation in Type 1 diabetes mellitus. Diabet Med 1998; 15:991–996.
27. Redmon JB, Teuscher AI, Robertson RP. Hypoglycemia after pancreas transplantation. Diabet Care 1998; 21:1944–1950.
28. Battezzati A, Benedini S, Caldara R, et al. Prediction of the long-term metabolic success of the pancreatic graft function. Transplantation 2001; 71:1560–1566.
29. Östman J, Bolinder, Gunnarsson R, et al. Effects of pancreas transplantation on metabolic and hormonal profiles in IDDM patients. Diabetes 1989; 38:88–91.
30. Light JA, Sasaki TM, Currier CB, Barhyte DY. Successful long-term kidney–pancreas transplants regardless of C-peptide status or race. Transplantation 2001; 71:152–154.
31. Sasaki TM, Gray RS, Rantner RE, et al. Successful long-term kidney pancreas transplants in diabetic patients with high C-Peptide levels. Transplantation 1998; 65:1510–1512.
32. Humar A, Parr E, Drangstveit MB, Kandaswamy R, Gruessner AC, Sutherland DER. Steroid withdrawal in pancreas transplant recipients. Clin Transplant 2000; 14:75–78.
33. Kaufman DB, Leventhal J, Koffron AJ, et al. A prospective study of rapid corticosteroid elimination in simultaneous pancreas–kidney transplantation: comparison of two maintenance immunosuppression protocols: tacrolimus/mycophenolate mofetil versus tacrolimus/sirolimus. Transplantation 2002; 73:169–177.
34. Drachenberg CB, Klassen DK, Weir MR, et al. Islet cell damage associated with tacrolimus and cyclosporine: morphological features in pancreas allograft biopsies and clinical correlation. Transplantation 1999; 68:396–402.
35. Gaber AO, Shokouh-Amiri MH, Hathaway DK. Pancreas transplantation with portal venous and enteric drainage eliminates hyperinsulinemia and reduces post operative complications. Transplant Proc 1993; 25:1176.
36. Philosophe B, Farney AC, Schweitzer EJ, et al. Superiority of portal venous drainage over systemic drainage in pancreas transplantation: a retrospective study. Ann Surg 2001; 234:689–696.

37. Martin X, Petruzzo P, Dawahra M, et al. Effects of portal versus systemic venous drainage in kidney–pancreas recipients. Transplant Int 2000; 13:64–68.
38. Egidi MF, Cowan PA, Naseer A, Gaber AO. Conversion to sirolimus in solid organ transplantation: a single-center experience. Transplant Proc 2003; 35(suppl 3A):131S–137S.
39. Adler G. Regulation of human pancreatic secretion. Digestion 1997; 58:39.
40. Luzi L, Battezzati A, Perseghini GL, et al. Lack of feedback inhibition of insulin secretion in denervated human pancreas. Diabetes 1992; 41:1632–1639.
41. Berry SM, Friend L, McFadden DW, Brodish RJ, Krusch DA, Fink AS. Pancreatic denervation does not influence glucose-induced insulin response. Surgery 1994; 116:67–75.
42. Robertson RP, Sutherland DER, Lanz KJ. Normoglycemia and preserved insulin secretory reserve in diabetic patients 10–18 years after pancreas transplantation. Diabetes 1999; 48:1737–1740.
43. Balsells FM, Esmatjes E, Ricart MJ, Casamitjana R, Astudillo E, Fernandez Cruz L. Successful pancreas and kidney transplantation: a view of metabolic control. Transplantation 1998; 12:582–587.
44. Petruzzo P, Andrelli F, McGregor B, et al. Evidence of recurrent type I diabetes following HLA-mismatched pancreas transplantation. Diabet Metab 2000; 26:218.
45. Esmajies E, Rodriquez-Villar C, Richart MJ, et al. Recurrence of immunological markers for type 1 (insulin-dependent) diabetes mellitus in immunosuppressed patients after pancreas transplantation. Transplantation 1998; 66:128–131.
46. Thivolet C, Abou-Amara S, Martin X, et al. Serological markers of recurrent beta cell destruction in diabetic patients undergoing pancreatic transplantation. Transplantation 2001; 69:99–103.
47. Braghi S, Bonifacio E, Secchi A, Di Carlo V, Pozza G, Bossi E. Modulation of humoral islet autoimmunity by pancreas allotransplantation influences allograft outcome in patients with type 1 diabetes. Diabetes 2000; 49:218–224.
48. Benz S, Bergt S, Obermaier R, et al. Impairment of microcirculation in the early reperfusion period predicts the degree of graft pancreatitis in clinical pancreas transplantation. Transplantation 2001; 71:759–763.
49. Klassen DK, Drachenberg CB, Papadimitriou JC, et al. CMV allograft pancreatitis: diagnosis, treatment, and histological features. Transplantation 2000; 69:1968–1971.
50. Stratta RJ, Taylor RJ, Lowell JA, et al. Selective use of sandostatin in vascularized pancreas transplantation. Am J Surg 1993; 166:598–604.
51. Letourneau JC, Maile CW, Sutherland DER, Feinberg SB. Ultrasound and computed tomography in the evaluation of pancreatic transplantation. Radiol Clin North Am 1987; 25:345–355.
52. Benedetti E, Najarian JS, Gruessner AC. Correlation between cystoscopic biopsy results and hypoamylasuria in bladder-drained pancreas transplants. Surgery 1995; 118:864–872.
53. Sugitani A, Egidi MF, Gritsch HA, Corry RJ. Serum lipase as a marker for pancreatic allograft rejection. Clin Transplant 1998; 12:175–183.
54. Gaber LW, Egidi MF. Surveillance and monitoring of pancreas allografts. Curr Opin Organ Transplant 2002; 7:191–195.
55. Egidi MF, Corry RJC. Simultaneous kidney–pancreas transplantation. Curr Opin Organ Transplant 1996; 1:44–50.
56. Marks WH, Borgstrom A, Sollinger H, Sollinger H, Marks C. Serum immunoreactive anodal trypsinogen and urinary amylase as biochemical marker for rejection of clinical whole organ pancreas allograft having exocrine drainage into the bladder. Transplantation 1990; 49:112–115.
57. Gruessner AC, Sutherland DER, Dunn D, et al. Pancreas after kidney transplants in posturemic patients with type I diabetes mellitus. J Am Soc Nephrol 2001; 12:2490–2499.
58. Humar A, Ramcharan T, Kandaswamy R, et al. Pancreas after kidney transplants. Am J Surg 2001; 182:155–161.
59. Fioretto P, Kim Y, Mauer M. Diabetic nephropathy as a model of reversibility of established renal lesions. Curr Opin Nephrol Hypertens 1998; 7:489–494.
60. Fioretto P, Steffes MW, Sutherland DER, Goetz FC, Mauer M. Reversal of lesions of diabetic nephropathy after pancreas transplantation. N Engl J Med 1998; 339:69–75.
61. Kreis HA, Ponticelli C. Causes of late allograft loss: chronic allograft dysfunction, death and other factors. Transplantation 2001; 71:SS5–SS9.
62. Hariharan S, Smith RD, Viero R, First R. Diabetic nephropathy after renal transplantation. Transplantation 1996; 62:632–635.
63. Burke G, Ciancio G, Cirocco R, et al. Microangiopathy in kidney and simultaneous pancreas/kidney recipients treated with tacrolimus: evident of endothelin and cytokine involvement. Transplantation 1999; 68:1336–1342.
64. Binet I, Nickeleit V, Hirsch HH. Polymavirus disease under new immunosuppressive drugs: a cause of renal graft dysfunction and graft loss. Transplantation 1999; 67:918–922.
65. Gaber L, Egidi MF, Reed L, Nezakatgoo N, Fisher J. Polyomavirus-nephropathy (PVN): determinants of graft loss. J Am Nephrol 2002; 13:178A.
66. Knight RJ, Bodian C, Rodriquez-Laiz G, Guy SR, Fishbein TM. Risk factors for intra-abdominal infection after pancreas transplantation. Am J Surg 2000; 179:99–102.
67. Stratta RJ. Ganciclovir/acyclovir and fluconazole prophylaxis after simultaneous kidney–pancreas transplantation. Transplant Proc 1998; 30:262.

68. Becker BN, Becker YT, Leverson GE, Simmons WD, Sollinger HW, Pirsch JD. Reassessing the cyto-megalovirus infection in kidney and kidney–pancreas transplantation. AJKD 2002; 39:1088–1095.
69. Stratta RJ, Shokouh-Amiri MH, Egidi MF, et al. A prospective comparison of simultaneous kidney–pancreas transplantation: with systemic-enteric versus portal-enteric drainage. Ann Surg 2001; 233:740–751.
70. Lassner D, Geissler F, Bosse S, et al. Diagnosis and monitoring of acute cytomegalovirus infection in peripheral blood of transplant recipients by nested reverse transcriptase polymerase chain reaction (RT-PCR). Transplant Int 2000; 13:S366–S371.
71. Tong CY, Cuevas LE, Williams H, Bakran A. Prediction and diagnosis of cytomegalovirus disease in renal transplant recipients using qualitative and quantitative polymerase chain reaction. Transplantation 2000; 9:985–991.
72. Nalesnik MA. Clinicopathologic characteristics of post-transplant lymphoproliferative disorders. Recent Results Cancer Res 2002; 159:9–18.
73. Egidi MF, Trofe J, Stratta RJ, et al. Post-transplant lymphoproliferative disorders: single center experience. Transplant Proc 2001; 33:1838–1839.
74. O'Dwyer ME, Launder T, Rabkin JM, Nichols CR. Successful treatment of aggressive post-transplant lymphoproliferative disorder using rituximab. Leuk Lymph 2000; 398:411–419.
75. Valensi PE, Johnson NB, Maison-Blanche P, Extramania F, Motte G, Coumel P. Influence of cardiac autonomic neuropathy on heart rate dependence of ventricular repolarization in diabetic patients. Diabet Care 2002; 25:918–923.
76. Gerritsen J, Dekker JM, Ten Voorde BJ, et al. Impaired autonomic function is associated with increased mortality, especially in subjects with diabetes, hypertension, or a history of cardiovascular disease: the Hoorn study. Diabet Care 2001; 24:1793–1798.
77. Taal MW, Brenner BM. Renoprotective benefits of RAS inhibition: from ACE I to angiotensin II antagonists. Kidney Int 2000; 57:1803–1817.
78. Stigant CE, Cohen J, Vivera M, Zaltman JS. Ace inhibitors and angiotensin II antagonist in renal transplantation: an analysis of safety and efficacy. AJKD 2000; 35:55–63.
79. Becker BN, Jacobson LM, Hullet DA. An antigen-independent important hormone: intrarenal angio-tensin II (AII) as a key to understanding chronic allograft nephropathy. Graft 2002; 5:199–203.
80. Hurst GC, Somerville KT, Alloway RR, Gaber AO, Stratta RJ. Preliminary experience with midodrine in kidney/pancreas transplant patients with orthostatic hypotension. Clin Transplant 2000; 14:42–47.
81. De Block CE, De Leeuw IH, Pelckmans PA, Callens D, Mayday E, van Gaal LF. Delayed gastric emptying and gastric autoimmunity in type 1 diabetes. Diabet Care 2002; 25:912–917.
82. Horowitz M, O'Donovan D, Jones KL, Feinle C, Rayner CK, Samsom M. Gastric emptying in diabetes: clinical significance and treatment. Diabet Med 2002; 19:177–194.
83. Camilleri M. Advances in diabetic gastroparesis. Rev Gastroenterol Dis 2000; 2:47–56.
84. Lyday WD II, Dibaise JK. Metoclopramide-simulated gastric emptying scintigraphy: does it predict symptom response to prokinetic therapy in chronic gastroparesis? Am J Gastroenterol 2002; 97:2474–2476.
85. Beard PL. Methods for treating diabetic gastroparesis. J Infus Nurs 2002; 25:105–108.
86. Prakash A, Wagstaff AJ. Domperidone. A review of its use in diabetic gastropathy. Drugs 1998; 56:429–445.
87. Foger B, Konigsrainer A, Ritsch A, et al. Pancreas transplantation modulates reverse cholesterol transport. Transplant Int 1999; 12:360–364.
88. Hughes TA, Gaber AO, Shokouh-Amiri H, et al. Kidney–pancreas transplantation: the effects of por-tal versus systemic venous drainage of the pancreas on the lipoprotein composition. Transplantation 1995; 60:1406–1412.
89. Bagdale JD, Teuscher AU, Ritter MC, Eckel RH, Robertson RP. Alteration in cholesterylester transfer, lipoprotein lipase, and lipoprotein composition after combined pancreas–kidney transplantation. Diabetes 1998; 47:113–118.
90. Fiorina P, La Rocca E, Venturini M, et al. Effects of kidney–pancreas transplantation on atherosclero-tic risk factors and endothelial function in patients with uremia and type I diabetes. Diabetes 2001; 50:496–501.
91. Carpentier A, Patterson BW, Uffelman KD, et al. The effects of systemic versus portal insulin delivery in pancreas transplantation on insulin action and VLDL metabolism. Diabetes 2001; 50:1402–1413.
92. Wierzbicki AS. The role of lipid lowering in transplantation. Int J Clin Pract 1999; 53:54–59.
93. Robertson RP, Davis C, Larsen J, Stratta RJ, Sutherland DER. Pancreas and islets transplantation for patients with diabetes. Diabet Care 2000; 23:112–116.
94. Gross CR, Limwattananon C, Matthee B, Zehrer JL, Savik K. Impact of transplantation on quality of life in patients with diabetes and renal dysfunction. Transplantation 2000; 70:1736–1746.
95. Sureshkumar KK, Mubin T, Mikhael N, Kashif MA, Nghiem DD, Marcus RJ. Assessment of quality of life after simultaneous pancreas–kidney transplantation. AJKD 2002; 39:1300–1306.
96. Odorico JS, Sollinger HW. Technical and immunosuppressive advances in transplantation for insu-lin-dependent diabetes mellitus. World J Surg 2002; 26:194–211.

# 10 | Immunobiology of Allograft Rejection

## Jennifer E. Woodward
*Department of Surgery, Thomas E. Starzl Transplantation Institute, University of Pittsburgh School of Medicine, Pittsburgh, Pennsylvania, U.S.A.*

## Abdul S. Rao
*Tampa General Hospital and University of South Florida School of Medicine, Tampa, Florida, U.S.A.*

## INTRODUCTION

Organ transplantation has become an increasingly effective option for treating end-stage diseases, and 26,539 transplants were performed in the United States in 2004. However, the number of patients awaiting transplantation has continued to exceed the number of available organs. During this time, 90,813 patients were on the waiting lists, and 7,306 died while waiting (1). Over the past 10 years, the development of potent immunosuppressive regimens has greatly reduced the incidence of acute cellular rejection, leading to remarkable improvements in short-term patient and allograft survival (2). However, there has been relatively little impact on long-term (>5 years) survival (3). Late organ deterioration and failure secondary to chronic rejection has made necessary the retransplantation of many organs, making further demands on the donor pool. Understanding the immunobiology of allograft rejection is therefore necessary and important to help develop novel and effective approaches to prevent the occurrence of acute and chronic rejection with the goal of prolonging patient and graft survival.

## T-CELL–MEDIATED ALLOGRAFT REJECTION

An allograft is an organ or tissue that is transplanted from one member of a species to a member of the same species. Except in the rare case of genetic identity between the donor and the recipient, it leads to an immune response. If this alloimmune response is allowed to proceed without any intervention (i.e., immunosuppression), the transplanted organ or tissue will be rejected after several days to a few weeks. During this rejection process, donor alloantigens are processed and presented by specialized antigen presenting cells (APCs) in the secondary lymphoid organs (i.e., draining lymph nodes and spleen), where naïve T-cells become activated by the recognition of donor alloantigens. These allospecific T-cells then begin to proliferate and differentiate into helper and cytotoxic T-cells (CTLs). Once the T-cells have differentiated into effector cells, the T-cells recirculate to the graft organ or tissue where they will either directly kill the allogeneic target cells or provide help for B-cell activation and the production of complement-fixing antibodies; both mechanisms eventually lead to the destruction of the graft. This T-cell–mediated allograft rejection involves both innate and adaptive immune events, specifically targeted to the microenvironment of the grafted tissue. The innate immune system regulates the activation of adaptive T- and B-cell responses.

### Major and Minor Histocompatibility Complex Antigens

Protein antigens from the polymorphic loci of the mammalian genome can trigger an immune response and lead to graft rejection, if the donor and recipient of the transplanted organ or tissue differ at any of these loci. The proteins encoded by these different alleles will be recognized as foreign, thereby initiating a T-cell response (4,5). The most prominent of these polymorphic genes are found on chromosome 6 in the major histocompatibility complex (MHC), designated in humans as human leukocyte antigens (HLAs) (6). In theory, matching both donor and recipient MHC could improve the success of organ transplantation; however, this does not prevent rejection unless the donor and the recipient are identical twins (7). Other polymorphic genes, known as minor histocompatibility antigens or minor H antigens can also be associated with rejection (5).

The MHC encodes polymorphic cell surface glycoproteins, termed class I and class II molecules. Class I molecules (HLAs A, B, and C) are expressed on most nucleated cells, while the expression of class II molecules (HLAs DP, DQ, and DR) is restricted to professional APCs, such as dendritic cells, B-cells, and macrophages. Exposure of these cells to inflammatory cytokines results in the induction of class II molecules on activated T-cells, and in humans on endothelial cells. T-cells require the recognition of both foreign antigen and the body's own self-MHC molecules for activation (8,9). The polymorphic nature of the MHC ensures the body's ability to recognize and generate an immune response against a wide range of pathogens, providing a survival advantage for the species (10). Transplant rejection is thus the consequence of this highly efficient and protective immune response.

APCs function to process and present exogenous and endogenous antigens as peptides to the MHC molecule (11). Exogenous antigens, such as bacteria and toxins, which are present in the extracellular fluid, are endocytosed by APCs, and the peptides derived from these exogenous antigens are expressed on MHC class II molecules. This antigen–MHC class II complex is subsequently recognized by $CD4^+$ T helper ($T_h$) cells. Upon activation, these $T_h$-cells participate in the elimination of these extracellular antigens by secreting cytokines, which stimulate B-cells to produce antibodies. In contrast, peptides from endogenous antigens (viruses and tumor antigens) are presented in the context of MHC class I molecules and are recognized by $CD8^+$ CTLs, resulting in the subsequent elimination of the virally infected cells or tumor cells. The activation of the CTLs induced by the antigen–MHC molecule is dependent on the aid of the $CD4^+$ $T_h$-cell.

## Direct and Indirect Pathways of Alloantigen Recognition

The recognition of MHC/peptide complexes during transplantation occurs via two distinct pathways (Fig. 1) (12). In the indirect pathway of allorecognition, for classical non-self peptides, donor non-self proteins (including both MHC and non-MHC peptides) that are shed from the graft are endocytosed by the recipient APCs, processed, and presented in the context of self-MHC molecules to the recipient T-cells. In the direct pathway, T-cells can recognize and respond to intact allogeneic MHC molecules expressed on the surface of the donor cells. Both mechanisms appear to be involved in allograft rejection. It has been suggested that the direct pathway may be preferentially involved in acute rejection, while the indirect pathway may be more

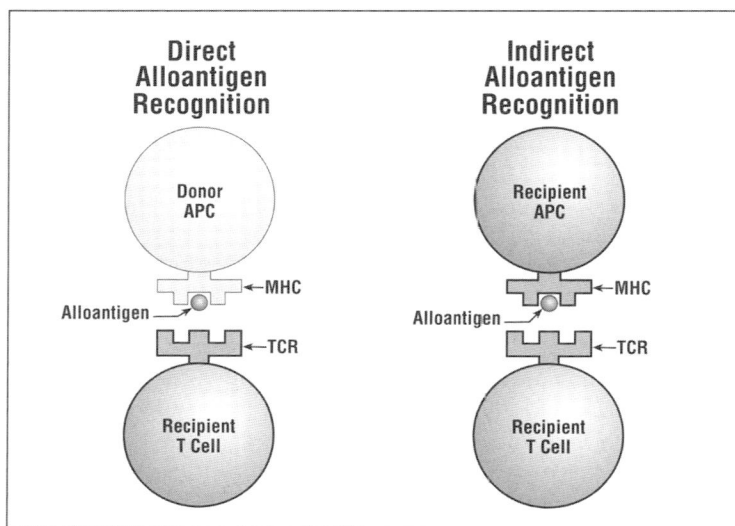

**Figure 1**  Direct and indirect alloantigen recognition. Two distinct pathways describe the recognition of the antigen–major histocompatibility complex (MHC). During direct alloantigen recognition, donor MHC molecules are presented by donor antigen presenting cells (APCs) to recipient T-cells. In contrast, indirect alloantigen recognition occurs when recipient APCs process and present donor non-self peptides to recipient T-cells. *Abbreviations*: APC, antigen presenting cells; MHC, major histocompatibility complex; TCR, T-cell receptor.

critical in the development of chronic rejection (13,14). During the early phase of acute allograft rejection, the allograft contains a significant number of donor-derived passenger leukocytes such as dendritic cells, which are particularly efficient in activating T-cells because of their high level of donor MHC and costimulatory molecule expression. When the number of passenger leukocytes is reduced, the allograft becomes less immunogenic, suggesting that the direct pathway of allorecognition is important during the initiation of acute allograft rejection (15). At the point when the donor APCs migrate from the graft and are cleared by the recipient immune system, the indirect pathway of allorecognition predominates and appears to be capable of eliciting the destruction of an allograft in the absence of direct allorecognition (16). However, the precise role of each pathway in allograft acceptance and rejection remains unclear.

## T-Cell Development and Maturation

T-cells are educated within the thymus during development to distinguish self from non-self. Those T-cells that exhibit too high an affinity for self-MHC molecules are deleted through negative selection, while those with the proper affinity are positively selected to proceed through maturation with subsequent export to the periphery (17,18). This stringent maturation process insures an affinity between the self-MHC and T-cell receptor (TCR) repertoire for the development of an immune system that is exceptionally competent in responding to a variety of foreign proteins. The non-self MHC molecules encountered by the recipient T-cells during transplantation suggest that the high-affinity T-cells for non-self MHC molecules are not eliminated during ontogeny but persist in the periphery, thereby maintaining the ability to mount an alloimmune response. The frequency of precursor T-cells for alloantigens is 100- to 1000-fold higher than for other antigens. In addition, unlike most immune responses, allogeneic immune responses are priming independent, rapid, and strong. It has been suggested that the aggressiveness of these responses is due to the natural affinity of TCR for MHC, the high density of alloantigens on the surface of the cells, the large number of potential MHC peptides recognized as non-self, and the potential molecular mimicry between self and non-self antigens; all of these factors can positively or negatively affect the strength of the immune responses (19).

## T-Cell Activation

The activation of naïve T-cells requires two signals (20). Signal 1, the antigen-specific signal, occurs when the TCR on the T-cell interacts with the appropriate antigen–MHC complex on the surface of the APCs. Signal 2 is an antigen-independent costimulatory signal that is required to initiate T-cell activation, and is mediated through coreceptor–ligand interactions (Fig. 2). Even though many costimulatory molecules (identified and unidentified) exist, the best characterized are the B7 molecules, B7-1 (CD80) and B7-2 (CD86), which are expressed on APCs and bind to the receptor CD28 on T-cells (21). Upon activation, the T-cell will also express cytotoxic T-lymphocyte-associated protein-4 (CTLA-4) (CD152), which exhibits high homology to CD28 and binds with 20× higher avidity to the B7 molecules than CD28. CTLA-4 is a negative regulator of T-cell activation, thereby signaling the termination of the immune response (22,23).

Another important T-cell costimulatory pathway is the CD40–CD40 ligand (CD40L = CD154) pathway. CD40 is constitutively expressed on APCs, whereas the CD40L is expressed on activated CD4$^+$ T-cells. The engagement of CD40 on dendritic cells upregulates the expression of B7-1 and B7-2 and induces the production of interleukin (IL)-12, enhancing the ability of dendritic cells to induce the proliferation of CD4$^+$ T-cells and the differentiation of CD8$^+$ T-cells into CTLs (24). In addition, the ligation of CD40 on B-cells by T-cells is necessary for isotype switching from IgM to IgG during humoral immune responses (25). T-cell ligation of CD40 on monocytes and macrophages enhances inflammation, and its subsequent engagement on endothelial cells upregulates the cell adhesion molecules, which are essential for the migration of leukocytes into the sites of inflammation (26).

In addition to the CD28 and CD40 T-cell costimulatory pathways, other costimulatory signals have been characterized and include the CD2/LFA-3, LFA-1/ICAM-1, and CD45 pathways; all of these enhance the activation of allospecific T-cells (27). More recently, several additional costimulatory molecules have been discovered that appear relevant to alloimmune

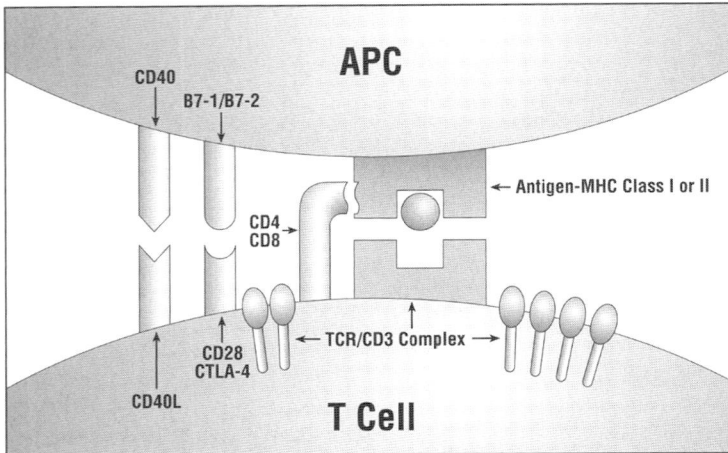

**Figure 2** T-cell activation. Two signals are required for the activation of naïve T-cells. Signal 1, the antigen-specific signal, is initiated when the T-cell receptor–CD3 complex interacts with the complex antigen–major histocompatibility complex. Signal 2 is a costimulatory signal that is mediated through coreceptor–ligand interactions such as the CD28/ B7 and CD40/CD40L pathways. Even though several additional costimulatory pathways have recently been discovered, their roles in transplantation remain ill defined. *Abbreviations*: APC, antigen presenting cells; MHC, major histocompatibility complex; CTLA-4, cytotoxic T-lymphocyte-associated protein 4; TCR, T-cell receptor.

responses. Both 4-1BB and heat-stable antigen have contributed to T-cell activation in the absence of CD28 costimulation (28). The 4-1BB (CD137) costimulatory signals preferentially induce CD8$^+$ T-cell proliferation and amplify in vivo CTL responses (29). Inducible costimulator (ICOS), a CD28-related molecule expressed preferentially on activated T-cells, binds to B7 homolog, a member of the B7 family found on B-cells and to some extent on monocytes. The ligation of B7 homolog by ICOS on activated T-cells leads to increased cytokine production and to the subsequent differentiation of B-cells into plasma cells and memory cells. In a murine model of allotransplantation, ICOS costimulation exhibits a critical role in the regulation of both acute and chronic allograft rejection (30). The in vivo roles of these recently discovered pathways in allograft rejection remains to be defined. Nonetheless, the evidence suggests that therapeutic intervention at these novel receptor–ligand interactions may be key in preventing graft injury and promoting long-term allograft survival.

T-cell stimulation through the TCR/CD3 complex and costimulatory pathways initiates a cascade of intracellular signals (31,32), which leads to the proliferation and differentiation of T-cells, both of which are important in T-cell activation and effector responses. The earliest T-cell activation signals include the activation of protein kinases (Lck, Fyn, Zap-70) that are responsible for phosphorylating the tyrosine residues of many cytoplasmic and membrane proteins. These signals lead to the activation of the enzyme phospholipase C-$\gamma$, which cleaves phosphatidylinositol biphosphate to yield inositol triphosphate and diacylglycerol. Inositol triphosphate increases intracellular calcium, which in turn activates the cytoplasmic calcium-dependent protein phosphatase, calcineurin, which subsequently dephosphorylates the transcription factor nuclear factor of activated T-cells (NFAT) (33). The activated NFAT translocates across the nucleus (possibly accompanied by calcineurin) to initiate IL-2 gene transcription. Additional kinase cascades within the cytoplasm result in the production of other transcription factors (AP-1, NF$_k$β), leading to the transcription of cytokine and cytokine receptor genes that are involved in cell proliferation and the subsequent generation of effector functions (34). This signaling is enhanced by the CD4 and CD8 molecules expressed on their respective T-cells, which bind to nonpolymorphic regions of the MHC class II and class I molecules, respectively (27). Within hours of activation, Th$_1$ [interferon (INF)-$\gamma$, IL-2, and tumor necrosis factor (TNF)-$\alpha$] and Th$_2$ (IL-4, IL-5, and IL-10) cells release cytokines, which act by both autocrine and paracrine mechanisms, to promote the proliferation and differentiation of T- and B-cells (35,36). The role of these cytokines in allograft rejection has been primarily determined in vitro, but has not necessarily correlated well with in vivo studies of rejection.

## Inflammation

Allograft rejection, triggered by the interaction of T-cells with alloantigens, is typically defined by cellular and humoral inflammatory responses that occur within the graft. Soluble mediators and by-products of inflammation are involved in regulating the rejection response, by promoting inflammatory cell accumulation, T-cell activation and modulation, and effector pathways of graft dysfunction and injury.

The classics signs of inflammation involved in acute rejection, which are often distorted and masked by immunosuppressive regimens, include redness, edema, pain, fever, and loss of function. Even though the precise mechanisms that initiate and regulate these inflammatory responses within the allograft remain ill defined, evidence suggests that delayed-type hypersensitivity (DTH) reactions contribute to the pathogenesis of rejection and graft injury. These inflammatory responses are characterized by edema, vascular permeability, the infiltration of antigen-specific and nonspecific T-cells, B-cells, and macrophages, and the release of cytokines and inflammatory mediators (IL-1β, IFN-γ, and TNF-α) (36). The tempo of the inflammation strongly affects the subsequent adaptive immune response not only by influencing the activation of T-cells but also by triggering counter-regulatory responses in order to minimize the antigen-specific damage. Such opposing proinflammatory and anti-inflammatory regulatory systems are instigated by IFN-γ for the recruitment of effector cells and the production of cytokine cascades (37).

The migration of T-cells into the allograft most likely occurs, at least initially, through both nonspecific and specific interactions with endothelial cells within the graft (38). Nonimmune–mediated ischemic injury originating from the transplant surgery may enhance these interactions. Clinical observations have suggested that ischemic injury and delayed graft function are associated with a higher incidence of acute rejection episodes, suggesting a link between nonimmune injury and the intensity of graft rejection.

These intragraft inflammatory responses require synchronized interactions between the endothelial cells, APCs, and immune cells of the recipient (Fig. 3) (37). The earliest of these events, trafficking and accumulation of inflammatory cells, requires activation and adhesion (38–40). First, the leukocytes begin rolling along the blood vessels, adhering loosely to the endothelium via the selectin family of adhesion molecules. L-selectin, which is expressed on leukocytes, binds to P- and E-selectin on the surface of the stimulated endothelium. Subsequently, the binding of the integrins enhances the adhesion of the leukocytes to the endothelial cells. Integrins (α4β1, αLβ2), expressed on inflammatory cells, interact with their ligands, VCAM-1, ICAM-1, and ICAM-2 on endothelial cells. The increase in the number of these

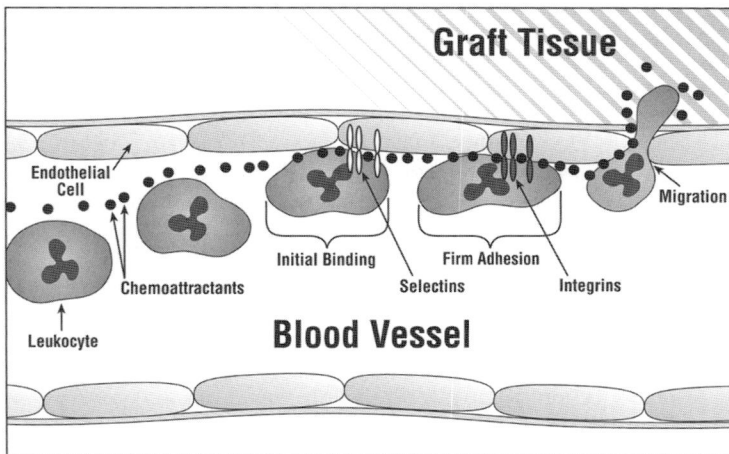

**Figure 3** Intragraft inflammatory responses. Trafficking and accumulation of inflammatory cells are initiated when the leukocytes begin rolling along the blood vessels, adhering loosely by selectins to the endothelium. Subsequently, the binding of integrins enhances the adhesion of the migrating leukocytes to the endothelial cells. Gradients of chemoattractants guide these inflammatory cells through the junctions between the endothelial cells into the graft interstitium.

ligands, by IL-1, TNF-α, and lipid mediators, facilitates this adhesion. This interaction is transient, but will lead to the migration of these inflammatory cells through the junctions between the endothelial cells; this migration is further guided by gradients of chemoattractants (chemokines) to the graft interstitium. Chemokines, the soluble factors involved in promoting chemoattraction during the homing, adhesion, and infiltration of lymphocytes into the inflamed graft site, have also been implicated in the pathogenesis of allograft rejection (41). Enhanced production of chemokines within rejecting grafts influences the recruitment and regulation of graft infiltrating T-cells and macrophages, thereby contributing to both acute and chronic rejection. Over 30 chemokines and eight chemokine receptors have been identified (with overlapping functions), and they have recently become the focus of investigation as potential therapeutic targets for the prevention of graft injury and rejection. Similarly, arachidonic acid metabolites (eicosanoids) also function in the pathogenesis of rejection. These proinflammatory mediators contribute to graft injury and dysfunction, and may modulate the inhibition of graft inflammation. Experimental models of allograft rejection have demonstrated enhanced production of eicosanoids in rejecting grafts and the beneficial effect of eicosanoid-specific antagonists on allograft function.

Unlike hyperacute rejection, the role for complement in both acute and chronic allograft rejection remains equivocal. Nevertheless, complement has been detected in the vascular lesions of several patients with acute allograft rejection. In addition, these rejection episodes have been associated with anti-donor antibodies and early graft loss, suggesting both a contribution of antibody and complement to allograft rejection (42,43).

## INITIATION OF ALLOGRAFT REJECTION

Through the use of in vivo and in vitro models, the immunological mechanisms of allograft rejection have been defined (15,37,39). Following transplantation, the graft-born APCs migrate from the graft to the draining lymph nodes. These passenger leukocytes provide donor MHC class I or class II and costimulatory molecules for the recognition and activation of recipient $CD4^+$ and $CD8^+$ T-cells. The alloantigens are presented via the direct pathway of antigen recognition for the efficient activation of antigen-specific T-cells. Following differentiation within the lymphoid tissue, the activated T-cells home to the graft via the circulation and survey the tissue for the target cells containing the specific antigen–MHC complex. The nonimmunological damage engendered by the transplant procedure and the infiltration of cells from the innate immune system into the graft initiates the activation of the graft endothelium and the secretion of chemokines, thereby facilitating the homing of activated T-cells to the transplanted organ or tissue. These migrating T-cells will mobilize from the blood into the graft parenchyma and effect graft destruction. Blocking of chemokines and adhesion molecules to prevent the migration of leukocytes into the graft have become attractive targets for therapeutic intervention in transplantation.

## MECHANISMS OF GRAFT DESTRUCTION

It is well known that T-cells are involved in graft rejection. However, the precise roles of the $T_h$-cells and CTLs in this process remain controversial. Two mechanisms, a secretory and nonsecretory mechanism for allograft destruction, have been proposed (Fig. 4) (44–46). In the first, CTLs mediate the destruction, while in the latter, the mechanism is similar to DTH in which activated macrophages and cytokines are responsible for the graft damage. Via several mechanisms of action, $CD8^+$ CTLs are directly responsible for the destruction of allografts. CTLs bind the specific allopeptide/MHC class I complex on the surface of the graft cell, and lytic granules containing the cytotoxins, perforin, and granzyme are released into the local environment between the CTL and the target cell. The pore-forming perforin polymerizes in the target cell membrane, leading to the osmotic lysis of the target cells. Granzymes are serine proteases, which degranulate the normal cellular processes by entering through the perforin-induced pores. This leads to DNA fragmentation, which is a characteristic of programmed cell death (apoptosis). Through this calcium-dependent process, the effector CTLs are themselves spared from being destroyed. CTLs can also utilize the nonsecretory Fas (CD95)/Fas ligand (FasL, CD95L) pathway for the induction of apoptosis (47). Upon activation, CTLs upregulate their expression of FasL, a member of the TNF family, on their cell surface. Fas, the ligand for

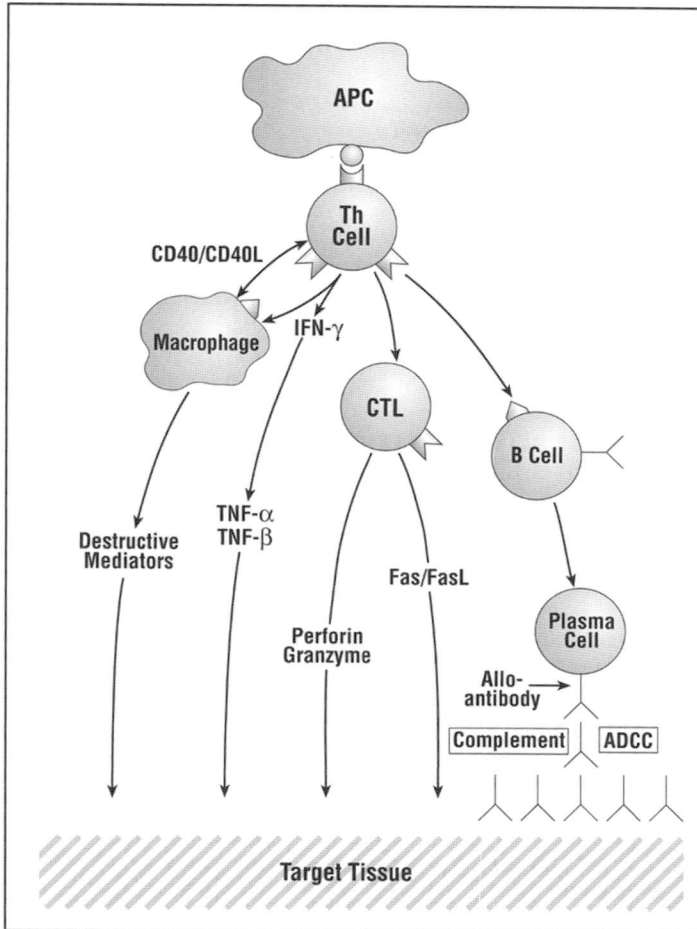

**Figure 4** Mechanisms of allograft destruction. At least four distinct, but not mutually exclusive, effector mechanisms are pivotal in allograft rejection: (1) Once activated by T-cells through the release of interferon (IFN)-γ and through the CD40/CD40L T-cell costimulatory pathway, macrophages release tissue-destructive mediators. (2) The secretion of IFN-γ, tumor necrosis factor (TNF)-α, and TNF-β by the T-cell directly damages the target tissue. (3) Lysis of the target tissue by cytotoxic T-cells occurs through the release of perforin and granzymes or through the induction of the Fas/FasL pathway. (4) The deposition of alloantibodies aids in the destruction of the target tissue by antibody-dependent cellular cytotoxicity or through the activation of the complement cascade. *Abbreviations*: APC, antigen presenting cells; IFN-γ, interferon-γ; CTL, cytotoxic T-cell; TNF-α, tumor necrosis factor-α; TNF-β, tumor necrosis factor-β; ADCC, antibody dependent cell-mediated cytotoxicity.

FasL, is expressed on a wide range of tissues, and its ligation by the FasL-positive CTL induces apoptosis in the target cell.

In addition to CTL-mediated damage, responses similar to DTH have been shown to be involved in allograft destruction (Fig. 4). The activated CD4$^+$ T$_h$1-cells activate macrophages through the release of INF-γ and through the CD40/CD40L T-cell costimulatory pathway (24,26). The macrophages, once activated, release a variety of destructive mediators, including nitric oxide, oxygen radicals, and proteases. Similarly, damage through the release of TNF-α, TNF-β, and INF-γ by the T$_h$1-cells can directly damage the graft. Even though the controversy concerning the relative importance of CTLs and DTH remains ongoing, allograft rejection most likely involves both mechanisms of destruction.

In addition to CTLs- and DTH-like responses, alloantibody responses can also play an important role in graft rejection (Fig. 4). However, the development of these anti-HLA antibodies posttransplantation is less understood. The production of alloantibodies against MHC is T-cell dependent, and requires the interaction and orchestration of APCs, CD4$^+$ T$_h$- and B-cells.

The interaction of the CD40 on activated B-cells with CD40L on activated T-cells plays a pivotal role in antibody production and isotype switching (24,25). Once the alloantibodies are produced, tissue damage results either from the activation of the complement cascade or secondary to antibody-dependent cellular cytotoxicity. During antibody-dependent cellular cytotoxicity, natural killer (NK) cells or macrophages bind to the Fc portion of the alloantibody and induce target cell lysis (48). The precise role of NK cells in transplant rejection remains ill defined, but it has been noted that both NK cells and granulocytes are present in the graft infiltrate and may be contributing to antigen nonspecific effector mechanisms of graft destruction.

Preformed antibodies against either HLA or blood group antigens can induce hyperacute rejection, a complement-dependent reaction, by binding to antigens on the graft vascular endothelium (49). Subsequently, complement and coagulation factors are activated, resulting in endothelial destruction, intravascular platelet and fibrin deposition, granulocyte and monocyte infiltration, fibrinoid necrosis of the vessel walls, and eventual ischemic necrosis of the allograft. These preformed antibodies are often found in recipients who have had a previous transplant, multiple transfusions, or pregnancies. The prescreening of the donor and recipient by cross-matching prior to transplantation has led to the near elimination of hyperacute rejection in allotransplantation. The extent to which alloantibodies are involved in both acute and chronic rejection remains largely ill defined.

## CHRONIC REJECTION

The development of potent immunosuppressive regimens has greatly reduced the incidence of acute cellular rejection, with important improvements in short-term patient and allograft survival (2). However, there has been less of an impact on long-term (>5 years) allograft survival. Chronic rejection, a major cause of late organ deterioration and failure, occurs months or years after transplantation, and remains poorly defined (3). While the etiology of this lesion is multifactorial, immunological processes have been postulated to be involved through both alloantigen-dependent and independent forms of injury. The immunological factors associated with the pathophysiology of chronic rejection include delayed graft function, acute cellular rejection, and posttransplant responses to donor antigens. However, the role of these major risk factors remains controversial. Nonimmunological influences, which may aggravate these alloantigen-dependent factors, include ischemia/reperfusion, cytomegalovirus, hyperlipidemia, diabetes, brain death, the use of marginal donors, donor/recipient size mismatch, and the nephrotoxic side effects of immunosuppressive regimens. Each of these alloantigen-independent factors intensifies the vascular and parenchymal alterations associated with alloimmune injury (2,3).

A significant number of transplant recipients experience a progressive decline in organ function, with eventual failure of the organ over a period of years secondary to chronic rejection. The graft vascular disease includes arterial fibrointimal hyperplasia, destruction of epithelial-lined vessels, and destruction and atrophy of organ-associated lymphoid tissue and lymphatics, ultimately leading to massive luminal narrowing and fibrosis of the parenchyma.

The development of this lesion can be divided into four inter-related phases (50): injury, immune cell recognition and activation, effector mechanisms amplifying the inflammatory response, and a regulatory phase comprised of fibrosis. Initially, a cascade of inflammatory events is instigated following injury. Once the T-cells become activated, either through alloantigen-specific or non-specific inflammatory stimuli, an increase in antigen presentation to the T-cells occurs through the upregulation of cell surface adhesion molecules, MHC class II, the costimulatory molecules, and the secretion of chemokines and cytokines. Upon activation, CD4$^+$ T-cells initiate DTH responses and provide the necessary help to B-cells to proliferate, differentiate, and produce cytokines, thereby amplifying the response. The effector phase of development is mediated by activated T-cells, macrophages, and B-cells for the production of cytokines, circulating antibodies, and adhesion molecules. These activated cells and their products propagate cell-mediated immune events between donor and recipient cells. As a result, the underlying donor parenchyma and vasculature become activated, leading to the regulatory phase of parenchymal remodeling. Nevertheless, the precise mechanisms responsible for these integrated responses and their role in chronic rejection remain largely unknown.

## CONCLUSIONS

Great strides have been made over the last 50 years in understanding the dynamic cascade of immune events that occur when the body recognizes non-self from self. Nonetheless, the immunobiology of allograft rejection still remains something of a mystery with respect to the underlying mechanisms involved. Only through continual exploration of these immune processes will the complexities of allograft rejection be unraveled, leading to the discovery of novel targets for developing safer and more effective strategies for the elimination of allograft rejection and for the preservation of allograft survival and function.

## REFERENCES

1. U.S. Scientific Registry of Transplant Recipients and the Organ Procurement and Transplantation Network 2005 Annual Report.
2. Matas AJ. Risk factors for chronic rejection: a clinical perspective. Transplant Immunol 1998; 6:1–11.
3. Nagano H, Tilney NL. Chronic allograft failure: the clinical problem. Am J Med Sci 1997; 313:305–309.
4. Benichou G, Takizawa PA, Olson CA, McMillan M, Sercarz EE. Donor major histocompatibility complex (MHC) peptides are presented by recipient MHC molecules during graft rejection. J Exp Med 1992; 275:305–308.
5. Warrens AN, Lombardi G, Lechler RI. Presentation and recognition of major and minor histocompatibility antigens. Transpl Immunol 1994; 2:103–107.
6. Campbell RD, Trowsdale J. Map of the human MHC. Immunol Today 1993; 14:349–352.
7. Martin S, Dyer PA. The case for matching MHC genes in human organ transplantation. Nat Genet 1993; 5:210–213.
8. Fremont DH, Rees WA, Kozono H. Biophysical studies of T cell receptors and their ligands. Curr Opin Immunol 1996; 8:93–100.
9. Zinkernagel RM, Doherty PC. Immunological surveillance against altered self components by sensitised T lymphocytes in lymphocyte choriomeningitis. Nature 1974; 251:547–548.
10. Zinkernagel RM, Doherty PC. Restriction of in vivo T-cell mediated cytotoxicity in lymphocyte choriomeningitis within a syngeneic or semiallogeneic system. Nature 1974; 248:701–702.
11. Morrison LA, Lukacher AE, Braciale VL, Fan DP, Braciale TJ. Differences in antigen presentation to MHC class I- and class II-restricted influenza virus-specific cytotoxic T-lymphocyte clones. J Exp Med 1986; 163:903–921.
12. Gould DS, Auchincloss H. Direct and indirect recognition: the role of MHC antigens in graft rejection. Immunol Today 1999; 20:77–82.
13. Benichou G, Valujskikh A, Heeger PS. Contributions of direct and indirect T cell alloreactivity during allograft rejection in mice. J Immunol 1999; 162:352–358.
14. Vella JP, Spadafora-Ferreira M, Murphy B, et al. Indirect allorecognition of major histocompatibility complex allopeptides in human renal transplant recipients with chronic graft dysfunction. Transplantation 1997; 64:795–800.
15. Lafferty KJ, Prowse SJ, Simeonovic CJ, Warren HS. Immunobiology of tissue transplantation: a return to the passenger leukocyte concept. Ann Rev Immunol 1983; 1:143–173.
16. Auchincloss H Jr, Lee R, Shea S, Markowitz JS, Grusby MJ, Glimcher LH. The role of "indirect" recognition in initiating rejection of skin grafts from major histocompatibility complex class II-deficient mice. Proc Natl Acad Sci 1993; 90:3373–3377.
17. Von Boehmer H. Positive selection of lymphocytes. Cell 1994; 76:219–228.
18. Nossal GJV. Negative selection of lymphocytes. Cell 1994; 76:229–239.
19. Krensky AM, Clayberger C. The nature of allorecognition. Curr Opin Nephrol Hypertens 1993; 2:898–903.
20. Liu Y, Janeway CA Jr. Cells that present both specific ligand and costimulatory activity are the most efficient inducers of clonal expansion of normal CD4 T cells. Proc Natl Acad Sci 1992; 89:3845–3949.
21. Rudd CE. Upstream–downstream: CD28 cosignaling pathways and T cell function. Immunity 1996; 4:527–534.
22. Tivol EA, Borriello F, Schweitzer AN, Lynch WP, Bluestone JA, Sharpe AH. Loss of CTLA-4 leads to massive lymphoproliferation and fatal multiorgan tissue destruction, revealing a critical negative regulatory role of CTLA-4. Immunity 1995; 3:541–547.
23. Waterhouse P, Penninger JM, Timms E, et al. Lymphoproliferative disorders with early lethality in mice deficient in CTLA-4. Science 1995; 270:985–988.
24. Foy TM, Aruffo A, Bajorath J, Buhlmann JE, Noelle RJ. Immune regulation by CD40 and its ligand gp39. Ann Rev Immunol 1996; 14:591–617.
25. Parker DC. T cell-dependent B-cell activation. Ann Rev Immunol 1993; 11:331–340.
26. Paulnock DM. Macrophage activation by T cells. Curr Opin Immunol 1992; 4:344–349.
27. Janeway CA Jr. The T cell receptor as a multi-component signaling machine: CD4/CD8 coreceptors and CD45 in T cell activation. Ann Rev Immunol 1992; 10:645–674.

28. Wang YC, Zhu L, McHugh R, Sell KW, Selvaraj P. Expression of heat-stable antigen on tumor cells provides co-stimulation for tumor-specific T cell proliferation and cytotoxicity in mice. Eur J Immunol 1995; 25:1163–1167.

29. Tan JT, Ha J, Cho HR, et al. Analysis of expression and function of the costimulatory molecule 4-1BB in alloimmune responses. Transplantation 2000; 15:175–183.

30. Ozkaynak E, Gao W, Shemmeri N, et al. Importance of ICOS-B7RP-1 costimulation in acute and chronic allograft rejection. Nature Immunol 2001; 2:591–596.

31. Crabtree GR, Clipstone NA. Signal transmission between the plasma membrane and nucleus of T lymphocytes. Ann Rev Biochem 1994; 63:1045–1083.

32. Cantrell D. T cell antigen receptor signal transduction pathways. Ann Rev Immunol 1996; 14:259–274.

33. Clipstone NA, Crabtree GR. Identification of calcineurin as a key signaling enzyme in T-lymphocyte activation. Nature 1992; 357:695–697.

34. Lindsten T, June CH, Ledbetter JA, Stella G, Thompson CB. Regulation of lymphokine messenger RNA stability by a surface-mediated T-cell activation pathway. Science 1989; 244:339–342.

35. Kamogawa Y, Minasi LA, Carding SR, Bottomly K, Flavell RA. The relationship of IL-4 and IFN-γ producing T cells studied by linease ablation of IL-4 producing cells. Cell 1993; 75:985–995.

36. Arai K, Lee F, Miyajima A, Miyatake S, Arai N, Yokota T. Cytokines: co-ordinators of immune and inflammatory responses. Ann Rev Biochem 1990; 59:783–836.

37. Fearon DT, Locksley RM. The instinctive role of innate immunity in the acquired immune response. Science 1996; 272:50–53.

38. Picker LJ, Butcher EC. Physiological and molecular mechanisms of lymphocyte homing. Ann Rev Immunol 1993; 10:561–591.

39. Springer TA. Traffic signals for lymphocyte recirculation and leukocyte emigration. The multi-step paradigm. Cell 1994; 76:301–304.

40. Hogg N, Landis RC. Adhesion molecules in cell interactions. Curr Opin Immunol 1993; 5:383–390.

41. Luster AD. Chemokines: chemotactic cytokines that mediate inflammation. N Engl J Med 1998; 388:436–445.

42. Tomlinson S. Complement defense mechanisms. Curr Opin Immunol 1993; 5:83–89.

43. Frank MM, Fries LF. The role of complement in inflammation and phagocytosis. Immunol Today 1991; 12:322–326.

44. Griffiths GM. The cell biology of CTL killing. Curr Opin Immunol 1995; 7:343–348.

45. Henkart PA. Lymphocyte-mediated cytotoxicology: two pathways and multiple effector molecules. Immunity 1994; 1:343–346.

46. O'Rourke AM, Mescher MF. Cytotoxic T lymphocyte activation involves a cascade of signaling and adhesion events. Nature 1992; 358:253–255.

47. Suda T, Takahashi T, Goldstein P, Nagata S. Molecular cloning and expression of the Fas ligand, a novel member of the tumor necrosis factor family. Cell 1993; 76:1169–1178.

48. Lanier LL, Ruitenberg JJ, Phillips JH. Functional and biochemical analysis of CD16 antigen on natural killer cells and granulocytes. J Immunol 1988; 141:3485–3487.

49. Kissmeyer Nielsen F, Olsen S, Petersen VP, Fjeldborg O. Hyperacute rejection of kidney allografts, associated with pre-existing humoral antibodies against donor cells. Lancet 1966; 2:662–665.

50. Russell ME, Raisanen-Sokolowski A, Koglin J, Glysing-Jensen T. Immunobiology of chronic rejection: effector pathways that regulate vascular thickening. Graft 1998; 1:7–10.

# 11 | Immunosuppressive Agents in Pancreatic Transplantation

**Seamus J. Teahan**
*Department of Urology and Transplantation, Beaumont Hospital, Dublin, Ireland*

**Angus W. Thomson**
*Thomas E. Starzl Transplantation Institute, University of Pittsburgh School of Medicine, Pittsburgh, Pennsylvania, U.S.A.*

Pancreas transplantation is now a well-accepted treatment option in selected uremic diabetic recipients of kidney transplants either simultaneously with or, less commonly, after the kidney transplantation, or in nonuremic diabetics undergoing solitary pancreas transplantation.

As the incidence of technical failure decreases, the relative importance of rejection as a cause of graft loss is increasing (1). Despite improvements in immunosuppression in the prevention and therapy of acute rejection, chronic rejection remains the leading cause of graft loss in patients who survive more than one year (2). It has also been shown that as the number of acute rejection episodes increases the likelihood of graft failure also increases (3). Therefore, a key element in improving graft survival is better immunosuppression, ideally with fewer side effects. This section will discuss the mechanisms of action of the agents currently in use and discuss their relative merits and drawbacks regarding pancreas transplantation. The potential role of newer immunosuppressive agents will also be discussed (Table 1).

## ADRENAL CORTICOSTEROIDS

Adrenal corticosteroids remain an integral part of the most immunosuppressive regimens used in pancreatic transplantation (4,5). Glucocorticoids are potent immunosuppressive agents and act at a number of levels. A marked leucopenia occurs within six hours of administration, as circulating lymphocytes become sequestered within lymphoid tissues; sessile lymphocytes are unaffected. Though circulating T- and B-lymphocytes are affected, the effect is more pronounced on T-cells.

Steroids inhibit cytokine gene transcription and secretion by macrophages and also suppress the production and effects of T-cell cytokines. These cytokines amplify the responses of macrophages and lymphocytes. Thus, steroids inhibit interleukin (IL)-2 production and binding of IL-2 to its receptor, while also interfering with the ability of macrophages to respond to lymphocyte-derived signals, specifically migration inhibition factor and macrophage activation factor. Steroids also inhibit the production of the cytokine IL-12. These effects may explain corticosteroid-induced impairment of dendritic cell development and function (6,7). Corticosteroids also suppress prostaglandin synthesis. The effect of glucocorticoid administration on antibody production is negligible.

Some of the molecular mechanisms by which glucocorticoids exert their effects have been elucidated. Much activity is initiated at the subcellular level by means of hormone receptors. Unlike polypeptide mediators with receptors on the surface of the cell, steroids move freely through the cell membrane and bind to cytoplasmic receptors. The steroid–receptor complexes move into the nucleus where they bind to DNA. They act on gene promoters causing either activation or depression of part of the genome, thereby affecting specific m-RNA transcription. Thus, protein synthesis may be either up- or down-regulated.

Though the efficacy of steroids in suppressing allograft rejection has been clearly established, specific problems are encountered more commonly in pancreatic transplantation, adding considerably to their side-effect profile. A normally functioning graft offsets the hyperglycemia associated with steroid use, but long-term damage to islet function may not

**Table 1**  Modes of Action of Immunosuppressive Drugs

| |
|---|
| *Alteration of gene expression* |
|   Cyclosporine A |
|   Tacrolimus |
| *Inhibition of cytokine action* |
|   Rapamycin |
|   Leflunomide |
| *Inhibition of DNA synthesis* |
|   Blockade of purine biosynthesis:- |
|   Mizoribine |
|   Mycophenolate mofetil |
|   Blockade of pyrimidine biosynthesis:- |
|   Brequinar |
| *Inhibition of cell maturation* |
|   Deoxyspergualin |

be reversible (8). An unexpectedly high incidence of pathological bone fractures has been reported in recipients of pancreas transplants (9), and though not entirely steroid related, steroids certainly contribute to the problem. Therefore, because of the side effects associated with their use, there is great interest in minimizing the use of or withdrawing steroids completely in pancreas transplant recipients.

## ANTIPROLIFERATIVE AGENTS

Antiproliferative agents prevent differentiation and division of immunocompetent lymphocytes after their encounter with antigen and thereby inhibit immune responses. They interfere with cell function late in the cell cycle by combining with certain cellular components, or by resembling, and competing with, essential metabolites.

### Azathioprine

Azathioprine (Imuran®, Burroughs Wellcome Kirkland, Quebec) interferes with DNA synthesis. It is cleaved to its active metabolite 6-mercaptopurine principally by erythrocyte glutathione. 6-Mercaptopurine is then cleaved into a series of mercaptopurine-containing nucleotides, which interfere with synthesis of DNA and polyadenylate-containing RNA. The synthesis and action of coenzymes are disrupted, and chromosomal breaks occur. By interfering with mitosis, azathioprine affects the division of both T- and B-lymphocytes; however, cells other than lymphocytes are also affected, resulting in bone marrow suppression and hepatic dysfunction.

As newer immunosuppressive agents have become available, the use of azathioprine in pancreas transplantation has diminished. However, because of its relatively low incidence of gastrointestinal toxicity, in a cohort of patients particularly susceptible to these effects, azathioprine remains widely used as a secondary agent in pancreas transplant recipients.

### Mycophenolate Mofetil

Lymphocyte proliferation is dependent on de novo purine biosynthesis. Mycophenolate mofetil (MMF) (Cellcept®, Roche, New Jersey, U.S.A.) is a prodrug, which is metabolized in the liver to its active form mycophenolic acid. Mycophenolic acid inhibits inosine monophosphate dehydrogenase and thus guanosine synthesis. In the absence of adequate levels of guanosine, lymphocyte proliferation cannot occur, and as levels of guanosine precursors rise proliferation is further inhibited. As lymphocytes do not contain enzymes of the salvage pathway to compensate for the depletion of guanosine nucleotides, DNA synthesis is suppressed. Unlike nucleoside analogues, the use of MMF has theoretical advantages, as DNA repair enzymes are not affected, and chromosomal breaks do not occur. Therefore, the patient is not exposed to the mutagenic effects associated with nucleoside analog rise.

MMF also inhibits the guanosine triphosphate (GTP)-dependent transfer of fructose and mannose to certain glycoproteins, some of which are adhesion molecules (10). Cell–cell interactions can therefore be affected. Some G proteins may be sensitive to GTP depletion, and this may account for the near complete inhibition of B-cell antibody formation by MMF. Antibody production by polyclonally activated human B-lymphocytes is almost completely inhibited. Interestingly, MMF does not deplete GTP in neutrophils and, consequently, the growth and responses of these cells to chemoattractants and their ability to produce superoxide and kill bacteria are not affected.

As a number of clinical trials demonstrated a significant reduction in the incidence of acute rejection in renal transplant patients treated with MMF versus azathioprine (11), the use of MMF in pancreas transplantation has increased. Recent data confirm these findings in simultaneous kidney–pancreas transplantation, where the incidence of acute renal and pancreas allograft rejection rates were significantly reduced (12). Although gastrointestinal side effects are common, particularly with high doses, most patients tolerate a reduction in dose of conversion to azathioprine-based immunosuppression without adverse effects (13).

## Mizoribine

Mizoribine, an antibiotic derived from *Eupenicillium brefeldianum*, is a potent suppressor of lymphocyte growth. It is activated to mizoribine-5-monophosphate (MZ-5-P) by adenosine kinase. Activated mizoribine acts in a fashion similar to MMF by targeting inosine monophosphate dehydrogenase and also GMP synthase. Guanosine nucleotide synthesis is almost completely inhibited with consequent inhibition in DNA synthesis. MZ-5-P is dephosphorylated intracellularly, and then exits the cell as extracellular mizoribine concentration falls. Extracellular mizoribine is inactive.

Mizoribine inhibits the passage of cells from the $G_0$ to the S phase of the cell cycle. T- and B-lymphocyte proliferation is suppressed, though not selectively. MZ-5-P can also interfere with DNA repair mechanisms and cause chromosome breaks.

Though clinical experience in pancreas transplantation is limited, mizoribine exhibits considerable synergism with both cyclosporine (CsA) and tacrolimus (TAC).

## Brequinar Sodium

Brequinar sodium acts by interfering with de novo pyrimidine synthesis. It is a noncompetitive inhibitor of the enzyme dihydro-orotate dehydrogenase (DHODH).

Lymphocytes cannot use the salvage pathway for pyrimidine biosynthesis, and therefore nucleotide precursors again become depleted with inhibition of DNA and RNA synthesis. Brequinar also inhibits IL-6–induced differentiation of human B-cells into IgM-secreting plasma cells (14). Like mizoribine and MMF, brequinar exhibits synergism with cyclosporine; however, because of significant side effects, it is no longer being evaluated as an immunosuppressive agent in clinical trials.

## T-CELL–DIRECTED IMMUNOSUPPRESSIVE AGENTS
## Cyclosporine

CsA (Sandimmune®, Neoral®, Novartis Pharmaceuticals Corp., New Jersey, U.S.A., Sang-CyA®, Sangstat) is a cyclic peptide fungal metabolite extracted from *Tolypocladium inflatum Gams*. It was responsible, possibly more than any other agent, for the rapid expansion of solid organ transplantation programs seen in the 1980s and for a significant improvement in pancreas graft survival rates (15). The suppressive effects of the drug on T-cells appear to be related to its selective inhibition of T-cell receptor–mediated activation events.

Cyclosporine inhibits cytokine production by CD4+ helper T-cells and blocks the development of CD4+ and CD8+ T-cells in the thymus. Unlike the antiproliferative agents, myelosuppression is not a problem because of its selectivity (16).

Cyclosporine affects T-lymphocytes on a number of levels:

1. Inhibition of both IL-2 producing and cytotoxic T-lymphocytes
2. Inhibition of IL-2 gene expression by activated T-lymphocytes
3. No inhibition of activated T-lymphocytes in response to exogenous IL-2
4. Inhibition of resting T-lymphocytes in response to alloantigen and exogenous cytokine
5. Inhibition of IL-1 production

The main side effect of cyclosporine is nephrotoxicity, which theoretically is a greater problem in pancreas transplantation alone. In addition to nephrotoxicity, cyclosporine may also cause hypertension, hyperkalemia, hirsutism, gingival hypertrophy, hepatotoxicity, tremor, and other neurotoxicities. Cyclosporine is also somewhat diabetogenic. As with other immunosuppressive agents, the risk of infection is increased, as is the incidence of neoplasia. Traditionally, the latter was believed to be related to a nonspecific impairment of the organ recipient's immune-surveillance system (16). Recent evidence suggests that CsA may also promote cancer progression directly, independently of its effect on the host's immune cells, by inducing the synthesis of transforming growth factor β (17).

## Tacrolimus

TAC (Prograf[R], Astellas Pharma US, Inc., Illinois, U.S.A.), a macrocyclic lactone previously known as FK-506, is a potent immunosuppressive agent that acts in a fashion similar to cyclosporine. Like cyclosporine, tacrolimus is a prodrug activated when it binds to a specific intracellular binding protein or immunophilin (FK-506 binding protein). The drug–immunophilin complex blocks the phosphatase activity of calcineurin, which inhibits dephosphorylation and nuclear translocation of the gene transcription regulatory protein, nuclear factor of activated T-cells. This results in inhibition of

1. IL-2 gene expression and IL-2 production,
2. T-lymphocyte proliferation in the mixed leucocyte reaction,
3. the appearance of IL-2 receptors on human lymphocytes.

In vivo, tacrolimus prolongs the survival of major histocompatibility complex (MHC) disparate grafts and exhibits approximately 100 times the potency of cyclosporine. Tacrolimus has a similar side-effect profile to cyclosporine although hirsutism and gum hypertrophy do not occur. Although one report suggested that TAC was more diabetogenic than CsA in renal transplant recipients (18), reports to date are somewhat at variance with respect to pancreas transplantation, where more recent studies have demonstrated a comparable incidence of posttransplant diabetes mellitus (19,20). However, because of lower rejection rates seen with TAC (21) and its usefulness in cases of CsA nephrotoxicity and CsA-resistant rejection (22), TAC is now often used as the T-cell–directed immunosuppressive agent of choice in pancreatic transplantation (23).

## Sirolimus

Sirolimus (Rapamycin[R], A.G. Scientific, Inc., San Diego, California, U.S.A.) is also a macrolide antibiotic, and is a close structural analogue of tacrolimus, binding to the same cytoplasmic receptor (FK506 binding protein; FKBP). Sirolimus does not block T-cell cytokine gene expression, but instead inhibits the transduction of signals from IL-2R to the nucleus. Binding of sirolimus to FKBP inhibits P70S6 protein kinase activity, which is essential for ribosomal phosphorylation and cell cycle progression. It is also a potent inhibitor of experimental allograft rejection and prevents chronic graft (heart) vessel disease (24). Sirolimus has been shown to act synergistically with cyclosporine, and with tacrolimus in the murine model of small bowel transplantation (25). It has also been shown to act synergistically with MMF to decrease the incidence of acute rejection in a rat model of pancreas transplantation (26). To date, there are essentially no clinical data available relating to the use of sirolimus in pancreas transplantation.

## LYMPHOCYTE-DEPLETING AGENTS

Anti-T-cell induction therapy became a part of standard immunosuppressive regimes in pancreas transplantation during the cyclosporine era, as convincing data accumulated demonstrating improved patient and graft survival (27). These agents function by nonselectively depleting or inactivating the host's lymphocytes. As newer and more potent immunosuppressive drugs have become available, the necessity for antibody induction therapy has been being questioned and, in certain situations, induction therapy has been safely withheld (28,29). In the view of some authors, antibody induction therapy may offer an advantage in the setting of posttransplant delayed graft function, where the administration of nephrotoxic agents such as CsA or tacrolimus is perhaps better avoided.

## Anti-Lymphocyte Globulin

Anti-lymphocyte globulins are produced when human lymphocytes are injected into animals of a different species, rabbit, goat, and horse being most commonly used. As anti-lymphocyte globulins (ALGs) ideally act on T-cells, the use of thymocytes for immunization results in the most potent sera. Administration of ALG interferes most with cell-mediated reactions, allograft rejection, tuberculin sensitivity, and the graft versus host response. Activated lymphocytes coated with ALG are either lyzed or cleared from the circulation by reticuloendothelial cells in the spleen and liver. ALG may be given prophylactically as a component of induction therapy, or it may be used to treat steroid-resistant rejection.

As ALG is prepared from heterologous serum raised against human tissue, there are inherent toxicities associated with its use. The degree of toxicity depends on

1. Cross reactivity of the serum with other tissue antigens, and
2. The ability of the patient to make antibodies against the foreign protein.

Side effects include anemia and thrombocytopenia because of a reaction between host erythrocytes and platelets and the ALG. Though there appears to be little difference in rejection rates between polyclonal (ALG) and monoclonal (OKT3) antibody induction therapy, a lower rate of opportunistic infection has been reported in ALG-treated patients (30).

## Monoclonal Antibody

Monoclonal antibodies to various subsets of T-cell populations are available. Muromonab-CD3 (OKT3, anti-CD3) reacts with all T-cell populations and is the monoclonal antibody used most frequently in clinical practice. Its clinical efficacy in pancreas transplantation has been well documented (31). Muromonab-CD3 binds to a site associated with the T-cell receptor (CD3) and functions to modulate the receptor and inactivate T-cell function (32). By engaging the T-cell receptor complex, muromonab-CD3 blocks not only the function of naïve T-cells but also the functions of established cytotoxic T-cells, and thus blocks cell-mediated cytotoxicity. After intravenous administration, OKT3 opsonizes or binds to T-cells. As these bound cells are removed by the reticuloendothelial system, circulating T-cell counts decrease abruptly within 30 to 60 minutes. Once administration of muromonab-CD3 is discontinued, T-cell counts rapidly return to normal.

## DEOXYSPERGUALIN

15-Deoxyspergualin (DSG) is a synthetic analogue of the antitumor antibiotic spergualin. Its mechanism of action is not clearly understood, but it appears to prevent differentiation of precursor cells and also impair antigen presentation and processing (33). This is achieved by inhibition of numerous enzymes necessary for the production of polyamides (spermine synthase, spermidine synthase, polyamine oxidase, spermidine-spermine N-acetyltransferase, and ornithine decarboxylase). The resulting depletion of polyamides prevents synthesis of cellular macromolecules necessary for normal differentiation and function.

DSG binds to heat shock protein (HSP) 70, a constitutively expressed member of the HSP family (34). HSPs contain peptide-binding grooves analogous to those of MHC molecules, and therefore may play a role in binding and intracellular transport of antigenic peptides in APCs. This may account for the impairment of antigen presentation to T-cells by monocytes exposed to DSG. HSP70 and HSP90 form complexes with steroid receptors and possibly cyclophilins, and are involved in translocation of proteins to the nucleus. Interference with the normal functions of these substances may account for the additional effects of this agent.

DSG inhibits proliferation and differentiation of cytotoxic T-lymphocytes, probably by preventing IL-2R expression (35). Helper T-cell functions are not affected, and neither are the mitogen responses nor are the early stages of the mixed leukocyte reaction (MLR). Release of IL-2 from T-lymphocytes and IL-1 from monocytes is not impaired. DSG inhibits the mitogenic stage of B-cells. It also suppresses differentiation of human B-cells into plasma cells, and,

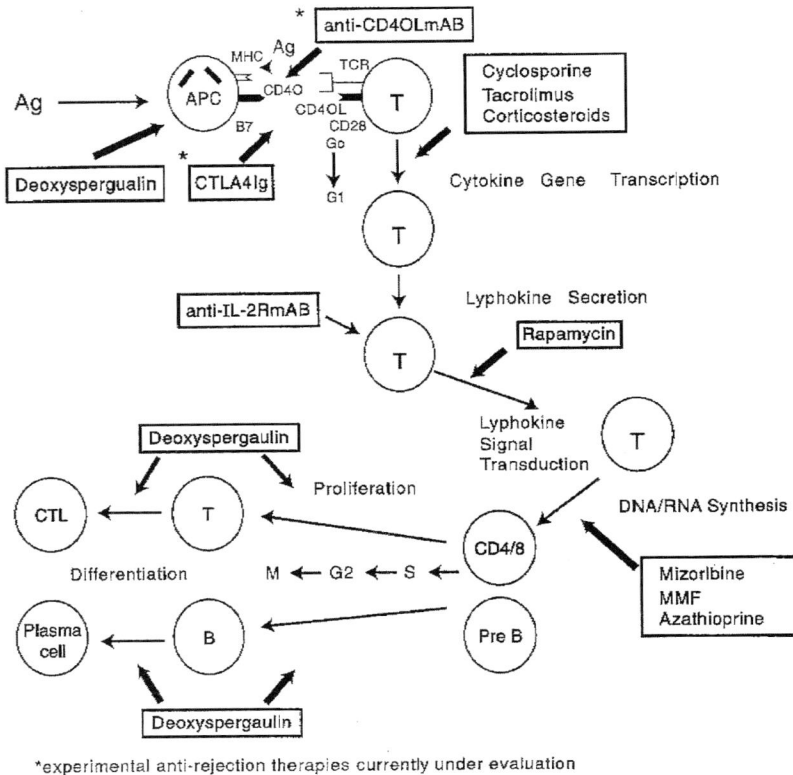

*experimental anti-rejection therapies currently under evaluation

**Figure 1**  Schematic representation of the sites of action of immunosuppressive drugs.

therefore, primary and secondary antibody responses are inhibited, as is production of xeno-phile antibodies. DSG suppresses the production of macrophage activating factor by murine cells stimulated with antigen. It impairs superoxide production in cells of the monocyte/macrophage lineage, and decreases MHC class II expression and IL-1 production in these cells. Antigen presentation by monocytes is inhibited. DSG inhibits lymphokine-activated killer cell activity and induces lymphocytopenia, granulocytopenia, and anemia (Fig. 1).

## New Developments in Anti-Rejection Therapy

An ideal immunosuppressive agent would selectively target T-cells that are destined to participate only in the immune reaction of interest and induce donor antigen-specific tolerance in the host. Monoclonal antibodies are uniquely suited for the realization of both of these goals because of their remarkable specificity (36). Transplantation of an allograft activates only a small fraction of the entire T-cell pool. Ideally, only this activated T-cell subset should be eliminated or modulated by mAb, resulting in tolerance by clone-specific anergy.

## Anti-Interleukin-2R Monoclonal Antibodies

Activation of the IL-2 receptor (IL-2R) marks a critical step in the activation of alloreactive T-cells. Blockade of this receptor interferes directly with the ability of activated T-cells to respond to normal growth and development signals. The receptor itself is a complex of three IL-2R subunits: IL-2Rα, IL-2Rβ, and IL-2Rγ. The α subunit is present only on activated T-cells, a subset of activated B-cells and APCs. Thus, anti-IL-2Rα mAb treatment targets a small population of cells enriched with antigen-activated T-cells. Two FDA-approved humanized mAbs are now available; Daclizumab (Zenapax®, Roche) and Basiliximab (Simulect®, Novartis) are of proven clinical efficacy in renal transplant recipients (37), although little data are available in pancreas transplant recipients. Unlike the high immunogenic rodent mAbs developed initially, these humanized mAbs do not induce production of neutralizing human anti-mouse antibodies.

## Anti-Adhesion Molecule Monoclonal Antibodies

Ligation of the T-cell receptor with the antigen and MHC is a prerequisite for T-cell activation. Blockade of T-cell adhesion molecules, such as lymphocyte function-associated antigen 1 (LFA-1, CD11a/CD18) or very late appearing antigen 4, is therefore another potentially useful method of immunosuppression. These molecules, in turn, bind to intercellular adhesion molecules, intercellular adhesion molecule-1 (ICAM-1; CD54), and vascular cell adhesion molecule-1 (CD106). Monoclonal antibodies against these adhesion molecules have the ability to prevent T-cells from homing to the allograft. ICAM-1 is constitutively expressed on about 20% of blood mononuclear cells, and on vascular endothelium. It is readily induced on many cell types, including endothelial and epithelial cells, by means of cytokine-induced activation. ICAM-1 functions as a ligand for LFA-1 antigen, which is expressed constitutively on T-cells. The LFA-1 antigen–ICAM-1 interaction provides a costimulatory signal for T-cell activation that is synergistic to the signal delivered via the T-cell receptor–CD3 complex.

## NOVEL EXPERIMENTAL IMMUNOSUPPRESSIVE AGENTS
### Costimulatory Molecule Blockade

Certain costimulatory signaling pathways are essential for the promotion of T-cell effector function and proliferation. Attempts are being made experimentally to induce specific T-cell clonal anergy by preventing T-cells from receiving these appropriate costimulatory signals. Potential targets include CD28 and its homologue cytotoxic T-lymphocyte antigen-4 (CTLA-4) on the T-cell surface. These molecules are involved because of their interaction with the B7 family proteins on APCs, with the delivery of the crucial second signal (in addition to antigen) that is essential to T-cell activation. Administration of soluble CTLA-4-Ig has been shown to prevent allograft rejection (38), possibly by down-regulating the T-cell IL-2 gene and thereby skewing the T-cell response to Th2 predominance. This results in specific T-cell unresponsiveness to donor antigens. Pancreas grafts have also been successfully transfected with a viral vector expressing the CTLA-4-Ig gene. The local increase in CTLA-4 production that ensued resulted in indefinite graft survival (39).

The interaction of CD40 and its T-cell–based ligand, CD40L (CD154), also plays an important role in T-cell activation by up-regulating CD80/86 (B7) (40). In addition, CD40 and CD40L play a fundamental role in establishing T-cell–dependent B-cell activity (41). Blockade of both CD28 and CD40/CD40L costimulatory pathways has been shown to act synergistically to decrease and reverse acute rejection in a primate model of renal transplantation (42). It has also been shown that blockade of CD40/CD40L, in a donor-specific transfusion presensitization model of islet allografts, leads to a state of alloantigen-specific tolerance (43). Recent studies demonstrated very promising results using a humanized monoclonal antibody against CD40L (hu5C8), which when used as monotherapy significantly improved graft and recipient survival in the primate model (44). Reported side effects were minimal using this therapy and rejection was not seen even when treatment was withdrawn. Interestingly, both this and another study have shown significantly poorer results when hu5C8 was used in conjunction with more traditional immunosuppressive agents (45).

## Leflunomide

Leflunomide (LFM) (Arava®, Aventis Pharmaceuticals, U.S.A.) is a novel immunosuppressive agent rapidly converted in vivo to its active metabolite A77 1726, which is a malononitrilamide. A77 1726 non-cytotoxically and reversibly inhibits proliferation of both T- and B-cells, and inhibits both T-cell–dependent and –independent antibody production. These actions are mediated via inhibition of IL-2R-associated tyrosine kinase activity (46) and inhibition of pyrimidine biosynthesis by inhibition of DHODH (47). The inhibition of DHODH is believed to be the more significant effect of leflunomide. LFM has also been shown to decrease chronic rejection, possibly due to its antiproliferative effect on vascular smooth muscle (48).

A77 1726 has also been shown in vitro to cause a Th2-type response by increasing transforming growth factor β-1 and decreasing IL-2 expression (49). This effect may explain the synergism displayed by CsA/LFM combinations (50).

The manufacturers of LFM have decided not to develop it further for transplantation, but to develop malononitralimide analogs for this purpose. Though LFM has many attractive properties, its long half-life (approximately 150 hours in humans) would prevent accurate titration of dosages in the clinical setting of organ transplantation. If these agents currently under investigation maintain the immunosuppressive properties of leflunomide with its relative lack of side effects, then these compounds may become an exciting addition to the immunosuppressive armamentarium.

## REFERENCES

1.  Stratta RJ, Sudan R, Sudan D. Long-term outcomes in simultaneous kidney–pancreas transplant recipients. Transplant Proc 1998; 30:1564–1565.
2.  Bruce DS, Newell KA, Josephson MA, et al. Long-term outcome of kidney–pancreas transplant recipients with good graft function at one year. Transplantation 1996; 62:451–456.
3.  Tesi RJ, Henry ML, Elkhammas EA, Davies EA, Ferguson RM. The frequency of rejection episodes after combined kidney–pancreas transplant—the impact of graft survival. Transplantation 1994; 58:424–430.
4.  Sollinger HW, Kalayoglu M, Hoffman RM, Deierhoi MH, Belzer FO. Quadruple immunosuppressive therapy in whole pancreas transplantation. Transplant Proc 1987; 19:2297–2299.
5.  Corry RJ, Egidi MF, Shapiro R, et al. Pancreas transplantation with enteric drainage under tacrolimus induction therapy. Transplant Proc 1997; 29:642.
6.  Moser M, De Smedt T, Sornasse T, et al. Glucocorticoids down-regulate dendritic cell function in vitro and in vivo. Eur J Immunol 1995; 25:2818–2824.
7.  Vieira PL, Kalinski P, Wierenga EA, Kapsenberg ML, de Jong EC. Glucocorticoids inhibit bioactive IL-12p70 production by in vitro generated human dendritic cells without affecting their T-cell stimulatory potential. J Immunol 1998; 161:5245–5251.
8.  Shapiro AM, Hao E, Lakey JR, Finegood D, Rajotte RV, Kneteman NM. Diabetogenic synergism in canine islet allografts from cyclosporine and steroids in combination. Transplant Proc 1998; 30:527.
9.  Smets YF, van der Pijl JW, de Fijter JW, Ringers J, Lemkes HH, Hamdy NA. Low bone mass and high incidence of fractures after successful simultaneous pancreas–kidney transplantation. Nephrol Dial Transplant 1998; 13:1250–1255.
10. Allison AC, Itoh H. MMF mode of action and effects on graft rejection. In: Thomson AW, Starzl TE, eds. Immunosuppressive Drugs: Developments in Anti-rejection Therapy. Boston, Brown, MA: Little, 1994:161–176.
11. Sollinger HW. Mycophenolate mofetil for the prevention of acute rejection in primary cadaveric renal allograft recipients. U.S. Renal Transplant Mycophenolate Mofetil Study Group. Transplantation 1995; 60:225–232.
12. Odorico JS, Pirsch JD, Knechtle SJ, D'Alessandro AM, Sollinger HW. A study comparing mycophenolate mofetil to azathioprine in simultaneous pancreas–kidney transplantation. Transplantation 1998; 66:1751–1759.
13. Gruessner RWG, Sutherland DER, Drangstveit MB, West M, Gruessner AC. mycophenolate mofetil and tacrolimus for induction and maintenance therapy after pancreas transplantation. Transplant Proc 1998; 30:518–520.
14. Tamura K, Woo J, Bakri MT, Thomson AW. Brequinar sodium inhibits IL-6 induced differentiation of a human B-cell line into IgM-secreting plasma cells. Immunology 1993; 79:587–593.
15. Sutherland DE, Moudry-Munns KC. International pancreas transplant registry report. Clin Transplants 1988:53–64.
16. Kahan BD. Cyclosporine. N Eng J Med 1989; 321:1725–1738.
17. Hojo M, Morimoto T, Maluccio M, et al. Cyclosporine induces cancer progression by a cell-autonomous mechanism. Nature 1999; 397:530–534.
18. Pirsch JD, Miller J, Deierhoi MH, Vincenti F, Filo RS. A comparison of tacrolimus (FK506) and cyclosporine for immunosuppression after cadaveric renal transplantation. FK506 Kidney Transplant Study Group. Transplantation 1997; 63:977–983.
19. El-Ghoroury M, Hariharan S, Peddi VR, et al. Efficacy and safety of tacrolimus versus cyclosporine in kidney and pancreas transplant recipients. Transplant Proc 1997; 29:649–651.
20. Elmer DS, Abdulkarim AB, Fraga D, et al. Metabolic effects of FK506 (tacrolimus) versus cyclosporine in portally-drained pancreas allografts. Transplant Proc 1998; 30:523–524.
21. Peddi VR, Demmy AM, Munda R, Alexander JW, First MR. Tacrolimus eliminates acute rejection as a major complication following simultaneous kidney and pancreas transplantation. Transplant Proc 1998; 30:509–511.
22. Gruessner RW, Burke GW, Stratta R, et al. A multicenter analysis of the first experience with FK-506 for induction and rescue therapy after pancreas transplantation. Transplantation 1996; 61:261–273.
23. Jordan ML, Shapiro R, Gritsch HA, et al. Long-term results of pancreas transplantation under tacrolimus immunosuppression. Transplantation 1999; 67:266–272.
24. Boyle MJ, Kahan BD. Immunosuppressive role of Rapamycin in allograft rejection. In: Thomson AW, Starzl TE, eds. Immunosuppressive Drugs: Developments in Anti-rejection Therapy. Boston, Brown, MA: Little, 1994:129–140.

25. Chen H, Qi S, Xu D, et al. Combined effect of Rapamycin and FK-506 in prolongation of small bowel graft survival in the mouse. Transplant Proc 1998; 30:2579–2581.
26. Vu MD, Qi S, Xu D, et al. Synergistic effects of mycophenolate mofetil and sirolimus in prevention of acute heart, pancreas, and kidney allograft rejection and in reversal of ongoing heart rejection in the rat. Transplantation 1998; 66:1575–1580.
27. Wadstrom J, Brekke B, Wrammer L, Ekberg H, Tyden G. Triple versus quadruple induction immunosuppression in pancreas transplantation. Transplant Proc 1995; 27:1317–1318.
28. Corry RJ, Egidi MF, Shapiro R, et al. Tacrolimus without anti-lymphocyte induction therapy prevents pancreas loss from rejection in 123 consecutive patients. Transplant Proc 1998; 30:521.
29. Gruessner RWG. Antibody induction therapy in pancreas transplantation. Transplant Proc 1998; 30:1556–1559.
30. Sollinger HW, Knectle SJ, Reed A, et al. Experience with 100 consecutive simultaneous kidney-pancreas transplants with bladder drainage. Ann Surg 1991; 214:703–711.
31. Peddi VR, Kamath S, Schroeder TJ, Munda R, First MR. Efficacy of OKT3 as primary therapy for histologically-confirmed acute renal allograft rejection in simultaneous kidney and pancreas transplant recipients. Transplant Proc 1998; 30:285–287.
32. Goldstein G. Overview of the development of Orthoclone OKT3: monoclonal antibody for therapeutic use in transplantation. Transplant Proc 1987; 19(2 suppl 1):1–6.
33. Suzuki S. Deoxyspergualin: mode of action and effects on graft rejection. In: Thomson Aw, Starzl TE, eds. Immunosuppressive Drugs: Developments in Anti-rejection Therapy. Boston, Brown, MA: Little, 1994:187–202.
34. Nadler SG, Tepper MA, Schacter B, Mazzucco CE. Interaction of the immunosuppressant deoxyspergualin with a member of the Hsp70 family of heat shock proteins. Science 1992; 258:484–486.
35. Tepper MA. Deoxyspergualin: mechanism of action studies of a novel immunosuppressive drug. Ann N Y Acad Sci 1993; 696:123–132.
36. Masroor S, Schroeder TJ, Michler RE, Alexander JW, First MR. Monoclonal antibodies in organ transplantation: an overview. Transplant Immunol 1994; 2:176–189.
37. Vincenti F, Kirkman R, Light S, et al. Interleukin-2-receptor blockade with Daclizumab to prevent acute rejection in renal transplantation. Daclizumab Triple Therapy Study Group. N Engl J Med 1998; 338:161–165.
38. Lin H, Wei RQ, Goodman RE, Bolling SF. CD28 blockade alters gene cytokine mRNA profiles in cardiac transplantation. Surgery 1997; 122:129–137.
39. Liu C, Deng S, Yang Z, et al. Local production of CTLA4-Ig by adenoviral-mediated gene transfer to the pancreas induces permanent allograft survival and donor specific tolerance. Transplant Proc 1999; 31:625–626.
40. Yang Y, Wilson JM. CD40 ligand-dependent T-cell activation: requirement of B7-CD28 signaling through CD-40. Science 1996; 273:1862–1864.
41. Lederman S, Yellin MJ, Krichevsky A, Belko J, Lee JJ, Chess L. Identification of a novel surface protein on activated CD4+ T cells that induces contact dependent B cell differentiation. J Exp Med 1992; 175:1091–1101.
42. Kirk AD, Harlan DM, Armstrong NN, et al. CTLA4-Ig and anti-CD40 ligand prevent renal allograft rejection in primates. Proc Natl Acad Sci 1997; 94:8789–8794.
43. Zheng XX, Li Y, Li C, et al. Blockade of CD40L/CD40 costimulatory pathway in a DS presensitization model of islet allograft leads to a state of allo-Ag specific tolerance and permits subsequent engraftment of donor strain islet or heart allografts. Transplant Proc 1999; 31:627–628.
44. Kirk AD, Burkly LC, Batty DS, et al. Treatment with humanized monoclonal antibody against CD154 prevents acute renal allograft rejection in nonhuman primates. Nat Med 1999; 5:686–693.
45. Larsen CP, et al. Long-term acceptance of skin and cardiac allografts after blocking CD40 and CD28 pathways. Nature 1996; 381:434–438.
46. Xu X, Williams JW, Bremer EG, Finnegan A, Chong AS. Inhibition of protein tyrosine phosphorylation in T cells by a novel immunosuppressive agent leflunomide. J Biol Chem 1995; 270:12,398–12,403.
47. Greene S, Watanabe K, Braatz-Trulson J, Lou L. Inhibition of dihydro-orate dehydrogenase by the immunosuppressive agent leflunomide. Biochem Pharmacol 1995; 50:861–867.
48. Nair RV, Cao WW, Morris RE. The anti-proliferative effect of leflunomide on vascular smooth muscle cells in vitro is mediated by selective inhibition of pyrimidine biosynthesis. Transplant Proc 1996; 28:3081.
49. Cao WW, Kao PN, Aoki Y, Xu JC, Shorthouse RA, Morris RE. A novel mechanism of action of the immunomodulatory drug, leflunomide: augmentation of the immunosuppressive cytokine, TGF-beta 1, and suppression of the immunostimulatory cytokine, IL-2. Transplant Proc 1996; 28:3079–3080.
50. Yeh LS, Gregory CR, Griffey SM, Lecouter RA, Hou SM, Morris RE. Combination leflunomide and cyclosporine prevents rejection in function of whole limb allografts in the rat. Transplantation 1997; 64:919–921.

# 12 | Immunosuppression for Pancreas Transplantation

**Amit Basu, Cynthia A. Smetanka, and Henkie P. Tan**
*Thomas E. Starzl Transplantation Institute, University of Pittsburgh School of Medicine, Pittsburgh, Pennsylvania, U.S.A.*

**Akhtar S. Khan**
*Milton S. Hershey Medical Center, Division of Transplantation, Hershey, Pennsylvania, U.S.A.*

**Ron Shapiro**
*Thomas E. Starzl Transplantation Institute, University of Pittsburgh School of Medicine, Pittsburgh, Pennsylvania, U.S.A.*

## INTRODUCTION

The aim of induction and maintenance immunosuppression is to prevent acute rejection and to allow long-term allograft function. The pancreatic allograft is more immunogenic than the kidney, and acute rejection rates of 75% were historically common (1) after pancreas transplantation. Advances in immunosuppression over the past decade have included the introduction of tacrolimus (TAC), mycophenolate mofetil (MMF), sirolimus (SRL), and antibody preparations such as Thymoglobulin (TMG) and the interleukin-2 (IL-2) receptor antagonists, basiliximab and daclizumab (DAC). A number of successful regimens have been evaluated in clinical trials of simultaneous pancreas–kidney (SPK) transplantation, pancreas after kidney transplantation (PAK), and pancreas transplantation alone (PTA). The ideal immunosuppressive regimen should be potent enough to prevent rejection, tailored to minimize immunosuppressive drug toxicity, and gentle enough to avoid the complications of over-immunosuppression. This chapter will discuss induction and maintenance immunosuppressive regimens after pancreas transplantation.

## SPK TRANSPLANTATION
### Evolution of Maintenance Immunosuppressive Agents

Most pancreas transplant surgery programs have utilized quadruple drug immunosuppression with antibody induction (Tables 1–3) (14). New immunosuppressive regimens have tended to focus on decreasing the incidence of acute rejection, with the goal of improving long-term outcomes (15).

The substitution of azathioprine (AZA) by MMF reduced the biopsy-proven kidney rejection rates in SPK patients from 75% to 31% (16). Withdrawal of steroids began with tacrolimus/MMF-based protocols (17,18), which demonstrated that prospectively planned steroid withdrawal was possible in 72% of patients within the first year after SPK (17). While International Pancreas Transplant Registry (IPTR) data have failed to show a significant survival benefit of pancreas transplants for TAC/MMF over cyclosporine (CsA)/MMF-based immunosuppression, a large prospective European randomized trial did show a pancreas graft survival advantage associated with TAC (see Chapter 34) (19). The utility of sirolimus in pancreas transplantation is still under investigation. Good preliminary results were reported in seven pancreas transplant patients (five SPK and two PAK), who were part of a larger study and treated with antithymocyte globulin (ATG), sirolimus, tacrolimus, and steroids (20).

**Table 1** Simultaneous Pancreas–Kidney Transplantation—Immunosuppression Trials (Retrospective)[a]

| Author(s) | Year | Reference | Induction | Maintenance immunosuppression | Duration of follow-up | Rejection rate (%) | Survival (%) 1 yr[a] | | | Survival (%) 5 yr | | |
|---|---|---|---|---|---|---|---|---|---|---|---|---|
| | | | | | | | P | K | Pt | P | K | Pt |
| Sutherland et al. | 1994–1998 | 2 | ATGAM | TAC + AZA; TAC + MMF | 1 yr | 34 | 70 | 87 | 87 | 73 | 81 | 81 |
| Sutherland et al. | 1998–2000 | 2 | DAC + ATGAM/RATG | TAC + MMF | 1 yr | 25 | 80 | 90 | 93 | 73 | 81 | 88 |
| Burke et al. | 2002 | 3 | DAC + RATG | ST + TAC + MMF | 1 yr | <10 | 100 | 100 | 100(6 m) | | | |
| | 2002 | 3 | DAC + RATG | ST + TAC + SRL | 1 yr | <10 | 95 | 100 | 100(6 m) | | | |
| Kaufman et al. | 2002 | 4 | Randomized no induction or anti IL-2 Ab | ST + TAC + MMF | 1 yr | 13 | 89 | 94 | 96 | | | |
| Kaufman et al. | 2002 | 4 | Thymoglobulin | ST (rapid withdrawal) + TAC + MMF or ST + TAC + SRL | 1 yr | 3.4 | 100 | 98 | 100 | | | |
| Saudek | 2001 | 5 | ATG (Fresenius), intra-op and three doses post-op | ST + MMF + TAC/CsA | 9.2 mo | 21 (K), 12.5 (P) | | | | | | |
| Stratta et al. | 2003 | 6 | DAC 1 mg/kg q14dX5 | ST + MMF + FK | 6 mo | 21 | | | | | | |
| Stratta et al. | 2003 | 6 | DAC 1 mg/kg q14dX2 | ST + MMF + FK | 6 mo | 17 | | | | | | |
| Sratta et al. | 2003 | 6 | No Ab | ST + MMF + FK | 6 mo | 32 | | | | | | |

[a]Except where follow-up is <1 year.

*Abbreviations:* P, pancreas; K, kidney; Pt, patient; ATGAM, antithymocyte globulin; TAC, tacrolimus; AZA, azathioprine; MMF, mycophenolate mofetil; ST, steroid; DAC, daclizumab; SRL, sirolimus; IL-2, interleukin-2; CsA, cyclosporine; ATG, antithymocyte globulin; Ab, antibody; RATG, rabbit antithymocyte globulin.

**Table 2** Simultaneous Pancreas–Kidney Transplantation—Immunosuppression Trials (Retrospective)[a]

| Author(s) | Year | Reference | Induction | Maintenance immunosuppression | Duration of follow-up | Rejection rate (%) | Survival (%) (1 yr)[a] | | | Survival (5 yr) | | |
|---|---|---|---|---|---|---|---|---|---|---|---|---|
| | | | | | | | P | K | Pt | P | K | Pt |
| Stratta et al. (portal-enteric) | 2003 | 7 | Daclizumab, basiliximab, thymoglobulin, no antibody | ST + MMF + TAC | 20 mo | 28 | 82 | 92 | 97.5 | | | |
| Woeste et al. | 2002 | 8 | ATG | ST + MMF + TAC | | 33 | | | | | | |
| | 2002 | 8 | ATG | ST + MMF + CsA | | 73 | | | | | | |
| Kaufman et al. | 2000 | 9 | ATGAM (bladder-drained) | MMF + TAC + ST (taper) | | 28 | 94 | 94 | 98 | | | |
| | 2000 | 9 | Anti-IL-2R antibody (enteric-drained) | MMF + TAC + ST (taper) | 1 yr | 6.1 | 89 | 97 | 97 | | | |
| | 2000 | 9 | No induction (enteric-drain) | MMF + TAC + ST (taper) | 1 yr | 23.5 | 89 | 97 | 97 | | | |

[a]Except where follow-up is >1 year.
*Abbreviations*: P, pancreas; K, kidney; Pt, patient; ST, steroid; ATGAM, antithymocyte globulin; TAC, tacrolimus; MMF, mycophenolate mofetil; IL-2, interleukin-2; CsA, cyclosporine; ATG, antithymocyte globulin; Ab, antibody.

**Table 3** Simultaneous Pancreas–Kidney Transplantation—Immunosuppression Trials (Prospective)[a]

| Author(s) | Year | Reference | Induction | Maintenance immunosuppression | Duration of follow-up (yr) | Rejection rate (%) | Survival (%) (1 yr)[a] | | | Survival (5 yr) | | |
|---|---|---|---|---|---|---|---|---|---|---|---|---|
| | | | | | | | P | K | Pt | P | K | Pt |
| Ciancio et al. | 2000 | 10 | IV FK 506 | MMF + TAC + ST | | 23 | | | | | | |
| Land et al. | 2002 | 11 | ATG | ST + MMF + CsA | 1 | | 73.9 | | | | | |
| | 2002 | 11 | ATG | ST + MMF + TAC | 1 | | 94.2 | | | | | |
| Vincenti and Stock | 2003 | 12 | RATG | TAC + MMF + SRL | | <10 | 90 | 90 | 90 | | | |
| Burke et al. | 2004 | 13 | No induction | TAC + MMF + ST | 3 | | 76 | 82 | 90 | | | |
| | 2004 | 13 | T-cell depleting agents, anti-IL-2 Ab | TAC + MMF + ST | 3 | | 76 | 92 | 94 | | | |

[a]Except where duration of follow-up >1 year.
*Abbreviations*: P, pancreas; K, kidney; Pt, patient; TAC, tacrolimus; AZA, azathioprine; MMF, mycophenolate mofetil; SRL, sirolimus; IL-2, interleukin-2; CsA, cyclosporine; ATG, antithymocyte globulin; Ab, antibody; ST, steroid.

Analyses of United Network of Organ Sharing data have focused on outcomes according to the maintenance immunosuppressive agents used. Since 1994, these have been one of TAC + MMF, TAC + AZA, CsA + MMF, or CsA + AZA (21). After Food and Drug Administration (FDA) approval of TAC in 1994 and MMF in 1995, TAC + MMF and CsA + MMF combinations were used with near equal frequency in SPK transplantation in the mid-1990s. Since 1997, TAC utilization has increased substantially, and is now being used in over 80% of SPK recipients.

## Antibody Induction

Antibody induction agents can be divided into two groups: T-cell depleting polyclonal (e.g., horse or rabbit antithymocyte globulin—ATGAM or Thymoglobulin) or monoclonal (e.g., muromonoab-CD3-OKT3, or alemtuzumab-Campath-1H) antibodies; or nondepleting [monoclonal anti-CD25 receptor—basiliximab (Simulect) or daclizumab (Zenapax)] antibodies. About 30% of SPK recipients have continued to receive no antibody induction since 1997. Anti-CD25 receptor antibodies began to be used as soon as they were introduced in 1998. In SPK transplantation, depleting antibodies were used slightly more frequently than nondepleting antibodies in 1998, but in 1999 and 2000 nondepleting antibodies were used slightly more frequently. In addition, approximately 10% of SPK recipients received both depleting and nondepleting antibodies in 2000. Overall pancreatic graft survival rates (GSRs) in patients receiving or not receiving antibody induction did not differ significantly at one year, and ranged from 82% to 86%. In the SPK bladder-drained subgroup, there was no significant difference in GSR according to whether or not induction therapy was given. In the SPK enteric-drained subgroup, GSR differences were small but significant ($p < 0.02$), at two years, ranging from 80% in patients not receiving antibody induction to 86% in those given nondepleting antibodies (22). In the logistic and Cox multivariate analysis of United Network of Organ Sharing data, induction therapy with anti-CD25 antibodies slightly decreased the risk of graft failure in SPK transplant recipients (22).

Analysis of individual components of immunosuppression is difficult because programs tend to utilize different combinations of agents, and it is easier, although perhaps less elegant, to approach the subject in terms of the evolution of multidrug regimens. What follows is an overview of different regimens from individual centers and multicenter trials (see also the single center chapters 27–34).

## Single- and Multicenter Experiences

In a report analyzing data from more than 1000 pancreas transplantations at the University of Minnesota, patients were divided into Eras 0 to 4, depending on the immunosuppression and duct management technique (2). In Era 0 (the Lillehei series) lasting from 1966–1973, only azathioprine and prednisone were used for immunosuppression. In Era 1, which lasted from July 1978 to June 1984, immunosuppression evolved from azathioprine and prednisone to cyclosporine and prednisone to cyclosporine, azathioprine, and prednisone (triple therapy) using Minnesota antilymphoblast globulin (MALG) in nearly all cases. Era 2 began in July 1986 and lasted till December 1993; the immunosuppressive regimen consisted of MALG or muromonoab-CD3 (OKT3) for induction and a combination of cyclosporine, azathioprine, and prednisone for maintenance. Era 3 began in 1994, when tacrolimus was approved by the U.S. FDA and begun to be used in clinical pancreas transplantation. A year later, when MMF was approved, it was immediately used with tacrolimus. The horse ATG (ATGAM) was used for induction immunosuppression, and OKT3 for the treatment of rejection episodes. Duct management in Era 3 was predominantly bladder drainage. Era 4 begin in March 1998, when DAC, alone or in combination with the polyclonal anti-T-cell antibody (ATGAM, initially; Thymoglobulin after it was approved by the FDA in 1999), was added to the induction immunosuppressive regimen. Anti-T-cell agents were started before graft revascularization. Enteric drainage was used as the principal exocrine drainage technique for deceased donor grafts in Era 4 (exceptions being some high-risk elderly or obese patients, or patients with chronic peritonitis from peritoneal dialysis). The principal difference between

Era 2 versus Eras 3 and 4 was the use of cyclosporine and azathioprine in the former, and tacrolimus and azathioprine or MMF in the latter for maintenance immunosuppression. [In the past year, the Minnesota program has changed yet again, using antibody induction and maintenance with alemtuzumab (Campath-1H) and a single dose of Thymoglobulin, followed by MMF monotherapy—see Chapter 27]. In primary SPK patients, pancreas and kidney graft survival rates were significantly higher in Eras 3 and 4 combined than in Era 2 (2). In Eras 3 and 4 combined, one-year patient, pancreas, and kidney survival rates were 92%, 79%, and 88%, respectively; at five years, the corresponding figures were 88%, 73%, and 81%. For technically successful cases (and with death with a functioning graft censored), the one-year rejection-associated graft loss rate was significantly lower in Eras 3 and 4 combined than in Era 2, 9% versus 19% (2). The cumulative incidence of rejection episodes by one year after transplantation was 34% in Era 3 and 25% in Era 4. After one year, the probability of having a rejection episode, if one had not previously occurred, was almost nonexistent (2). The one-year patient, pancreas, and kidney graft survival rates for SPK re-transplants were 87%, 70%, and 87%, versus 93%, 80%, and 90% for primary transplants, in Eras 3 and 4, respectively.

In a report on 500 SPK transplants from the University of Wisconsin (1), immunosuppressive therapy also evolved over the 12-year time span of the series. From 1985–1989, the immunosuppressive protocol consisted of a quadruple sequential regimen of azathioprine, prednisone, cyclosporine A, and a 14-day course of MALG. From January 1991 to January 1996, a 14-day course of OKT3 replaced MALG. From January 1996 to December 1997, ATGAM was used for induction therapy, the duration of which varied from 6–15 days. In May 1995, when MMF became commercially available, it replaced azathioprine at a dosage of 1500 mg twice daily. The use of induction therapy was associated with superior outcomes. No differences were noted between MALG/ATGAM and OKT3. However, the cytokine release syndrome associated with OKT3 led to its abandonment in favor of ATGAM in the latter part of the series. After the introduction of MMF, the course of ATGAM therapy was shortened from 12 to 14 days to four to eight days. More recently, DAC has been used. The introduction of MMF for maintenance immunosuppression led to a marked reduction in the incidence of rejection in the first year, as well as a reduction in the incidence of steroid-resistant rejection. Two-year kidney and pancreas survival rates with MMF were superior to those associated with azathioprine maintenance therapy. MMF use also allowed for more aggressive steroid tapering (1).

The rate of acute rejection in SPK transplantation has been falling over the past decade at the University of Miami Medical Center, from nearly 100% to < 10% in the first year following transplantation (3). In a prospective, randomized trial, 42 SPK recipients received Thymoglobulin and daclizumab induction, with TAC and steroids as baseline immunosuppression. Twenty-two patients were randomized to receive MMF, and 20 patients received SRL, in addition to TAC and steroids. Actuarial patient, kidney, and pancreas allograft survivals, with six-month's follow-up, were 100%, 100%, and 95% in the SRL group, and 100%, 100%, and 100% in the MMF group. The incidence of acute rejection was <10% and limited to those instances where recipient immunosuppression was significantly reduced (3).

A prospective study of combined TAC, MMF, and steroids without antibody induction was carried out in 17 SPK transplant patients at Miami. These patients received low-dose intravenous TAC as induction therapy. Clinical and biopsy-proven rejection was seen in four (23%) patients. Leukopenia, gastroparesis, and gastrointestinal side effects, leading to discontinuation of MMF or low TAC levels, were present in those patients who developed rejection. All rejection episodes were responsive to steroids (10).

Ciancio et al., from Miami, also have reported on the use of intravenous tacrolimus and mycophenolate mofetil for induction and maintenance immunosuppression in simultaneous pancreas–kidney or kidney retransplant recipients (23). Group A consisted of six patients with previous transplants who underwent SPK, and Group B consisted of four patients with previous SPK who underwent deceased donor kidney transplants. With a mean follow-up of 20.4 months (range 12–27 months) in all Group A and B patients, the kidneys and pancreases were functioning, although one patient in Group A developed type II diabetes. Two patients in Group A developed three rejection episodes that responded to steroid treatment.

At Northwestern University, immunosuppression for SPK transplantation was divided into four eras over a period of 8.5 years (4). In Era 1 (March 1993 to February 1997), three immunosuppression combinations were used: CsA/azathioprine/steroids ($n = 28$), CsA/MMF/steroids ($n = 8$), or tacrolimus/MMF/steroids ($n = 10$); bladder drainage was used. In Era 2 (July 1995 to February 1998), the combination of tacrolimus, MMF, and corticosteroids was used with bladder drainage. In Era 3, combinations of TAC (target 12-hour trough concentrations 10–12 ng/mL by immunoassay) and MMF (target dose 3 g/day) were used along with corticosteroids for maintenance immunosuppression; enteric drainage was utilized. Immunosuppression in Era 4 was distinct from the earlier eras in that steroids were eliminated within six days of transplantation and TAC was combined with either MMF ($n = 20$) or SRL ($n = 38$); again enteric drainage was utilized. TAC target 12-hour trough concentrations were 10–12 ng/mL, MMF target dosing was 3 g/day, and SRL target 24-hour trough concentrations were 4–8 ng/mL. In Eras 1 and 2, all recipients received induction therapy with ATGAM for 7–14 days after transplantation. Induction therapy in Era 3 had 17 patients randomized to a noninduction therapy arm and 37 patients randomized to an anti-IL-2 receptor monoclonal antibody (daclizumab, $n = 35$; basiliximab, $n = 2$). In Era 4, induction therapy consisted of Thymoglobulin 1.0 mg/kg intraoperatively and on postoperative days 1, 2, 4, 6, 8, 10, 12, and 14. The one-year actuarial patient survival rates in Eras 3 and 4 were 96.3% and 100%, respectively; the one-year actuarial kidney survival rates in Eras 3 and 4 were 94.4% and 97.7%, respectively, and the one-year actuarial pancreas survival rates were 88.9% and 100%, respectively. The one-year rejection-free rate was 87.1% for Era 3 and 96.6% for Era 4. The quality of kidney function significantly improved in the three eras in which modern immunosuppressive agents were used, compared to Era 1. In Era 4, the rapid elimination of corticosteroids was successful in all recipients, and patient and graft survival rates were higher than those observed in the previous three eras (4). Rejection rates further decreased in Era 4. The improved results were not associated with an increase in infectious complications. The Northwestern group concluded that corticosteroids could be rapidly eliminated prospectively in all recipients, without a decrease in graft survival rates or an increase in the rate of rejection (4). Most recently, the Northwestern group has explored the use of alemtuzumab instead of Thymoglobulin in pancreas recipients.

In a report of SPK transplants from the Northwestern University, the results of 50 patients with bladder-drained pancreas allografts were compared with the next 50 recipients who had enterically drained pancreas allografts, and included a subgroup of patients ($n = 17$) who were randomized to receive no induction immunotherapy (9). Maintenance immunosuppression was with MMF and tacrolimus. Corticosteroids were used and tapered over one year to 5–7.5 mg/day. In the bladder-drained group all 50 patients received induction therapy with ATGAM, while in the enteric-drained group induction therapy consisted of anti-IL-2 receptor monoclonal antibody (daclizumab, 31 cases; basiliximab, two cases). The one-year actuarial patient, kidney, and pancreas survival rates in the bladder-drainage group were 98%, 94%, and 94%, and in the enteric-drainage group were 97%, 97%, and 89%, respectively. In the bladder-drained group, the rates of rejection at 1, 6, and 12 months after transplantation were 6%, 18%, and 28%, respectively; in the enteric-drained group, the incidences of acute rejection at 1, 6, and 12 months after transplantation were 12%, 12%, and 16%, respectively. In the enteric-drained group, the 33 patients who received induction therapy with anti-IL-2 receptor antibody had a 6.1% incidence of acute rejection at 12 months compared to a 23.5% incidence of acute rejection at 12 months in 17 patients randomized to noninduction therapy group (9). Significantly reduced rates of readmission and the mean number of readmission days per patient were observed in recipients with enteric drainage. Within the group that received enteric drainage, 48% of recipients who received induction therapy avoided readmission, and only 29% of recipients who did not receive induction therapy avoided readmission.

In a study done on 24 SPK transplant patients from the Czech Republic, immunosuppressive therapy consisted of 2 g/day MMF started preoperatively, 500 mg intravenous methylprednisone, followed by 20 mg/day prednisone, a calcineurin inhibitor beginning six hours after surgery, and intraoperative ATG 8 mg/kg (Fresenius) administered prior to revascularization and followed by an additional three doses of 3 mg/kg over the next three days (5). Recipients were randomized to receive either cyclosporine or tacrolimus. With a mean follow-up of 9.2 months, kidney rejection was observed in five (20.8%) and pancreas rejection in three recipients (12.5%). The most important side effect of ATG administration was thrombocytopenia.

In a study done using DAC and ATG versus ATG alone from Ruhr University, Germany, in 31 SPK transplant patients maintained on triple immunosuppression, no difference was noted between the ATG and ATG/DAC groups with regard to acute rejection episodes, infectious complications, and patient and graft survival (24). The combination of TAC, MMF, and steroids with ATG induction had an incidence of acute rejection of 33% compared with an incidence of 73% using ATG induction followed by cyclosporine, azathioprine, and steroids in another randomized trial reported from Ruhr University, Germany (8). The incidence of infections, including cytomegalovirus, and malignancies was not higher using FK/MMF compared to CsA/AZA regimen with five year's follow-up.

A study comparing DAC to horse ATGAM induction was performed at the Washington Hospital Center in Washington, D.C., in 24 SPK transplant patients between September 1995 and September 1998 (25). Maintenance immunosuppression consisted of cyclosporine or TAC, mycophenolate mofetil, and steroids. DAC induction, coupled with triple immunosuppressive therapy, was associated with a reduced incidence of rejection and a longer time to acute rejection, compared to ATGAM induction.

A prospective multicenter, open-labeled study was undertaken to evaluate different doses of DAC induction in SPK transplantation (6). Of the 297 SPK transplant patients enrolled, 107 patients (Group I) received DAC 1 mg/kg per dose every 14 days for five doses, 112 patients (Group II) received DAC 2 mg/kg per dose every 14 days for two doses, and 78 patients (Group III) received no antibody induction (6). All patients received tacrolimus, MMF, and steroids as maintenance immunosuppression. The probability of kidney or pancreas allograft rejection at six months was 21%, 17%, and 32% in Groups I, II, and III, respectively ($p = 0.042$). At six months, the actuarial event-free survival (no acute rejection, allograft loss, or death) rates were 66%, 77%, and 56% in Groups I, II, and III, respectively (Group I vs. III, $p = 0.119$, Group II vs. III, $p = 0.002$). There was no difference in the incidence of serious adverse events, including infectious complications, among the groups. Daclizumab was safe and effective in reducing the incidence of acute rejection in SPK recipients compared with no antibody induction. The two-dose regimen of daclizumab (2 mg/kg on days 0 and 14) compared favorably with the standard five-dose regimen (6).

A study was performed at the University of Tennessee on 67 SPK patients using portal-enteric drainage with maintenance immunosuppression consisting of TAC, MMF, and steroids. No antibody induction therapy was given in 33 patients; the others received DAC ($n = 15$), basiliximab ($n = 2$), or Thymoglobulin ($n = 14$) induction. Of the patients, 14.5% were African-American (7). Patient, kidney, and pancreas graft survival rates were 97%, 93%, and 82%, respectively, with a mean follow-up of 20 months (range 1–56). Five kidney graft losses and 12 pancreas graft losses occurred. The incidence of acute rejection was 28%, but no grafts were lost to acute rejection. The composite end point of no rejection, graft loss, or mortality was attained by 63% of patients, suggesting excellent intermediate term outcome.

In a report from Pittsburgh (26), 123 patients (106 in combination with a kidney transplant) received pancreas transplants over a three-year period. No antibody induction was used. Maintenance immunosuppression consisted of intravenous TAC for the first five to seven days, followed by oral TAC twice a day. Patients also received tapering steroid doses and azathioprine during the first half of the series, and MMF during the second half. With an 18-month follow-up, patient, kidney, and pancreas survival rates were 98%, 94%, and 83%, respectively. Three patients lost graft function to chronic rejection, and one patient lost the graft to antibody-mediated rejection. No grafts were lost to acute cellular rejection (26); antibody induction therapy was not necessary to prevent early graft loss from rejection.

In a multicenter trial that assessed the effect of antibody induction in SPK transplant recipients receiving tacrolimus, mycophenolate mofetil, and corticosteroids (13), 174 SPK transplant recipients were randomized to induction ($n = 87$) or noninduction ($n = 87$), and followed for three years. Induction agents included T-cell depleting or IL-2 receptor antibodies. At three years, actual patient (94.3% and 89.7%) and pancreas (75.9% and 75.9%) survivals were similar between the induction and noninduction groups, respectively. Actual kidney survival was significantly better in the induction group compared to the noninduction group at three years (92% vs. 82%; $p = 0.04$) (13). The odds of kidney rejection were 4.6 times greater in African-Americans, regardless of whether they had received antibody induction ($p = 0.004$). There were significantly higher rates of cytomegalovirus infection and disease in those receiving depleting antibody induction (36.1%), compared to those receiving IL-2 receptor antibodies (2%) or no induction (8.1%).

The EuroSPK study group reported its one-year results of a large multicenter trial comparing tacrolimus versus cyclosporine in primary simultaneous pancreas–kidney transplantation (11). Two hundred five patients were enrolled in this study. After ATG induction, patients were randomized to receive either TAC or CsA microemulsion together with MMF and steroids. At one year posttransplant, patient and kidney survival were excellent in both treatment arms. There was a significant difference in pancreas graft survival: 94.2% for TAC and 73.9% for CsA ($p = 0.00048$). There were significantly fewer grade 2 and 3 rejections with TAC-based therapy. In another publication (19) reporting on results of the same study, the EuroSPK study group presented data showing that 34 patients were switched from CsA to TAC, but only six patients receiving TAC required conversion to alternative therapy during the course of the study. Mean doses of MMF at one year were also lower in the TAC group (1.36 vs. 1.67 g/day; $p = 0.007$).

Thymoglobulin induction, followed by MMF, sirolimus, and low-dose tacrolimus for maintenance therapy has been used in 30 simultaneous pancreas–kidney transplants at the University of California at San Francisco (12). Using this steroid-free maintenance regimen, rejection rates were less than 10% for either the kidney or the pancreas. Kidney and pancreas allograft survival at one year was 90%. With two years' follow-up, there were no admissions for opportunistic infections and no cases of posttransplant lymphoproliferative disorder (12).

Eleven type I diabetic patients with end-stage renal disease received SPK transplants from 11 donors in Halifax, Nova Scotia (Group 1). The 11 mate kidneys from the same donors were transplanted into 11 nondiabetic patients (Group 2) (27). Immunosuppression in Group 1 was induced with thymoglobulin; maintenance immunosuppression was with TAC, sirolimus, and prednisone 25 mg on postoperative day 1, tapered by 5 mg every other day to 10 mg/day, with discontinuation by six months. In Group 2, antibody induction was used in four patients; maintenance therapy was with CsA, MMF, and prednisone. At a mean follow-up of 16 months, no patient or graft was lost in either group, but there were differences in renal function, acute rejection rates, and side effects, which favored TAC–SRL compared to the CsA–MMF. It is likely that the 20% to 30% difference in GFR were attributable to the low trough levels of tacrolimus, made possible by the addition of sirolimus (27).

## PAK TRANSPLANTATION

According to data from the IPTR, the current nearly uniform use of TAC + MMF in PAK transplant makes comparison with other regimens difficult, although GSRs have been significantly better than in the preceding era when CsA + AZA was used (Table 4) (22). By 2001, only 20% of PAK transplant recipients were not receiving antibody induction. The proportion of recipients given no induction, depleting antibody alone, a nondepleting antibody alone, or both for induction have been about the same since 1998. In the overall analysis of TAC + MMF-treated primary PAK transplant recipients, GSR did not differ significantly whether or not antibody induction was given, although it tended to be numerically higher in PAK recipients given depleting or nondepleting antibodies than in those not given antibody induction (22). In the PAK category, the relative risk (RR) of pancreas graft failure was reduced by the use of TAC and MMF for immunosuppression (22).

Between July 1, 1978, and April 30, 2000, 406 PAK transplants were performed at the University of Minnesota (28). Immunosuppression was divided into eras. In Era 1, only azathioprine and prednisone were used for induction and maintenance immunosuppression; only one patient received antibody therapy with MALG. In Era 2, CsA was added for induction and maintenance therapy; all recipients received antibody induction therapy

**Table 4** Pancreas After Kidney Transplants—Immunosuppression Trials (Retrospective)

| Author(s) | Year | Reference | Induction | Maintenance immunosuppression | Duration follow-up (yr) | Rejection rate (%) | Survival (%) (1 yr) | | | Survival (%) (3 yr) | | |
|---|---|---|---|---|---|---|---|---|---|---|---|---|
| | | | | | | | P | K | Pt | P | K | Pt |
| Gruessner et al. | 2001 | 28 | ATGAM (99%) or OKT3 (1%) × 5 day | TAC + ST + AZA/MMF | 3 | 43 | 78 | | 97 | 60 | | 90 |
| Gruessner et al. | 2001 | 28 | DAC alone (21%), or DAC + ATGAM/RATG (79%) × 3 day | TAC + ST + MMF | 1 | 51 | 77 | | 96 | | | |

*Abbreviations*: P, pancreas; K, kidney; Pt, patient; ATGAM, antithymocyte globulin; TAC, tacrolimus; AZA, azathioprine; MMF, mycophenolate mofetil; ST, steroids; RATG, rabbit antithymocyte globulin.

(MALG or ATGAM in 88% and OKT3 in 12% of recipients). In Era 3, TAC was used in combination with prednisone, and initially AZA. MMF replaced AZA once it was approved by the FDA. Polyclonal antibody induction therapy with ATGAM was used in 99% and monoclonal antibody (OKT3) in only 1% of patients; the median duration of antibody therapy was five days. In Era 4, TAC, MMF, and prednisone were the principal maintenance immunosuppressive agents. For induction, DAC was used, either alone (21%) or in combination (79%) with a polyclonal antibody (ATGAM or Thymoglobulin). The median duration of antibody therapy was three days. Overall patient survival rates (cadaveric and living donor) at one and three years in Era 3 were 97% and 90%, respectively, and at one year in Era 4 was 96%. Overall pancreas graft survival rates (cadaveric and living donor) at one and three years in Era 3 were 78% and 60%, respectively, and in Era 4 at one year was 77%. Upon analyzing technically successful transplants, pancreas graft loss rates to rejection in Era 3 at one and three years were 10% and 19%, respectively; in Era 4, at one year, it was 9%. The rates of first reversible rejection episodes at one and three years in Era 3 were 43% and 52%, respectively, in primary transplants, and 38% and 38% in re-transplants. The rate in Era 4 was 51% in primary transplants and 47% in re-transplants. The rate of first rejection episodes at one year in Eras 3 and 4 combined, according to the type of induction therapy, was 42% for polyclonal induction therapy only, 36% for monoclonal antibody induction therapy only, and 59% for combined monoclonal and polyclonal induction therapy. This difference is statistically significant ($p = 0.05$). PAK transplants can now be performed almost as successfully as SPK transplants; the introduction of TAC and MMF in the mid-1990s contributed to this development. The introduction of newer anti-T-cell agents such as the monoclonal interleukin-2 receptor blockers has not resulted in further improvement in post-transplant outcome. Combining monoclonal and polyclonal antibodies in Era 4 for an overall shorter antibody induction period did not increase graft survival. Using TAC- and MMF-based immunosuppression, only 20% of recipients experiencing rejection episodes ultimately lost their pancreas graft to irreversible rejection. In Eras 3 and 4, when TAC was being used, there no longer existed a difference in outcome between primary transplants and re-transplants. In addition, with the use of TAC, the advantage of living donor PAK transplants over deceased donor PAK transplants no longer existed (28). Again, the most recent regimens at the University of Minnesota have included alemtuzumab, Thymoglobulin, and MMF or SRL monotherapy.

The IPTR analysis suggested that the use of anti-T-cell antibody induction therapy was associated with higher one-year pancreas graft survival rates. The maintenance combination of MMF and TAC demonstrated a trend toward higher one-year pancreas graft survival rates (29). Virtually, all patients reported to the IPTR received corticosteroids, at least during the induction and early maintenance phases of immunosuppression.

## SOLITARY PANCREAS TRANSPLANTS

Some of the reported studies have combined data on PAK and PTA transplantation together in analysis of solitary pancreas (SP) transplants, and these are presented here.

Data from 29 patients who received 30 solitary pancreas transplants (17 PTA, 13 PAK) at the Mayo Clinic between January 1998 and February 2000 were reviewed. Maintenance immunosuppression was with TAC, MMF, and prednisone (30). Antibody induction therapy consisted of one of three regimens: DAC, 1 mg/kg on day 0, 7, 14; OKT3, 5 mg daily on days 0 to 7; or thymoglobulin, 1.5 mg/kg on days 0 to 10. The primary end point of the study was biopsy-proven acute rejection in the first six months after pancreas transplantation. The mean follow-up time was 14.8 months. Biopsy-proven acute rejection in the first six months was significantly lower in the Thymoglobulin group (7.7%), compared with the OKT3 group (60%) or the daclizumab group (50%). The one-year pancreas graft survival was 89.3% overall and 91.7% in the thymoglobulin group (31).

Eighteen pancreas after kidney transplants and four pancreas transplants alone were performed between January 1998 and October 2000 at McGill University, Canada. One-year patient and graft survival rates of 100% and 96% were obtained, with a one-year acute rejection rate of 27.3%. Induction therapy with TMG, at a starting dose of 1.5 mg/kg/day, was started 12 hours postoperatively (32). The daily dose of TMG was held if the total leukocyte count was $< 2500/\text{min}^3$ or if the lymphocyte count was $< 100/\text{min}^3$. Maintenance therapy was with steroids, tacrolimus, and MMF. Monitoring the total leukocyte and lymphocyte counts resulted in a 43% reduction in the amount of TMG used, compared with recommended dosing; patient and graft survivals were excellent, with acute rejection rates comparing favorably with other published series.

Twenty-eight patients underwent solitary pancreas transplantation at the University of Tennessee, with 13 patients undergoing PTA and 15 patients undergoing PAK transplantation (33). Solitary pancreas transplantation was done with portal-enteric drainage in 18 patients and systemic-enteric drainage in 10 patients. Thirteen patients received DAC induction, while the next 15 received TMG induction. Patient and pancreas graft survival rates were 96% and 79%, respectively, with a mean follow-up of 22 months. The incidence of acute rejection was 54%, including 50% in PTA and 58% in PAK recipients. Patients receiving TMG induction had a lower rate of rejection than those receiving DAC induction (43% vs. 70%). Portal-enteric drainage was associated with a slightly lower rate of acute rejection [44% portal-enteric vs. 75% systemic-enteric; $p = \text{NS}$ (not significant)]. Solitary pancreas transplants with portal-enteric drainage and TMG induction may be associated with improved intermediate-term outcomes and possible immunological advantages (33).

A report from the University of Wisconsin emphasized improved solitary pancreas graft survival in the modern immunosuppressive era (31). Twenty-three SP transplants (14 PAK, four PTA, five pancreas after SPK) performed after January 1997 were compared to 56 SP transplants (53 PAK, one PTA, two pancreas after SPK) performed before 1994. In the earlier era, immunosuppressive therapy included CsA, AZA, corticosteroids, and, in half the patients, antilymphocyte globulin or OKT3. The newer SP transplants received TAC, MMF, corticosteroids, and induction with antithymocyte globulin ($n = 9$), OKT3 ($n = 1$), daclizumab ($n = 5$), or basiliximab ($n = 8$). The one-year patient survival was 85% in the early era and 100% in the more recent era. The one-year graft survival in the early era was 19%; in the recent era, it was 87% ($p = 0.0001$). Of the early SP transplants, 76% experienced at least one rejection episode within the first year, whereas only 35% of recent SP transplants experienced acute rejection during the first year ($p = 0.04$) (31).

## PANCREAS TRANSPLANTATION ALONE

According to the IPTR, in the PTA category, the nearly uniform use of TAC + MMF immunosuppression made comparison with other regimens difficult, although graft survival rates were significantly higher than in preceding eras when maintenance was with cyclosporine and azathioprine (Table 5) (22). By 2001, the percentage of PTA patients receiving no antibody induction therapy was 15%. The proportion of patients given a depleting antibody, a nondepleting antibody, or both, was about equal in 1998, but by 2001 nondepleting antibodies were seldom used alone. More than a third of PTA recipients received both depleting and nondepleting antibodies. In the overall analysis of TAC + MMF-treated PTA recipients, graft survival rates did not differ significantly by type of induction therapy. The RR of rejection was decreased in patients given TAC. The use of TAC also decreased the RR for technical failure of PTA.

In the report analyzing results of more than 1000 pancreas transplants at the University of Minnesota, the time period was divided into eras, depending on immunosuppressive protocol and duct drainage (2). Immunosuppression in the different eras has been described in the section under SPK transplant. In Eras 3 and 4 combined, for PTA transplants, patient and pancreas graft survival rates at one-year were 95% and 76%; at five years, they were 78% and 57%. The rejection graft loss rates in Eras 3 and 4 were 35% and 9%, respectively.

The lower rejection rate in PAK than in PTA recipients may be related to the fact that PAK patients are chronically immunosuppressed prior to transplantation. Based on this reasoning, in March 1998, the Minnesota program began to give immunosuppression (TAC and MMF) to PTA candidates while they were on the waiting list (35). The average waiting time (and thus the duration of immunosuppression) was 6.5 months. TAC and MMF were given pre- and posttransplant, and DAC as well as TMG were given for induction with the first doses given prior to revascularization and the next four doses given posttransplantation. The PTA GSR improved significantly ($p < 0.0001$) from era to era, and was 80% at one year in

**Table 5**  Pancreas Transplants Alone—Immunosuppression Trials (Retrospective)

| Author(s) | Year | Reference | Induction | Maintenance immunosuppression | Duration follow-up (yr) | Rejection rate (%) | Survival (%) (1 yr) | | | Survival (%) (5 yr) | | |
|---|---|---|---|---|---|---|---|---|---|---|---|---|
| | | | | | | | P | K | Pt | P | K | Pt |
| Sutherland et al. | 1994–1998 | 2 | ATGAM | TAC + AZA/TAC+MMF | | 35 | 78 | | 95 | 57 | | 76 |
| Sutherland et al. | 1998–2000 | 2 | DAC+ATGAM/RATG | TAC+MMF | | 9 | 78 | | 95 | 57 | | 76 |
| Bartlett et al. | 1996 | 34 | | TAC | 1 | | 90.1 | | | | | |
| Bartlett et al. | 1996 | 34 | | CsA | 1 | | 53.4 | | | | | |

*Abbreviations*: P, pancreas; K, kidney; Pt, patient; ATGAM, antithymocyte globulin; DAC, daclizumab; TAC, tacrolimus; AZA, azathioprine; MMF, mycophenolate mofetil; CsA, cyclosporine; RATG, rabbit antithymocyte globulin.

**Table 6**  Sirolimus in Pancreas Transplantation—Immunosuppression Trials[a]

| Author(s) | Year | Reference | Induction | Maintenance immunosuppression | Duration of follow-up | Rejection rate (%) | Survival (%) (1 yr)[a] | | | Survival (5 yr) | | |
|---|---|---|---|---|---|---|---|---|---|---|---|---|
| | | | | | | | P | K | Pt | P | K | Pt |
| Burke et al. | 2002 | 3 | RATG + DAC | ST + TAC + MMF | 6 mo | <10 | 100 | 100 | 100 | | | |
| Burke et al. | 2002 | 3 | RATG + DAC | ST + TAC + SRL | 6 mo | <10 | 95 | 100 | 100 | | | |
| Kaufman et al. | 2002 | 4,38 | RATG | ST (rapid taper) + TAC + MMF, ST (rapid taper) + TAC + SRL | 1 yr | | 100 | 95 | 100 | | | |
| Vincenti and Stock | 2003 | 12 | RATG | TAC + MMF + SRL | 1 yr | <10 | 90 | 90 | | | | |
| Friese et al. | 2003 | 39 | RATG | TAC + MMF + SRL (ST discontinued by 1 wk post-op) | 3 mo | 2.5 | 100 | | | | | |

[a]Unless duration of follow-up <1 year.
*Abbreviations*: P, pancreas; K, kidney; Pt, patient; DAC, daclizumab; TAC, tacrolimus; MMF, mycophenolate mofetil; SRL, sirolimus; ST, steroids.

Era 4. The risk of having at least one reversible rejection episode in recipients of technically successful grafts was also slightly lower ($p = 0.06$) in Era 4 than in Era 3. With the protocol of pretransplant immunosuppression for PTA recipients, one-year results for 1998–2000 (Era 4) cases are similar to those of SPK and PAK results in Eras 3 and 4 (1994–2000). More recently, alemtuzumab and Thymoglobulin induction, with MMF or SRL monotherapy, has been employed by the Minnesota group.

Twenty-seven pancreas transplant alone recipients prospectively were treated with TAC-based immunosuppression (PA-TAC) at the University of Maryland (34). Percutaneous biopsy was performed for hyperamylasemia, hyperlipasemia, hypoamylasuria, or unexplained fever. One-year pancreas graft survival in these patients was compared with 15 cyclosporine-treated pancreas transplant alone cases (PA-CsA) and 113 SPK patients. The one-year pancreas graft survival rate of 90.1% in technically successful PA-TAC patients was better than the 53.4% rate in PA-CsA recipients ($p = 0.0002$) and no different from the 87.4% pancreas graft survival rate in SPK recipients (34).

## STEROID WITHDRAWAL/STEROID AVOIDANCE

Reduction of steroid use is extremely desirable in pancreas transplantation, given the association between chronic steroid therapy and hypertension, hyperlipidemia, and glucose intolerance (36).

In a report from the University of Pittsburgh, complete steroid withdrawal was achieved in 58 (47%) of 124 patients, with a mean time to steroid withdrawal of $15.2 \pm 8.0$ months (18). Patient, pancreas, and kidney survival rates at one year were 100%, 100%, and 98% (off steroids), versus 97%, 91%, and 96% (on steroids, all NS). The cumulative risk of rejection was 74% for patients off steroids versus 76% for patients on steroids. The mean glycosylated hemoglobin levels were $5.2 \pm 0.9\%$ (off steroids) and $6.2 \pm 2.1\%$ (on steroids, $p = 0.02$). The Pittsburgh group concluded that steroid withdrawal could be achieved in pancreas transplant patients under tacrolimus-based immunosuppression and was associated with excellent patient and graft survival (18). More recently, the Pittsburgh group has utilized alemtuzumab preconditioning with tacrolimus monotherapy in pancreas recipients (see Chapter 1).

The Minnesota group reported a prospective trial of steroid withdrawal in pancreas transplantation (37). Only recipients with functioning grafts $\geq 6$ and $\leq 36$ months after simultaneous pancreas–kidney or pancreas after kidney transplants were enrolled. All patients received triple therapy for maintenance immunosuppression using tacrolimus and MMF, with the following inclusion criteria: (1) low maintenance steroid dose 0.075 mg/kg, (2) MMF $\geq 750$ mg orally twice a day, and (3) tacrolimus levels $\geq 8$ ng/mL. Fifty-five patients (29 SPK, 26 PAK) were randomized to standard immunosuppression or steroid withdrawal after four to eight weeks. The median follow-up after transplantation was 27 months in the SPK category and 26 months in the PAK category, and from randomization, 10 months in both categories. Steroid withdrawal $\geq 6$ months after a successful pancreas transplant was not associated with a decrease in patient or graft survival, nor was it associated with an increase in the rate of graft loss from rejection or in the incidence of rejection. There was a better quality of life and reduction in serum cholesterol levels in the steroid withdrawal group with a six-month follow-up (37).

A trial of rapid corticosteroid elimination (RCE) was reported in 40 simultaneous kidney–pancreas transplant patients from Northwestern University in Chicago (38). Induction was with anti-Thymocyte globulin. Maintenance immunosuppression was with tacrolimus/ MMF in 20 patients and tacrolimus/sirolimus in 20 patients. Patient and graft survival rates and rejection rates were compared to historical controls ($n = 86$). One-year actuarial patient, kidney, and pancreas survival rates in the RCE group were 100%, 100%, and 100%, and in the historical control group were 97%, 93%, and 97%, respectively (38). The one-year rejection-free survival rate in the RCE recipients was 97%, versus 80% in the historical control group. At 6 and 12 months posttransplant, the serum creatinine remained stable in all of the groups.

Excellent short-term results have been reported with steroid-free immunosuppression in low-risk pancreas–kidney transplantation recipients from the University of California at San Francisco (39). Forty patients underwent pancreas–kidney transplantation from November

2000 to July 2002. Thymoglobulin induction was combined with MMF, TAC, and sirolimus for maintenance immunosuppression. Steroids were used as pretreatment only, given with Thymoglobulin and discontinued by the end of the first postoperative week. Patient, kidney and pancreas survival rates were 95%, 92.5%, and 87.5%, respectively. Biopsy-proven pancreas rejection rates at one and three months posttransplantation were 2.5%, and kidney rejection rates at one and three months were 2.5%.

Based upon experimental studies, it was found that preconditioning with a depleting antibody and low-dose posttransplant immunosuppression could lead to partial tolerance (40). T-lymphocyte-depletional strategies using alemtuzumab (Campath-1H) (41), or Thymoglobulin (42) administered as preconditioning agents are based on this principle. Fourteen patients received pancreatic allografts at the University of Pittsburgh, which were transplanted alone ($n = 4$) or with kidneys from the same donor ($n = 10$). Two of the four pancreas alone recipients and 6 of the 10 pancreas–kidney recipients also had donor bone marrow infusion (42). The immunosuppression regime consisted of pretreatment with 5 mg/kg of Thymoglobulin (Sangstat, Menlo Park, California, U.S.A.) over several hours preceding transplantation; participants also received 1–2 g intravenous methylprednisone concomitantly to minimize cytokine reactions. Twice-daily monotherapy with tacrolimus was begun the day after transplantation, with a target trough concentration level of 10 µg/L. Other agents, e.g., prednisone, sirolimus, or muromonoab-CD3, were added as necessary for control of rejection and for as brief a period as possible. At four months, patients on tacrolimus monotherapy were considered for consolidation to once-daily tacrolimus and eventually spaced weaning. At 13 to 18 months of follow-up, patient survival was 100%, and pancreas graft survival was 86%. Five of 12 patients with functioning pancreas grafts were on spaced doses of TAC monotherapy, ranging from every other day ($n = 6$) to three times a week ($n = 2$) and once a week ($n = 2$) (42). More recently, alemtuzumab has been used for preconditioning (see Chapter 1).

## SIROLIMUS IN PANCREAS TRANSPLANTATION

The use of sirolimus with TAC in SPK transplantation has been alluded to earlier in the chapter (Table 6) (3,4,12,20,37–39). The use of SRL with TAC often enables successful corticosteroid elimination (38,39).

An immunosuppressive protocol using Thymoglobulin induction in combination with SRL and steroids, followed by markedly reduced exposures to cyclosporine, was used in 14 SPK and four PAK transplant recipients at Houston, Texas (43). With a mean follow-up of $13.6 \pm 4.7$ months, patient, kidney, and pancreas graft survivals were 100%, 100%, and 94%, respectively. One pancreas graft was lost to thrombosis. There were no acute rejection episodes and no opportunistic infections (43). There was a high incidence of incisional hernias related to the combination of SRL and steroids in a cohort of patients with other risk factors for poor wound healing (i.e., diabetes and renal failure).

## CONCLUSIONS

The general tendency of the pancreas allograft to elicit a greater immunologic response than a liver or a kidney allograft has made the pancreas transplant an important model for testing the efficacy of immunosuppressive agents and their combinations. Although requirements of immunosuppressive agents vary among SPK, PAK, and PTA transplants, some general conclusions may be drawn from the studies reported.

The use of TAC in maintenance immunosuppression is associated with a lower incidence of rejection episodes and higher graft survival rates than CsA. Similarly, the use of MMF gives better results than the use of AZA in maintenance immunosuppression protocols. Overall, the combination of TAC + MMF maintenance immunosuppression gives the best results at present and allows for rapid corticosteroid elimination.

Antibody induction therapy is important. Use of a nondepleting antibody such as daclizumab in SPK transplantation gives good results in terms of the composite end points of rejection, graft loss, and mortality even when only two doses are administered (2 mg/kg on days 0 and 14). Readmission rates may be significantly reduced in enteric-drained pancreas transplants in patients receiving induction therapy with nondepleting antibodies. The use of

TAC–SRL combination in SPK transplantation is associated with low rejection rates and, at the same time, preserved renal function.

The use of TAC + MMF for maintenance immunosuppression in PAK transplantation has resulted in success rates almost as good as those seen with SPK transplants. The use of anti-T-cell antibody therapy was associated with a higher one-year pancreas graft survival rate. The introduction of newer anti-T-cell agents, such as the monoclonal IL-2 receptor blockers, has not resulted in further improvements in posttransplantation outcomes in PAK transplantation. Solitary pancreas transplants with portal-enteric drainage and depleting antibody (e.g., Thymoglobulin) induction may be associated with improved intermediate-term outcome and immunologic advantages.

PTA transplantation is being performed with antibody induction therapy and TAC + MMF + steroids as maintenance immunosuppression. The current trend is to use depleting antibodies (alone or in combination with nondepleting antibodies) for induction therapy. Pretransplant immmunosuppression may be an important strategy to improve results of PTA transplants.

Among steroid avoidance protocols, T-cell depletion strategies followed by TAC monotherapy may be particularly attractive, although long-term outcomes need to be assessed.

## ACKNOWLEDGMENT

We are grateful to Ms. Judy Canelos, M.A., for assistance with the manuscript.

## REFERENCES

1. Sollinger HW, Odorico JS, Knechtle SJ, et al. Experience with 500 simultaneous pancreas–kidney transplants. Ann Surg 1998; 228(3):284–296.
2. Sutherland DER, Gruessner RWG, Dunn DL, et al. Lessons learned from more than 1000 pancreas transplants at a single institution. Ann Surg 2001; 233(4):463–501.
3. Burke GW, Ciancio G, Figueiro J, et al. Can acute rejection be prevented in SPK transplantation? Transplant Proc 2002; 34(5):1913–1914.
4. Kaufman DB, Leventhal JR, Gallon LG, et al. Technical and immunologic progress in simultaneous pancreas–kidney transplantation. Surgery 2002; 132(4):545–554.
5. Saudek F, Adamec M, Koznarova R, et al. Low rejection rate with high-dose ATG bolus therapy in simultaneous pancreas and kidney transplantation. Transplant Proc 2001; 33(3):2304–2306.
6. Stratta R, Alloway RR, Lo A, Hodges E. Two-dose daclizumab regimen in simultaneous kidney–pancreas transplant recipients: primary end-point analysis of a multicenter, randomized study. Transplantation 2003; 75(8):1260–1266.
7. Stratta RJ, Shokouh-Amiri MH, Egidi MF, et al. Long-term experience with simultaneous kidney–pancreas transplantation with portal-enteric drainage and tacrolimus–mycophenolate-based immunosuppression. Clin Transplant 2003; 17(suppl 9):69–77.
8. Woeste G, Wullstein C, Dette K, et al. Tacrolimus/mycophenolate versus cyclosporine A/azathioprine after simultaneous pancreas and kidney transplantation: five-year results of a randomized study. Transplant Proc 2002; 34(5):1920–1921.
9. Kaufman DB, Leventhal JR, Kaffron A, et al. Simultaneous pancreas–kidney transplantation in the mycophenolate mofetil/tacrolimus era: evolution from induction therapy with bladder drainage to noninduction therapy with enteric drainage. Surgery 2000; 128(4):726–737.
10. Ciancio G, LoMonte A, Buscemi G, Miller J, Burke G. Use of tacrolimus and mycophenolate mofetil as induction and maintenance in simultaneous pancreas–kidney transplantation. Transplant Int 2000; 13(15):S191–S194.
11. Land W, Malaise J, Sandberg J, et al. Tacrolimus versus cyclosporine in primary simultaneous pancreas-kidney transplantation: preliminary results at one-year of a large multicenter trial. Transplant Proc 2002; 34(5):1911–1912.
12. Vincenti F, Stock P. De novo use of sirolimus in immunosuppression regimens in kidney and kidney–pancreas transplantation at the University of California, San Francisco. Transplant Proc 2003; 35:S183–S186.
13. Burke GW, Kaufman DB, Millis JM, et al. Prospective, randomized trial of the effect of antibody induction in simultaneous pancreas and kidney transplantation: three year results. Transplantation 2004; 77(8):1269–1275.
14. Sollinger HW, Stratta RJ, Kalayoglu M, et al. Pancreas transplantation with pancreatico-cystostomy and quadruple immunosuppression. Surgery 1987; 102:614–679.
15. Stratta RJ. Review of immunosuppressive usage in pancreas transplantation. Clin Transplant 1999; 13(1):1–12.

16. Odorico JS, Pirsch JD, Knechtle SJ, et al. A study comparing mycophenolate mofetil to azathioprine in simultaneous pancreas–kidney transplantation. Transplantation 1998; 66:1751–1759.
17. Kahl A, Bechstein WO, Lorenz F, et al. Long-term prednisone withdrawal after pancreas and kidney transplantation in patients treated with ATG, tacrolimus, and mycophenolate mofetil. Transplant Proc 2001; 33:1694–1695.
18. Jordan ML, Chakrabarti P, Luke P, et al. Results of pancreas transplantation after steroid withdrawal under tacrolimus immunosuppression. Transplantation 2000; 69:265–271.
19. Bechstein WO, Malaise J, Saudek F, et al. Efficacy and safety of tacrolimus compared with cyclosporin microemulsion in primary simultaneous pancreas–kidney transplantation: 1-year results of a large multicenter trial. Transplantation 2004; 77:1221–1228.
20. McAlister VC, Gao Z, Peltekian K, et al. Sirolimus–tacrolimus combination immunosuppression. Lancet 2000; (355):376–377.
21. Gruessner AC, Sutherland DE. Analysis of United States (U.S.) and non-U.S. pancreas transplants reported to the United Network for Organ Sharing (UNOS) and the International Pancreas Transplant Registry (IPTR) as of October 2001. In: Cecka JM, Terasaki PI, eds. Clinical Transplants 2001. Los Angeles: UCLA Tissue Typing Laboratory, 2002:41–72.
22. Gruessner AC, Sutherland DER. Pancreas transplant outcomes for United States (U.S.) and non-U.S. cases as reported to the United Network for Organ Sharing (UNOS) and International Pancreas Transplant Registry (IPTR) as of October 2002. In: Cecka JM, Terasaki PI, eds. Clinical Transplants 2002. Los Angeles: UCLA Tissue Typing Laboratory, 2003:41–77.
23. Ciancio G, Miller J, Burke GW. The case of intravenous tacrolimus and mycophenolate mofetil as induction and maintenance immunosuppression in simultaneous pancreas–kidney recipients with previous transplants. Clin Transplant 2001; 15(2):142–145.
24. Dette K, Woeste G, Schwarz R, et al. Daclizumab and ATG versus ATG in combination with tacrolimus, mycophenolate mofetil and steroids in simultaneous pancreas–kidney transplantation: an analysis of outcome. Transplant Proc 2002; 34(5):1909–1910.
25. Rasaiah SB, Light JA, Sasaki TM, et al. A comparison of daclizumab to ATGAM induction in simultaneous pancreas–kidney transplant recipients on triple maintenance immunosuppression. Clin Transplant 2000; 14(4):209–212.
26. Corry RJ, Egidi MF, Shapiro R, et al. Tacrolimus without antilymphocytic therapy prevents pancreas loss from rejection in 123 consecutive patients. Transplant Proc 1998; 30(2):521.
27. Salazar A, McAlister VC, Kiberd BA, et al. Sirolimus–tacrolimus combination for combined kidney–pancreas transplantation: effect on renal function. Transplant Proc 2001; 33(1–2):1038–1039.
28. Gruessner AC, Sutherland DER, Dunn DL, et al. Pancreas after kidney transplants in posturemic patients with type I diabetes mellitus. J Am Soc Nephrol 2001; 12(11):2490–2499.
29. Hariharan S, Pirsch JD, Lu CY, et al. Pancreas after kidney transplantation. J Am Soc Nephrol 2002; 13(4):1109–1118.
30. Stegall MD, Kim DY, Prieto M, et al. Thymoglobulin induction decreases rejection in solitary pancreas transplantation. Transplantation 2001; 72(10):1671–1675.
31. Odorico JS, Becker YT, Groshek M, et al. Improved solitary pancreas transplant graft survival in the modern immunosuppressive era. Cell Transplant 2000; 9:919–927.
32. Tan M, Cantarovich M, Mangel R, Paraskevas S, Fortier M, Metrakos P. Reduced dose Thymoglobulin, tacrolimus, and mycophenolate mofetil results in excellent solitary pancreas transplant outcome. Clin Transplant 2002; 16(6):414–418.
33. Stratta RJ, Lo A, Shokouh-Amiri MH, Egidi MF, Gaber LW, Gaber AO. Improving results in solitary pancreas transplantation with portal-enteric drainage, Thymoglobulin induction and tacrolimus/mycophenolate mofetil-based immunosuppression. Transplant Int 2003; 16(3):154–160.
34. Bartlett ST, Schweitzer EJ, Johnson LB, et al. Equivalent success of simultaneous pancreas kidney and solitary pancreas transplantation: a prospective trial of tacrolimus immunosuppression with percutaneous biopsy. Ann Surg 1996; 224(4):440–452.
35. Sutherland DER, Gruessner RWG, Humar A, et al. Pretransplant immunosuppression for pancreas transplants alone in nonuremic diabetic recipients. Transplant Proc 2001; 33:1656–1658.
36. Humar A, Parr E, Drangstveit MG, Kandaswarmy R, Gruessner AC, Sutherland DER. Steroid withdrawal in pancreas transplant recipients. Clin Transplant 2000; 14:75–78.
37. Gruessner RWG, Sutherland DER, Parr E, Humar A, Gruessner AC. A prospective, randomized open labeled study of steroid withdrawal in pancreas transplantation—a preliminary report with six months' follow up. Transplant Proc 2001; 33:1663–1664.
38. Kaufman DB, Leventhal JR, Koffron AJ, et al. A prospective study of rapid corticosteroid elimination in simultaneous pancreas–kidney transplantation. Transplantation 2002; 73:169–177.
39. Friese CE, Sang-Mo K, Feng S, et al. Excellent short-term results with steroid-free maintenance immunosuppression in low-risk simultaneous pancreas–kidney transplantation. Arch Surg 2003; 138:1121–1126.
40. Calne R, Friend P, Moffatt S, et al. Proper tolerance, peri-operative Campath 1H, and low-dose cyclosporine monotherapy in renal allograft recipients. Lancet 1998; 351:1701–1702.
41. Calne R, Soffatt SD, Friend PJ, et al. Campath-1H allows low-dose cyclosporine monotherapy in 31 cadaveric renal allograft recipients. Transplantation 1999; 68:1613–1616.

42. Starzl TE, Murase N, Abu-Elmagd K, et al. Tolerogenic immunosuppression for organ transplantation. Lancet 2003; 361:1502–1510.
43. Knight RJ, Kerman RH, Scott Z, et al. Thymoglobulin, sirolimus, and reduced-dose cyclosporine provides excellent rejection prophylaxis for pancreas transplantation. Transplantation 2003; 75: 1301–1306.

# 13 | Pancreas Transplant Rejection

**Liise K. Kayler and Henkie P. Tan**

*Thomas E. Starzl Transplantation Institute, University of Pittsburgh School of Medicine, Pittsburgh, Pennsylvania, U.S.A.*

Acute rejection is the most important cause of graft loss in patients who undergo technically successful pancreas transplantation (1). By one year after transplantation, the incidence of acute rejection is approximately 25% in simultaneous pancreas–kidney (SPK) recipients, 35% in pancreas after kidney (PAK) recipients, and 40% in pancreas transplant alone (PTA) recipients (2,3). In most cases, acute rejection does not lead to immediate allograft loss. With current immunosuppressive regimens, the one-year rates of immunologic graft loss are 2% after SPK, 9% after PAK, and 16% after PTA (1). Acute rejection, however, can impact long-term allograft survival and has been demonstrated to be an important risk factor for the development of chronic rejection (2,4,5).

## IMMUNOSUPPRESSION

To prevent rejection, most pancreas transplant programs initially use quadruple drug immunosuppression consisting of an induction agent, a calcineurin inhibitor, an antiproliferative agent, and corticosteroids (see Chapter 12) (6,7). In the past, induction with antilymphocyte antibodies, such as muromonab-CD3 or antithymocyte globulin, and maintenance therapy with cyclosporine, azathioprine, and corticosteroids were the cornerstones of therapy; this regimen was associated with acute rejection rates of 50% to 80% (6,7). The introduction of tacrolimus (FK) and mycophenolate mofetil (MMF) in the mid-1990s improved the quality of maintenance immunosuppression by lowering rejection rates.

Induction therapy is used with greater frequency for pancreas recipients than for any other solid organ recipients (8). Between 1988 and 1996, the proportion of pancreas recipients who received induction therapy exceeded 86% in each of the three recipient categories (SPK, PAK, PTA). Since no Food and Drug Administration-approved antibodies are on the market with a labeled indication to reduce rejection rates specifically in pancreas recipients, the use of antibody induction therapy in pancreas transplant recipients has been guided by practical experience and varies greatly. The anti-T-cell agents available include depleting polyclonal (Thymoglobulin, antithymocyte globulin) and monoclonal (OKT3, Campath) antibodies and nondepleting monoclonal (daclizumab and basiliximab) antibodies. According to the 2003 International Pancreas Transplant Registry report (9), between 2000 and 2003, depleting antibodies were used most frequently in all three categories (PTA 43%, PAK 42%, and SPK 37%), followed by nondepleting antibodies (SPK 32%, PAK 19%, PTA 9%) or a combination of depleting and nondepleting antibodies (PTA 28%, PAK 16%, SPK 7%), and no antibody induction therapy (SPK 24%, PAK 24%, PTA 20%) (9).

The incidence of pancreas rejection varies by recipient category: it is highest in nonuremic PTA recipients, next highest in posturemic PAK recipients, and lowest in uremic SPK recipients. Therefore, the greatest amount of immunosuppression is usually given to PTA and PAK patients. According to data from the International Pancreas Transplant Registry, graft survival rates in all three recipient categories were highest for recipients given antibody induction therapy and maintained on FK and MMF. For transplants between 2000 and 2004, recipients given any type of anti-T-cell induction therapy and maintained on TAC and MMF had the highest one- and three-year pancreas graft survival rates: SPK ($n = 2500$), 88% and 81%; PAK ($n = 712$), 82% and 67%; and PTA ($n = 278$), 82% and 65% ($P < 0.0001$) (9).

Individualized immunosuppressive therapy may be beneficial in several types of recipients. More potent immunosuppression is needed for recipients who are at higher risks for rejection such as young recipients, African-American recipients, recipients with high panel reactive antibody levels, and retransplant recipients. The highest graft loss rate from rejection in all three pancreas recipient categories is seen in those $\leq 18$ years (9). African-Americans also have a higher risk of immunological graft loss compared to Whites (10). Less potent immuno-suppressive protocols may benefit older recipients ($\geq 60$ years of age) who have a significantly lower risk of graft loss from rejection (10), recipients with certain infections such as hepatitis C, and those with previous histories of posttransplant lymphoproliferative disease. FK is currently utilized in $> 90\%$ of all pancreas recipients (9), in spite of its well-known toxic effects on the kidney. SPK recipients with delayed renal allograft function may benefit from delayed introduction or lower dose calcineurin inhibitors. Steroids remain a standard component of immunosuppressive regimens after pancreas transplantation at many transplant centers. However, the long-term side effects are harmful to both adult and pediatric recipients.

Several studies have demonstrated that different combinations of immunosuppressive agents, such as induction avoidance and steroid withdrawal, can be successful; other strategies, like calcineurin inhibitor avoidance, may have a role in certain recipients. The results of SPK without anti-T cell induction are comparable to treatment regimens employing polyclonal or monoclonal antibody induction (3,6,7,11–14). Steroid withdrawal has been successfully employed in SPK recipients within the first week after transplantation (i.e., near avoidance) (15,16) and by six months after transplantation (10,15,17). In small studies, these regimens have resulted in similar outcomes in terms of patient survival, pancreas survival, and graft loss from rejection (15,17). One observational study examining alemtuzumab for induction and maintenance, with MMF monotherapy, avoiding calcineurin inhibitors and steroids, found no differences in patient, pancreas, and kidney survival rates or graft loss from rejection, compared to a historical group who had received Thymogloublin induction and FK maintenance. The incidence of a first reversible rejection episode in SPK recipients was, however, higher in the alemtuzumab/MMF group than in the Thymoglobulin/FK group (41% vs. 9%, respectively; $P \leq 0.0003$), but not in PAK and PTA recipients.

## ACUTE REJECTION

The majority of rejection episodes occur early (in the first six months posttransplant) (2). The diagnosis of pancreas rejection is problematic, in that clinical findings and biochemical markers correlate poorly with rejection (18,19). Clinical criteria consistent with rejection include fever, allograft swelling and tenderness, ileus, abdominal pain, or hematuria (in bladder-drained pancreas allografts). Laboratory findings can include an increase in the serum creatinine (after SPK), serum amylase, lipase or anodal trypsinogen, pancreas-specific protein (20–24), a reduction in urine amylase or pH (25), or positive urine cytology (if bladder drained) (26). However, as diagnostic tools, these parameters lack specificity (27–29). An elevated blood sugar is a late manifestation of acute rejection and portends a poor prognosis, but can also be elevated with chronic rejection, high-dose steroids, or FK toxicity (30). Most centers monitor serum amylase, lipase, and creatinine (for SPK) because of their universal availability. In SPK recipients with both grafts from a single donor, monitoring the serum creatinine for signs of renal allograft rejection has proven to be a valuable marker of rejection. Rejection of the pancreas graft in the absence of concurrent kidney graft rejection is possible but uncommon; in any event, the diagnosis based only on clinical criteria can be inaccurate, and histopathology remains the gold standard. For PAK and PTA recipients, a definitive diagnosis of rejection can only be made with a pancreas biopsy (31).

A number of techniques of pancreas allograft biopsy have been described. Percutaneous biopsy under ultrasound or CT guidance is performed most often, and is associated with a very low complication rate. In patients with bladder drainage, cystoscopic transduodenal needle biopsy with ultrasound guidance has also been performed successfully (32). Both techniques utilize a semiautomated instrument such as the Biopty$^{\circledR}$ gun, which sets a predetermined length of needle penetration to obtain an adequate tissue sample for diagnosis. In cases where a radiologic window cannot be identified, open or laparoscopic biopsy is an alternative (33).

The most widely used grading scheme for pancreas allograft biopsy specimens was published in 1997 and helped standardize interpretation of pancreas transplant biopsies (Table 1) (see Chapter 14) (34). The degree of septal and acinar inflammation, eosinophils, and the presence of endothelitis or vasculitis determine the severity of rejection. With this classification, biopsy specimens are graded on a scale from 0 to V, reflecting normal histology to

**Table 1** Grading Scheme for Pancreas Transplant Biopsies

| Grade | Severity | Histopathologic finding |
|---|---|---|
| 0 | Normal | Unremarkable pancreatic parenchyma without inflammatory infiltrates |
| I | Inflammation of undetermined significance | Sparse, purely septal mononuclear inflammatory infiltrates |
| | | No venous endotheliitis or acinar involvement |
| II | Minimal rejection | Purely septal inflammation with venous endotheliitis |
| | | In absence of endotheliitis, a constellation of at least three of the following four histologic features must be present: |
| | | • Septal inflammatory infiltrates composed of mixed population of small and large lymphocytes |
| | | • Eosinophils |
| | | • Acinar inflammation in rare (up to two) foci |
| | | • Ductal inflammation (permeation of inflammatory cells through the ductal basement membrane) |
| III | Mild rejection | Septal inflammatory infiltrates with three or more foci of acinar inflammation |
| | | Eosinophils, venous endotheliitis, ductal inflammation, and acinar cell injury |
| IV | Moderate rejection | Arterial endotheliitis and/or necrotizing arthritis (vasculitis), usually together with Grade III features |
| V | Severe rejection | Extensive acinar lymphoid or mixed inflammatory infiltrates with multicellular focal or confluent acinar cell necrosis |
| | | Vascular and ductal lesions may be demonstrated. |

*Source*: From Ref. 34.

severe rejection, respectively. Although the advanced grades of rejection correlate strongly with immunologic graft loss, it is unclear how lower grades impact graft outcome and, consequently, how they should best be managed (35). Very mild forms of rejection may respond to boluses of corticosteroids alone, but for more severe forms of rejection (grade III and higher); antilymphocyte therapy is necessary to reverse rejection (19). High-grade or vascular rejections may be refractory to either form of treatment (36,37). In the immunologically more favorable SPK category, pancreas rejection episodes graded as minimal or mild can be reversed with steroid boluses and with recycling of the steroid taper and/or with increases in the dosage of the maintenance immunosuppressive agents. In SPK recipients, antibody therapy is frequently reserved for moderate or severe rejection episodes. In contrast to the SPK category, even minimal or mild pancreas rejection episodes in the immunologically less favorable PTA and PAK categories are usually responsive only to antibody treatment, and this is currently considered standard therapy at most centers (10). Different therapeutic strategies according to the histologic severity of pancreas rejection episodes have yet to be studied in prospective randomized trials (10).

## CHRONIC REJECTION

With decreased rejection rates, an increasing number of pancreas allografts are continuing to function beyond the first year after transplantation, and allograft loss to chronic rejection is becoming increasingly common. In one of the largest series (500 SPKs) reported to date, rejection accounted for 44% of long-term graft failures (38). In large analyses, the most common cause of allograft loss, after technical failure, is chronic rejection (8.8%) (2). The strongest risk factor for graft loss to chronic rejection is a previous episode of acute rejection (2). Other risk factors include repeated episodes of acute rejection (4,5), higher grades of acute rejection (5), and late (>1 year) acute rejection (5). The type of transplant is also an independent risk factor for chronic rejection, with PAK or PTA recipients having a significantly higher risk (11%) compared with SPK recipients (3.7%). Other risk factors are cytomegalovirus infection, retransplantation, and mismatches at the B loci (2).

No clear, uniformly accepted definition of chronic rejection exists for pancreas transplant recipients. The clinical course is characterized by a gradual deterioration in pancreas graft function beginning two months or more after transplantation. The exocrine component is usually affected first (manifested by falling urine amylase levels in bladder-drained grafts), followed by the endocrine component (manifested by episodes of hyperglycemia and the need for insulin therapy). Histologically, chronic rejection is characterized by arteriopathy with concentric narrowing of the small vessels and by parenchymal fibrosis with atrophy of acini (34,39). The atrophy is initially of the acinar component, followed by atrophy or disruption of the endocrine component (islet cells) (39). Clinical/pathological studies have shown that, in addition to the presence of progressive fibrosis and proportional acinar loss, vascular changes characterized by narrowing of arterial lumina and concentric fibroproliferative endarteritis are an integral part of the pattern of chronic rejection of the pancreas. These vascular changes are similar to those observed in kidney and heart transplants. An additional important histological feature associated with pancreas graft sclerosis (chronic rejection) is the presence of recent and organized thrombosis in the arteries and veins (35). Radiologic imaging with computed tomographic scan of grafts with extensive chronic rejection may demonstrate a small shrunken mass of tissue, consistent with significant parenchymal fibrosis and atrophy.

## CONCLUSION

Since the introduction of new immunosuppressive agents in the mid-1990s, acute rejection rates have decreased substantially. Individualization of immunosuppressive therapy after pancreas transplantation will become more important in the future to improve outcomes, minimize side effects, and decrease infectious complications. Therapy for rejection has also been increasingly individualized and now depends primarily on the severity of the rejection episode. The type and success of rejection therapy may have an impact on allograft loss to chronic rejection. Different therapeutic strategies have yet to be studied in prospective randomized trials.

## REFERENCES

1. Gruessner AC, Sutherland DER. Analysis of pancreas transplants for United States (US) and non-US pancreas transplants as reported to the International Pancreas Transplant Registry (IPTR) and to the United Network for Organ Sharing (UNOS). In: Cecka JM, Terasaki PI, eds. Clinical Transplants 2000. Los Angeles: Tissue Typing Laboratory, 2001:45–72.
2. Humar A, Khwaja K, Ramcharan T, et al. Chronic rejection: the next major challenge for pancreas transplant recipients. Transplantation 2003; 76:918–923.
3. Reddy KS, Stratta RJ, Shokouh-Amiri H, et al. Simultaneous kidney–pancreas transplantation without antilymphocyte induction. Transplantation 2000; 69:49.
4. Tesi RJ, Henry ML, Elkammas EA, Davies ED, Ferguson FM. The frequency of rejection episodes after combined kidney–pancreas transplant—the impact on graft survival. Transplantation 1994; 58:424–430.
5. Papadmitriou JC, Drachenberg CB, Klassen DK. Histological grading of chronic pancreas allograft rejection/graft sclerosis. Am J Transplant 2003; 3:599–605.
6. Gruessner AC, Sutherland DER. Analysis of pancreas transplant outcomes for United States cases reported to the United Network for Organ Sharing (UNOS) and non-US cases reported to the International Pancreas Transplant Registry (IPTR). In: Cecka JM, Terasaki PI, eds. Clinical Transplants 1999. Los Angeles: UCLA Immunogenetics Center, 2000:51.
7. Stratta RJ. Immunosuppression in pancreas transplantation: progress, problems and perspective. Transplant Immunol 1998; 6:69.
8. Kaufman DB. Immunosuppression in pancreas transplantation: induction therapy. In: Gruessner RWG, Sutherland DER, eds. Transplantation of the Pancreas. New York: Springer-Verlag, 2004:267.
9. Gruessner AC, Sutherland DE. Pancreas Transplant Outcomes for United States (US) and Non-US Cases as Reported to the United Network for Organ Sharing (UNOS) and the International Pancreas Transplant Registry (IPTR) as of May 2003. Los Angeles, CA: UCLA Immunogenics Center, 2004:21.
10. Gruessner RWG, Sutherland DER, Parr E, Humar A, Gruessner AC. A prospective, randomized, open-label study of steroid withdrawal in pancreas transplantation—a preliminary report with 6-month follow-up. Transplant Proc 2001; 33:1663–1664.
11. Gruessner RWG. Antibody induction therapy in pancreas transplantation. Transplant Proc 1998; 30:1556.
12. Stratta RJ, Alloway RR, Lo A, et al. Two dose daclizumab regimen in simultaneous kidney–pancreas transplant recipients: primary endpoint analysis of a multicenter, randomized study. Transplantation 2003; 75:1260.
13. Trofe J, Stratta RJ, Egidi MF, et al. Thymoglobulin for induction or rejection therapy in pancreas allograft recipients: a single centre experience. Clin Transplant 2002; 16(7):34–44.

14. Shultz T, Papapostolou G, Schenker P, Kapischke M. Single-shot antithymocyte globulin (ATG) induction for pancreas/kidney transplantation: ATG-Fresenius versus Thymoglobulin. Transplant Proc 2005; 37:1301–1304.
15. Kandaswamy R, Khwaja K, Gruessner AC, et al. A prospective randomized trial of steroid-free maintenance vs. delayed steroid withdrawal, using a sirolimus/tacrolimus regimen in simultaneous pancreas–kidney transplants (SPK). Am J Transplant 2003; 3:530.
16. Kaufman DB, Leventhal JR, Koffron AJ, et al. A prospective study of rapid corticosteroid elimination in simultaneous pancreas–kidney transplantation: comparison of two maintenance immunosuppression protocols: tacrolimus/mycophenolate mofetil versus tacrolimus/sirolimus. Transplantation 2002; 73:169–177.
17. Kandaswamy R, Khwaja K, Gruessner A, et al. A prospective, randomized trial of steroid withdrawal with mycophenolate mofetil (MMF) vs. sirolimus (SRL) in pancreas after kidney (PAK) transplants. Am J Transplant 2003; 3:292.
18. Gruessner RWG, Sutherland DER. Clinical diagnosis in pancreas allograft rejection. In: Solez K, Racusen LC, Billingham ME, eds. Solid Organ Transplant Rejection: Mechanisms, Pathology and Diagnosis. New York: Marcel Dekker, 1996:455.
19. Papadmitriou JC, Drachenberg CB, Wiland A, et al. Histologic grading of acute allograft rejection in pancreas needle biopsy. Transplantation 1998; 66:1741.
20. Sutherland DER, Gruessner RWG, Gores PF. Pancreas and islet transplantation: an update. Transplant Rev 1994; 8:185.
21. Marks WH, Borgstrom A, Marks CR, et al. Serum markers for pancreas rejection: long term behavior following clinical pancreatico-duodenal transplantation. Transplant Proc 1991; 23:1596.
22. Perkal M, Marks C, Lorber MI, Marks WH. A three-year experience with serum anodal trypsinogen as a biochemical marker for rejection in pancreatic allografts: false positives, tissue biopsy, comparison with other markers, and diagnostic strategies. Transplantation 1992; 53:415.
23. Fernstad R, Tyden G, Brattstrom C, et al. Pancreas-specific protein: a new marker for graft rejection in pancreas transplant recipients. Diabetes 1989; 38(1):55.
24. Nyberg G, Olaavsson M, Norden G, et al. Pancreas-specific protein monitoring in pancreas transplantation. Transplant Proc 1991; 23:1604.
25. Prieto M, Sutherland DER, Fernandez-Cruz L, et al. Experimental and clinical experience with urine amylase monitoring for early diagnosis of rejection in pancreas transplantation. Transplantation 1987; 43:71.
26. Tyden G, Rienholt F, Brattstrom SO, et al. Diagnosis of pancreas graft rejection by pancreatic juice cytology. Transplant Proc 1989; 21:2780.
27. Nankivell BJ, Allen RDM, Bell B, et al. Urinary amylase measurement for detection of bladder-drained pancreas allograft rejection. Transplant Proc 1990; 22:2158.
28. Munn SR, ENgen DE, Barr D, et al. Differential diagnosis of hypoamylasuria in pancreas allograft recipients with urinary exocrine drainage. Transplantation 1990; 49:359.
29. Moukarzel M, Benoit G, Charpentier B, et al. Is urinary amylase a reliable index for monitoring whole pancreas endocrine graft function? Transplant Proc 1992; 24:925.
30. Gruessner RWG, Nakhieh R, Tzardis P, et al. Differences in rejection grading after simultaneous pancreas and kidney transplantation in pigs. Transplantation 1994; 57:1021.
31. Kuo PC, Johnson LB, Schweitzer EJ, et al. Solitary pancreas allografts: the role of percutaneous biopsy and standardized histologic grading of rejection. Arch Surg 1997; 132(1):52.
32. Lowell JA, Bynon JS, Nelson N, et al. Improved technique for transduodenal pancreas transplant biopsy. Transplantation 1994; 57(5):752.
33. Kayler LK, Maraschio M, Punch JD, et al. Evaluation of pancreatic allograft dysfunction by laparoscopic biopsy. Transplantation 2002; 74:1287–1289.
34. Drachenberg CB, Papadimitriou JC, Klassen DK, et al. Evaluation of pancreas transplant needle biopsy: reproducibility and revision of histologic grading system. Transplantation 1997; 63:1579–1586.
35. Drachenberg CB, Papadimitriou JC, Farney A, et al. Pancreas transplantation: the histologic morphology of graft loss. Transplantation 2001; 71:1784–1791.
36. Papadimitriou JC, Wiland A, Drachenberg CB, Klassen DK, Bartlett ST. Effectiveness of immunosuppressive treatment for recurrent or refractory pancreas allograft rejection: correlation with histologic grade. Transplant Proc 1998; 30:3945.
37. Boonstra JG, Wever PC, Laterveer JC. Apoptosis of acinar cells in pancreas allograft rejection. Transplantation 1997; 64(8):1211–1213.
38. Sollinger HW, Odorico JS, Knechtle SJ, D'Alessandro AM, Kalayoglu M, Pirsch JD. Experience with 500 simultaneous pancreas-kidney transplants. Ann Surg 1998; 288:284.
39. Drachenberg CB, Papadimitriou JC, Klassen DK, et al. Chronic pancreas allograft rejection: morphologic evidence of progression in needle biopsies and proposal of a grading scheme. Transplant Proc 1999; 31(1–2):614.

# 14 | Pathology of the Allograft Pancreas

Parmjeet S. Randhawa and Anthony J. Demetris

*Department of Pathology, University of Pittsburgh Medical Center, Pittsburgh, Pennsylvania, U.S.A.*

## INTRODUCTION

Among the factors that have contributed to improved outcomes after pancreatic transplantation, the ability to diagnose rejection, and to differentiate it from nonimmunologic causes of allograft injury, has been of great importance. The tissue biopsy remains the gold standard for the diagnosis of rejection (1,2). It minimizes the risk of graft loss due uncontrolled rejection, while sparing the patient from unnecessary and potentially harmful increases in immunosuppression for other causes of graft malfunction. In most cases, the concomitantly transplanted kidney has been used as a marker for the pancreas, because of the greater safety associated with renal biopsy. However, in the case of solitary pancreas transplantation, and pancreas after kidney transplantation, use of the pancreatic allograft biopsy becomes necessary to optimize clinical management and enhance graft survival (2). This chapter will discuss the principal graft dysfunction syndromes seen after pancreatic transplantation, with special reference to the corresponding pathologic findings seen in biopsy material.

### Tissue Sampling Considerations

As noted above, in simultaneous kidney–pancreas transplant recipients, most rejection episodes can be diagnosed by a renal allograft biopsy guided by serial determinations of serum creatinine (3). Nonetheless, it is advisable to simultaneously monitor pancreatic allograft function by monitoring the urinary amylase (bladder-drained pancreas grafts) or serum lipase (enteric-drained pancreas grafts) (4). In approximately 7% of patients, we have found significant rejection in renal allograft biopsies performed solely for a rise in the serum lipase. The lipase level in these patients returned to normal after treatment with steroids and augmentation of tacrolimus dosage. A renal rather than a pancreatic biopsy was performed in these cases, as it is technically easier and less prone to complications.

In patients who have received an isolated pancreas transplant, direct sampling of the pancreas allograft may become necessary when clinical or biochemical evidence of graft dysfunction develops. Histologic documentation of rejection is very desirable, since biochemical abnormalities of pancreatic function can be due to nonimmune causes in up to 53% of cases (3). Biopsy tissue may be obtained cystoscopically in bladder-drained grafts or percutaneously in enterically drained grafts (5–7). In the case of pancreaticoduodenal grafts, endoscopic biopsy of the allograft duodenum has been shown to be as reliable as a biopsy of the pancreas itself (6,8,9). Ultrasound-guided percutaneous biopsies of the pancreas graft are usually performed with an 18 gauge automated biopsy needle, and result in successful sampling in up to 93% of cases (10,11). Biopsy-related complications are infrequent, and include gross hemorrhage without graft loss in 3%, and mild pancreatitis in 7% of cases (12). In simultaneous pancreas–kidney recipients with histologically proven renal rejection, concurrent pancreatic rejection can be found in 69% (10,11,13). Pancreas rejection is said also to occasionally occur in the absence of renal rejection, although concomitant renal biopsies have not always been performed in this setting.

Even though conventional core biopsy has been shown to be generally safe, some clinicians continue to be concerned about the possibility of biopsy-induced enzyme leakage and tissue necrosis. To minimize this possibility, some centers advocate fine needle aspiration cytology for monitoring isolated pancreas transplant recipients, particularly in the early postoperative phase, when the graft is relatively mobile and more difficult to biopsy (14). Technical complications of fine needle aspiration are limited to occasional instances of transient hematuria, and elevations in serum amylase, which return to baseline within three days. The diagnosis of acute rejection is based on obtaining aspirates rich in activated mononuclear cells. The diagnostic sensitivity of an aspirate, 59.1%, for documenting clinically suspected rejection, is lower than that achieved by conventional biopsy, 75% (15). Another serious limitation of the fine needle aspiration technique is that it cannot document arteritis or chronic rejection. A final caveat to be kept in mind is that aspiration of peritoneal macrophages in patients with ascites or graft infarction may occasionally lead to a false positive diagnosis of rejection (16).

In an effort to avoid trauma to the allograft pancreas altogether, pancreatic juice cytology has been suggested as a method for the diagnosis of acute rejection in the early postoperative phase (17,18). Samples are collected via a pancreatic duct catheter passed through the enteric wall, and further through the abdominal wall. Rejection is diagnosed if an increase in the number of activated lymphocytes is found with at least two blast-transformed cells seen per specimen. By serial monitoring, a diagnosis can be made at a very early stage even before a decrease in the pancreatic juice amylase activity manifests itself. Unfortunately, the need for percutaneous catheter drainage limits the use of this method to the first few weeks after transplantation, and it is not possible to diagnose vasculitis or chronic rejection by this technique. In addition, the catheter has been associated with the development of graft pancreatitis. For bladder-drained grafts, urine cytology can be used instead of pancreatic juice analysis (19).

In actual practice, the most commonly used method to obtain diagnostic tissue material from an isolated pancreas allograft is a core biopsy performed by the percutaneous or endoscopic route.

We will now discuss the clinicopathologic characteristics of various graft dysfunction syndromes seen after pancreatic transplantation.

## NONSPECIFIC BIOPSY CHANGES

Pancreatic biopsies from patients with well-functioning grafts typically show no significant inflammation or only minor inflammatory infiltrates. Some biopsy cores include peripancreatic collagenous, adipose, and skeletal muscle tissue with fat necrosis, foreign body giant cell reaction, or degenerative changes. Reactive lymph nodes can be occasionally sampled and confused with rejection-associated infiltrates.

## DONOR DISEASE

Organs harvested from elderly donors can show arteriosclerosis and arteriolar hyalinosis in the pancreatic arterial tree. A history of alcoholism, liver disease, or gallstones in the donor may be associated with changes of acute or chronic pancreatitis. When clinically suspected, such changes can be identified by performing a pretransplant donor biopsy (Fig. 1) and taken into consideration when evaluating the suitability of the donor pancreas for transplantation.

## ISCHEMIC/PRESERVATION INJURY

Nearly all pancreas transplant recipients have elevated serum amylase or lipase levels in the first few postoperative days, reflecting perioperative ischemic injury to the pancreatic parenchyma. The biopsy findings of pancreatic ischemia include acinar cytoplasmic swelling, microvesicular steatosis, apoptosis, cytolysis, focal coagulative necrosis, and a variable polymorphonuclear infiltrate (20). More severe ischemic insults occur during vascular thrombosis, which is discussed separately below.

## VASCULAR THROMBOSIS

Thrombosis of the pancreatic vessels is still the leading cause of nonimmunologic pancreatic graft failure. The overall thrombosis rate at the University of Minnesota is 12%. Occlusion of the venous system is reported more commonly than the arterial system (21). Ischemic injury sustained during harvesting and implantation, surgical manipulation of the organ during surgery, poor postoperative perfusion, and kinking of the pancreatic vessels can all play a role in the pathogenesis of this catastrophic complication. The clinical presentation is a sudden loss of graft function, usually occurring within the first few days of transplantation. Histopathologic examination shows varying degrees of ischemic injury in the form of nuclear pyknosis,

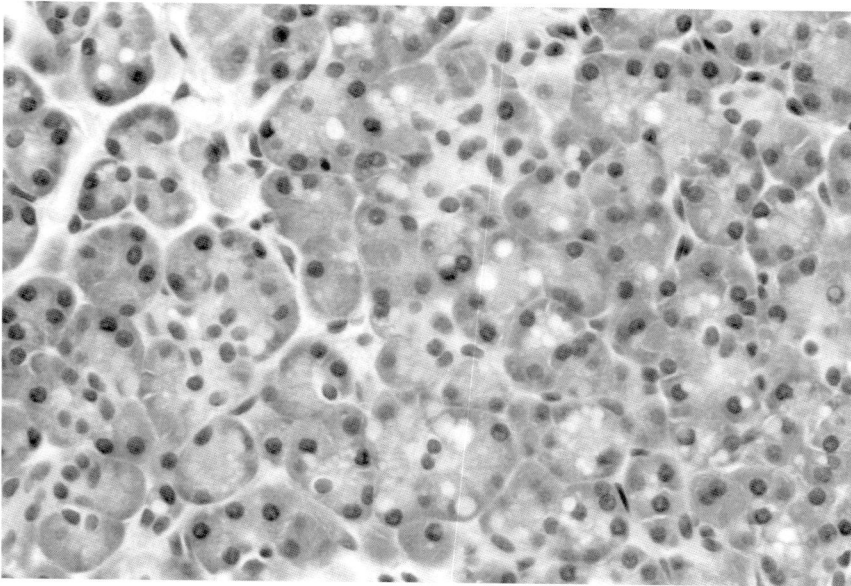

**Figure 1** Wedge biopsy from donor pancreas taken prior to transplantation. The acinar epithelium shows focal cytoplasmic vacuolation and fatty change related to the harvesting operation and subsequent cold preservation of the organ (H & E ×500).

cytoplasmic eosinophilia, or frank coagulative necrosis (20,22). In some cases, diffuse proliferation of the islet cells (nesidioblastosis) has also been reported (23). When examining an infarcted graft, it is important not to miss an underlying cellular or antibody-mediated rejection, either of which can secondarily lead to thrombosis of the pancreatic vascular tree. Vascular thrombosis can also complicate acute pancreatitis and chronic vascular rejection. Most grafts with vascular thrombosis are lost, but early diagnosis can reportedly lead to successful anticoagulation, thrombolytic therapy, or thrombectomy (24,25).

## ACUTE ANTIBODY-MEDIATED REJECTION

Hyperacute rejection is described in experimental pancreas transplantation (25), but is rare in clinical practice, because of the efficacy of currently available immunologic screening techniques for detecting preformed antibodies in sensitized patients. Milder forms of antibody-mediated rejection probably exist, as have been documented in the kidney, but are yet to be formally defined. It has been noted that low titer anti-donor antibodies detected by flow cytometric cross-matching do not necessarily lead to an adverse graft outcome (26). Conversely, antibody-mediated rejection (27) has been reported in a patient with a panel reactive antibody level of 80%, but a negative pretransplant cross-match. Histopathologic examination in this case showed margination of neutrophils, and frequent small vessel fibrin thrombi.

## ACUTE CELLULAR REJECTION

Acute cellular rejection is the result of cell-mediated immune injury directed against the allograft pancreas. It is a relatively common cause of graft dysfunction, particularly in the early post-transplant period. The initial clinical manifestation can be an elevation of the serum amylase or lipase. In the combined kidney–pancreas transplant program at the University of Pittsburgh, these abnormalities have been respectively seen in 54% and 71% of cases with biopsy-proven renal allograft rejection (4). False positive elevations of amylase and lipase can occur in ischemic injury or graft pancreatitis; less common causes include renal disease, perforated gastric or duodenal ulcer, intestinal obstruction, and diseases of the native pancreas and salivary gland (28–30). In allografts drained into the urinary bladder, a decrease in urinary amylase excretion may precede a rise in the serum amylase.

Another biochemical marker for acute rejection is a 25% or greater rise in blood glucose levels (27). The underlying mechanism is believed to be an immune-mediated isletitis leading to release of IL-1 (by macrophages or inflamed endothelial cells), and inhibition of insulin secretion by the beta cells of Langerhans, with resulting hyperglycemia (27). When an elevated blood sugar is seen with little alteration in the serum amylase or lipase, the possibility of steroid, cyclosporine, or tacrolimus toxicity to the endocrine pancreas should also be kept in mind.

A histologic diagnosis of acute cellular rejection depends on demonstrating a predominantly mononuclear inflammatory infiltrate containing lymphocytes, immunoblasts, and plasma cells, accompanied by a variable number of neutrophils or eosinophils (31,32). This infiltrate invades and damages acinar cells (33), ductal epithelium, and the islets of Langerhans (Figs. 2–4). Vascular lesions, such as venous endothelialitis and intimal arteritis occur in the more serious forms of rejection (Fig. 5) (34,35). Intra- and peripancreatic nerves can become a target for alloimmune injury, and rejection-associated inflammation may also extend into the peripancreatic fat (Figs. 6,7). Involvement of the islets of Langerhans is in the form of a lymphocytic infiltrate producing a lesion termed isletitis or insulitis. Immunohistochemical staining for insulin and glucagon usually demonstrates a normal distribution of insulin- and glucagons-producing cells (23). A biopsy is generally a reliable tool for the diagnosis of acute cellular rejection. Nonetheless, if clinically suspected rejection is not confirmed by histopathologic examination, repeat biopsy should be considered to rule out sampling error. In a study from the University of Baltimore, repeat biopsy documented rejection missed on the first specimen in 2/7 cases (35).

Histologic criteria to assess the severity of rejection in allograft biopsies have been proposed (36,37). The schema of Drachenberg and colleagues, which defines the use of five clinically validated grades of rejection, is outlined below (37).

Grade 0 or normal refers to pancreatic parenchyma without inflammatory infiltrates. Grade I acute cellular rejection, also designated as inflammation of undetermined significance, is characterized by sparse, mononuclear infiltrates of mostly small lymphocytes, located within the fibrous septae. The veins, arteries, and acini are free of inflammatory change. Mild ductal inflammation may occur, but is not considered to be significant, in the absence of accompanying acinar injury and venous endotheliitis. Grade I rejection, defined by these parameters, is observed in protocol biopsies obtained in the setting of normal graft function,

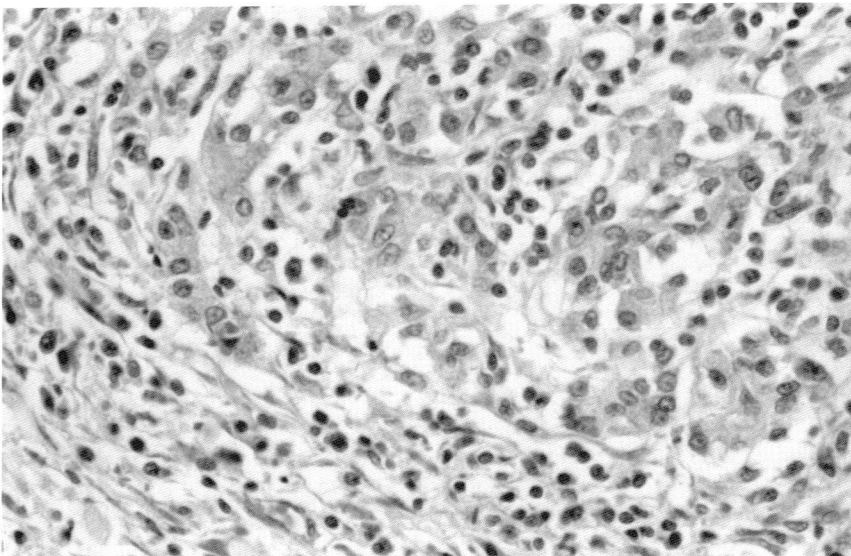

**Figure 2** Pancreas allograft tissue biopsied during an episode of acute cellular rejection. There is an interstitial infiltrate of activated mononuclear cells that focally invades the pancreatic glandular epithelium (H & E ×500).

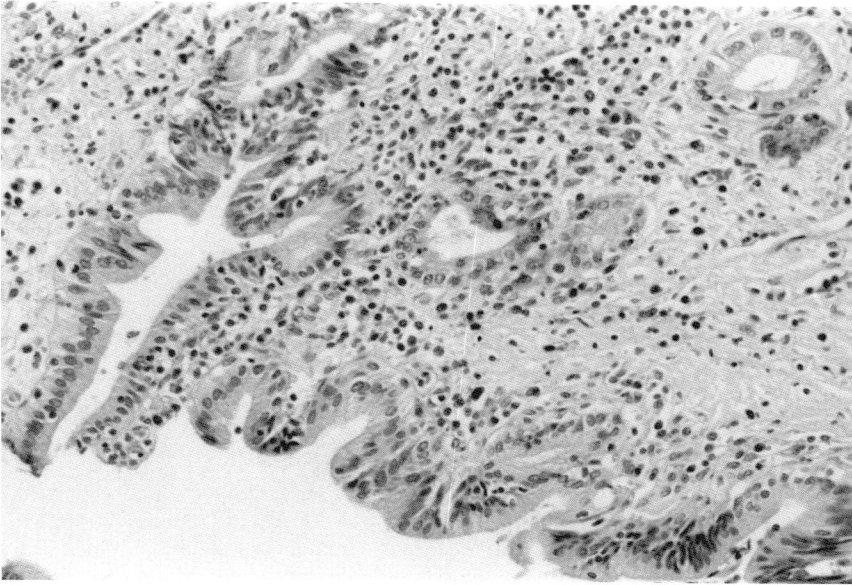

**Figure 3** The same case as illustrated in Figure 2. A pancreatic duct is infiltrated by lymphocytes and plasma cells. Some of these cells extend into the epithelium and are associated with cytoplasmic vacuolization (H & E ×250).

and in follow-up biopsies performed after successful anti-rejection treatment of higher grades of rejection.

Grade II acute cellular rejection, or minimal acute rejection, is defined by the presence of septal mononuclear infiltrates with superimposed venous endothelialitis, i.e., subendothelial infiltration of venous channels by lymphocytes. In the absence of venous endothelialitis, grade II rejection can be also defined as the presence of any three of the following four features: (1) septal inflammation composed of "activated" lymphocytes, (2) presence of eosinophils, (3)

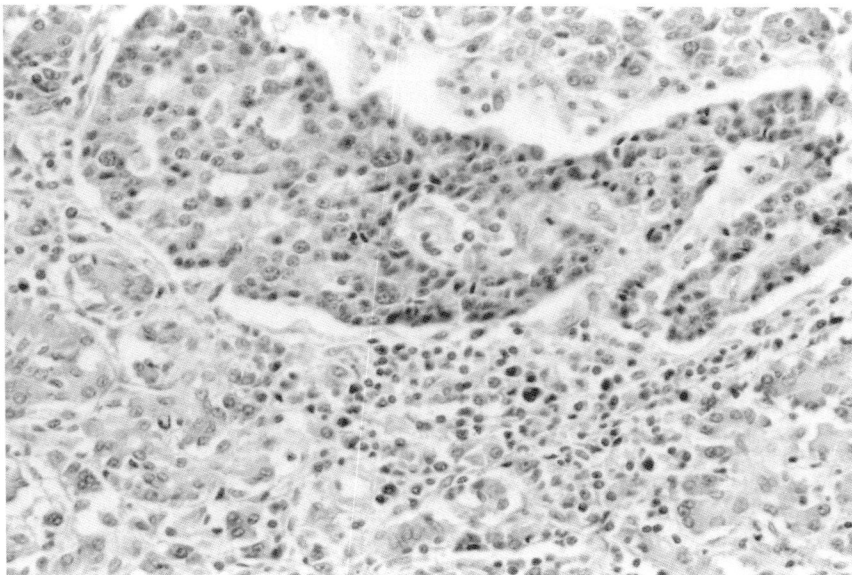

**Figure 4** The cellular infiltrates associated with acute cellular rejection may extend into the islets of Langerhans producing a lesion variously termed isletitis or insulitis (H & E ×250).

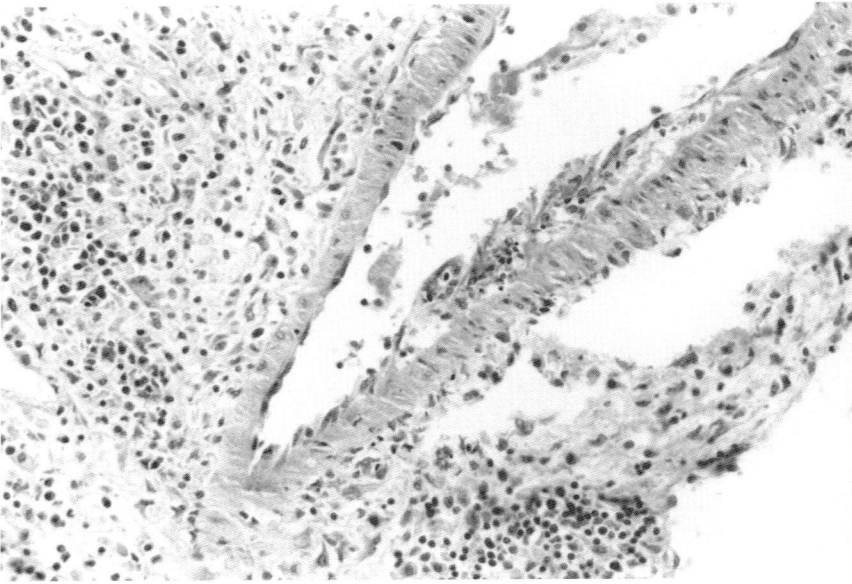

**Figure 5** Moderate acute cellular rejection characterized by intimal arteritis. The artery in this illustration shows sub-endothelial lymphocytic infiltrates, which lift the endothelial cells from the underlying media (H & E ×250).

focal acinar inflammation with presence of one or two foci of at least 10 inflammatory cells each, and (4) ductal inflammation with permeation of inflammatory cells through the ductal basement membranes.

Grade III, or mild acute rejection, is defined by the presence of septal inflammation and three or more foci of acinar inflammation, each focus of acinar inflammation being comprised of at least 10 cells. Neutrophilic infiltrates and focal microabscess formation are seen in some cases. These findings are typically accompanied by acinar cell damage in the form of cytoplasmic vacuolization, apoptosis, necrosis, or cell dropout.

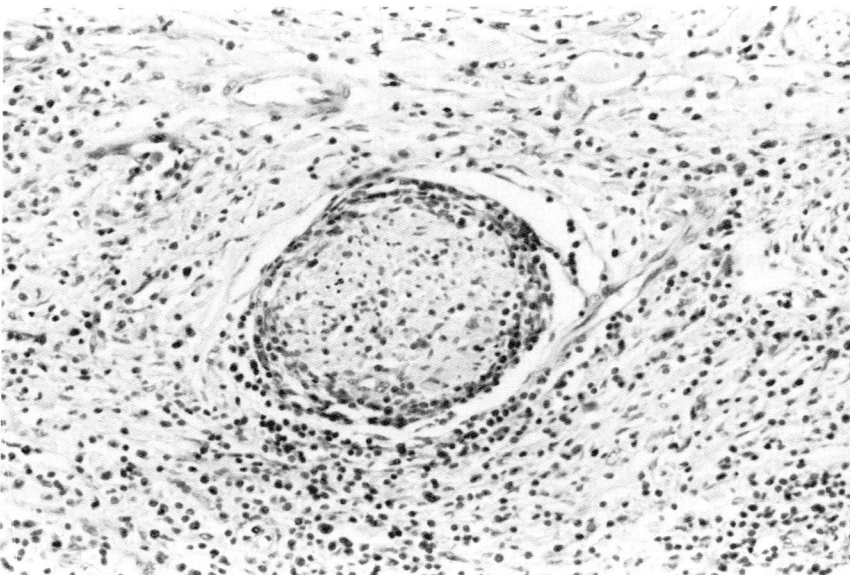

**Figure 6** A nerve running within an allograft pancreas with acute rejection is seen infiltrated by lymphocytes in different stages of maturation (H & E ×250).

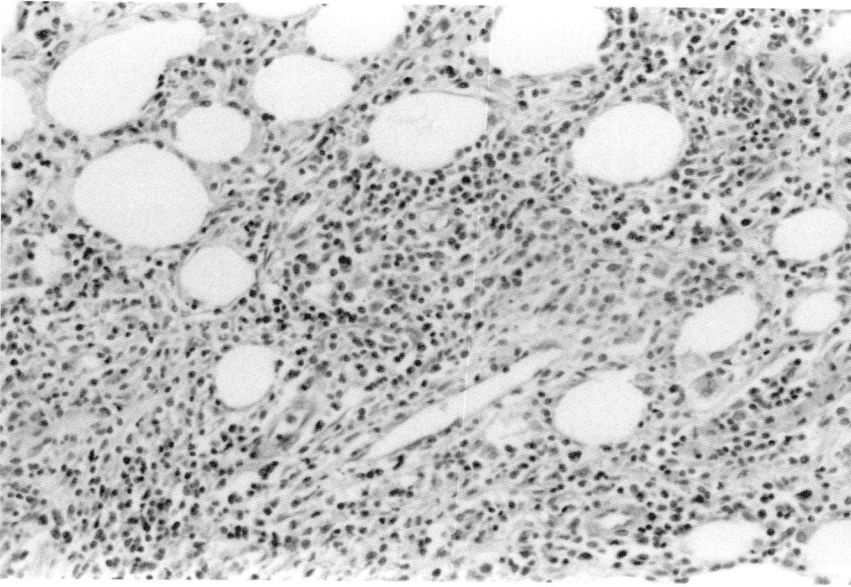

**Figure 7** During acute cellular rejection lymphocytes, plasma cells, and imunoblasts may spill into the peripancreatic fat. These cells are probably targeting donor-specific antigens in the peripancreatic vessels, nerves, and perhaps, also in the adipocytes (H & E ×250).

Grade IV, or moderate acute rejection, requires the presence of arterial involvement manifested as endothelialitis or necrotizing arteritis. Generally, morphological features described for grades II and III rejection are also present in the background.

Grade V, or severe acute rejection, is diagnosed in the presence of multifocal or confluent parenchymal necrosis accompanied by features of grade II, III, or IV rejection.

The reproducibility of this grading system has been formally studied (35). Among the five pathologists who participated in this study, the overall interobserver kappa statistic was 0.83, while the kappa scores for individual grades were 0.9 for grade 0, 0.85 for grade I, 0.66 for grade II, 0.72 for grade III, 0.79 for grade IV, and 0.9 for grade V. The clinical relevance of using this grading schema has been validated by data showing a correlation between rejection grade and ultimate graft outcome (34,35). After a mean follow-up of 19.3 ± 1.9 months, the rates of graft loss associated with rejection grades 0–I, II, III, IV, and V were 0%, 11.5%, 17.3%, 37.5%, and 100%, respectively. In this study, treatment for rejection was given in 0/7 patients with grade 0, 3/12 patients with grade I, 22/31 patients with grade II, 27/27 patients with grade III, 8/8 patients with grade IV, and 7/7 patients with grade V rejection. The biochemical response rates in these groups were 0%, 17%, 71%, 75%, and 50%, respectively. Notably, cases designated as minimal rejection (grade II) also frequently responded to pulse steroids.

## CHRONIC REJECTION

Chronic rejection is a multifactorial process that results in a slow, progressive graft deterioration that culminates in graft loss. On histopathological examination, biopsies of grafts with early chronic rejection show ongoing cellular rejection with superimposed septal fibrosis, acinar atrophy, and focal loss of acinar parenchyma. In advanced chronic rejection, the most diagnostic lesion is a concentric fibro-obliterative vasculopathy involving the major pancreatic arteries and its medium- and small-sized branches (Fig. 8). The intima of these vessels is thickened, and contains mucopolysaccharide-like deposits accompanied by variable numbers of mononuclear cells and foam cells (27). Marked intimal proliferation, thrombotic luminal occlusion, and recanalization are seen in later cases. Completely occluded arteries blend intimately with the surrounding fibrous tissue, and are not readily recognized unless highlighted

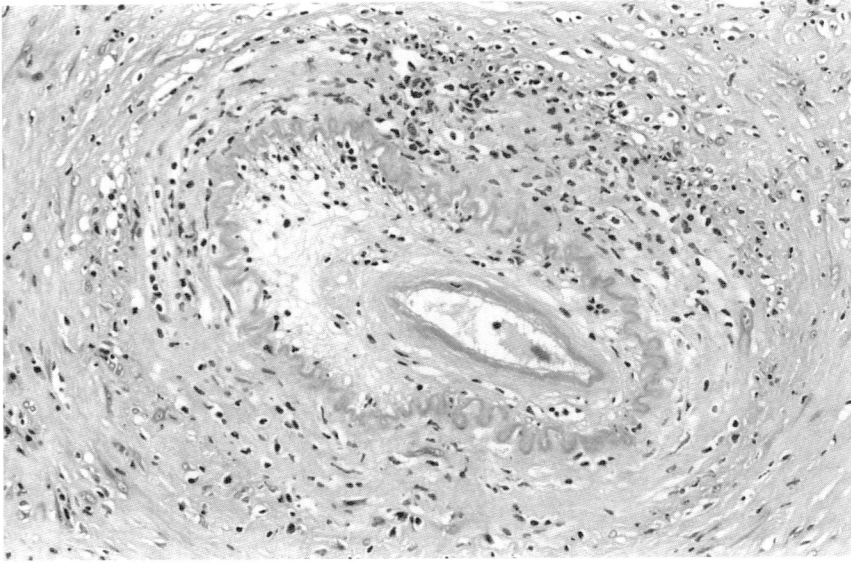

**Figure 8** Chronic vascular rejection involving a major branch of the pancreatic artery. The intima is markedly thickened by accumulated mucopolysaccharide and collagen. A transmural arteritis is superimposed on this chronic lesion (H & E ×250).

by elastic stains. The pancreatic lobules in late chronic rejection show extensive fibrosis accompanied by relatively sparse mononuclear infiltrates. Pancreatic ducts can become thick, fibrous, and infiltrated by lymphocytes. The islets of Langerhans may be normal, architecturally disorganized, atrophic, or hyperplastic (23). Even when there is loss of glycemic control, immunoperoxidase stains can demonstrate insulin staining within the residual islets. The hyperglycemia in this clinical setting is likely due to a combination of reduced total beta cell mass and an insulin secretory defect.

The vascular changes of chronic rejection may not always be seen at needle biopsy due to sampling error. In these cases, chronic pancreatitis may be difficult to exclude on histologic grounds alone. A prior history of recurrent episodes of acute rejection argues against pancreatitis or duct obstruction, but the absence of such a history does not rule out chronic rejection developing in an insidious fashion. The severity of chronic rejection in a biopsy should be graded according to the schema formulated by Papadimitriou et al. (38). In this schema, biopsies are assigned grades I, II, or III, depending on whether fibrous tissue occupies < 30%, 30% to 60%, or > 60%, respectively, of the sampled parenchyma. This classification is clinically relevant, because the predicted graft survivals corresponding to these three grades of chronic rejection were 24.6, 9.7, and 1.6 months, respectively.

## GRAFT VERSUS HOST DISEASE

Incompatibility between donor and host immune cells most often results in a host versus graft reaction, which is referred to as rejection and has been discussed in the preceding sections. However, sometimes graft-derived mononuclear cells migrate into the recipient circulation in large enough numbers to result in host organ damage referred to as graft versus host disease (39). The commonest clinical manifestations are skin rash, hepatitis, gasterointestinal symptoms, and pancytopenia. Donor lymphocyte-derived antibodies directed against host ABO blood group antigens can result in an immune-mediated hemolytic anemia. A definitive diagnosis of graft versus host disease requires demonstration of donor T-cells at the site of tissue injury.

## ACUTE PANCREATITIS

Acute graft pancreatitis develops in up to 16% of pancreatic allograft recipients (40–42). Risk factors include sepsis, ischemia-reperfusion injury, surgical trauma, the use of steroids or

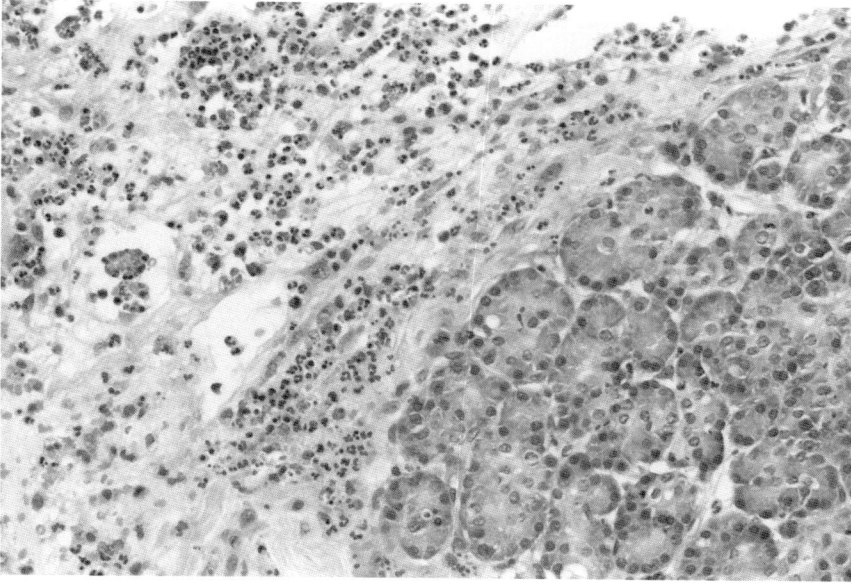

**Figure 9**   The presence of numerous neutrophils in the interstitium and within the glandular lumen is a typical finding in graft pancreatitis. Associated acute cellular or humoral rejection should be kept in mind, since neutrophils can migrate secondarily into tissue damaged primarily by immunologic mechanisms (H & E ×250).

alcohol, stones, and viral infections. Clinically, patients present with fever, epigastric pain, and vomiting. Functional impairment of the pancreas leads to hyperamylasemia and hyperglycemia. Histologic examination shows septal and ductal neutrophilic infiltrates with focal necrosis in the acini and peripancreatic adipose tissue (Fig. 9). Therapy may consist of reduction in immunosuppression, since steroids, azathioprine, tacrolimus, and cyclosporine can all potentiate injury to the pancreatic parenchyma. Somatostatin can also be useful in cases occurring in the early post-transplantation period.

## CHRONIC PANCREATITIS

Recurrent or persistent acute pancreatitis may lead to chronic pancreatitis. Calculus obstruction of a major pancreatic duct can produce a similar clinical picture. The pathology in these cases includes chronic duct inflammation, epithelial proliferation, squamous metaplasia, concentric periductal fibrosis with compressed, dilated, or angulated ducts, dystrophic parenchymal calcification, and islet cell atrophy or hyperplasia.

A unique form of chemical pancreatitis is seen in grafts in which liquid synthetic polymer has been injected into the ducts (43). The rationale behind this technique is to let the injected polymer harden into a solid cast, which reduces the incidence of anastomotic leakage, retroperitoneal fluid collection, and pancreatic fistula formation. Although the ensuing complete blockage of the secretory system leads to obstructive atrophy of the pancreatic acini, the islets of Langerhans remain functionally intact, and continue insulin secretion. Unfortunately, prolonged tissue contact with these polymers excites a foreign-body reaction, with acute or chronic inflammation, fat necrosis, and extensive fibrosis in the graft parenchyma (27).

## BACTERIAL INFECTIONS

Urinary tract infections occur in virtually all bladder-drained patients (44), while surgical site infections have been reported in up to 30% of cases (45), and other miscellaneous infections in 5% of individuals (40). The diagnosis is primarily based on clinical examination and microbiologic cultures. The clinical manifestations include wound dehiscence, bacterial peritonitis, intra-abdominal abscess, urinary tract infection, pneumonia, systemic sepsis, and arterioenteric fistula formation (46). It is important for the pathologist to realize that intra-abdominal infections can cause reactive changes in the pancreas, which may be confused with acute or chronic rejection. The graft biopsy typically shows mixed or mononuclear septal infiltrates and proliferation of immature fibroblasts. In chronic infections, paraseptal fibrous bands may give a cirrhotic appearance to the exocrine lobules. The presence of relatively minimal acinar inflammation and absence of vascular injury usually allows the pathologist to distinguish this from rejection. However, if immunosuppression is reduced to facilitate recovery from infection, biopsies with overlapping features may be encountered, and this may lead to difficulty in interpretation.

## CMV INFECTION

Cytomegalovirus (CMV) inclusions can be seen in up to 13% of pancreatic grafts (27,45). CMV infection can be a part of a multisystemic viral syndrome or can represent disease localized to the graft. Concomitant acute rejection or silicone-associated pancreatitis may be present in some cases. The clinical presentation includes acute pancreatitis and gastrointestinal hemorrhage. On histopathologic examination, CMV-infected cells show marked cytomegaly, and contain large prominent eosinophilic intranuclear inclusions surrounded by a clear halo. Viral inclusions can occur in epithelial, endothelial, or stromal cells (Fig. 10). Immunoperoxidase stains for CMV can be performed if viral cytopathic changes are equivocal on light microscopy. In the setting of CMV infection, the diagnosis of a concurrent mild rejection may be difficult on morphologic grounds. Mild focal venous endothelialitis and acinar damage can probably be secondary to virus-mediated injury, and do not call for anti-rejection treatment. The proper management is to reduce immunosuppression (47). Early initiation of ganciclovir therapy is successful in most cases. Delayed treatment can lead to pancreatic abscess formation and graft loss (48).

## POSTTRANSPLANT LYMPHOPROLIFERATIVE DISORDERS

The incidence of post-transplant lymphoproliferative disorders (PTLDs) in pancreas and pancreas–kidney transplant recipients has ranged from 2.2% to 12% (49). This disease is a complication of Epstein–Barr virus (EBV) infection in immunosuppressed patients, wherein virally

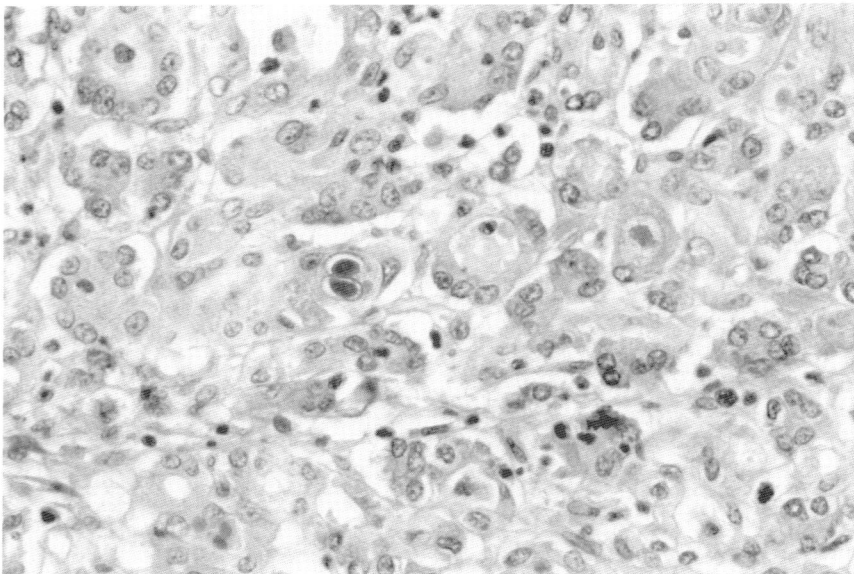

**Figure 10**  Acinar epithelium showing intranuclear cytomegalovirus inclusions surrounded by a clear halo. Granular cytoplasmic inclusions of varying size can also be seen in some cells. The associated inflammatory response is quite sparse: this is not an infrequent finding in immunosuppressed individuals (H & E ×500).

infected B-lymphocytes escape normal immune surveillance mechanisms and initiate unrestrained proliferation of lymphoid cells. PTLD can involve the allograft with or without disease in other organ systems, such as lymph nodes and gastrointestinal tract (50). Discontinuation or significant reduction of immunosuppression and administration of gancyclovir produces a good therapeutic response in many cases, while other patients succumb to disseminated disease despite additional treatment with alpha-interferon, radiation, and/or chemotherapy. Surgical excision can be quite effective in managing patients with localized lesions.

Based on histologic features, most PTLD lesions can be categorized as early lesions (showing plasmacytic hyperplasia or an infectious mononucleosis-like picture), polymorphic PTLDs (showing architectural effacement of the affected organ by a pleomorphic lymphoid infiltrate), or monomorphic PTLDs (showing a predominance of transformed cells) (51). Although early lesions and polymorphic PTLDs tend to have a better prognosis, morphologic appearances cannot always reliably predict the ultimate clinical prognosis.

Making a distinction between PTLD and severe acute rejection is critical, because the correct treatment is discontinuation or reduction of immunosuppression for PTLD, but aggressive anti-T-cell therapy for acute rejection. PTLD characteristically shows a nodular infiltrates with irregular foci of geographic necrosis. These nodular infiltrates must be distinguished from lymphoid hyperplasia occurring in rejection due to allogeneic stimulation. The infiltrates in PTLD generally show significant nuclear atypia exceeding 25% of the total population (49,52). Some biopsies present a monotonous appearance that closely resembles conventional lymphomas. Acinar injury is not prominent in PTLD, but venous endothelialitis is common, and lesions may center on the connective tissue septae in the pancreas. Arterial endothelialitis or necrotizing vasculitis was not found in one series of four PTLD specimens affecting the allograft pancreas (49). However, in renal allografts, we have found that rare interlobular arteries entrapped within PTLD lesions can show vasculitis (52). Infiltration of the hilar soft tissues or nerves can be seen in PTLD as well as in severe acute rejection, although some observers feel that this is less prominent in the setting of rejection (49).

While the aforementioned observations provide helpful criteria for the separation of PTLD from severe acute rejection by routine light microscopy, difficulties can be encountered with limited biopsy material. In the latter circumstance, the final diagnosis must await the results of immunophenotyping, and EBV in situ hybridization. With rare exceptions, PTLD lesions contain predominantly B-cells and are EBV positive, while rejection is associated with a primarily T-cell infiltrate that is EBV negative (52). In lesions with significant numbers of plasma cells, staining for kappa and lambda light chains is a convenient way of identifying lesions that are clearly clonal. If sufficient fresh tissue is available, immunoglobulin gene rearrangement and oncogene studies can be performed to help in diagnosis, and to generate information relevant to the ultimate prognosis (53). It is also worth remembering that PTLD and severe acute rejection are not always mutually exclusive diagnoses. Since PTLD frequently arises in the setting of severe acute rejection, evidence of both processes can be found in some specimens.

## UROLOGIC COMPLICATIONS

In bladder-drained organs, proteolytic enzymes secreted by the allograft come into direct contact with the bladder mucosa. These enzymes are secreted in an inactive form, and normally do not get activated, since the required enterokinases are lacking in the bladder lumen. However, infections may promote conditions favorable for in situ digestion of the urothelium. This may result in hemorrhagic cystitis, urethritis, urethral diverticulosis, or penile necrosis (54,55).

## RECURRENT INSULIN-DEPENDENT DIABETES MELLITUS

Type I diabetes mellitus is believed to be an autoimmune disorder directed against the islets of Langerhans. Many investigators believe that cell-mediated immunity plays an important role in the beta cell destruction characteristic of this disease (56–58). Furthermore, serologic and tissue immunofluorescence data suggest an additional role for the humoral limb of the immune system in this process (59–61). Consistent with the autoimmune nature of the disease, recurrence of type I diabetes in the allograft pancreas has been reported. Initial reports were confined to human leucocyte antigen (HLA)-identical siblings or monozygous twins (27), but it has since been shown that sharing of HLA alleles is not a prerequisite for recurrence (62). The low frequency with which recurrent disease is documented in clinical practice may be related to inhibition of autoimmune reactions by routine post-transplant immunosuppression, or perhaps by donor T-cell chimerism (63,64).

Clinically, recurrent diabetes manifests as hyperglycemia occurring 1 to 32 months after transplantation, with progression to insulin dependence 2.5 to 58 months later. Rising titers of antibodies to glutamate decarboxylase and tyrosine phosphatase may be demonstrable (65). Allograft biopsy performed at the time of initial hyperglycemia shows "isletitis," characterized by architectural disarray and mononuclear infiltrates in the islets of Langerhans, with associated degranulation and destruction of the beta cells (66). Following the onset of insulin dependence, inflammatory infiltrates become less prominent or disappear, and some biopsies show complete absence of beta cells. In cases with only sparse lymphocytic infiltrates, immunoperoxidase stains using antibodies for T-cells are helpful in demonstrating subtle lesions of isletitis. The infiltrating lymphocytes in recurrent diabetes are said to be mostly CD8-positive T-lymphocytes (31). No immunoglobulin or complement deposits are seen, but islet cells do show strong expression of Class I major histocomplexity complex (MHC) antigens on the cell surface. Immunohistochemistry is also a very useful method of demonstrating that immune injury to the islets in recurrent type I diabetes is selective for beta cells. The majority of islets in advanced cases show less than 20% beta cells and greater than 60% alpha cells (32). In contrast, the isletitis occurring in association with acute or chronic rejection is not associated with any alteration in the relative proportion of insulin- and glucagon-producing cells. Calculation of the ratio of insulin islet units to glucagon islet units permits a diagnosis of recurrent diabetes even when isletitis has subsided completely or is felt to be related to coexisting rejection (67). A ratio of insulin islet units to glucagon islet units below 1.00 is said to be highly suggestive of recurrent diabetes.

## SUMMARY

Pancreatic transplantation has now become a relatively successful surgical procedure, although additional research is needed to further improve long-term outcomes. When episodes of allograft dysfunction occur in the post-transplant phase, a biopsy plays a critical role in recognizing various forms of rejection, and to differentiate these from nonimmunologic causes of graft malfunction, such as donor disease, ischemia/preservation injury, vascular thrombosis, pancreatitis, infections, Epstein-Barr virus-associated post-transplant lymphoproliferative disease, technical complications, drug toxicity, and recurrence of diabetes mellitus. In most patients with simultaneous kidney and pancreas transplantation, the pancreatic graft can be adequately monitored by renal allograft biopsy. In cases where only the pancreas has been transplanted, the most practical way of obtaining allograft tissue for study is a percutaneous needle biopsy performed under ultrasound guidance. The histologic diagnosis of acute cellular rejection is based on the presence of a predominantly mononuclear inflammatory infiltrate, damage to the acinar cells or ductal epithelium, and the occurrence of vascular lesions such as venous endothelialitis or intimal arteritis. Most episodes of acute rejection are readily reversed by an increase in immunosuppression. Grading the severity of acute rejection can guide the intensity of anti-rejection therapy and help determine the prognosis of the graft. Chronic rejection is characterized by ongoing low-grade acute rejection with superimposed septal fibrosis, acinar atrophy, and focal loss of acinar parenchyma. The most diagnostic lesion is a concentric fibro-obliterative vasculopathy, but this is not always present at needle biopsy, and may only be appreciated at allograft pancreatectomy or autopsy. As with other solid organ allografts, chronic rejection remains a significant obstacle to the long-term success of pancreatic transplantation.

## REFERENCES

1. Laftavi MR, Gruessner AC, Bland BJ, et al. Significance of pancreas graft biopsy in detection of rejection. Transplant Proc 1998; 30:642–644.
2. Kuo PC, Johnson LB, Schweitzer EJ, et al. Solitary pancreas allografts. The role of percutaneous biopsy and standardized histologic grading of rejection. Arch Surg 1997; 132:52–57.

3. Tesi RJ, Henry ML, Elkhammas EA, Davies EA, Ferguson RM. The frequency of rejection episodes after combined kidney–pancreas transplant—the impact on graft survival. Transplantation 1994; 58:424–430.
4. Sugitani A, Egidi MF, Gritsch HA, Corry RJ. Serum lipase as a marker for pancreatic allograft rejection. Transplant Proc 1998; 30:645.
5. Carpenter HA, Engen DE, Munn SR, et al. Histologic diagnosis of rejection by using cystoscopically directed needle biopsy specimens from dysfunctional pancreaticoduodenal allografts with exocrine drainage into the bladder. Am J Surg Pathol 1990; 14:837–846.
6. Nakhleh RE, Benedetti E, Gruessner A, et al. Cystoscopic biopsies in pancreaticoduodenal transplantation. Transplantation 1995; 60:541–546.
7. Stratta RJ, Taylor RJ, Grune MT, et al. Experience with protocol biopsies after solitary pancreas transplantation. Transplantation 1995; 60:1431–1437.
8. Nghiem DD. Role of duodenal biopsy in bladder-drained pancreas transplants. Transplant Proc 1992; 24:1247–1248.
9. Nakhleh RE, Gruessner RWG, Tzardis PJ, Dunn DL, Sutherland DER. Pathology of transplanted human duodenal tissue: a histologic study, with comparison to pancreatic pathology in resected pancreaticoduodenal transplants. Clin Transplant 1991; 5:241–247.
10. Allen RDM, Wilson TG, Grierson JM, et al. Percutaneous pancreas transplant fine needle aspiration and needle core biopsies are useful and safe. Transplant Proc 1990; 22:663–664.
11. Allen RDM, Wilson TG, Grierson JM, et al. Percutaneous biopsy of bladder-drained pancreas transplants. Transplantation 1991; 51:1213–1216.
12. Laftavi MR, Gruessner AC, Bland BJ, et al. Diagnosis of pancreas rejection: cystoscopic transduodenal versus percutaneous computed tomography scan guided biopsy. Transplantation 1998; 65:528–532.
13. Klassen DK, Hoehn-Saric EW, Weir MR, et al. Isolated pancreas rejection in combined kidney pancreas transplantation. Transplantation 1996; 61:974–976.
14. Egidi MF, Corry RJ, Sugitani A, et al. Enteric-drained pancreas transplants monitored by fine-needle aspiration biopsy. Transplant Proc 1997; 29:674–675.
15. Gray DWR, Richardson A, Hughes D, et al. A prospective randomized, blind comparison of three biopsy techniques in the management of patients after renal transplantation. Transplantation 1991; 53:1226–1232.
16. Greene CL, Fehrman I, Tillery GW, Husberg BS, Klintmalm GB. Transplant aspiration cytology detects entities other than acute cellular rejection in liver allografts. Transplant Proc 1988; 20:692–694.
17. Kubota K, Reinholt FP, Tyden G, Groth CG. Pancreatic juice cytology for monitoring pancreatic grafts in the early postoperative period. Transplant Int 1992; 5:133–138.
18. Radio SJ, Stratta RJ, Taylor RJ, Linder J. The utility of urine cytology in the diagnosis of allograft rejection after combined pancreas-kidney transplantation. Transplantation 1993; 55:509–516.
19. Mittal VK, Toledo-Pereyra LH. Urinary cytology as a complementary marker of rejection in combined kidney and pancreatic transplants with urinary drainage. Transplant Proc 1990; 22:629–663.
20. Matsukuma S, Suda K, Abe H. Histopathological study of pancreatic ischemic lesions induced by cholesterol emboli: fresh and subsequent features of pancreatic ischemia. Hum Pathol 1998; 28:41–46.
21. Troppmann C, Gruessner AC, Benedetti E, et al. Vascular graft thrombosis after pancreatic transplantation: univariate and multivariate operative and nonoperative risk factor analysis. J Am Coll Surg 1996; 182:285–316.
22. Sutherland DER, Goetz C, Najarian JS. Pancreas transplantation at the University of Minnesota: donor and recipient selection, operative and postoperative management, and outcome. Transplant Proc 1987; 19:63–74.
23. Drachenberg CB, Papadimitriou JC, Klassen DK, Bartlett ST. Distribution of alpha and beta cells in pancreas allograft biopsies: correlation with rejection and other pathologic processes. Transplant Proc 1998; 30:665–666.
24. Kuo PC, Wong J, Schweitzer EJ, Johnson LB, Lim JW, Bartlett ST. Outcome after splenic vein thrombosis in the pancreas allograft. Transplantation 1997; 64:933–935.
25. Drachenberg CB, Papadimitriou JC, Farney A, et al. Pancreas transplantation: the histologic morphology of graft loss and clinical correlations. Transplantation 2001; 71:1784.
26. Pelletier RP, Orosz CG, Adams PW, et al. Clinical and economic impact of flow cytometry crossmatching in primary cadaveric kidney and simultaneous pancreas–kidney transplant recipients. Transplantation 1997; 63:1639–1645.
27. Sibley RK. Pancreas transplantation. In: Sale GE, ed. The Pathology of Organ Transplantation. Stoneham, MA: Buttersworth Publishers, 1990:179–216.
28. Prieto M, Sutherland DER, Fernandez-Cruz L, Heil J, Najarian JS. Experimental and clinical experience with urine amylase monitoring for early diagnosis of rejection in pancreas transplantation. Transplantation 1987; 43:73–79.
29. Dafoe DC, Campbell DA, Rocher L, Schwartz R, Turcotte JG. Diagnosis of rejection in simultaneous renal/pancreas (urinary bladder drained) transplantation. Transplant Proc 1987; 19:2345–2347.
30. Moss DW, Henderson RA. Digestive enzymes of pancreatic origin. In: Burtis CA, Ashwood ER, eds. Tietz Textbook of Clinical Chemistry. Philadelphia, PA: W.B. Saunders Company, 1994:852–871.

31. Sibley RK, Sutherland DER. Pancreas transplantation. An immunohistologic and histopathologic examination of 100 grafts. Am J Pathol 1987; 128:151–170.
32. Nakhleh RE, Gruessner RWG, Swanson PE, et al. Pancreas transplant pathology. Am J Surg Pathol 1991; 15:246–256.
33. Boonstra JG, Wever PC, Laterveer JC, et al. Apoptosis of acinar cells in pancreas allograft rejection. Transplantation 1997; 64:1211–1213.
34. Boonstra JG, van der Pijl JW, Smets YF, et al. Interstitial and vascular pancreas rejection in relation to graft survival. Transplant Int 1997; 10:451–456.
35. Drachenberg CB, Papadimitriou JC, Klassen DK, et al. Evaluation of pancreas transplant needle biopsy: reproducibility and revision of histologic grading system. Transplantation 1997; 63:1579–1586.
36. Nakhleh RE, Sutherland DER. Pancreas Rejection. Significance of histopathologic findings with implications for classification of rejection. Am J Surg Pathol 1992; 16:1098–1107.
37. Drachenberg C, Klassen D, Bartlett S, et al. Histologic grading of pancreas acute allograft rejection in percutaneous needle biopsies. Transplant Proc 1996; 28:512–513.
38. Papadimitriou JC, Drachenberg CB, Klassen D, et al. Histologic grading of chronic pancreas allograft rejection/graft sclerosis. Am J Transplant 2003; 3:599.
39. Kimball P, Ham J, Eisenberg M, et al. Lethal graft-versus-host disease after simultaneous kidney–pancreas transplantation. Transplantation 1997; 63:1685–1688.
40. Moudry-Munns KC, Gillingham K, Dunn D, Sutherland DER. Mortality risk for technically successful vs technically failed bladder drained pancreas transplants and causes of death. Transplant Proc 1992; 24:863–865.
41. Fernandez-Cruz L, Sabater L, Gilabert R, Ricart MJ, Saenz A, Astudillo E. Native and graft pancreatitis following combined pancreas-renal transplantation. Br J Surg 1993; 80:1429–1432.
42. Grewal HP, Garland L, Novak K, Gaber L, Tolley EA, Gaber AO. Risk factors for postimplantation pancreatitis and pancreatic thrombosis in pancreas transplant recipients. Transplantation 1993; 56:609–612.
43. Cantarovich D, Traeger J, LaRocca E, et al. Evolution of metabolic and endocrine function in ten neoprene-injected segmental pancreas allografts at 3 to 54 months after transplantation, versus preliminary results in nine whole pancreas allografts with enteric diversion. Transplant Proc 1987; 19:2310–2313.
44. Van der Pijl JW, Smets YFC, de la Fuente R, Ringers J, Lemkes HHPJ, van der Woude FJ. Urologic infections and problems after 50 simultaneous pancreas-kidney transplantations. Transplant Proc 1995; 27:3105.
45. Smets YF, van der Pijl JW, van Dissel JT, Ringers J, de Fijter JW, Lemkes HH. Infectious disease complications of simultaneous pancreas kidney transplantation. Nephrol Dial Transplant 1997; 12:764–771.
46. Gritsch HA, Shapiro R, Egidi F, Randhawa PS, Starzl TE, Corry RJ. Spontaneous arterioenteric fistula after pancreas transplantation. Transplantation 1997; 63:903–904.
47. Margreiter R, Schmid T, Dunser M, Tauscher T, Hengster P, Konigsrainer A. Cytomegalovirus (CMV)–pancreatitis: a rare complication after pancreas transplantation. Transplant Proc 1991; 23:1619–1622.
48. Backman LC, Brattstrom C, Reinholt FP, Andersson J, Tyden G. Development of intrapancreatic abscess—a consequence of CMV pancreatitis? Transplant Int 1991; 4:116–121.
49. Drachenberg CB, Abruzzo LV, Klassen DK, et al. Epstein-Barr virus-related post-transplantation lymphoproliferative disorder involving pancreas allografts: histological differential diagnosis from acute allograft rejection. Hum Pathol 1998; 29:569–577.
50. Nalesnik MA, Jaffe R, Starzl TE, et al. The pathology of posttransplant lymphoproliferative disorders occurring in the setting of cyclosporine A–prednisone immunosuppression. Am J Pathol 1988; 133:173–192.
51. Harris NT, Ferry J, Swerdlow S. Post-transplant lymphoproliferative disorders: summary of Society of Hematopathology Workshop. Semin Diag Pathol 1997; 14:8–14.
52. Randhawa PS, Demetris AJ, Pietrzak B, Nalesnik M. Histopathology of renal posttransplant lymphoproliferation: comparison with rejection using the Banff Schema. Am J Kidney Dis 1996; 28:578–584.
53. Seiden MV, Sklar J. Molecular genetic analysis of post-transplant lymphoproliferative disorders. Hematol Oncol Clin North Am 1993; 7:447–465.
54. Konigsrainer A, Feichtinger H, Waitz W, et al. Does pancreatic juice have a detrimental effect on the bladder mucosa? Transplant Proc 1990; 22:1600–1601.
55. Kaplan AJ, Rames R, Bromberg JS. Multiple giant urethral diverticula—an unusual complication of combined kidney/pancreas transplantation. Transplantation 1995; 59:910–912.
56. Gepts W, Lecompte PM. The pancreatic islets in diabetes. Am J Med 1981; 70:105–115.
57. Foulis AD, Stewart JA. The pancreas in recent-onset type I (insulin-dependent) diabetes mellitus; insulin content of islets, insulitis and associated changes in the exocrine acinar tissue. Diabetologia 1984; 26:456–461.
58. Gepts W. Pathological anatomy of the pancreas in juvenile diabetes mellitus. Diabetes 1965; 1:619–633.

59. Bottazzo GF, Dean BM, McNally JM, MacKay EH, Swift PGF, Gamble DR. In situ characterization of autoimmune phenomena and expression of HLA molecules in the pancreas in diabetic insulitis. N Engl J Med 1985; 313:353–360.
60. Bottazzo GF, Dean BM, Gorsuch AN, Cudworth AG, Doniach D. Complement-fixing islet-cell antibodies in type I diabetes: possible monitors of active beta cell damage. Lancet 1980; 1:668–672.
61. Irvine WJ, McCallum CJ, Gray RS, et al. Pancreatic islet-cell antibodies in diabetes mellitus correlated with the duration and type of diabetes, coexistent autoimmune disease, and HLA type. Diabetes 1977; 26:138–147.
62. Tyden G, Reinholt FP, Sundkvist G, Bolinder J. Recurrence of autoimmune diabetes mellitus in recipients of cadaveric pancreatic grafts. N Engl J Med 1996; 335:860–863.
63. Drachenberg CB, Papadimitriou JC, Weir MR, Klassen DK, Hoehn-Saric E, Bartlett ST. Histologic findings in islets of whole pancreas allografts: lack of evidence of recurrent cell-mediated diabetes mellitus. Transplantation 1996; 62:1770–1773.
64. Bartlett ST, Chin T, Dirden B, Quereshi A, Hadley G. Inclusion of peripancreatic lymph node cells prevents recurrent autoimmune destruction of islet transplants: evidence of donor chimerism. Surgery 1995; 118:392–397.
65. Thivolet CH, Abou-Amara S, Martin X, et al. Serological markers of recurrent beta cells destruction in diabetic patients undergoing pancreatic transplantation. Transplantation 2000; 69:99.
66. Sibley RK, Sutherland DER, Goetz F, Michael AF. Recurrent diabetes mellitus in the pancreas iso- and allograft. A light and electron microscopic and immunohistochemical analysis of four cases. Lab Invest 1985; 53:132–144.
67. Nakhleh RE, Gruessner RWG, Tzardis PJ, Brayman K, Dunn DL, Sutherland DER. Pancreas transplant pathology: an immunohistochemical comparison of allografts with rejection, syngeneic grafts, and chronic pancreatitis. Transplant Proc 1991; 23:1598–1599.

# 15 | Fine Needle Aspiration Biopsy in Kidney and Pancreas Transplantation

**M. Francesca Egidi**

*The University of Tennessee Health Science Center, Methodist University, Transplant Institute, Memphis, Tennessee, U.S.A.*

## INTRODUCTION

In the past 20 years, numerous attempts have been made to develop noninvasive procedures for monitoring rejection episodes in solid organ transplantation. Although new activation markers detected from blood and urine specimens have shown accuracy and reliability (1,2), these tests are still research tools and have not been utilized in routine clinical practice. A needle biopsy is still the only reliable method to assess intragraft events and is considered the "gold standard" in clinical practice. However, in spite of increasingly accurate ultrasonographic techniques and safer needles, biopsies are still associated with a risk of bleeding, fistula formation (either arteriovenous or parenchymal), and infection.

Fine needle aspiration biopsy (FNAB) was introduced by Pasternack et al. (3) in 1968 for monitoring after kidney transplantation. The technique was then improved by Häyry and Willebrand (4) to the point where its clinical utility could be assessed (5). In the 1970s, the Helsinki group worked extensively on animal models and on specimens from rejected human kidneys in order to characterize the heterogeneous population of white cells infiltrating the grafts (6). Those discoveries provided the basis for the transplant cytology used to define and quantify the type and degree of inflammation. Further studies analyzing the cell traffic from the graft and the recipient, such as peripheral blood, spleen, or lymph nodes, proved that immuno-activation is initiated in the graft, where the lymphocytes and monocytes are transformed from immature precursors (blasts) that are actively replicating and secreting immunoglobulins and cytokines (7,8). The rationale for FNAB resides in detecting blasts and other activated cells that are considered markers for active acute rejection. FNAB, initially performed in the kidney, has been extended to the liver (9), and more recently to pancreas transplants (10–13). Sequential follow-up of transplanted recipients with frequent FNAB allows for

- Monitoring of the onset, type, severity, and duration of inflammatory episodes of rejection,
- Analysis of the impact of inflammation and other unrelated factors (such as drug toxicity) on the graft parenchymal components,
- Analysis of the impact of treatment on these parameters (5,14).

Unlike needle biopsy, FNAB is a safe and fast procedure that can be performed on outpatients, often repeatedly, on a daily basis, and processed in a very short time. Thus, the great power of the FNAB is a frequent assessment of the intragraft events with good reproducibility and reliability. FNAB has been proven to be less traumatic and better accepted by children for whom the core biopsy procedure might require general anesthesia and hospitalization (15).

FNAB is based on cytological findings, so the information derived from the aspirate is different, when compared to tissue biopsies. However, several studies reported a high degree of concordance between histopathological and cytological findings in samples taken simultaneously (16,17).

The possible etiologies for graft dysfunction identified by FNAB and compared to core biopsy findings are summarized in Table 1. Although not without potential limitations, FNAB can be a useful tool for monitoring rejection or other causes of graft dysfunction in the immediate posttransplant period, when the main issues are related to acute issues, such as immunoactivation or drug toxicity. The utility of FNAB for late posttransplant follow-up is more limited.

**Table 1**  Comparison of Fine Needle Aspiration Biopsy and Core Biopsy Findings

|  | FNAB | | Core biopsy | |
|---|---|---|---|---|
|  | **Kidney** | **Pancreas** | **Kidney** | **Pancreas** |
| Acute cellular rejection | ++ | ++ | +++ | +++ |
| Humoral/vascular rejection | +(?) | +(?) | +++ | ++ |
| Parenchymal cell damage (acute) |  |  |  |  |
|     Tubular cell damage (ATN) | +++ | NA | +++ | NA |
|     Acinar cell damage | NA | +++ | NA | ++(?) |
|     Cyclosporine/tacrolimus toxicity | +++ | +++ | ++ | ++(?) |
| Parenchymal cell damage (chronic) | ? | ? | Fibrosis | Fibrosis |
| Infections | ++ | ++ | Pyelonephritis | Pancreatitis |
| Recurrent diseases | NA | NA | +++ | +++ |

*Abbreviations*: FNAB, fine needle aspiration biopsy; ATN, acute tubular necrosis; NA, not applicable.

In addition to its clinical utility, FNAB provides a unique research tool for culturing and categorizing viable intragraft cells and their possible significance (18).

## FNAB TECHNIQUE AND SPECIMEN EVALUATION

Under ultrasound guidance, without local anesthesia, a 22 to 25 gauge spinal needle connected to a 10 to 20 mL syringe loaded with 5 mL of sterile medium containing RPMI 1640, heparin (25,000 I.U. per 1000 mL), and human albumin 20% (50 mL per 1000 mL) is inserted percutaneously into the graft. Suction is applied and 10 to 20 μL specimens are obtained (Fig. 1). The content of the FNAB is gently flushed in 1 to 2 mL medium and adjusted to approximately $1 \times 10$ nucleated cells per milliliter. In order to obviate the variable contamination of the aspirate by blood, a peripheral blood sample of similar size is taken from the fingertip. Both specimens are processed onto microscopic slides by cytocentrifugation and stained, usually by May-Grünwald-Giemsa (4,19). Immunofluorescence, immunoperoxidase, and other staining techniques for further cell characterization with monoclonal antibodies can also be performed (20,21).

### Quantification of the Inflammation

Before the infiltrating cell evaluation can be performed, the sample adequacy must be determined by the presence of at least 7 to 10 parenchymal cells per 100 leucocytes within the aspirate. Immunoactivation and the diagnosis of acute rejection are determined by a wide spectrum of cells at different stages of activation, including T- and B-lymphocytes, lymphoblasts, plama cells, and monoblasts (Fig. 2). The intense presence of plasma cells and their transformation from plasmablasts seems to be more related to antibody-mediated rejection. A rapid maturation of blood-borne monocytes into tissue macrophages is frequently seen in advanced and possibly irreversible rejection. To quantify the severity of the inflammation,

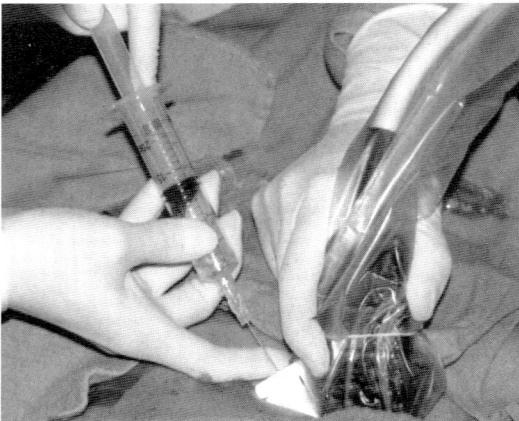

**Figure 1**  Fine needle aspiration biopsy procedure under ultrasound guidance.

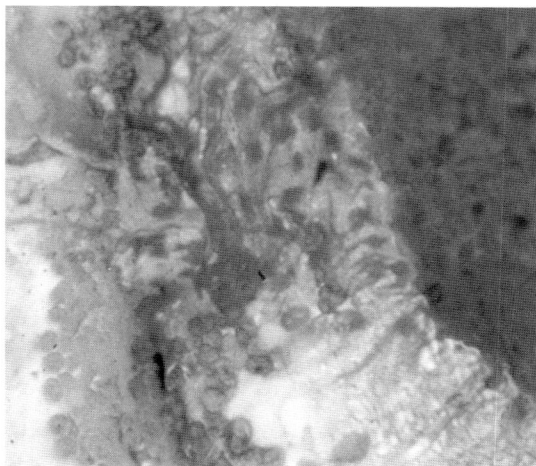

**Figure 2** Acute rejection with lymphoblast and macrophage infiltrate (May-Grünwald-Giemsa, ×325).

the "corrected increment" method has been established (19). In brief, 100 inflammatory mononucleated cells are categorized and counted in the aspirates and the peripheral blood. The numerical difference between the two specimens and their sum gives a numerical score. The diagnostic impact of the score is based on the fact that each cell category has a different value, according to the maturation stage, so the more immature cells (blasts) will increase the total score and consequently the likelihood of rejection. The response to anti-rejection therapy can be assessed by repeated FNAB (3,4,14). Recently, advanced immunological techniques have shown that cytokines and other substances released by the inflammatory population are affected by different immunosuppressive regimens (22).

## Parenchymal Cells

Parenchymal cells belonging to kidney, liver, and pancreas grafts express similar lesions and are qualitatively evaluated as a part of the overall interpretation of FNAB (Figs. 3 and 4). The degree of cellular damage depends on the extent and origin of the injury. The different cellular components of tubuloepithelial, endothelial, and glomerular cells have been extensively established in native and transplanted kidneys. In acute tubular necrosis, the graft tubular cells (small basophilic and large, clear, or granulated tubular cells) appear swollen and vacuolated. The severity of tubular cell damage correlates with the clinical dysfunction. These changes disappear with the recovery of renal function (19,23). Similar findings detected in pancreatic acinar cells might represent a sign of early injury, although the pancreatic parenchyma appears

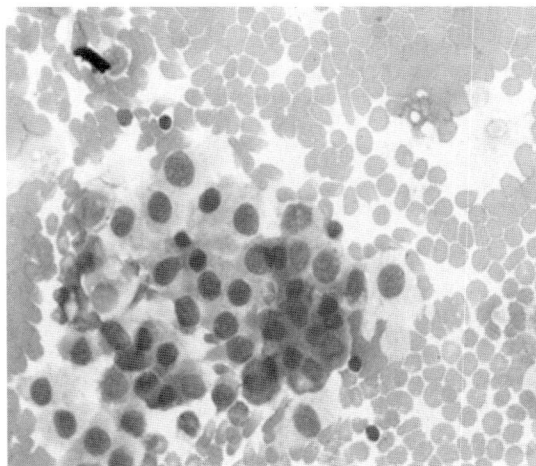

**Figure 3** Normal parenchymal acinar pancreatic cells (May-Grünwald-Giemsa, ×325).

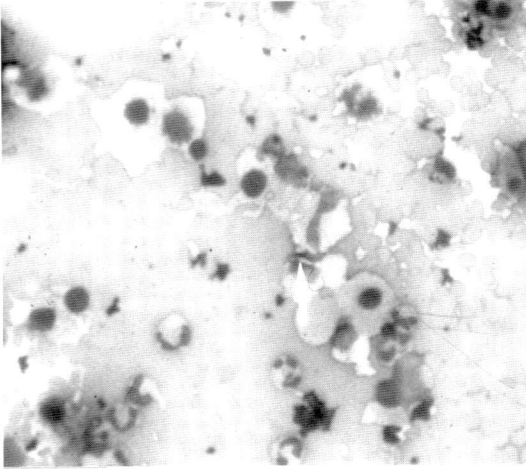

**Figure 4**  Normal parenchymal acinar pancreatic cells (May-Grünwald-Giemsa, ×325).

to be normal in most cases. Cyclosporine and tacrolimus induce characteristic changes common to all the graft types. These abnormalities, which are potentially reversible after dosage reduction, include isometric vacuolization, foamy changes, and ingestion of amorphous material (Fig. 5). Light and electron microscopy of percutaneous pancreatic biopsies have shown similar morphological abnormalities in islet cells (24). Aspiration cytology seems to be a more sensitive test than core biopsies for the detection of acute and reversible parenchymal cell changes; this may be related to the simplicity of the procedure that may allow a better preservation of the cellular components. The detection of late findings documented by core biopsy, such as interstitial fibrosis, is difficult if not impossible, and limits the utility of FNAB to the early posttransplant phases (25–27). However, ischemic and picnotic cells can be related to chronic cellular damage (19,23).

## Other Findings

The detection of blasts as a sign of immunoactivation and the acute parenchymal cell lesions represent the real utility for the FNAB in clinical practice; however, other findings may also be useful (23). Acute infection can be identified in FNAB by the number of neutrophils in the aspirate exceeding that counted in the peripheral blood. These findings may be diagnostic of acute pyelonephritis or pancreatitis in FNAB performed in renal or pancreatic grafts, respectively. Aspirate samples can also be cultured for microorganisms representing bacterial or fungal infections. In addition, cytomegalovirus and Epstein-Barr virus infections have been

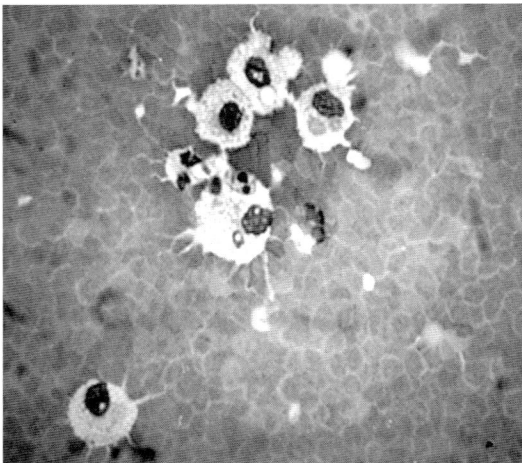

**Figure 5**  Isometric vacuolization of pancreatic acinar cells, typical of calcineurin inhibitor-related toxicity (May-Grünwald-Giemsa, ×325).

detected by immunochemical staining and monoclonal antibodies directed against specific viral membrane proteins or viral genomes (28,29).

## THE ROLE OF FNAB IN RESEARCH

FNAB can provide an adequate number of parenchymal and infiltrating cells for further cyto-morphological characterization, gene expression by RNA extraction, reverse transcription polymerase chain reaction, flow-cytometry, immunophenotyping, and cultures (30). Oliveira et al. (20) have reported that FNAB sample cultures have significant proliferative abilities and synthesize a large array of cytokines that reflect different immunological reactions and pathways. The same group has reported significant differences in cytokine production related to different immunosuppressive drugs (22). Taken together, these studies might be useful not only for elucidating processes and mechanisms of engraftment and rejection but also for monitoring immunosuppressive management.

## REFERENCES

1.  Li B, Hartono C, Ding R, et al. Non invasive diagnosis of renal-allograft rejection by measurement of messenger RNA for perforin and granzyme B in urine. NEJM 2001; 344(13):947–954.
2.  Strom TB, Suthanthiran M. Prospects and applicability of molecular diagnosis of allografts rejection. Semin Nephrol 2002; 20(2):103–107.
3.  Pasternack A, Virolainen M, Häyry P. Fine-needle aspiration biopsy of human renal allografts rejection. J Urol 1973; 109:167–172.
4.  Häyry P, von Willebrand E. Practical guidelines for fine needle aspiration biopsy of human renal allografts. Ann Clin Res 1981; 13:288–306.
5.  Häyry P, von Willebrand E. Transplant aspiration cytology. Transplantation 1984; 38:7–12.
6.  von Willebrand E. Fine-needle aspiration cytology of human renal transplants. Clin Immunol Immunopathol 1980; 17:309–322.
7.  von Willebrand E Soots A, Häyry P. In situ effector mechanisms in rat kidney allograft rejection. I. Characterization of host cellular infiltrate in rejecting allograft parenchyma. Cell Immunol 1979; 46:309–326.
8.  Häyry P, von Willebrand E, Soots A. In situ effector mechanisms in rat kidney allograft rejection. III. Kinetics of the inflammatory response and generation of donor-directed killer cells. Scan J Immunol 1979; 10:95–108.
9.  Lautenschlager I, Höckerstedt J, Ahonen J, et al. Fine-needle aspiration biopsy in the monitoring of liver allografts. Applications to human liver allografts. Transplantation 1988; 46:47–52.
10. Ekberg H, Allen RDM, Greenberg ML, et al. Early diagnosis of rejection of canine pancreas allografts by fine needle aspiration cytology. Transplantation 1988; 46:485–489.
11. Egidi MF, Shapiro R, Khanna A, Fung JJ, Corry RJ. Fine-needle aspiration biopsy in pancreatic transplantation. Transplant Proc 1995; 27:3055–3056.
12. Egidi MF, Corry RJ, Sugitani A, et al. Enteric-drained pancreas transplants monitored by fine-needle aspiration cytology. Transplant Proc 1997; 29:674–675.
13. Egidi MF, Corry RJ. Simultaneous kidney–pancreas transplantation. Curr Opin Organ Transplant 1996; 1:44–50.
14. Kreis HA. Use of the fine needle aspiration cytology to diagnose rejection. Transplant Proc 1984; 16:1569–1572.
15. Their M, von Willebrand E, Taskinen E, Rönnholm K, Holmberg C, Jalanko H. Fine-needle aspiration biopsy allows early detection of acute rejection in children after renal transplantation. Transplantation 2001; 71:736–743.
16. Egidi MF, Banfi G, Bogetic J, Passerini P, Ponticelli C. Correlation between fine needle aspiration biopsy and renal biopsy in renal transplantation. Transplant Proc 1988; 20:589–591.
17. Boshkos C, Steinmuller D, Novick A, Streem ST, Cunningham R, Dlugosz B. Fine needle aspiration biopsy and core biopsy in renal allografts recipients. Transplant Proc 1988; 20:592–595.
18. Oliveira GG, Xavier P, Mendes A, Guerra LE. Cultures of aspiration biopsy specimens in the immunological monitoring of renal transplants. Nephron 1996; 76:310–314.
19. Egidi MF. Fine-needle aspiration biopsy in renal transplantation: a review of cytologic features. Diagn Cytopathol 1990; 6:330–335.
20. Oliveira GG, Xavier P, Neto S, Menfdes A, Guerra LE. Monocytes-macrophages and cytokines/chemokines in fine-needle aspiration biopsy cultures. Transplantation 1997; 63:1751–1756.
21. Nast CC, Zuo XJ, Prehn J, Danovitch GM, Wilkinson A, Jordan SC. Gamma-interferon gene expression in human renal allograft fine-needle aspirates. Transplantation 1994; 57:498–502.
22. Oliveira GG, Xavier P, Sampaio S, et al. Compared to mycophenolate mofetil, Rapamycin induces significant changes in growth factors and growth factor receptors in the early days post kidney transplantation. Transplantation 2002, 73:915–920.

23. Hammer C. In: Schulz RS, ed. Cytology in Transplantation. Germany: Kempfenhausen, 1989.

24. Drachenberg CB, Klassen DK, Weir M, et al. Islet cell damage associated with tacrolimus and cyclosporine: morphological features in pancreas allografts biopsies and clinical correlation. Transplantation 1999; 68:396–402.

25. Sibley RK, Sutherland DE. Pancreas transplantation: an immunohistologic and histopathologic examination of 100 grafts. Am J Pathol 1987; 128:151–170.

26. Drachemberg CB, Papadimitriou JC, Klassen DK, et al. Evaluation of pancreas transplant needle biopsy: reproducibility and revision of histologic grading system. Transplantation 1997; 63:1579–1586.

27. Gaber LW, Egidi MF. Surveillance and monitoring of pancreas allografts. Curr Opin Organ Transplant 2002; 7:191–195.

28. Nast CC, Wilkinson A, Rosenthal JT, et al. Differentiation of cytomegalovirus infection from acute rejection using renal allograft fine needle aspirates. J Am Soc Nephrol 1991; 1:1204–1211.

29. Solez K, Williams GM, eds. Kidney Transplant Rejection. New York: Marcel Dekker, 1992:419.

30. Oliveira GG, Ramos JP, Xavier P, Magalhães M, Mendes A, Guerra LE. Analysis of fine-needle aspiration biopsies by flow cytometry in kidney transplant recipients. Transplantation 1997; 64:97–102.

# 16 | Surgical Complications After Pancreatic Transplantation

**Cynthia A. Smetanka, Ron Shapiro, and Amit Basu**
*Thomas E. Starzl Transplantation Institute, University of Pittsburgh School of Medicine, Pittsburgh, Pennsylvania, U.S.A.*

**Akhtar S. Khan**
*Milton S. Hershey Medical Center, Division of Transplantation, Hershey, Pennsylvania, U.S.A.*

**Amadeo Marcos and Henkie P. Tan**
*Thomas E. Starzl Transplantation Institute, University of Pittsburgh School of Medicine, Pittsburgh, Pennsylvania, U.S.A.*

The first pancreas transplant was performed by Kelly and Lillehei in 1966. Since that time, the technical aspects of the procedure have been modified, resulting in improved outcomes with fewer complications. As of October 2001, over 17,000 pancreatic transplants had been performed, of which 11,500 were carried out in the United States (1). The most common procedure performed is simultaneous kidney and pancreas (SPK) transplantation (Fig. 1), although the number of pancreas after kidney (PAK) and pancreas transplants alone (PTA) has also increased (Fig. 2). Currently, SPK transplantation is the procedure of choice for patients with diabetes mellitus and end-stage renal failure. The benefits of pancreas transplantation extend far beyond the maintenance of normal glucose homeostasis. Numerous recent reports have shown evidence for the arrest, prevention, and possible reversal of the secondary complications of diabetes, such as retinopathy, neuropathy, nephropathy, and vasculopathy.

Despite these great benefits, there are still significant complications associated with the procedure. Pancreas transplantation is associated with the highest complication rate of all of the routinely performed solid organ transplants (4). The pancreas is somewhat predisposed to these complications because of its low microcirculatory blood flow and the management of its exocrine drainage. In addition, performing a major abdominal and vascular operation in patients with long-standing diabetes adds to the morbidity.

## VASCULAR COMPLICATIONS

The leading technical cause of pancreatic graft failure is vascular thrombosis. The overall thrombosis rate is reported to range between 6% and 12% (5,6), and can be either arterial or venous. There are several factors that predispose the pancreas to thrombosis.

One of the reasons that the pancreas is more susceptible to thrombosis, more than any other transplanted solid organ, is its low microvascular flow. Also, in donors where the liver is used, the gastroduodenal artery is ligated, and this decreases the vascular supply to the head of the pancreas and the duodenum. Specific risk factors for thrombosis include the following: Cerebrovascular cause of donor death, increased donor age, use of an aortic Carrel patch, and graft reconstruction using a splenic artery to superior mesenteric artery anastomosis or an interposition graft between the splenic artery and the superior mesenteric artery (5). Additional risk factors include use of a portal vein extension graft, graft pancreatitis (hyperamylasemia exceeding five days posttransplantation), or left-sided implantation (5).

In a study comparing the different types of pancreas transplants (5), the PAK category was found to be an independent risk factor for thrombosis, having a thrombosis rate of up to 20%. A possible explanation may be that in this group of patients, the kidney, which was transplanted first, was most likely placed on the right side (the anatomically preferred side), leaving the left side for the pancreas. In diabetic end-stage renal failure patients, it may be prudent to place the kidney on the left side, if a pancreatic transplant is a future possibility.

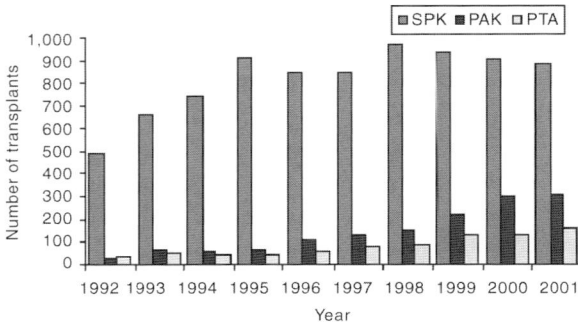

**Figure 1** Pancreas transplant numbers by category (1992–2001). *Abbreviations*: PAK, pancreas after kidney; PTA, pancreas transplants alone; SPK, simultaneous kidney and pancreas. *Source*: From Ref. 2.

Additionally, older donors, those with a long preservation time (6), and those with cerebrovascular disease should be considered to be at increased risk for whole organ pancreas donation. Routine portal vein extension grafts and arterial reconstructions other than the Y-graft should be avoided.

The key to possible graft salvage for vascular complications is early diagnosis. There are several methods of diagnosis: duplex ultrasound, radionuclide perfusion scanning, and arteriography. Using duplex sonography, the reversal of diastolic flow in the arteries supplying the pancreas was found to be extremely specific for the detection of venous graft thrombosis during the first 12 days posttransplantation (7). In a radiological study that attempted to determine if elevated arterial resistive indices and absence of venous flow correlated with venous thrombosis (7), the findings suggested that a resistive indices of 1.0 with an absence of venous flow was highly sensitive and specific for the diagnosis of venous thrombosis in the pancreatic graft.

Besides thrombosis, there are other vascular complications that can occur, such as pseudoaneurysms. Pseudoaneurysms can be mycotic (infectious), or noninfectious. Mycotic pseudoaneurysms usually occur as a result of an intra-abdominal infection and may not present until late in the postoperative course. They may present as a thrombosis, a pulsatile mass, or even with life-threatening sepsis. The treatment is usually graft pancreatectomy with ligation and division of the recipient iliac artery and revascularization using an extra-anatomic bypass.

Noninfected pseudoaneurysms are fairly unusual. If they are not recognized and adequately treated, they may be associated with significant patient morbidity and graft loss. However, if promptly diagnosed and managed surgically, noninfected pseudoaneurysms can be repaired without graft loss. Some of these pseudoaneurysms may be diagnosed incidentally following an ultrasound examination. Using standard vascular techniques, surgical repair can be performed without loss of the pancreatic graft (8).

Another vascular complication that can occur is fistula formation. Fistulae may be arteriovenous or arterioenteric. In the case of arteriovenous fistulae, patients can present with severe endocrine insufficiency and hematuria (9). Significant arteriovenous fistulae can occur in the transplanted mesenteric bundle. They can also occur as a consequence of a biopsy (10). Clinical presentation may be suggested by physical examination, which is usually followed by duplex ultrasonography and/or radionuclide perfusion scanning. Arteriography can then be used to confirm the diagnosis. The treatment of these fistulae is surgical correction, usually ligation, which can reverse the endocrine insufficiency (11).

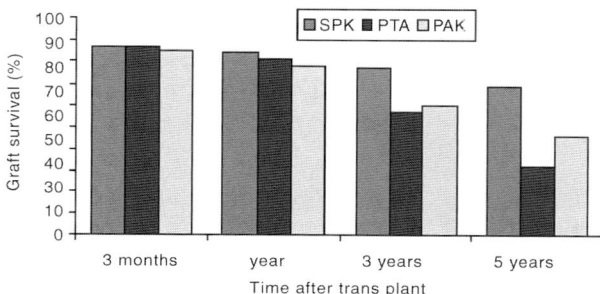

**Figure 2** Pancreas graft survival among pancreas transplant recipients. Cohorts are transplants preformed during 1999–2000 for three months and one year; 1997–1998 for three years; and 1995–1996 for five year survival. *Abbreviations*: PAK, pancreas after kidney; PTA, pancreas alone transplants; SPK, simultaneous kidney and pancreas. *Source*: From Ref. 3.

Arterioenteric fistulae are most often related to mycotic pseudoaneurysms. A previous intra-abdominal infection can predispose patients to these fistulae. The presentation may be late and may eventually lead to overwhelming sepsis. To avoid these additional serious complications, several groups are now recommending elective removal of nonfunctioning, enterically drained pancreatic allografts (10).

These complications can be further compounded by the onset of hemorrhage. The graft can become friable, which can lead to significant bleeding. A significant risk factor for bleeding is the use of anticoagulant or antiplatelet agents, which are used to try to prevent thrombosis. Additionally, patients who are diabetic with renal failure may be coagulopathic because of platelet dysfunction and vitamin K deficiency. In a report of a small series of kidney–pancreas patients who developed significant bleeding associated with vitamin K deficiency (12), their coagulopathy was resolved following parenteral administration of vitamin K. The authors of this study (12) recommended that vitamin K treatment should be considered in those patients who had a prolonged prothrombin or partial thromboplastin time during the first postoperative week, to try to avoid hemorrhagic complications.

A final vascular complication deserves a brief discussion. Chronic diabetic patients are very prone to vasculopathies of various types. Following transplantation, these patients may suffer from distal limb ischemia on the side of the transplant secondary to a "steal" syndrome. Because of this, it is always prudent to assess the patients' pulses prior to transplantation, immediately after, and periodically throughout the early postoperative period. Revascularization, if necessary, can be accomplished using standard vascular techniques.

## INTRA-ABDOMINAL COMPLICATIONS

Intra-abdominal complications represent an important source of morbidity after pancreatic transplantation. They may range from mild to life threatening. Relatively straightforward complications include ileus, partial small bowel obstruction, wound infection, gastroparesis, hematomas, seromas, and wound infections. These complications are fairly common, and respond to the usual appropriate therapies.

Intra-abdominal infections have a high potential for morbidity and mortality. These infections can occur early, in the form of leaks or duodenal rupture, or they can present late (>3 months posttransplant), in the case of a delayed abscess.

The risk factors for the development of intra-abdominal complications have been studied; these include body weight and body mass index, serum glucose, donor age, vasopressor requirements in the donor, and peak donor serum amylase. Additional risk factors include the cause of death, recipient age, cold ischemia time, surgical technique, and peak recipient amylase (5). Elevated donor body mass index, body weight, and the peak recipient serum amylase in the first postoperative week have been found to be significant risk factors for the development of intra-abdominal infection (5). Analyzing these factors from several studies suggests that pancreatic grafts from obese donors may be more susceptible to abscess formation secondary to ischemia-reperfusion injury (5).

An additional, independent risk factor for the development of intra-abdominal infection in diabetics with renal failure is the dialysis modality. Peritoneal dialysis has been widely used in diabetics with end-stage renal disease (6). In a study comparing kidney/pancreas transplant patients undergoing hemodialysis versus peritoneal dialysis, a significant difference was observed in the incidence of abdominal infections (6). Although graft-related complications were high in both groups (which led to a reoperation rate of 60% and a re-hospitalization rate of 55%), the rate of abdominal infections was significantly higher in the peritoneal dialysis group, 44%, compared to 34% in hemodialysis recipients (6).

An important factor in these intra-abdominal infections is the incidence of duodenal complications. Duodenal complications can manifest as leaks, rupture, ulceration, or necrosis. These complications can be fairly common; however, with early diagnosis and treatment, graft loss can be minimized to as low as 9%, with a mortality rate of 0% (7). The key factor is early and accurate diagnosis.

An accurate method of diagnosing duodenal leaks in bladder-drained patients is with computed tomography (CT) cystography. In a patient with abdominal pain, fever, and the suspicion of a leak or abscess, it is prudent to do a CT scan of the abdomen and pelvis. Initially, a plain CT can be done. Then a CT cystogram with the bladder fully distended using air and contrast can be performed. If these images are negative, a postvoiding image can then be completed. If no leak is identified, the remainder of the scan can be done with contrast to evaluate the rest of the abdomen.

In a radiological study using CT cystography (8), bladder leaks were identified in 11 out of 12 studies: one by plain CT, seven by full CT cystography, and three by post-voiding CT. One leak was missed by CT cystography because of a large amount of pelvic fluid (8). Overall, the sensitivity of this study for duodenal leaks was 92%, accuracy 96%, and specificity 100% (8).

In addition to the risk of a leak, additional duodenal complications may occur. The duodenum can rupture, which can lead to bleeding, or the duodenum can undergo necrosis, which can lead to bacterial translocation. This can further progress to sepsis, and even multi-organ failure. Once again, the key to minimizing morbidity and mortality is early diagnosis and treatment. In the past, many grafts were lost because of a delay in treatment. In many cases, if early treatment via percutaneous drainage or operative exploration takes place, graft loss and mortality can be minimized.

In a study of 40 pancreas transplants, the overall incidence of intra-abdominal infection was 27.5% ($n = 11$) (9). Five of these patients underwent a pancreatectomy (12.5%). The remaining six grafts were rescued by aggressive necrosectomy and radical drainage of the abscess (in five patients) or by percutaneous drainage in one patient (9). One of these patients had a duodenal leak secondary to ischemia (9). The authors of this study concluded that early postoperative intra-abdominal infection was the major risk factor for graft loss; however, an aggressive diagnostic approach could maximize the likelihood of graft salvage (9).

In addition to intra-abdominal infections, another common cause of abdominal pain and significant morbidity is graft pancreatitis. Graft pancreatitis can be related to several factors, including donor characteristics, reperfusion injury, hypotension, and organ recovery issues. Most episodes of pancreatitis will resolve uneventfully; however, some may lead to secondary complications such as pseudocysts, fluid collections, and fistulae.

Pancreatic fistulae can occur rather frequently. These fistulae may be drained percutaneously with the insertion of a catheter. A serous fluid with a high amylase concentration is usually seen. Additionally, patients may be treated with octreotide, which is administered subcutaneously at a dose of 300 to 750 µg/day. In a study using octreotide (11), a progressive reduction in fistula output occurred at a mean of $16 \pm 2$ days. Drainage continued to decrease, and follow-up sonography did not show any recurrence.

Some peripancreatic collections can occur late, i.e., greater than three months after transplantation. These collections can also be indicative of a delayed presentation of a peripancreatic abscess, which may or may not be associated with a duodenal leak. These late complications are usually less likely to be reported and also less likely to be understood. In one of the studies that looked at late complications (10), eight out of 44 SPK patients who had an uneventful early postoperative course were re-hospitalized because of delayed intra-abdominal complications. The timing after transplantation ranged from four to 43 months, with a mean of 16 months (10). Exocrine drainage was re-established by a Roux-en-y conversion. Two of these patients had a mechanical small bowel obstruction, but the other six were treated for delayed anastomotic leaks or perigraft abscesses (10). Management of these complications consisted of surgical drainage ($n = 5$), graft tube duodenostomy ($n = 2$), or percutaneous drainage ($n = 1$) (10). These patients secondarily developed a pancreaticocutaneous fistula, which resolved within a few weeks to months. One patient died of sepsis (10). This last study demonstrates that, even in patients with a smooth early postoperative course, significant life-threatening complications may occur later. A high index of suspicion is necessary. Early diagnosis is the key in both early and late complications. Once an accurate diagnosis is made, expeditious treatment, in the form of surgical intervention, percutaneous drainage, or other therapy can take place. Favorable outcomes can still be achieved with late complications if they are promptly treated.

## UROLOGICAL COMPLICATIONS

In bladder-drained pancreatic transplants, the incidence of urological complications has been reported to be as high as 83% to 85% (13,14). The most common complication is urinary tract infection (14). Dysuria and urethritis (which may sometimes lead to stenosis) are also common and can be irritating to the patient. Inflammation and/or infection can spread along the urinary tract to cause epididymitis, prostatitis, and even pyelonephritis, which may be life threatening in the immunosuppressed patient. Reflux pancreatitis can also occur because of inadequate emptying of the bladder, and this can add to the irritation and inflammation, which occur secondary to drainage of the exocrine secretions. Ulcerations and stone formation may also occur.

Overall, the most common complications reported have been urinary tract infections, metabolic acidosis and dehydration, duodenal leaks, hematuria, urethritis (sometimes complicated by strictures) (15), and duodenovesical fistulae (14).

Unfortunately, the duodenum can be involved in many of the urological complications. These duodenal complications can cause fistula formation and significant morbidity secondary to perforation and leakage. Some of these complications can present in an atypical fashion. In an unusual report of a duodenal rupture, a patient presented with refractory hematuria (16). Usually, hematuria is mild and self-limited. However, in this case, the patient began having refractory hematuria 17 days after solitary pancreas transplantation (16). The patient had developed severe duodenal swelling with mucosal rupture, which required operative intervention (16).

Because of these duodenal complications, various centers have studied the technique of duodenocystostomies, to determine if there were any differences that could decrease the number of complications. Stapled and hand-sewn duodenocystostomies were compared (17). Both techniques resulted in a similar incidence of complications and similar graft survival rates (17).

Other centers have looked at using urodynamic testing to try to predict and possibly to avoid long-term urological complications. Preoperative urodynamic assessments were done in a group of bladder-drained kidney–pancreas recipients (18). The patients who were found to have abnormal urodynamics had a much higher rate of urological complications, 79% (relative risk 5:1) (18). Preoperative evaluation might identify the patients at risk to develop these problems, and this information could then be used to plan the operative approach in these patients.

Management of these complications can be a challenge. Fortunately, many of them will respond to conservative treatment (19). More complex treatments include percutaneous and operative procedures. For the treatment of a transplant pseudocyst (20), the authors of an interesting study described a percutaneous drainage procedure from the pseudocyst to the bladder. The catheter was capped following the procedure to allow pancreatic secretions to drain into the bladder (20). Following this drainage, the patient's amylase and lipase normalized and the pseudocyst resolved (20). The tube was subsequently removed after a prolonged period of time without any evidence of recurrence and a normal amylase (20).

Unfortunately, some of these patients require operative intervention, which usually requires conversion to enteric drainage. Early operative intervention has been found to result in superior outcomes in terms of quality of life and allograft survival (21,22). In one cohort of patients (22), 32% required early cystoenteric conversions for complications such as leaks and refractory metabolic acidosis. The graft salvage rate was 96.1%, with 0% mortality and a definite improvement in the quality of life (22).

## COMPARISON BETWEEN SURGICAL TECHNIQUES

Because of these urological and metabolic complications, in the mid-late 1990s, many centers began to revisit enteric drainage. Many centers found enteric drainage to be safe, without an increase in intra-abdominal complications or graft loss (23). Intestinal leaks were rare and were managed straightforwardly in most cases, particularly if a Roux-en-y reconstruction had been used (23).

Another issue that has been actively investigated has been the use of portal venous versus systemic venous drainage to see if there have been any differences in patient or graft survival. Although portal drainage is more physiological, many groups report no significant differences with regard to patient and graft survival and complications (24,25). There have been, however, several centers that have shown a decreased number of surgical complications with portal venous drainage (26,27). These issues will to need to be studied further in order to determine the techniques that will result in the best endocrine function with the lowest number of complications.

The biggest technical issue that has been studied is the comparison in outcomes over time between enteric- and bladder-drained pancreas transplants. A number of studies have investigated this issue. In an interesting study comparing three techniques, segmental graft with duct obstruction, whole graft with bladder drainage, and whole graft with enteric drainage, the best results were obtained with enteric drainage (28). After three years, overall graft survival was 47% for duct obstruction, 60% for bladder drainage, and 65% for enteric drainage (28).

Most of the other studies, however, have not shown a clear advantage for one technique over another. Many centers have shown similar complication rates between bladder and enterically drained pancreatic grafts (29–32), although the specific type and severity of the complication differed between the two techniques.

In a German study (29), 90% of the transplants were performed using bladder drainage, with an enteric conversion rate of 10% to 20%. They reported no anastomotic leaks and an equivalent patient and graft survival rate (29). Stratta and colleagues (31,32) compared the differences in complications between the two techniques. The incidence of readmission for dehydration was significantly less in the enterically drained group (31). The bladder-drained group had a slight increase in readmissions, urinary tract infections and other urological complications, metabolic acidosis, and dehydration (32). In an overall comparison, both techniques yielded excellent results (31,32).

In another comparison that involved 123 pancreas patients (33), no statistically significant difference was found in patient or graft survival; bladder drainage was associated with an increased rate of surgical complications compared to enteric drainage, and enteric drainage was associated with a higher intra-abdominal infection rate (Table 1) (33). A flexible approach may be necessary; certain situations may result in a more favorable outcome with one technique over the other. For example, bladder drainage may be more beneficial in those who are receiving a solitary pancreas graft and also those requiring left-sided placement (33).

An excellent and more detailed comparison was done in a subsequent study by Corry and colleagues (34), who studied 243 pancreas recipients transplanted between 1994 and 2000. Differences in outcomes between these two techniques can vary depending on the type of transplant (SPK, PAK, and PTA) (Fig. 3). Overall, the enterically drained group showed a slightly better pancreas survival rate (Fig. 4) (34). However, the survival curves were reversed for solitary pancreas and pancreas after kidney transplants (Fig. 5) (34). Complications such as fistulae and anastomotic bleeds requiring transfusions were higher in the bladder-drained pancreas patients (34). Current IPTR/UNOS data are similar to the Pittsburgh experience, and shows a technical failure rate of 12% for bladder drainage and 13% for enteric drainage (1).

Although comparisons of these complications are important, a comparison of their severity should also be examined. Bladder drainage is associated with an increased complication rate, but these complications may be less morbid than those seen with enteric drainage. For example, the anastomotic bleeds in the bladder-drained group usually stopped without requiring a laparotomy (34); some patients required transfusions, while others needed cystoscopic fulguration (34).

Fistulae usually can be managed with ultrasound-guided percutaneous drainage and bladder catherization (34). Some fistulae, which were related to a small duodenal staple line disruption, could be managed conservatively; however, with an anastomotic breakdown of the duodenoenterostomy, the morbidity was more severe and usually required reoperation, with conversion to Roux-en-y drainage (34).

The interpretation of these data is not completely straightforward and suggests a more flexible approach for the method of exocrine drainage. Some centers tend to lean more toward enteric drainage for SPK and bladder drainage for PAK/PTA (34). Currently, there is a progressive increase in the use of enteric drainage (1). This method is gaining increased support, as the technical aspects of the procedure have become more refined and the complication rates have decreased. With better immunosuppressive regimens, the use of urinary amylase as a sign of rejection is not as critical as it was in the past. Enteric drainage is a more physiological approach that avoids the urinary tract complications, dehydration, and metabolic acidosis associated with bladder drainage. This can significantly affect quality of life after pancreas transplantation.

## RELAPAROTOMY

The most serious surgical complications are those that result in relaparotomy and sometimes allograft pancreatectomy. Relaparotomy is performed because of vascular, urological, or

**Table 1** Major Complications and Graft Losses Within Each Group

| BD-related | Patients (26) | Graft loss | ED-related | Patients (97) | Graft loss | Drainage unrelated | Patients (123) | Graft loss |
|---|---|---|---|---|---|---|---|---|
| Reflux pancreatitis | 2 | 1 | Duodenal fistula | 5 | 2 | Thrombosis | 10 | 10 |
| Bladder fistula | 2 | 0 | Intra-abdominal abscess | 3 | 1 | Pancreatitis | 4 | 2 |
| Anastomotic bleeding | 1 | 0 | Anastomotic bleeding | 3 | 1 | Chronic rejection | 3 | 3 |
| Severe acidosis | 1 | 0 | Intestinal perforation | 2 | 0 | Arterial rupture | 2 | 1 |
| | | | Intestinal obstruction | 1 | 0 | Peripancreatic bleeding | 2 | 0 |
| | | | Wound obstruction | 1 | 0 | Ligation of IPDA | 1 | 1 |
| | | | | | | Iliac artery thrombosis | 1 | 0 |
| | | | | | | Intestinal perforation | 1 | 0 |
| | | | | | | Ab-mediated rejection | 1 | 1 |
| Total | 6 | 1 | | 15 | 4 | | 25 | 18 |

*Abbreviations*: BD, bladder drainage; ED, enteric drainage; IPDA, inferior pancreaticoduodenal artery; Ab, antibody.
*Source*: From Ref. 33.

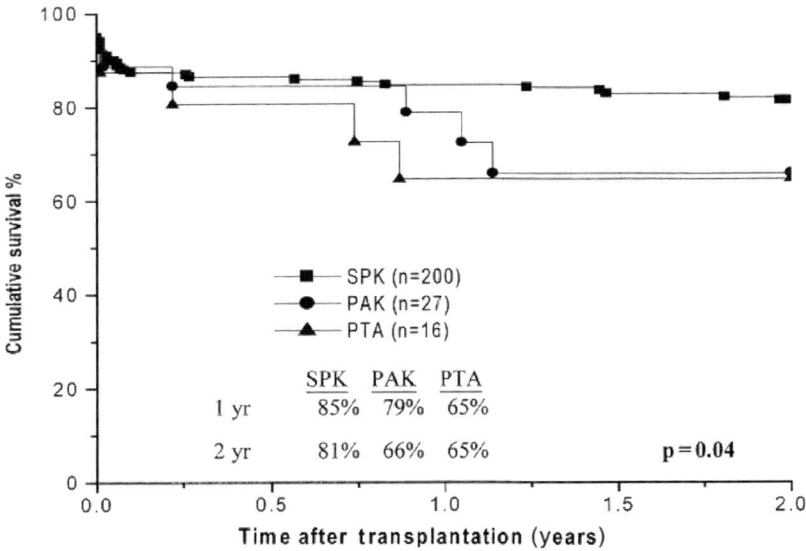

**Figure 3** Kaplan–Meier pancreas survival. *Abbreviations*: PAK, pancreas after kidney; PTA, pancreas alone transplants; SPK, simultaneous kidney and pancreas. *Source*: From Ref. 34.

intra-abdominal complications. In a review of patients with bladder-drained transplants, the relaparotomy rate was 32% (35). The most common causes were intra-abdominal infection/ graft pancreatitis (38%), thrombosis (27%), and anastomotic leak (15%) (35). The relaparotomy mortality rate was 9%, with a transplant pancreatectomy rate of 57% (35). Overall, the long-term graft loss was 80% in recipients who had a relaparotomy. Patient survival rates were significantly lower if a relaparotomy was required (35).

Relaparotomy may also be required for vascular complications. In these situations, a high index of suspicion, early recognition, and treatment are key to possible graft salvage. The most common vascular complication that can lead to relaparotomy and graft loss is thrombosis. Graft salvage can be very difficult. However, some venous thromboses involving

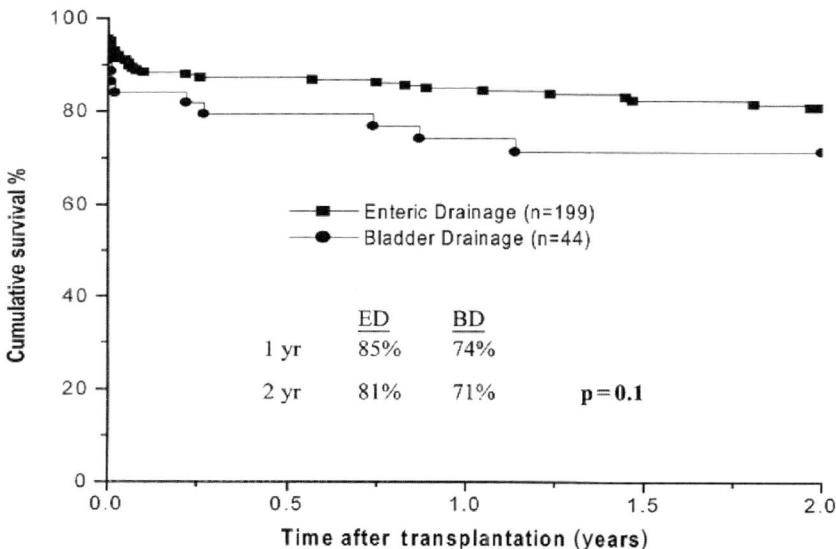

**Figure 4** Kaplan–Meier pancreas survival. *Abbreviations*: ED, enteric drainage; BD, bladder drainage. *Source*: From Ref. 34.

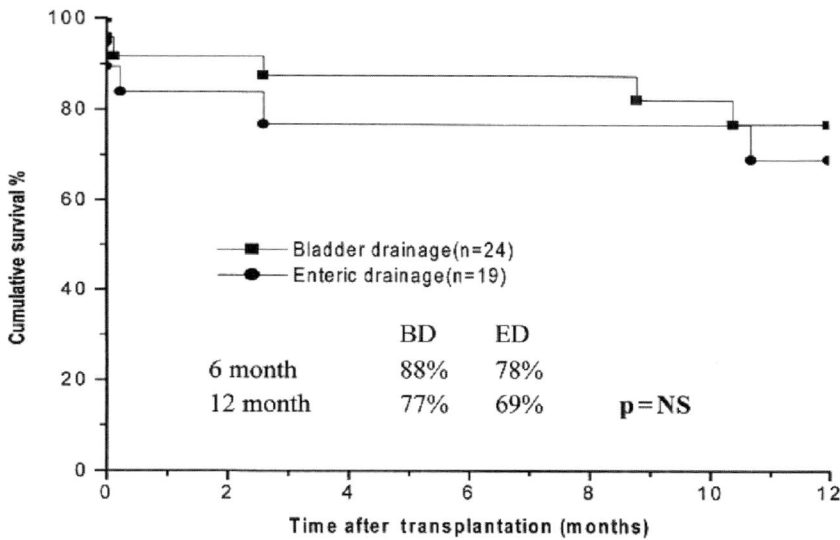

**Figure 5**  Kaplan-Meier pancreas survival (pancreas after kidney/panereas alone transplants). *Abbreviations*: BD, bladder drainage; ED, enteric drainage; NS, not specified. *Source*: From Ref. 34.

the splenic and superior mesenteric veins can be treated by thrombectomy followed by heparin and oral anticoagulation (36). Some early arterial thromboses may also be salvaged by thrombectomy and revascularization. Repairs of noninfected pseudoaneurysms and arteriovenous fistulae can usually be performed with salvage of allograft function (36).

In enterically drained patients, a higher rate of intra-abdominal infections can occur, with a higher rate of relaparotomy and subsequent graft loss (33). Anastomotic breakdown of the duodenoenterostomy in the enterically drained group can lead to increased morbidity, relaparotomy, and graft loss (34). A substantial perioperative mortality can occur if treatment is delayed (35). In cases where the anastomotic breakdown and subsequent infection are severe and require relaparotomy, the focus needs to shift from graft salvage to preservation of the patient's life (35). In these cases, the threshold for pancreatectomy should be low (35).

There are an increasing number of cases where early detection through better diagnostic testing leads to earlier intervention with a higher graft salvage rate, and without placing the patient's life in undue jeopardy. In a recent study (37), five out of seven allografts (71%) were salvaged without major impairment of endocrine function. This surgical salvage technique consisted of pancreaticoduodenectomy with conversion from a whole organ transplant with bladder or enteric drainage to a segmental graft with duct injection (in three cases), and a duodenectomy and conversion to a whole graft with duct occlusion in the other four cases (37). In four of these cases, it was technically impossible to perform a re-anastomosis because of duodenal ischemia (37). Initial attempts at repair were unsuccessful requiring duodenectomy with duct occlusion (37). In the other three cases, a pancreaticoduodenectomy was performed because the head of the pancreas and duodenum were ischemic in two cases and a huge pseudoaneurysm that involved the pancreatic head was present in the third (37). Overall, in the five cases that were salvaged, there were no differences in endocrine function after one year (37). This technique may be an example of one of the ways in which graft salvage rates can be improved, especially with prompt diagnosis and aggressive management.

## PANCREAS RETRANSPLANTATION

A brief mention should be made about retransplantation and its risks and complications. The increased success of pancreas transplantation has resulted in an increased number of patients who desire retransplantation. An interesting question that occurs is whether these patients are at a higher risk of complications and if these complications would be similar or different compared to those undergoing primary transplantation.

**Table 2**  Organ Procurement and Transplantation Network Pancreas: Kaplan–Meier Graft Survival Rates for Transplants Performed: 1996–2001 in the United States

| Primary vs. repeat transplant | Years posttransplant (yr) | Number functioning/alive | Survival rate | 95% Confidence interval |
|---|---|---|---|---|
| Primary transplant | 1 | 663 | 79.1 | (76.6, 81.7) |
| Repeat transplant | 1 | 148 | 73.5 | (67.0, 70.2) |
| Primary transplant | 3 | 356 | 61.1 | (57.5, 64.6) |
| Repeat transplant | 3 | 85 | 54.1 | (47.1, 61.0) |

*Note*: Based on OPTN data as of July 11, 2003. Data subject to change based on future data submission or correction.
[a]Denotes that a graft survival was not computed to *N* less than 10. One-year survival is based on 1999–2001 transplants, and three-year survival is based on 1996–1999 transplants.
*Source*: Based on OPTN data as of July 11, 2003.

Two groups of patients were compared, those with primary transplants versus retransplants (38), to analyze the incidence of surgical complications and patient and graft survival rates. Complications such as thrombosis and bleeding were slightly more common in the retransplanted group, but this was not statistically significant (38). The number of leaks and infections was equivalent between the two groups (38), but the incidence of acute rejection and early graft loss was higher in the retransplanted group (38). Retransplantation appears to be an appropriate treatment, and can be performed with only a slightly higher risk of surgical complications. However, because of the decreased graft survival (Table 2), it may require a more aggressive approach to immunosuppression.

## CURRENT TRENDS: THE DECREASING RATE OF SURGICAL COMPLICATIONS

In numerous analyses at various centers worldwide, there is increasing evidence that the incidence of surgical complications after pancreatic transplantation has significantly decreased in the modern era (39). In a European study comparing two eras (1988–1996 and 1998–2001), 87% of patients suffered surgical complications requiring laparotomy in the first era, versus 57% in the second era (4). In this first group, pancreatectomy was necessary in 57%, versus 37% in the second group (4). In addition, patient survival increased from 63% to 92% (4).

Studies in American centers have also demonstrated these findings. The Minnesota group noted a significant decrease in the incidence of surgical complications between two eras (1985–1994 and 1994–1997) (Table 3) (40). The relaparotomy rate decreased from 32% to 19% (40). The authors felt that the main reason for this was the decreased incidence of thrombosis related to their use of postoperative low-dose heparin and aspirin in the second era (40). An additional discovery was that the incidence of intra-abdominal infections decreased, which might have been related to improved prophylactic regimens in the newer era (40). Improvements in the identification of risk factors and refinements in technique probably also played a role in the overall decrease in surgical complications.

These findings were also reported by Reddy et al. (30), who compared surgical complications (which they defined as the need for relaparotomy within the first three months posttransplantation) between two eras: 1990–1995 and 1996–1997. They found that the incidence of surgical complications was 45% in the first era, and 29% in the second one (30). The rate of

**Table 3**  Incidence and Reasons for Relaparotomy

|  | Era 1 | Era 2 | *p* Value |
|---|---|---|---|
| Total transplants (*n*) | 367 | 213 | – |
| Relaparotomy rate | 32.4% | 18.8% | 0.001 |
| Reasons for relaparotomy: |  |  |  |
|    Thrombosis | 10.1% | 5.6% | 0.06 |
|    Infections | 12.0% | 3.8% | 0.001 |
|    Bleeding | 4.9% | 6.6% | 0.14 |
|    Leaks | 3.8% | 6.1% | NS |
|    Other | 6.5% | 1.3% | 0.001 |

*Abbreviation*: NS, not specified.
*Source*: From Ref. 40.

vascular thrombosis decreased from 17% to 10%, the rate of intra-abdominal infection decreased from 12% to 7%, and the rate of duodenal leaks decreased from 5% to 2% (30).

## CONCLUSIONS

Pancreas transplantation is an important therapy for diabetes, which is a very destructive and expensive disease. Because of the high impact this disease has on society, there is a tremendous amount of interest and funding devoted to its treatment and ultimate cure. Currently, the best long-term method of restoring normal glucose homeostasis is pancreas transplantation. Earlier in the history of this operation, a high incidence of serious complications were associated with this treatment. With advances in immunosuppression, postoperative care, antibiotic prophylaxis, and surgical techniques, the complication rate has declined, and pancreas transplantation has become more successful, with continuing improvements in patient and graft survival rates and reductions in morbidity and mortality.

## REFERENCES

1. Gruessner AC, Sutherland DE. Analysis of United States (US) and non-US pancreas transplants reported to the United Network for Organ Sharing (UNOS) and the International Pancreas Transplant Registry (IPTR) as of October 2001. Clin Transplant 2001: 41–72.
2. OPTN/SRTR Annual Report. Tables 6.4, 7.8, 8.4.
3. OPTN/SRTR Annual Report. Tables 6.4, 7.8, 8.8.
4. Michalak G, Xzerwinski J, Kwiatkowski A, et al. Surgical complications observed in simultaneous pancreas–kidney transplantation: thirteen years of experience of one center. Transplant Proc 2002; 34:661–662.
5. Troppman C, Gruessner AC, Benedetti E, et al. Vascular graft thrombosis after pancreatic transplantation: univariate and multivariate operative and nonoperative risk factor analysis. J Am Coll Surg 1996; 182:285–316.
6. Humar A, Kandaswamy R, Drangstveit MB, Parr E, Gruessner AG, Sutherland DE. Prolonged preservation increases surgical complications after pancreas transplants. Surgery 2000; 127:545–551.
7. Foshager MC, Hedlund LJ, Troppmann C, Benedetti E, Gruessner RW. Venous thrombosis of pancreatic transplants: diagnosis by duplex ultrasonography. Am J Roentgenol 1997; 169:1269–1273.
8. Verni MP, Leone JP, DeRoover A. Pseudoaneurysm of the Y-graft/iliac artery anastomosis following pancreas transplantation: a case report and review of the literature. Clin Transplant 2001; 15:72–76.
9. Lowell JA, Byron JS, Stratta RJ, Taylor RJ. Superior mesenteric arteriovenous fistula in vascularized whole organ pancreatic allografts. Surg Gynecol Obstet 1993; 177:254–258.
10. Gritsch HA, Shapiro R, Egidi F, Randhawa PS, Starzl TE, Corry RJ. Spontaneous arterioenteric fistula after pancreas transplantation. Transplantation 1997; 63:903–904.
11. Lowell JA, Stratta RJ, Taylor RJ, Bynon JS. Mesenteric arteriovenous fistula after vascularized pancreas transplantation resulting in graft dysfunction. Clin Transplant 1996; 10:278–281.
12. Prasad GV, Abidi SM, McCauley J, Johnston JR. Vitamin K deficiency with hemorrhage after kidney and combined kidney–pancreas transplantation. Am J Kidney Dis 1999; 33:963–965.
13. Baktavatsalam R, Little DM, Connolly EM, Farrell JG, Hickey DP. Complications relating to the urinary tract associated with bladder-drained pancreatic transplantation. Br J Urol 1998; 81:219–223.
14. Gutierrez del Pozo R, Ricart BMJ, Bacque MC, Fernandez-Cruz, Talbot-Wright R, Carretero Gonzalez P. Renopancreatic transplant. Urologic complications. Actas Urol Esp 1997; 21:950–955.
15. Sollinger HW, Messing EM, Eckhoff DE, et al. Urological complications in 210 consecutive simultaneous pancreas-kidney transplants with bladder drainage. Ann Surg 1993; 218:561–568.
16. Esterl RM, Stratta RJ, Taylor RJ, Radio SJ. Rejection with duodenal rupture after solitary pancreas transplantation: an unusual cause of severe hematuria. Clin Transplant 1995; 9(3 Pt 1):155–159.
17. Douzdjian V, Gugliuzza KK, Fish JC. Urologic complications after simultaneous pancreas-kidney transplantation: hand-sewn versus stapled duodenocystostomy. Clin Transplant 1995; 9:396–400.
18. Blanchet P, Droupy S, Eschwege P, et al. Urodynamic testing predicts long-term urological complications following simultaneous pancreas–kidney transplantation. Clin Transplant 2003; 17:26–31.
19. Eckhoff DE, Sollinger HW. Surgical complications after simultaneous pancreas–kidney transplant with bladder drainage. Clin Transplant 1993:185–191.
20. Shlansky-Goldberg R, Cope C, McGuckin J, et al. Percutaneous management of a bladder-drained pancreas transplant pseudocyst by a transcystic approach. Transplantation 1997; 15(64):1568–1571.
21. Gettman MT, Levy JB, Engen DE, Nehra A. Urological complications after kidney-pancreas transplantation. J Urol 1997; 159:38–42.
22. Kaplan AJ, Valente JF, First MR, Demmy AM, Munda R. Early operative intervention for urologic complications of kidney-pancreas transplantation. World J Surg 1998; 22:890–894.
23. Badosa F, Mital D, Sands L, et al. Our experience with Roux-Y intestinal drainage in simultaneous kidney and pancreas transplantation. Transplant Int 1994; 7(suppl 1):S412–S413.

24. Petruzzo P, DaSilva M, Feitosa LC, et al. Simultaneous pancreas–kidney transplantation: portal versus systemic venous drainage of the pancreas allografts. Clin Transplant 2000; 14(4 Pt 1):287–291.

25. Dawahra M, Petruzzo P, Lefrancois N, et al. Portal drainage of pancreas allograft: surgical complications and graft survival. Transplant Proc 2002; 34:817–818.

26. Gaber AO, Shokouk-Amiri H, Hathaway DK, et al. Results of pancreas transplantation with portal venous and enteric drainage. Ann Surg 1995; 221:613–624.

27. Bartlett ST, Kuo PC, Johnson LB, Lim JW, Schweitzer EJ. Pancreas transplantation at the University of Maryland. Clin Transplant 1996:271–280.

28. Feitosa Tajra LC, Dawhara M, Benchaib M, Lefrancois N, Martin X, Dubernard JM. Effect of the surgical technique on long-term outcome of pancreas transplantation. Transplant Int 1998; 11:295–300.

29. Busing M, Martin D, Schulz T, Heimes M, Klempnauer J, Kozuschek W. Pancreas transplantation with bladder and intestinal drainage technique with systemic-venous and initial experiences with portal venous drainage. Which technique can be recommended today? Chirurg 1998; 69:291–297.

30. Reddy KS, Stratta RJ, Shokouh-Amiri MH, Alloway R, Egidi MF, Gabe AO. Surgical complications after pancreas transplantation with portal enteric drainage. J Am Coll Surg 1999; 189:305–313.

31. Lo A, Stratta RJ, Hathaway DK, et al. Long-term outcomes in simultaneous kidney–pancreas transplant recipients with portal-enteric versus systemic-bladder drainage. Am J Kidney Dis 2001; 38:132–143.

32. Stratta RJ, Gaber AO, Shokouh-Amiri MH, et al. A prospective comparison of systemic-bladder versus portal-enteric drainage in vascularized pancreas transplantation. Surgery 2000; 127:217–226.

33. Sugitani A, Gritsch HA, Shapiro R, Bonham CA, Egidi MF, Corry RJ. Surgical complications in 123 consecutive pancreas transplant recipients: comparison of bladder and enteric drainage. Transplant Proc 1998; 30:293–294.

34. Corry RJ, Chakrabarti P, Shapiro R, Jordan ML, Scantlebury VP, Vivas CA. Comparison of enteric versus bladder drainage in pancreas transplantation. Transplant Proc 2001; 33(1–2):1647–1651.

35. Troppmann C, Gruessner AC, Dunn DL, Sutherland DE, Gruessner RW. Surgical complications requiring early relaparotomy after pancreas transplantation: a multivariate risk factor and economic impact analysis of the cyclosporine era. Ann Surg 1998; 227:255–268.

36. Ciancio G, Lo Monte A, Julian JF, Romano M, Miller J, Burke GW. Vascular complications following bladder drained, simultaneous pancreas–kidney transplantation: the University of Miami experience. Transpl Int 2000; 13(suppl 1):S187–S190.

37. Orsenigo E, Cristallo M, Socci C, et al. Successful surgical salvage of pancreas allograft. Transplantation 2003; 75:233–236.

38. Humar A, Kandaswamy R, Drangstveit MB, Parr E, Gruessner AG, Sutherland DE. Surgical risks and outcome of pancreas retransplants. Surgery 2000; 127:634–640.

39. Humar A, Ramcharan T, Kandaswamy R, et al. Pancreas after kidney transplants. Am J Surg 2001; 182:155–161.

40. Humar A, Kandaswamy R, Granger D, Gruessner RW, Gruessner AG, Sutherland DE. Decreased surgical risks of pancreas transplantation in the modern era. Ann Surg 2000; 231:269–275.

# 17 | Medical Complications Following Pancreas Transplantation

**Joao Seda Neto, Jerry McCauley, Henkie P. Tan, and Ron Shapiro**
*Thomas E. Starzl Transplantation Institute, University of Pittsburgh School of Medicine, Pittsburgh, Pennsylvania, U.S.A.*

## INTRODUCTION

Improvements in immunosuppression and the refinement of surgical techniques have made pancreas transplantation an established therapeutic modality for patients with type I diabetes mellitus.

Unfortunately, a variety of complications can occur following pancreas transplantation. This chapter will focus on medical complications (see Chapters 16 and 18 through 20 for surgical, infectious, oncologic, and neurologic complications).

## BONE DISEASE

Osteonecrosis of the hip, bone pain, and a fracture rate of 3% per year are the main manifestations of bone disease after pancreas transplantation (1). Development of uremic osteodystrophy before simultaneous pancreas–kidney transplantation, exacerbation immediately after transplantation because of high doses of immunosuppressive therapy, stabilization secondary to immunosuppressive dose reduction, and return of uremic osteodystrophy caused by failing graft function are the four phases that can occur (1).

The fracture rate is higher among diabetics and in patients receiving a simultaneous kidney–pancreas transplant, amounting 11% to 13% per year (2–4). Other factors predicting a greater risk of fracture are age, history of pretransplant fracture, duration of pretransplant renal failure, and female gender (5,6).

Osteopenia after transplantation is multifactorial. Glucocorticoids have many osteoporotic effects (7,8). They decrease intestinal calcium absorption and increase calcium excretion, with consequent secondary or tertiary hyperparathyroidism, decrease the effect of insulin-like growth factor 1, suppress gonadal hormone secretion, and inhibit proteoblast to osteoblast transformation. Cyclosporine may also contribute to bone loss following transplantation by stimulating bone resorption (9) and by blunting parathyroid hormone (PTH) effects (10). Tacrolimus has similar actions to cyclosporine, and osteotoxic effects can be expected to be similar (11–13).

Hyperparathyroidism is present in up to 30% of patients after renal transplantation in the presence of normal renal function and vitamin D metabolism, and should be considered a significant cause of bone loss (1). Glucocorticoid therapy (14), relative hypovitaminosis D (15,16), hypercalciuria (17), and cyclosporine are possible related causes.

Osteonecrosis, most commonly affecting the femoral head and neck, occurs in 6% to 8% of patients. Other sites include the knee, shoulder, and elbow. The pre-existence of damaged bone, trauma, intravenous steroids, hyperparathyroidism, and low bone mass are associated with a greater incidence of osteonecrosis.

### Management of Posttransplant Bone Disease

Management should be directed at reducing risk factors. Early ambulation and physical exercise should be encouraged. After recovering from the operation, all patients should be recommended to begin a weight-bearing exercise program that maintains muscle mass, analogous to recommendations for steroid-induced osteoporosis (18).

Bone density should be screened before or immediately after transplantation and then annually with dual energy X-ray absorptiometry (19), and osteodystrophy prophylaxis should be optimized preoperatively.

Hyperphosphatemia should be controlled with phosphate binders and hyperparathyroidism with alphacalcidol or calcitriol therapy while maintaining normocalcemia (20,21). Calcium and vitamin D supplements are recommended in the prophylaxis of steroid-induced osteoporosis (22). Hypercalciuria should be avoided if the glomerular filtration rate is less than 30 mL/min, and vitamin D should be given to normalize 1,25-D levels (23).

Parathyroidectomy is indicated in patients with tertiary hyperparathyroidism or persistent severe hypercalcemia (>12.5 mg/dL for more than a year), persistent metabolic bone disease, nephrolithiasis, symptomatic hypercalcemia, vascular calcification, and calcium-related renal allograft dysfunction. Most patients with moderate hypercalcemia related to secondary hyperparathyroidism do not require parathyroidectomy. The classic approach has been to delay surgery for approximately one year to allow involution of the glands. If, however, the hypercalemia that persists beyond one year is severe (>12.5 mg/day), or causes severe bone disease, surgery should be performed earlier. The new calcimimetic agent (cinacalcet) may offer a new approach to control of hypercalcemia and reduction of PTH levels after transplantation. A recent report by Kruse et al. demonstrated that this agent could normalize the serum calcium in most renal transplant patients with persistent hyperparathyroidism, but some continued to have persistent hypercalcemia (24). A subsequent report demonstated that it could be used to treat symptomatic hypercalcemia in renal transplant recipients with improvement in symptoms and PTH levels (25). This promising agent may become very useful in managing persistent hypercalcemia after renal and pancreas transplantation, but confirmation of its efficacy should await larger well-designed studies in transplant patients.

There are no published studies of bone loss prevention in pancreas transplant recipients. The inhibition of bone resorption by biphosphonates is effective in steroid-induced osteoporosis. Studies regarding the use of biphosphonates in the transplant population are controversial. One dose of pamidronate before liver transplantation was ineffective at preventing bone loss 12 months after transplant (26). Intravenous pamidronate infusions every three months decreased the fracture rate after lung transplantation (27). Biphosphonate therapy may be justifiable in potential high-risk candidates: patients with diabetes mellitus, postmenopausal women, and recipients of kidney/pancreas transplants (28).

The effectiveness of calcitonin after transplantation has yet to be determined. One study after liver transplantation (29) showed its effectiveness for the treatment of osteoporosis but, in two other studies (30,31), calcitonin had no impact on bone histomorphometry, bone mass, and bone fractures after liver transplant. It is probably not more effective than biphosphonates (1).

In summary, pancreas transplant recipients should be screened for osteoporosis, hyperparathyroidism, and vitamin D status, and should receive calcium and vitamin D replacement (19). Patients at high risk may benefit from biphosphonate treatment. Although the trend toward steroid sparing immunosuppressive regimens posttransplantation may reduce the risks of osteoporosis and fractures, calcineurin inhibitors also have osteotoxic effects, and it remains to be seen whether steroid-free protocols will prevent bone loss after transplantation (19).

## HYPOGLYCEMIA

Hypoglycemia is unusual after pancreas transplantation, although symptoms of hypoglycemia have been reported in as many as 30% to 50% of pancreas and kidney–pancreas transplant recipients (32–34).

Patients with long-standing diabetes mellitus have a decreased to absent glucagon response to hypoglycemia, followed by a diminished epinephrine response to hypoglycemia over time. Glucose recovery in response to insulin-induced hypoglycemia is markedly improved after pancreas transplantation compared to nontransplanted diabetic controls (35,36).

The presence of autoantibodies (37), excessive postprandial insulin levels occurring as a result of systemic, as opposed to portal, drainage of the graft (32,38), or the presence of counter-regulatory abnormalities in type I diabetes after pancreas transplantation (33,39,40) have been proposed as reasons for hypoglycemia, but do not account for every case. Gastroparesis and the acute effects of corticosteroids on insulin secretion in the early posttransplant period have also been proposed as contributing factors to the hypoglycemic symptoms reported in some patients after pancreas transplantation (19). Hypoglycemic symptoms and documented events are uncommon and tend to diminish over time. In recurrent and severe hypoglycemic episodes, in order to suppress endogenous hyperinsulinemia, diaxozide could be an option

(41). In order to increase the peripheral and hepatic insulin resistance, increasing or adding steroids to the immunosuppressive regimen could promote hyper- or normoglycemia. Although not proven, somatostatin analogues could suppress beta-cell function. As a last option, partial or total pancreatectomy may be considered (41).

## MACROVASCULAR DISEASE

The most common cause of death in diabetes and transplant patients is vascular disease. Pre-existing vascular disease severely reduces patient survival following simultaneous pancreas–kidney transplantation (42). Individual vascular risk factors may increase or decrease depending on genetic predispositions, differences in behaviors (weight gain, persistent smoking), specific immunosuppressive agents, type of procedure, and allograft function after transplantation (19).

The factors that best predict rate of progression include pre-existing vascular disease, older age, ongoing smoking, hyperphosphatemia, hypoalbuminemia, and longer duration of pretransplant dialysis (43). In addition to cardiovascular events, amputation remains an ongoing concern and a significant cause of morbidity after transplantation (19).

In one study, 11 patients receiving simultaneous pancreas–kidney transplantation were compared to 10 diabetic patients undergoing kidney transplantation alone. The first group of patients had lower hemoglobin $A_{1C}$ and lower triglyceride levels, but similar cholesterol concentrations and blood pressures, compared to the patients receiving kidney transplant alone. No difference between the two groups was found in progression to macrovascular and coronary heart disease or in the progression of peripheral vascular disease (44).

Carotid intimal thickness correlates with future vascular disease risk. Carotid intima media thickness improved by two years after simultaneous pancreas–kidney transplant, independent of significant changes in lipids, blood pressure, or use of hypolipidemic agents in this cohort (45,46). La Rocca et al. (47) showed that diastolic dysfunction normalized by four years in simultaneous pancreas–kidney transplant recipients but not in kidney transplant alone recipients. Fewer cardiovascular events, specifically acute myocardial infarction and acute pulmonary edema, have been reported to occur after simultaneous pancreas–kidney transplantation compared with type I diabetes recipients receiving kidney transplant alone (48).

Altogether, macrovascular disease improves in most patients after simultaneous pancreas–kidney transplant, but not enough data are available to assess macrovascular disease after pancreas alone or pancreas after kidney transplant.

### Hypertension

An excess of cardiovascular disease and cardiac mortality is well established in patients with type I diabetes mellitus. Hypertension is causally related to this excessive cardiovascular risk, and is a nearly constant finding in type I diabetics with diabetic nephropathy (49). Despite the restoration of normal renal function, hypertension remains a significant issue for diabetics who have undergone successful kidney transplantation, with persistent hypertension occurring in up to 60% to 80% of patients (50,51).

The pathogenesis of posttransplantation hypertension is multifactorial and may include chronic allograft nephropathy, use of calcineurin inhibitors, corticosteroids, and posttransplant renal artery stenosis.

Elliott et al. (49) demonstrated a substantial decrease in blood pressure after successful kidney–pancreas transplantation despite a marked reduction in the use of antihypertensive therapy. Noteworthy is that this improvement in hypertension occurred despite the addition of immunosuppressive agents known to aggravate hypertension. Naf et al. (52) observed an important reduction in the percentage of patients with hypertension (48.6%) without a change in the prevalence of dyslipemia (19.9%) after transplantation. Hypertension after transplantation was clearly associated with the appearance or persistence of macrovascular events.

Another factor that can impact blood pressure changes after pancreas transplantation is enteric versus bladder drainage of the allograft pancreas. Blood pressure decreases after simultaneous pancreas–kidney transplant with bladder drainage, even with cyclosporine- and steroid-based immunosuppression, in part because of salt and water loss that accompanies bladder drainage of the exocrine duct (49,53,54). On the other hand, enteric drainage may not improve blood pressure at all (55).

Management of hypertension after transplantation is often complicated by autonomic neuropathy causing orthostatic hypotension. These patients commonly develop severe supine hypertension and upright hypotension complicating the pharmacologic management of their hypertension. Such patients usually describe the absence of orthostatic hypotension during the period on dialysis. They are typically hypervolemic while on dialysis, but develop hypovolemia after a bladder-drained pancreas transplant because of excessive urinary losses of sodium, bicarbonate and water. In patients with enteric drainage, the volume losses are minimized, but pooling of splanchnic blood characteristic of diabetic autonomic neuropathy persists, leading to orthostatic hypotension. Orthostatic hypotension can be minimized by avoiding agents that cause or exacerbate it. These include diuretics, sympathetic antihypertensive agents such as clonidine, antidepressants, and antianginal agents (if possible). In addition, custom-fitted elastic stockings may be particularly useful if the above agents cannot be discontinued. These stockings must extend to the waist since splanchnic blood pooling is the major cause of this disorder. Compression of the lower extremities alone will have little impact. Patients should be instructed to rise slowly from lying and supine positions and elevate the head of their bed to approximately 20° to 30° while sleeping. First-line pharmacologic measures include the use of fludrocortisone to increase intravascular volume, possibly increase sensitivity of blood vessels to catecholamine, and increase norepinephrine release. The use of sympathomimetic agents such as ephedrine and pseudoephedrine is not recommended because of the increased potential for stroke. The selective alpha-1 adrenergic agonist midodrine has also been demonstrated to be effective in minimizing orthostatic hypotension by both arterial and venous vasoconstriction, and should be considered to be second-line treatment. Interestingly, clonidine may be used to treat orthostatic hypotension despite its known side effect of orthostatic hypotension in patients with intact autonomic activity. It is a centrally acting alpha-2 adrenergic agonist, and patients with autonomic neuropathy may have minimal central sympathetic efferent activity, with postsynaptic receptors predominating, leading to hypertension. The effect of clonidine, however, has been unpredictable, so it is typically avoided in this setting. Great care must be exercised in managing hypertension in patients with autonomic neuropathy causing orthostatic hypotension, since many blood pressure determinations are performed only in the supine position in the early postoperative period by the nursing staff. Normalization of supine pressures alone will usually result in severe upright hypotension, limiting the patient's ability to ambulate and increasing the risk of falls. Blood pressures should be monitored in supine, sitting, and standing positions to assess accurately the patient's response to treatment and to avoid delayed rehabilitation.

## RECURRENT AUTOIMMUNE PANCREATITIS

Insulin-dependent diabetes mellitus is an autoimmune disease in which the beta cells of the islets of Langerhans are selectively destroyed. In a patient with this disease, a transplanted pancreas should be as susceptible to the autoimmune process as the native pancreas. Usually, however, the degree of immunosuppression required to prevent rejection is sufficient to prevent autoimmune damage of the pancreatic graft (56).

Tyden et al. reported two patients who underwent pancreatic transplantation with poor human leukocyte antigen (HLA) matching, in whom the beta cells in the transplants were subsequently destroyed despite standard immunosuppressive therapy. They showed that the first sign of deterioration was a decline in the rise in the serum C-peptide concentration after a meal, followed by a decrease in the serum C-peptide concentration in the fasting state. This gradual decline in beta-cell secretory capacity was similar to that which occurs in adults with insulin-dependent diabetes mellitus. The excised grafts showed selective destruction of beta cells without evidence of rejection, with preservation of alpha and delta cells, resembling pancreatic islets from patients with long-standing insulin-dependent diabetes mellitus. Furthermore, in one of their patients, serum tests for antibodies against islet cells and glutamic acid decarboxylase were initially negative, but were detected at high titers at the time of overt beta-cell dysfunction. Association between the reappearance of islet-cell antibodies and the failure of a deceased donor pancreatic graft have been suggested elsewhere (57).

Sutherland et al., in a series of 200 pancreas transplants with follow-up of six months to almost nine years, identified recurrent disease as the cause of graft failure in eight cases, all in non- or minimally immunosuppressed recipients of transplants from identical twin ($n = 3$) or HLA-identical sibling ($n = 5$) donors. Recurrence of disease was defined as selective loss of beta cells; other endocrine cell types persisted and appeared normal within the islets of the graft (58).

Selective destruction of beta cells may occur despite sustained immunosuppressive therapy. Poor HLA matching between the donor and recipient may reduce the risk of recurrent autoimmune diabetes after pancreatic transplantation (58), although the donor and recipient do not have to share HLA alleles for autoimmune destruction of the graft to occur, as shown in the Tyden et al. report.

## FLUID AND ACID–BASE DISTURBANCES

Urinary diversion of exocrine secretions of pancreas allografts may result in acid–base and electrolyte disorders after pancreas transplant.

Excessive urinary loss of bicarbonate and concomitant metabolic acidosis are exacerbated during periods of renal dysfunction (acute cellular rejection, immunosuppression-induced renal toxicity, urological complications) in bladder-drained pancreas allografts. Hyperkalemia, volume depletion, and urinary obstruction are other factors that can exacerbate metabolic acidosis. Poorly controlled metabolic acidosis also increases the risk of severe hyperkalemia related to intracellular shifts of hydrogen ions for potassium. Cyclosporine and tacrolimus may also contribute to hyperkalemia, which may cause these patients to be particularly vulnerable to life-threatening hyperkalemia. Since bladder-drained pancreas transplant patients require large amounts of oral sodium bicarbonate, ensuring compliance with this agent is often difficult. Avoidance of calcineurin inhibitor toxicity and careful management to metabolic acidosis should be maintained to avoid hyperkalemic deaths.

Volume depletion occurs more frequently during the first three postoperative months, when metabolic acidosis is more problematic (59). This is primarily related to the loss of sodium, which is excreted in conjunction with bicarbonate and water in the bladder-drained patients. In addition, patients with renal insufficiency have obligatory urinary sodium losses, which may compound the problem. Diarrhea related to diabetic enteropathy, mycophenolate mofetil, or other causes results in often massive volume losses and severe nonrenal bicarbonate losses. This leads to severe volume depletion, metabolic acidosis, and hypomagnesemia, but the hyperkalemia may be attenuated by the hypomagnesemia.

Bruce et al. reported 37 episodes of readmission for rehydration or metabolic acidosis among 50 patients with BD (60). Newell et al. also described a higher rate of postoperative complications, with more metabolic acidosis (9/12 vs. 1/12) and dehydration (7/12 vs. 0/12) noted in patients with bladder drainage than with enteric drainage (61).

In another review of 150 combined kidney–pancreas transplants with systemic venous and exocrine bladder drainage, Elkhammas et al. reported that 36% of readmissions were related to one or all of a triad of dehydration, acidosis, or hyperkalemia (62).

Treatment options include correction of any underlying cause, bicarbonate supplementation with or without acetazolamide (63), or surgical conversion from bladder drainage to enteric drainage (63–65).

### Diabetic Gastroparesis and Enteropathy

Autonomic neuropathy involving the upper gastrointestinal tract is common in diabetics and has been estimated to be prevalent in approximately 50% of patients with long-standing type I or type II diabetes. Following pancreas transplantation, delayed gastric emptying persists and may be exacerbated in the early postoperative period. The medication most commonly used in the United States is metaclopromide (Reglan®), since cisapride use has been proscribed because of potential life-threatening cardiac complications. Patients with pre-existing diabetic gastroparesis usually present to hospital taking metaclopromide at the time of transplantation. In most cases, it is withheld during the early postoperative period when the patients are not eating. Thereafter, it should be restarted orally at the pretransplant dose to avoid clinically evident delayed gastric emptying. Dosing should, however, be guided by the patient's renal function. For patients with a creatinine clearance $< 40 \text{ cm}^3/\text{min}$, 50% of the manufacturer's usual starting dose should be used. Intravenous metaclopromide can be used for patients with severe delayed gastric emptying occurring before oral medications can be used. Although this agent is effective in controlling the symptoms of gastroparesis, major side effects may limit its use. Potential adverse reactions include cardiovascular (A-V block, supraventricular tachycardia, bradycardia, and congestive heart failure among others), neurologic (acute dystonic reactions, akathisia, parkinsonian-like symptoms, hallucinations, depression, and others), and many other less common complications. The long-term use of erythromycin is not recommended, but it may be useful as short-term therapy in patients unable to take metaclopromide.

Diabetic enteropathy may develop in approximately 25% of all diabetics and presents usually with diarrhea and uncommonly with steatorrhea. It is also predominately related to diabetic autonomic neuropathy. The usual pharmacologic treatment is with loperamide (Imodium$^{R}$) as needed. This is usually discontinued in the early postoperative period and restarted if the diarrhea recurs. Clonidine may decrease intestinal transit time, but may also decrease secretions, leading to decreased stool volume, and can be used cautiously in the setting. It may exacerbate or improve the orthostatic hypotension, in addition to causing neurologic symptoms among others.

## CONCLUSION

Although pancreas/kidney transplantation has evolved to become a widely accepted therapeutic option for patients with end-stage renal disease secondary to type I diabetes mellitus, preventing and improving transplant-associated complications will improve the quality of life in this cohort of patients.

Pancreas transplantation has become more common, as the long-term success rates have improved and risks have decreased. Fracture rates and bone disease are higher among diabetics and in patients receiving a simultaneous pancreas transplant. These patients should receive prophylaxis and treatment for osteoporosis. Ongoing monitoring for cardiovascular and peripheral vascular complications should continue after pancreas transplantation. Hypertension also needs to be aggressively treated, as it can increase cardiovascular morbidity and mortality after transplantation. The risks of autoimmune recurrence of diabetes have yet to be established, as there are few reports in the literature.

## REFERENCES

1. Heaf JG. Bone disease after renal transplantation. Transplantation 2003; 75(3):315.
2. Ramsey-Goldman R, Dunn JE, Dunlop DD, et al. Increased risk of fracture in patients receiving solid organ transplants. J Bone Miner Res 1999; 14(3):456.
3. Chiu MY, Sprague SM, Bruce DS, Woodle ES, Thistlethwaite JR Jr., Josephson MA. Analysis of fracture prevalence in kidney–pancreas allograft recipients. J Am Soc Nephrol 1998; 9(4):677.
4. Smets YF, van der Pijl JW, de Fijter JW, Ringers J, Lemkes HH, Hamdy NA. Low bone mass and high incidence of fractures after successful simultaneous pancreas–kidney transplantation. Nephrol Dial Transplant 1998; 13(5):1250.
5. O'Shaughnessy EA, Dahl DC, Smith CL, Kasiske BL. Risk factors for fractures in kidney transplantation. Transplantation 2002; 74(3):362.
6. Durieux S, Mercadal L, Orcel P, et al. Bone mineral density and fracture prevalence in long-term kidney graft recipients. Transplantation 2002; 74(4):496.
7. Lukert BP, Raisz LG. Glucocorticoid-induced osteoporosis: pathogenesis and management. Ann Intern Med 1990; 112(5):352.
8. Canalis E. Clinical review 83: mechanisms of glucocorticoid action in bone: implications to glucocorticoid-induced osteoporosis. J Clin Endocrinol Metab 1996; 81(10):3441.
9. Movsowitz C, Epstein S, Fallon M, Ismail F, Thomas S. Cyclosporin-A in vivo produces severe osteopenia in the rat: effect of dose and duration of administration. Endocrinology 1988; 123(5):2571.
10. Stewart PJ, Green OC, Stern PH. Cyclosporine A inhibits calcemic hormone-induced bone resorption in vitro. J Bone Miner Res 1986; 1(3):285.
11. Cvetkovic M, Mann GN, Romero DF, et al. The deleterious effects of long-term cyclosporine A, cyclosporine G, and FK506 on bone mineral metabolism in vivo. Transplantation 1994; 57(8):1231.
12. Leidig-Bruckner G, Hosch S, Dodidou P, et al. Frequency and predictors of osteoporotic fractures after cardiac or liver transplantation: a follow-up study. Lancet 2001; 357(9253):342.

13. Park KM, Hay JE, Lee SG, et al. Bone loss after orthotopic liver transplantation: FK 506 versus cyclosporine. Transplant Proc 1996; 28(3):1738.
14. Nowacka-Cieciura E, Durlik M, Cieciura T, et al. Positive effect of steroid withdrawal on bone mineral density in renal allograft recipients. Transplant Proc 2001; 33(1–2):1273.
15. Reinhardt W, Bartelworth H, Jockenhovel F, et al. Sequential changes of biochemical bone parameters after kidney transplantation. Nephrol Dial Transplant 1998; 13(2):436.
16. Lucas PA, Woodhead JS, Brown RC. Vitamin D3 metabolites in chronic renal failure and after renal transplantation. Nephrol Dial Transplant 1988; 3(1):70.
17. Suzuki Y, Ichikawa Y, Saito E, Homma M. Importance of increased urinary calcium excretion in the development of secondary hyperparathyroidism of patients under glucocorticoid therapy. Metabolism 1983; 32(2):151.
18. Grotz WH, Mundinger FA, Rasenack J, et al. Bone loss after kidney transplantation: a longitudinal study in 115 graft recipients. Nephrol Dial Transplant 1995; 10(11):2096.
19. Larsen JL. Pancreas transplantation: indications and consequences. Endocr Rev 2004; 25(6):919.
20. Heaf J. Causes and consequences of adynamic bone disease. Nephron 2001; 88(2):97.
21. Hyodo T, Kumano K, Endo T, et al. Clinical evaluation of bone metabolism after renal transplantation to support the theory to perform 1,25(OH)2D3 pulse therapy before transplantation. Nephron 1996; 73(4):723.
22. American College of Rheumatology Task Force on Osteoporosis Guidelines. Recommendations for the prevention and treatment of glucocorticoid-induced osteoporosis. Arthritis Rheum 1996; 39(11):1791.
23. Hamdy NA, Kanis JA, Beneton MN, et al. Effect of alfacalcidol on natural course of renal bone disease in mild to moderate renal failure. BMJ 1995; 310(6976):358.
24. Kruse AE, Eisenberger U, Frey FJ, Mohaupt MG. The calcimimetic cinacalcet normalizes serum calcium in renal transplant patients with persistent hyperparathyroidism. Nephrol Dial Transplant 2005; 20(7):1311–1314.
25. Leonard N, Brown JH. Persistent and symptomatic post-transplant hyperparathyroidism: a dramatic response to cinacalcet. Nephrol Dial Transplant 2006; 21(6):1736.
26. Ninkovic M, Love S, Tom BD, Bearcroft PW, Alexander GJ, Compston JE. Lack of effect of intravenous pamidronate on fracture incidence and bone mineral density after orthotopic liver transplantation. J Hepatol 2002; 37(1):93.
27. Cahill BC, O'Rourke MK, Parker S, Stringham JC, Karwande SV, Knecht TP. Prevention of bone loss and fracture after lung transplantation: a pilot study. Transplantation 2001; 72(7):1251.
28. Weber TJ, Quarles LD. Preventing bone loss after renal transplantation with bisphosphonates: we can. But should we? Kidney Int 2000; 57(2):735.
29. Valero MA, Loinaz C, Larrodera L, Leon M, Moreno E, Hawkins F. Calcitonin and bisphosphonates treatment in bone loss after liver transplantation. Calcif Tissue Int 1995; 57(1):15.
30. Schwarz C, Mitterbauer C, Heinze G, Woloszczuk W, Haas M, Oberbauer R. Nonsustained effect of short-term bisphosphonate therapy on bone turnover three years after renal transplantation. Kidney Int 2004; 65(1):304.
31. Guichelaar MM, Malinchoc M, Sibonga JD, Clarke BL, Hay JE. Bone histomorphometric changes after liver transplantation for chronic cholestatic liver disease. J Bone Miner Res 2003; 18(12):2190.
32. Redmon JB, Teuscher AU, Robertson RP. Hypoglycemia after pancreas transplantation. Diabet Care 1998; 21(11):1944.
33. Kendall DM, Teuscher AU, Robertson RP. Defective glucagon secretion during sustained hypoglycemia following successful islet allo- and autotransplantation in humans. Diabetes 1997; 46(1):23.
34. Cottrell DA, Henry ML, O'Dorisio TM, Tesi RJ, Ferguson RM, Osei K. Hypoglycemia after successful pancreas transplantation in type I diabetic patients. Diabet Care 1991; 14(11):1111.
35. Diem P, Redmon JB, Abid M, et al. Glucagon, catecholamine and pancreatic polypeptide secretion in type I diabetic recipients of pancreas allografts. J Clin Invest 1990; 86(6):2008.
36. Bolinder J, Wahrenberg H, Persson A, et al. Effect of pancreas transplantation on glucose counterregulation in insulin-dependent diabetic patients prone to severe hypoglycaemia. J Intern Med 1991; 230(6):527.
37. Tran MP, Larsen JL, Duckworth WC, et al. Anti-insulin antibodies are a cause of hypoglycemia following pancreas transplantation. Diabet Care 1994; 17(9):988.
38. Sutherland DE, Gruessner AC, Gruessner RW. Pancreas transplantation: a review. Transplant Proc 1998; 30(5):1940.
39. Gupta V, Wahoff DC, Rooney DP, et al. The defective glucagon response from transplanted intrahepatic pancreatic islets during hypoglycemia is transplantation site-determined. Diabetes 1997; 46(1):28.
40. Battezzati A, Luzi L, Perseghin G, et al. Persistence of counter-regulatory abnormalities in insulin-dependent diabetes mellitus after pancreas transplantation. Eur J Clin Invest 1994; 24(11):751.
41. Osei K. Post-transplantation hypoglycaemia in type 1 diabetic pancreas allograft recipients. Acta Diabetol 1998; 35(4):176.
42. Sutherland DE, Gruessner RW, Dunn DL, et al. Lessons learned from more than 1,000 pancreas transplants at a single institution. Ann Surg 2001; 233(4):463.

43. Nankivell BJ, Lau SG, Chapman JR, O'Connell PJ, Fletcher JP, Allen RD. Progression of macrovascular disease after transplantation. Transplantation 2000; 69(4):574.
44. Biesenbach G, Margreiter R, Konigsrainer A, et al. Comparison of progression of macrovascular diseases after kidney or pancreas and kidney transplantation in diabetic patients with end-stage renal disease. Diabetologia 2000; 43(2):231.
45. Larsen JL, Colling CW, Ratanasuwan T, et al. Pancreas transplantation improves vascular disease in patients with type 1 diabetes. Diabet Care 2004; 27(7):1706.
46. Larsen JL, Ratanasuwan T, Burkman T, et al. Carotid intima media thickness decreases after pancreas transplantation. Transplantation 2002; 73(6):936.
47. La Rocca E, Fiorina P, di Carlo V, et al. Cardiovascular outcomes after kidney–pancreas and kidney-alone transplantation. Kidney Int 2001; 60(5):1964.
48. La Rocca E, Fiorina P, Astorri E, et al. Patient survival and cardiovascular events after kidney–pancreas transplantation: comparison with kidney transplantation alone in uremic IDDM patients. Cell Transplant 2000; 9(6):929.
49. Elliott MD, Kapoor A, Parker MA, Kaufman DB, Bonow RO, Gheorghiade M. Improvement in hypertension in patients with diabetes mellitus after kidney/pancreas transplantation. Circulation 2001; 104(5):563.
50. Najarian JS, Fryd DS, Strand M, et al. A single institution, randomized, prospective trial of cyclosporin versus azathioprine-antilymphocyte globulin for immunosuppression in renal allograft recipients. Ann Surg 1985; 201(2):142.
51. Ponticelli C, Montagnino G, Aroldi A, Angelini C, Braga M, Tarantino A. Hypertension after renal transplantation. Am J Kidney Dis 1993; 21(5 suppl 2):73.
52. Naf S, Jose Ricart M, Recasens M, Astudillo E, Fernandez-Cruz L, Esmatjes E. Macrovascular events after kidney–pancreas transplantation in type 1 diabetic patients. Transplant Proc 2003; 35(5):2019.
53. Kaufman DB, Leventhal JR, Stuart J, Abecassis MM, Fryer JP, Stuart FP. Mycophenolate mofetil and tacrolimus as primary maintenance immunosuppression in simultaneous pancreas–kidney transplantation: initial experience in 50 consecutive cases. Transplantation 1999; 67(4):586.
54. Markowski DM, Larsen JL, McElligott MC, et al. Diet after pancreas transplantation. Diabet Care 1996; 19(7):735.
55. Hricik DE, Chareandee C, Knauss TC, Schulak JA. Hypertension after pancreas–kidney transplantation: role of bladder versus enteric pancreatic drainage. Transplantation 2000; 70(3):494.
56. Tyden G, Reinholt FP, Sundkvist G, Bolinder J. Recurrence of autoimmune diabetes mellitus in recipients of cadaveric pancreatic grafts. N Engl J Med 1996; 335(12):860.
57. Bosi E, Bottazzo GF, Secchi A, et al. Islet cell autoimmunity in type I diabetic patients after HLA-mismatched pancreas transplantation. Diabetes 1989; 38(suppl 1):82.
58. Sutherland DE, Goetz FC, Sibley RK. Recurrence of disease in pancreas transplants. Diabetes 1989; 38(suppl 1):85.
59. Ketel B, Henry ML, Elkhammas EA, Tesi RJ, Ferguson RM. Metabolic complications in combined kidney/pancreas transplantation. Transplant Proc 1992; 24(3):774.
60. Bruce DS, Newell KA, Josephson MA, et al. Long-term outcome of kidney–pancreas transplant recipients with good graft function at one year. Transplantation 1996; 62(4):451.
61. Newell KA, Bruce DS, Cronin DC, et al. Comparison of pancreas transplantation with portal venous and enteric exocrine drainage to the standard technique utilizing bladder drainage of exocrine secretions. Transplantation 1996; 62(9):1353.
62. Elkhammas EA, Henry ML, Tesi RJ, Ferguson RM. Combined kidney/pancreas transplantation at the Ohio State University Hospitals. Clin Transplant 1992:191.
63. Stephanian E, Gruessner RW, Brayman KL, et al. Conversion of exocrine secretions from bladder to enteric drainage in recipients of whole pancreaticoduodenal transplants. Ann Surg 1992; 216(6):663.
64. Munda R, Tom WW, First MR, Gartside P, Alexander JW. Pancreatic allograft exocrine urinary tract diversion. Pathophysiology. Transplantation 1987; 43(1):95.
65. Burke GW, Gruessner R, Dunn DL, Sutherland DE. Conversion of whole pancreaticoduodenal transplants from bladder to enteric drainage for metabolic acidosis or dysuria. Transplant Proc 1990; 22(2):651.

# 18 | Infectious Complications in Pancreas Transplant Recipients

**Eun Jeong Kwak**
*Division of Infectious Diseases, Department of Medicine, Thomas E. Starzl Transplantation Institute, University of Pittsburgh School of Medicine, Pittsburgh, Pennsylvania, U.S.A.*

**Shimon Kusne**
*Mayo Medical School, Mayo Clinic Scottsdale, Scottsdale, Arizona, U.S.A.*

## INTRODUCTION

Pancreas transplantation has become an accepted treatment modality for type 1 diabetes mellitus, especially for patients with poorly controlled disease and end-stage renal disease. The U.S. Organ Procurement and Transplantation Network and the Scientific Registry of Transplant Recipients reported that there were 9579 pancreas transplants performed, including 957 solitary transplants and 8622 pancreas with or after a kidney transplantation, from 1993 to 2002. Infectious complications, together with rejection, are the two main concerns of transplantation in general. In this review, the infectious complications reported in the literature after pancreas transplantation are summarized. It is the purpose of this review to concentrate on infectious disease issues that are unique to pancreas transplantation.

## GENERAL PRINCIPLES

It is very important to understand the underlying medical condition of this transplant population before describing the different infectious complications. Poorly controlled diabetics are prone to infection, and these candidates usually have a significant history of infection. The initial period after transplantation is crucial most because the organ is both recovering from perioperative ischemia-reperfusion injury and is at the highest risk for rejection. These patients may also have a new kidney that is subject to these issues, and renal failure is also a risk for infection.

The details of the surgical technique used in this operation are crucial to understanding the potential infectious complications (1). When the infection rate is compared between kidney transplantation alone and kidney–pancreas transplantation, the latter has a higher incidence of infectious complications (2). This is related to the nature of the organ, specifically the need to deal with the exocrine secretions, and the associated increased technical complexity. There are two alternative exocrine drainage techniques, bladder or enteric. The infections seen with the two techniques are likely to involve different flora. The pancreatic juices secreted in the bladder can irritate the mucosa and lead to urinary tract infection (UTI). With enteric drainage, the gastrointestinal flora are involved in abdominal infections associated with leaking of material from the gut.

## BACTERIAL INFECTIONS

The authors reviewed their own data regarding bacterial infections after pancreas transplantation (3). Between April 1994 and February 1998, 132 patients underwent pancreas transplant at the University of Pittsburgh Medical Center. Eight (6%) patients had pancreas transplant alone (PTA), 12 (9%) had pancreas transplant after kidney (PAK) and 112 (85%) underwent simultaneous pancreas and kidney transplant (SPK). Of these 132 patients, 103 (78%) had enteric drainage, 27 (20.5%) had bladder drainage, and two (1.5%) had bladder drainage that was converted to enteric later. Some of the bacterial infections in this population were mixed together with fungal organisms, and originated after the development of a bowel leak. The rates of

**Table 1**  Types of Severe Bacterial and Fungal Infections After Adult
Pancreas Transplantation in 44 Cases

| | |
|---|---:|
| Peritonitis | 12 |
| Peripancreatic infected collection | 10 |
| Abdominal wound infection | 5 |
| Pancreatic abscess | 4 |
| Other abdominal abscess | 4 |
| *Clostridium difficile* colitis | 4 |
| Pyelonephritis | 2 |
| Others | 3 |

bacterial and fungal infections were 75%, 25%, and 37.5% after PTA, PAK, and SPK, respectively ($p = 0.06$). The higher rate of infections after PTA was because of UTIs. All eight patients undergoing PTA had bladder drainage. In this series there were 44 severe infections. These infections are shown in Table 1. Simple UTIs without bacteremia were not included.

## Type of Anastomosis and Infection

When clinicians assess pancreas transplant recipients for infection, it is crucial to know the type of exocrine drainage used. UTIs are more commonly seen when bladder drainage is used (4), while enteric drainage may be associated with both chemical and infectious peritonitis (5). With bladder drainage, the pancreatic enzymes irritate the mucosa of the bladder (4), while with enteric drainage, leakage of pancreatic enzymes into the peritoneal cavity together with enteric organisms from the bowel may be the cause of peritonitis and intra-abdominal abscess formation (5).

## Surgical Complications and Infection

Surgical and technical complications are associated with an increased incidence of infectious complications. In our experience, both bacterial and fungal infections were more frequent in the 18 patients who developed surgical complications, compared to the 114 patients without any surgical complications (15/18, 83.5% vs. 36/114, 31.6%; $p < 0.0001$). Examples of urological complications reported after bladder-drained pancreas transplantation are hematuria and urethral strictures. Severe hematuria may be an indication for conversion from bladder to enteric drainage (6,7). Infections reported with bladder drainage are recurrent UTIs, prostatitis, epididymitis, and pyelonephritis (6). Since the pancreas is being transplanted with a duodenal segment, complications may also involve an infection of the duodenum (8,9), which can lead to leak, ulceration, and necrosis (9). In one institution, of 140 consecutive pancreas transplantations with bladder drainage, 21% required conversion to enteric drainage (7). Indications for enteric conversion included hematuria from duodenitis, recurrent pancreatitis, bladder calculi, and retained sutures (7).

## Urinary Tract Infections

A number of studies have confirmed that UTIs are more commonly seen in bladder-drained pancreas transplant recipients (3,7,10). In our own series, the rate of UTIs in patients with bladder drainage was 29.6%, while the rate of UTIs with enteric drainage was only 5.8% ($p = 0.0001$). The pancreatic enzymes entering the bladder cause inflammation of the urothelium. Sutures and staples are a good nidus for formation of calculi and for bacteria (7). Frequently, urological complications are associated with these UTIs. In one series, recurrent UTIs occurred in 36% of the patients (7), and the most common organisms involved were *Escherichia coli* (24%), *Staphylococcus epidermidis* (21%), and *Enterobacter cloacae* (12%).

## Wound Infections

Wound infections usually occur during the first month after pancreas transplantation and are related to technical events (2). Mittal and Toledo-Peryera found that culture of the duodenal loop might predict the etiology of wound infection after bladder-drained pancreas transplantation (11). In their series, seven of 10 patients with a positive duodenal culture developed infection after transplantation, five of which were with the same organism (11). The authors suggested irrigation of the duodenal loop with betadine and amphotericin B (11). Other authors argue with this practice and found no correlation between the bacteriology of the duodenum and infection (12). In a series of 40 bladder-drained SPKs (8), the overall incidence of wound infection was 16%. Four of these episodes were deep and were associated with allograft pancreatitis and bladder leaks. The cultures of the duodenal segment were sterile in 32% of wound infections, and the authors suggested that other factors might be important in development of wound infection after pancreas transplantation (8). When midline and transverse incisions were compared in bladder-drained SPK transplant patients, there was no significant difference in the infection rate (13). Deep abscesses were more common when a midline incision was used (14). Independent risk factors for development of wound infection included older age (≥40 years), bladder leak, and serum amylase ≥1000 IU/L during the first week (14).

## Intra-Abdominal Infections

Most of the intra-abdominal infections occur during the first month after transplantation and are related to anastomotic leakage. They may lead to death or graft loss and may portend problems after retransplantation. In one series, 12 of 13 patients who developed intra-abdominal infection that resulted in the loss of the pancreatic allograft developed recurrence of their intra-abdominal infection after a second pancreas transplant (14). Some feel that intra-abdominal infection represents a relative contraindication for pancreas retransplantation (14). Deep intra-abdominal wound infection, including peritonitis and intra-abdominal abscesses, are often an indication for removal of the allograft (15). Risk factors identified for the development of superficial and deep abdominal infections included prolonged operating time, older donors, and enteric drainage (15). An important type of intra-abdominal infection in this population is the formation of a peripancreatic abscess, which has a higher incidence in pancreas transplant recipients who were maintained on peritoneal dialysis prior to transplantation than in those on hemodialysis (16).

## VIRAL INFECTIONS

The most common viral infection in pancreas transplant recipients is cytomegalovirus (CMV), which causes clinical disease in 8% to 55% of solid organ transplant recipients, depending on the risk factors (17). Epstein-Barr virus (EBV), while an uncommon cause of viral syndrome in this population, plays a major role in development of posttransplant lymphoproliferative disease (PTLD). Other herpesviruses, such as herpes simplex virus (HSV) and varicella-zoster virus (VZV) are responsible for a wide spectrum of symptoms, from minor oral ulcers to fulminant multisystem disease. Recently, there has been increasing interest in HHV-6 and HHV-8 infections in transplant patients.

## CYTOMEGALOVIRUS

CMV is a double-stranded DNA virus of the herpesviridiae family, and is capable of causing latent infection and clinical disease through either reactivation, or as a primary infection. It can present in a variety of ways in a transplant recipient, ranging from asymptomatic infection to disseminated disease and death. The frequency and severity of the infection is most striking in a mismatched transplant, i.e., a CMV seronegative patient receiving a CMV seropositive organ, as this causes a primary infection that often leads to invasive disease. Rarely, a seronegative individual can acquire infection from blood transfusions. Reactivation of the virus in a seropositive individual also occurs, especially when a patient is treated with antilymphocyte antibodies such as OKT3 or thymoglobulin.

### Clinical Presentation

Primary infection in the setting of a CMV seropositive donor/CMV seronegative recipient usually occurs in the first one to four months after transplantation. Asymptomatic early infection can sometimes be diagnosed when a preemptive strategy is used by detecting the viral load in the blood. Low-grade fever and other constitutional symptoms such as fatigue and anorexia can occur as the viral load increases. Pancytopenia is often seen as the result of bone marrow suppression. Other than serological mismatch and augmented immunosuppression, bladder drainage of pancreas allograft appears to increase the rate of CMV reactivation (18).

Organ-specific invasive CMV disease usually involves the transplanted organ. However, in the pancreas transplant population, CMV pancreatitis is uncommon. Klassen et al.'s report (19) of four patients with CMV allograft pancreatitis showed that three out of the four cases involved a seropositive donor/seronegative recipient. Three patients received OKT3 for rejection prior to the onset of CMV disease. All patients presented with increased amylase and lipase, which was clinically difficult to distinguish from rejection, and required a biopsy for clarification. Only one patient had fever.

Invasive disease can also involve sites other than the transplanted organ. One of the most common sites is the upper gastrointestinal tract, in the form of CMV esophagitis and gastro-duodenitis. The presence of fever is variable. Common symptoms include malaise, anorexia, nausea, vomiting, and heartburn, although the presentation can be subtle, requiring a high index of suspicion. CMV can also cause invasive disease in the lungs, eyes, liver, and colon.

## Diagnosis

Transplant recipients often shed CMV in their bodily fluids. The spectrum of CMV infection runs from asymptomatic infection, in which the virus is isolated in a bodily fluid without signs of invasive disease, to symptomatic CMV disease with or without tissue invasion (20).

The traditional CMV culture that requires detection of cytopathic effects on cell lines is of no clinical use because of prolonged turnover time. Although the use of the Shell-vial culture and detection of p72 protein via stain with monoclonal antibody reduced the turnover time to 72 hours, this technique was replaced by the CMV antigenemia (pp65) test, which uses a monoclonal antibody staining against the pp65 lower matrix phosphoprotein of leukocytes (21,22), the result of which is reported as the number of positively staining leukocytes per 200,000 cells. This test is usually completed in five hours. The newer polymerase chain reaction (PCR) technique can yield comparable results within a much shorter time frame, using less sample volume (23). Although PCR is a very sensitive test, there have been concerns that it is too sensitive to be useful in the diagnosis of CMV disease. This problem could, in theory, be addressed by predetermination of a viremia level for which an action would be taken, based on prior studies on correlation of CMV viremia and disease (24). Other methods for CMV detection include hybrid capture system (25) and testing for messenger RNA.

The definitive diagnosis of invasive CMV disease requires demonstration of tissue invasion, usually in the form of CMV inclusion bodies seen in tissue, in the appropriate clinical setting. A positive tissue immunostain for CMV is also accepted.

## Therapy and Prevention

Strategies for the prevention and treatment of invasive CMV disease in transplant recipients vary from center to center. One approach is to treat only symptomatic and proven disease; this has fallen out of favor because of the potential severity of CMV disease. Another is universal prophylaxis, in which all transplant recipients are given an antiviral agent immediately post-transplantation for a fixed period of time (usually three to six months). Although effective, universal prophylaxis carries with it the disadvantage of the cost and inconvenience. The third is preemptive strategy, in which the patients are monitored by a sensitive blood test (e.g., CMV antigenemia or PCR), and an antiviral agent is given only when the virus is detected (26). The aim of preemptive therapy is to detect the virus and treat it before it causes symptomatic infection. Although there are no specific studies in pancreas transplant recipients, the preemptive strategy has been shown to be efficient and cost-effective in prevention and treatment of CMV infection in renal transplant (27) and liver transplant recipients (28,29). The disadvantage of preemptive therapy is that it depends on intensive monitoring and close followup, which may not be realistic in a large program, and which may cost more than universal prophylaxis.

The most commonly used antiviral agent for CMV infection is ganciclovir, an acyclic nucleoside analog that inhibits viral replication. Its intravenous (IV) formulation is still the first-line therapy for documented CMV infection, and it is well tolerated except for the known side effect of bone marrow suppression. The newly available oral formulation, valganciclovir, has both excellent bioavailability and efficiency, but clinical experience with this drug is still being acquired. The other two antivirals used for CMV are foscarnet, a direct DNA polymerase inhibitor, and cidofovir, a nucleotide analog. Although effective, both agents are profoundly nephrotoxic, and are reserved for those who are intolerant of or unresponsive to ganciclovir. CMV immunoglobulin has been shown to have benefit in the reduction of CMV disease, according to a meta-analysis of 18 prophylaxis trials (30).

Ganciclovir needs to be converted to a triphosphate form before it can be active in vivo, and mutations in the gene controlling the protein kinase enzyme that performs phosphorylation (*UL97* gene) result in resistance to the drug. Another path of resistance comes from mutations in viral DNA polymerase gene (*UL54*), which confers cross-resistance to foscarnet. Ganciclovir resistance usually presents as rising CMV viremia despite treatment with full-dose ganciclovir, often in the setting of prior prolonged therapy or of subtherapeutic dosing. A prompt recognition of clinical resistance and modification of therapy is important, as genotyping for mutations can take weeks.

## EBV AND PTLD

EBV, like CMV, belongs to the herpesviridiae family, and is thus capable of causing latent infection. Most adult transplant recipients are seropositive for the virus, with EBV-associated disease occurring as the consequence of viral reactivation. In pediatric transplant recipients, primary EBV infection is a major problem, as a larger proportion of pediatric transplant recipients are EBV-naive. EBV infection has a close association with PTLD, which is thought to occur as the consequence of uncontrolled proliferation of EBV-infected lymphocytes overwhelming the suppressive effects of EBV-specific cytotoxic T-lymphocytes. However, not all PTLD is associated with EBV.

### Clinical Presentation

The incidence of PTLD varies among the different organ transplant populations, ranging from 1% in renal transplantation (31) to as high as 28% in small bowel transplant (32). In a single-center experience, Keay et al. (33) reported an 8.2% (4/49) incidence of PTLD in their pancreas transplant recipients. Traditional risk factors associated with development of PTLD in solid organ transplant patients include (i) EBV infection, especially primary infection in seronegative patients who have received seropositive organs, (ii) augmented immunosuppression, particularly with antilymphocyte antibodies, and (iii) coinfection with CMV.

A common presentation among younger patients is with infectious mononucleosis-like symptoms. Nonspecific constitutional symptoms and lymphadenopathy can be the presenting symptoms in adults as well. PTLD limited to the allograft is common in early stages of PTLD, and often presents as allograft dysfunction, which can mimic rejection. Distinguishing PTLD from rejection is of obvious importance, as an incorrect diagnosis of rejection can easily lead to inappropriate augmentation of immunosuppression and exacerbation of PTLD (34).

### Diagnosis

The diagnosis of PTLD requires histopathological examination of tissue. In EBV-associated PTLD, EBV viral antigen can be frequently demonstrated by in situ hybridization (EBER).

Various methods for EBV detection in the blood are supportive of the diagnosis when present, but insufficient on their own for the diagnosis of PTLD. A de novo EBV infection or reactivation is likely when serological testing reveals a high IgM titer or a greater than four-fold increase in IgG viral capsid antigen. Recently, quantitative EBV PCR has been widely adopted to help diagnose EBV-associated lymphoproliferation before it becomes full-blown PTLD (35). However, many aspects of this test need to be further studied, such as the cut-off for significance in viral load, difference between various PCR techniques, the exact indication for EBV PCR monitoring, and its use in follow-up after treatment of PTLD.

### Therapy

The mainstay of PTLD therapy is temporary discontinuation or profound reduction of immunosuppression. Spontaneous regression of PTLD occurs in many patients after decrease in immunosuppression (36), although it is often done at the risk of precipitating rejection.

There is no clear evidence that antivirals are of any utility in treatment of PTLD and their role is controversial. However, many early PTLDs, particularly in children, appear to behave more like EBV infections and respond quickly to a combination of temporary cessation of immunosuppression and IV ganciclovir. PTLD has also occurred in patients receiving both acyclovir and ganciclovir prophylaxis (37,38). Chemotherapy and radiotherapy can be effective but have their own associated toxicities (39). More work is needed to clarify the role of other possible therapies, such as cytotoxic T-cell infusion, interferon-α, and immunoglobulins.

Preliminary data show that rituximab, a humanized anti-CD20 monoclonal antibody, can be a promising tool in treatment of PTLD (40). In an ongoing study, Morrison et al. (41) showed a response rate of 75% in eight patients with PTLD who were treated with rituximab. More information is needed in order to determine the subgroup of patients with PTLD most likely to respond to therapy, as well as the utility of rituximab in the treatment of relapsed PTLD.

## HERPES SIMPLEX VIRUS

The seroprevalence of HSV is about 62% for HSV-1 and 22% for HSV-2 (42,43) in the adult population in the United States. HSV-1 most frequently presents as herpes labialis (cold sores), and HSV-2 most commonly presents with genital lesions, although asymptomatic shedding of the virus is common. Most of clinical HSV infection in transplant recipients results from reactivation of endogenous latent virus, rather than from a primary infection from an outside source.

In patients not receiving antiviral prophylaxis, HSV disease usually occurs within the first 30 days of transplantation. The initial presentation of mucocutaneous HSV disease in transplant recipients does not differ significantly from that seen in immunocompetent patients. However, HSV infection in this population tends to heal more slowly and disseminate more readily (44). Among solid organ transplant recipients in Pittsburgh, 9% of clinical infection was associated with widespread infection (45). HSV hepatitis, in particular, is associated with significant morbidity and a 67% mortality, according to one review (46). Other non-mucocutaneous manifestations of the infection include HSV esophagitis and HSV pneumonitis.

Oral acyclovir or valacyclovir is the therapy of choice for mild cases of HSV infection. Full dose of IV acyclovir (10–12 mg/kg q8h for patients with normal renal function) should be used for more fulminant cases, and a reduced dose of 5 mg/kg q8h for mild cases. Low-dose acyclovir (200 mg po b.i.d) used in prophylaxis effectively prevented HSV recurrence posttransplantation in the renal transplant population (47), and subsequent widespread use of antiviral prophylaxis has decreased the incidence of HSV infection substantially. Ganciclovir, an agent widely used for CMV prophylaxis, has good activity against HSV, and can be used for HSV prophylaxis as well.

## VARICELLA-ZOSTER VIRUS

VZV infection more frequently manifests as reactivation in the form of herpes zoster-associated rash (shingles) than as a primary VZV infection in the form of chickenpox, as most adults receiving a transplant are already seropositive for VZV. Once the diagnosis of either primary or reactivation VZV infection is made, the treatment is straightforward: IV acyclovir 10–12 mg/kg IV q8h for primary VZV, multi-dermatomal shingles, or herpes zoster opthalmicus (herpes zoster infection involving the ophthalmic branch of the trigeminal nerve). In fact, IV acyclovir is recommended for most cases of VZV infection in immunosuppressed individuals, as the likelihood of a simple shingles rash evolving into disseminated zoster infection is higher in transplant recipients.

Of particular concern with VZV infection in a transplant recipient is the issue of infection control. Determination of VZV IgG serologic status is recommended for all transplant candidates. The family members and household contacts of seronegative candidates should be considered for VZV vaccination prior to the transplant. Any seronegative recipient with possible exposure to individuals with active VZV infection should be given VZV immunoglobulin, and started on IV acyclovir if recipient develops a VZV-like rash until two days after all lesions are crusted. All hospitalized patients with VZV disease should be placed under airborne precautions until the lesions have crusted (48).

## FUNGAL INFECTIONS

There is not much information available in the literature regarding fungal infections in pancreas transplant recipients. The reported rate of fungal infection in this population ranges from 9.2% when only intra-abdominal infections have been included (49), up to 38% (50), although the rate may be lower in this era of improved surgical technique and antifungal prophylaxis (51). *Candida* species are by far the most common pathogen implicated, causing peritonitis, wound infection, UTI, and fungemia (52).

## CANDIDIASIS

Most of the invasive candidiasis seen in this population occurs during the early postoperative phase. The most common sites involved are surgical wounds and the abdominal cavity, followed by the urinary tract and bloodstream infections, which are often associated with urinary and central venous catheters (52). Intra-abdominal fungal infection in this population is facilitated by various factors, including (i) postreperfusion pancreatitis, (ii) contamination from the donor duodenum, (iii) anastomotic leaks, (iv) postoperative bleeding, (v) graft necrosis because of vascular thrombosis or rejection, and (vi) poor healing and compromised vascular supply because of underlying diabetes mellitus.

In a study of 445 pancreatic transplant recipients, Benedetti et al. (49) found 41 cases of intra-abdominal candidiasis (9.2%), 38 of which were by *Candida albicans*, five by *C. glabrata*, and one by *C. krusei*. An increased incidence of candidiasis was significantly associated with increased donor age. There was also a slightly higher rate of candidiasis in enterically drained than in bladder-drained patients, 21% versus 10%, although this was not statistically significant. Intra-abdominal candidiasis was significantly associated with increased mortality and decreased graft survival. Fifty-eight percent of the patients required transplant pancreatectomy before the infection could be resolved. In 20% of the cases, the infected patients died despite the removal of the pancreatic allograft. The patients with fungal infection alone or with mixed bacterial and fungal infection were three times more likely to die than those with bacterial infection alone.

The mainstay of treatment for invasive *Candida* infection has traditionally been amphotericin B, the dosage of which is limited because of its nephrotoxicity, especially in the presence of other nephrotoxic agents such as calcineurin inhibitors, which are the cornerstones of immunosuppression in most institutions. Fluconazole can be substituted for infections with *C. albicans*, although the drug interaction with immunosuppressive medications makes its use problematic. The clinical use of new azole medications such as voriconazole needs to be studied further, but may be a promising alternative, especially for infections with the non-albicans *Candida* species (53). Lastly, a well-controlled, recently published study suggests that a new echinocandin antifungal agent caspofungin, which acts on a novel target site, may be superior to amphotericin B in both efficacy and side-effect profile for bloodstream *Candida* infections (54).

## ASPERGILLOSIS

Although little is known of the rate of aspergillosis in the pancreatic transplant population, it is still one of the most dreaded complications after any solid organ transplantation. A high index of suspicion and prompt diagnosis are critically important because of the highly aggressive nature of the infection. Traditionally, the treatment of choice for invasive aspergillosis has been amphotericin B, with its attendant toxicity, but more recently, better-tolerated antifungal regimens have become available, including the liposomal formulation of amphotericin B, the echinocandin antifungal caspofungin, and new azoles with increased activity against *Aspergillus* species, such as voriconazole. Caspofungin, a glucan synthase inhibitor, has shown excellent in vitro activity against *Aspergillus*, but has not been extensively studied in the transplant population (55). Voriconazole, a newer generation azole antifungal, has undergone a controlled trial in patients with documented invasive disease (including solid organ transplant recipients) and was found to be superior to conventional amphotericin B both in its efficacy and toxicity profile (56). However, the issue of interaction with immunosuppressive medications is still problematic. The use of combination antifungal therapy may be the next logical step, but clinical data to support their routine use are lacking thus far.

## CRYPTOCOCCOSIS

Unlike candidiasis and aspergillosis, infection with *Cryptococcus neoformans* usually occurs late in the posttransplant course. In a review examining cryptococcal infection in solid organ transplant patients, Husain et al. (57) showed that the median time to the onset of the disease was 1.6 years. The central nervous system was the most common site involved (72%), followed by the lungs (25%), and other miscellaneous sites such as skin, soft tissue, and joints. The overall mortality was 42%.

The definitive diagnosis of cryptococcal meningitis requires the sampling of cerebrospinal fluid for culture. Cryptococcal antigen is usually positive in both serum and cerebrospinal fluid, and is useful in facilitating a quick diagnosis. The current recommended therapy for cryptococcal meningitis is combination of amphotericin B and 5-fluorocytosine, followed by oral fluconazole after several months. Cryptococcosis limited to the lungs or skin has been successfully treated with oral fluconazole alone (58).

## PREVENTIVE STRATEGIES

To date, there have not been any prospective controlled studies, nor any clearly established guidelines regarding the use of antifungal prophylaxis in pancreas transplantation, although several institutions have utilized a regimen of prophylactic fluconazole of variable duration. In one retrospective study, the patients who received fluconazole 400 mg/day IV for one week and postoperative oral nystatin for an indefinite duration had a rate of intra-abdominal *Candida* infection of 6%, compared to 10% in those who did not receive antifungal prophylaxis (49). However, the difference was not statistically significant. In another report, an 11% incidence of invasive fungal infection was observed in a cohort of 106 pancreas–kidney transplant recipients who received two to three months of oral fluconazole 200 mg once or twice a day (59). Further studies are needed to determine the utility of antifungal prophylaxis in pancreatic transplant recipients.

There are no clear guidelines for the prevention of *Aspergillus* and cryptococcal infections. Maintenance of a high index of suspicion in the care of patients at risk and close microbiological surveillance may facilitate early diagnosis and treatment of these infections.

## MISCELLANEOUS INFECTIONS

Protozoan infections such as *Pneumocystis carinii* and *Toxoplasma gondii* have become relatively uncommon in the transplant population because of the widespread use of prophylaxis with trimethoprim–sulfamethoxazole. *Mycobacterium tuberculosis* is an important potential pathogen in transplant recipients from TB-endemic areas. A pretransplant Mantoux skin test is often routinely performed, with the recommendation of a regimen of isoniazid (INH and B6) for 6 to 12 months posttransplantation in those with a positive skin test. INH has been used to reduce the rate of reactivation TB in lung transplant patients (60), but data are lacking in pancreas transplant recipients.

## CONCLUSIONS

Several factors, such as the nature of the surgery, underlying diabetes mellitus, and relatively intensive immunosuppressive regimens, play a role in putting pancreas transplant recipients at a higher risk of infectious complication, compared to recipients of organs such as the kidney and the heart. However, improvement in surgical techniques and the development of novel anti-infective agents in the past few years may contribute to a reduction in the infection rate. Careful examination of risk factors, diligent surveillance for early signs of infection, and prompt intervention are necessary to minimize serious infectious complications, which often contribute to death and graft loss in this population.

# REFERENCES

1. Corry RJ, Chakrabarti PK, Shapiro R, et al. Simultaneous administration of adjuvant donor bone marrow in pancreas transplant recipients. Ann Surg 1999; 23(3):372–379.
2. Brayman KL, Stephanian E, Matas AJ, et al. Analysis of infectious complications occurring after solid-organ transplantation. Arch Surg 1992; 127(1):38–47.
3. Kusne S, Chakrabarti P, Akhavan-Heidari M, Corry RJ. Association of bacterial and fungal infections with surgical complications in pancreas transplantation (Abstract). The 17th Annual Scientific Meeting of the American Society of Transplant Physicians, Chicago, May 1998.
4. Sollinger HW, Geffner SR. Pancreas transplantation. Horizons Organ Transplant 1994; 74(5): 1183–1194.
5. Hesse UJ, Sutherland DE, Simmons RL, Najarian JS. Intra-abdominal infections in pancreas transplant recipients. Ann Surg 1986; 203(2):153–162.
6. Baktavatsalam R, Little DM, Connolly EM, Farrell JG, Hickey DP. Complications relating to the urinary tract associated with bladder-drained pancreatic transplantation. Br J Urol 1998; 81(2): 219–223.
7. Del Pizzo JJ, Jacobs SC, Barlett ST, Sklar GN. Urological complications of bladder-drained pancreatic allografts. Br J Urol 1998; 81(4):543–547.
8. Barone GW, Hudec WA, Sailors DM, Ketel BL. Prophylactic wound antibiotics for combined kidney and pancreas transplants. Clin Transplant 1996; 10(4):386–388.
9. Hakim NS, Gruessner AC, Papalois BE, et al. Duodenal complications in bladder-drained pancreas transplantation. Surgery 1997; 121(6):618–624.
10. Smith JL, See WA, Piper JB, Corry RJ. Lower urinary tract complications in patients with duodeno-cystostomies for exocrine drainage of the transplanted pancreas. Transplant Proc 1991; 23(1 Pt 2):1611–1612.
11. Mittal VK, Toledo-Peryera LH. Effect of duodenal culture and postoperative infection on the long-term function of pancreaticoduodenal grafts. Transplant Proc 1991; 23(5):2469.
12. Sollinger HW, Knechtle SJ, Reed A, et al. Experience with 100 consecutive simultaneous kidney–pancreas transplants with bladder drainage. Ann Surg 1991; 214(6):703–711.
13. Douzdjian V, Gugliuzza KK. The impact of midline versus transverse incisions on wound complications and outcome in simultaneous pancreas–kidney transplants: a retrospective analysis. Transplant Int 1996; 9(1):62–67.
14. Benedetti E, Troppmann C, Gruessner AC, Sutherland DE, Dunn DL, Gruessner WG. Pancreas graft loss caused by intra-abdominal infection. A risk factor for a subsequent pancreas retransplantation. Arch Surg 1996; 131(10):1054–1060.
15. Everett JE, Wahoff DC, Statz C, et al. Characterization and impact of wound infection after pancreas transplantation. Arch Surg 1994; 129(12):1310–1316.
16. Douzdjian V, Abecassis M. Deep wound infections in simultaneous pancreas–kidney transplant recipients on peritoneal dialysis. Nephrol Dial Transplant 1995; 10(4):533–536.
17. Ho M. Advances in understanding cytomegalovirus infection after transplantation. Transplant Proc 1994; 26:7–11.
18. Keay S. CMV infection and disease in kidney and pancreas transplant recipients. Transplant Infect Dis 1999; 1(suppl):19–24.
19. Klassen D, Drachenberg C, Weir MR, et al. CMV allograft pancreatitis: diagnosis, treatment, and histological features. Transplantation 2000; 69(9):1968–1971.
20. Ljungman P, Plotkin SA. Workshop on CMV disease, definitions, clinical severity scores, and new syndromes. Scand J Infect Dis Suppl 1995; 99:87–89.
21. Revello MG, Percivalle E, Matteo AD, Morini F, Erna G. Nuclear expression of the lower matrix protein of human cytomegalovirus in peripheral blood leukocytes of the immunocompromised viremic patients. J General Virol 1992; 73:437–442.
22. Van der Ploeg M, Van den Berg AP, Vileger AN, Van der Giessen WJ. Direct detection of cytomegalovirus in peripheral blood leukocytes—a review of the antigenemia assay and polymerase chain reaction. Transplantation 1992; 54:193–198.
23. Guiver M, Fox AJ, Egan JJ, et al. Evaluation of CMV viral load using Taqman CMV quantitative PCR and comparison with CMV antigenemia in heart and lung transplant recipients. Transplantation 2001; 71:1609–1615.
24. Humar A, Gregson D, Caliendo AM, et al. Clinical utility of quantitative cytomegalovirus viral load determination for predicting cytomegalovirus disease in liver transplant recipients. Transplantation 1999; 68(9):1305–1311.
25. Imbert-Marcille BM, Cantarovich D, Ferre-Aubineau V, Richet B, Soulillou JP, Billaudel S. Usefulness of DNA viral load quantification for cytomegalovirus disease monitoring in renal and pancreas/renal transplant recipients. Transplantation 1997; 63(10):1476–1481.
26. Rubin RH. Preemptive therapy in immunocompromised hosts. N Engl J Med 1991; 324:1057–1059.
27. Gotti E, Suter F, Baruzzo S, Perani V, Moioli F, Remuzzi G. Early ganciclovir therapy effectively controls viremia and avoids the need for cytomegalovirus (CMV) prophylaxis in renal transplant patients with cytomegalovirus antigenemia. Clin Transplant 1996; 10(6 Pt 1):550–555.

28. Grossi P, Kusne S, Rinaldo C, et al. Guidance of ganciclovir therapy with pp65 antigenemia in cyto-megalovirus-free recipients of livers from seropositive donors. Transplantation 1996; 61(11):1659–1660.
29. Kusne S, Grossi P, Irish W, et al. Cytomegalovirus PP65 antigenemia monitoring as a guide for pre-emptive therapy: a cost effective strategy for prevention of cytomegalovirus disease in adult liver transplant recipients. Transplantation 1999; 68(8):1125–1131.
30. Glowacki LS, Smaill FM. Use of immune globulin to prevent symptomatic cytomegalovirus disease in transplant recipients—a meta-analysis. Clin Transplant 1994; 8:10–18.
31. Cockfield SM, Preikasaitis JK, Jewell LD, Parfrey NA. Post-transplant lymphoproliferative disorder in renal allograft recipients. Clinical experience and risk factor analysis in a single center. Transplan-tation 1993; 56:88–96.
32. Reyes J, Green M, Rowe D, et al. Spectrum of Epstein-Barr virus disease after intestinal transplan-tation in humans [abstr #21]. Int Congress Transplant Soc 1996.
33. Keay S, Oldach D, Bartlett S, et al. Posttransplant lymphoproliferative disorder associated with OKT3 and decreased antiviral prophylaxis in pancreas transplant recipients.
34. Rosendale N, Youseum SA. Discrimination of Epstein-Barr virus-related posttransplant lymphopro-liferation from acute rejection in lung allograft patients. Arch Pathol Lab Med 1995; 119:418–423.
35. Riddler SA, Breining MC, McKnight JLC. Increased level of Epstein-Barr virus infected-lymphocytes and decreased level of EBV nuclear antigen antibody responses are associated with the development of posttransplant lymphoproliferative disease in solid-organ transplant recipients. Blood 1994; 84:972–984.
36. Starzl TE, Porter KA, Iawtsuki S, et al. Reversibility of lymphomas and lymphoproliferative lesions developing under cyclosporine-steroid therapy. Lancet 1984; 1:583–587.
37. Pirsch JD, Stratta RJ, Sollinger HW, et al. Treatment of severe Epstein-Barr virus-induced lymphopro-liferative syndrome with ganciclovir: two cases after solid organ transplantation. Am J Med 1989; 86(2):241–244.
38. Hanto DW, Frizzera G, Gajl-Peczalska KJ, et al. Epstein-Barr virus-induced B-cell lymphoma after renal transplantation: acyclovir therapy and transition from polyclonal to monoclonal B-cell prolifer-ation. N Engl J Med 1982; 306(15):913–918.
39. Garrett TJ, Chadburn A, Barr ML, et al. Posttransplantation lymphoproliferative disorders treated with cyclophosphamide–doxorubicin–vincristine–prednisone chemotherapy. Cancer 1993; 72(9):2782–2785.
40. Verschuuren EA, Stevens SJ, van Imhoff GW, et al. Treatment of posttransplant lymphoproliferative disease with rituximab: the remission, the relapse, and the complication. Transplantation 2002; 73(1):100–104.
41. Morrison VA, Bartlett N, Dunn DL, Peterson BA. Rituximab Therapy for Post-Transplant Lympho-proliferative Disorders (PTLD): Preliminary Outcome Results. [abstract #1277]. American Society of Clinical Oncology.
42. Fleming DT, McQuilan GM, Johnson RE, et al. Herpes simplex virus type 2 in the United States, 1976 to 1994. N Engl J Med 1997; 337:1105–1111.
43. Resenthal SL, Stanberry LR, Biro FM, et al. Seroprevalence of herpes simplex virus type 1 and 2 and cytomegalovirus in adolescents. Clin Infect Dis 1997; 24:135–139.
44. Whitle RJ, Levin M, Barton N, et al. Infections caused by herpes simplex virus in the immuno-compromised hosts; natural history and topical acyclovir therapy. J Infect Dis 1984; 150:323–329.
45. Kusne S, Dummer JS, Singh N, et al. Infection after liver transplantation: an analysis of 101 consecu-tive cases. Medicine 1988; 67:132–143.
46. Kusne S, Schwartz M, Breinig MK, et al. Herpes simplex virus hepatitis after solid organ transplan-tation in adults. J Infect Dis 1991; 163(5):1001–1007.
47. Pettersson E, Hovi T, Ahonen J, et al. Prophylactic oral acyclovir after renal transplantation. Trans-plantation 1985; 39:279–281.
48. Sullivan KM, Dykewicz CA, Longworth DL, et al. Preventing opportunistic infections after hemato-poietic stem cell transplantation: the Centers for Disease Control and Prevention, Infectious Diseases Society of America, and American Society for Blood and Marrow Transplantation practice guidelines and beyond. Hematology (Am Soc Hematol Educ Program) 2001:392–421.
49. Benedetti E, Gruessner AC, Troppmann C, et al. Intra-abdominal fungal infections after pancreatic transplantation: incidence, treatment, and outcome. J Am Coll Surg 1996; 183(4):307–316.
50. Tollemar J. Fungal infections in solid organ transplant recipients. In: Bowden RA, Ljungman P, Paya CV, eds. Transplant Infections. Philadelphia: Lippincott-Raven, 1998:339–349.
51. Humar A, Kandaswamy R, Granger D, Gruessner RW, Gruessner AC, Sutherland DE. Decreased surgical risks of pancreas transplantation in the modern era. Ann Surg 2000; 231(2):269–275.
52. Hagerty JA, Ortiz J, Reich D, Manzarbeitia C. Fungal infections in solid organ transplant patients. Surg Infect (Larchmt) 2003; 4(3):263–271.
53. Lewis RE, Kontoyiannis DP, Darouiche RO, Raad II, Prince RA. Antifungal activity of amphotericin B, fluconazole, and voriconazole in an in vitro model of *Candida* catheter-related bloodstream infec-tion. Antimicrob Agents Chemother 2002; 46(11):3499–3505.
54. Mora-Duarte J, Betts R, Rotstein C, et al. Comparison of caspofungin and amphotericin B for invas-ive candidiasis. N Engl J Med 2002; 347(25):2020–2029.

55. Bowman JC, Hicks PS, Kurtz MB, et al. The antifungal echinocandin caspofungin acetate kills growing cells of *Aspergillus fumigatus* in vitro. Antimicrob Agents Chemother 2002; 46(9):3001–3012.
56. Herbrecht R, Denning DW, Patterson TF, et al. Voriconazole versus amphotericin B for primary therapy of invasive aspergillosis. N Engl J Med 2002; 347(6):408–415.
57. Husain S, Wagener MM, Singh N. *Cryptococcus neoformans* infection in organ transplant recipients: variables influencing clinical characteristics and outcome. Emerg Infect Dis 2001; 7(3):375–381.
58. Saag MS, Graybill RJ, Larsen RA, et al. Practice guidelines for the management of cryptococcal disease. Infectious Diseases Society of America. Clin Infect Dis 2000; 30(4):710–718.
59. Stratta RJ. Ganciclovir/acyclovir and fluconazole prophylaxis after simultaneous kidney–pancreas transplantation. Transplant Proc 1998; 30(2):262.
60. Roman A, Bravo C, Levy G, et al. Related isoniazid prophylaxis in lung transplantation. J Heart Lung Transplant 2000; 19(9):903–906.

# 19 | Malignancy After Pancreas Transplantation

Michael J. Hanaway, Joseph F. Buell, Jennifer Trofe, Thomas M. Beebe,
M. Roy First, V. Ram Peddi, Thomas M. Gross, Rita Alloway, and E. Steve Woodle
*The Israel Penn International Transplant Tumor Registry, University of Cincinnati,
Cincinnati, Ohio, U.S.A.*

An increased risk of cancer is a well-recognized complication of organ transplantation (1). In 1968, Dr. Israel Penn et al. described the first series of de novo malignancies in organ transplant recipients (2), and over the next 30 years, compiled the largest collection of data on posttransplant malignancies in the world. Dr. Penn's registry, originally known as the Cincinnati Transplant Tumor Registry, was renamed the Israel Penn International Transplant Tumor Registry (IPITTR) in memory of Dr. Penn shortly following his death in 2000. In general, organ transplant recipients do not exhibit an increase in the incidence of tumors commonly found in the general population (such as colon, breast, prostate, and lung cancer) (2–5). The most common malignancies in the IPITTR include cancers of the skin and lips (3075 patients), post-transplant lymphoproliferative disease (PTLD) (1080 patients), Kaposi's sarcoma (537 patients), and renal cell cancers (532 patients).

The largest number of organ transplants performed over the past 40 years has been renal transplants, and the greatest experience in posttransplant malignancies has thus been observed in renal transplant recipients. The distribution of tumors among renal transplant recipients in the IPITTR included cancers of the skin or lips (39%), PTLD (12%), renal tumors (4%), Kaposi's sarcoma (4%), cervical cancer (4%), and vulvar/perineal cancer (3%). When hepatic transplant recipients were examined, a different pattern of malignancy was discovered. While skin cancer and PTLD were again the two most common tumors after liver transplant, PTLD (57%) was much more common than cutaneous cancer (15%) (6,7). It has been hypothesized that increased immunosuppression in nonrenal transplant recipients and the delayed presentation of some tumors in renal transplant patients may explain this trend.

While much has been written about posttransplant malignancies in renal and hepatic allograft recipients, the existing literature on malignancy after pancreas transplantation is substantially smaller, with less than 20 patients reported to date. Martinenghi et al. reported on cancer in 99 diabetic end-stage renal disease patients who had undergone either simultaneous pancreas/kidney (SPK) transplantation or kidney transplantation (8). In this study, there was a 12% incidence of malignancy in the SPK group and 0% in the kidney transplant group. The most common cancers among pancreas transplant recipients were cutaneous cancers and PTLD, with incidences of 5.5% and 2.6%, respectively. However, the applicability of this report to pancreas transplant patients is limited by its retrospective nature and the small number of patients. Keay et al. reported on four cases of early onset PTLD after pancreas transplantation between 1994 and 1995, after initiating a protocol of intense induction immunosuppression and aggressive treatment of rejection (9). This report suggested that heightened immunosuppression in pancreas transplant recipients resulted in an increased incidence of PTLD.

In this study, the IPITTR experience with recurrence of pre-existing cancers, de novo malignancies, and donor-associated cancers after pancreas transplantation is described. De novo malignancies after pancreas transplantation will be divided into two groups: de novo PTLD and de novo solid (non-PTLD) tumors.

## MATERIALS AND METHODS

A retrospective review was conducted of over 15,000 cancer cases reported to the IPITTR between 1965 and 2001. The IPITTR data were supplemented by patient information from five pancreas transplant centers (University of Chicago, Northwestern University, University of Tennessee—Memphis, University of Cincinnati, and Ohio State University). A total of 137 pancreas transplant recipients were identified, with a history of cancer prior to transplantation (pre-existing, $n = 20$), cancer after transplantation (de novo, $n = 113$), or potential or actual donor-transmitted cancer after transplantation (donor-associated, $n = 4$). Recipient demographics were examined, as well as tumor type and subtype (when available), site(s) of cancer presentation at diagnosis, recipient immunosuppression, treatment modalities, and survival.

Follow-up was calculated for each subject as the number of months from date of diagnosis to date of last follow-up (death or survival). Kaplan–Meier survival curves of time to death were plotted for various categories [immunosuppression, chemotherapy, liver, central nervous system (CNS), spleen, gastrointestinal (GI), lymph nodes (LNs)]. Additionally, a log-rank test was performed to test for differences in survival within each category.

## RESULTS
### Pre-Existing Cancers

Twenty patients were reported to the IPITTR with pre-existing tumors prior to pancreas transplantation. This group consisted of 12 patients transplanted after the diagnosis (and presumed successful treatment) of solid tumors, and eight patients who underwent liver and pancreas transplantation for pre-existing hepatobiliary malignancy. Solid tumors included basal cell Ca (BCCa) (three), squamous cell Ca (SCCa) (one), malignant melanoma (two), bladder Ca (two), breast Ca (one), colon Ca (one), thyroid Ca (one), and osteogenic sarcoma (one). Average waiting times prior to transplant were 8.8 months for basal cell Ca, 32.5 months for squamous cell Ca, 57.5 for malignant melanoma, 22 months for bladder Ca, 55 months for breast Ca, 5.1 months for colon Ca, 249 months for thyroid, and 259 months for osteogenic sarcoma. There were no recurrences of solid tumors and no deaths secondary to malignancy.

### Cancer After Transplantation: PTLD

Fifty-two recipients of pancreas transplants who developed PTLD were reported to the IPITTR between 12/21/89 and 5/4/01 (Fig. 1). Fifty patients were diagnosed with PTLD while alive, and two were diagnosed post-mortem. Forty-four patients were recipients of SPK transplants, while eight received solitary pancreas transplants. The mean age of the patients at the time of PTLD diagnosis was 38.5 years, with a median time to PTLD diagnosis of seven months (range $= 0.9$–91) after transplantation. Sixty-eight percent of patients presented with PTLD within the first year post transplant and 78% presented within the first two years posttransplant. PTLD characteristics included Epstein-Barr virus (EBV) seropositivity of patients (24/26–93%), B-cell phenotype (25/28–89%), and monoclonal morphology (13/14–93%) (Table 1).

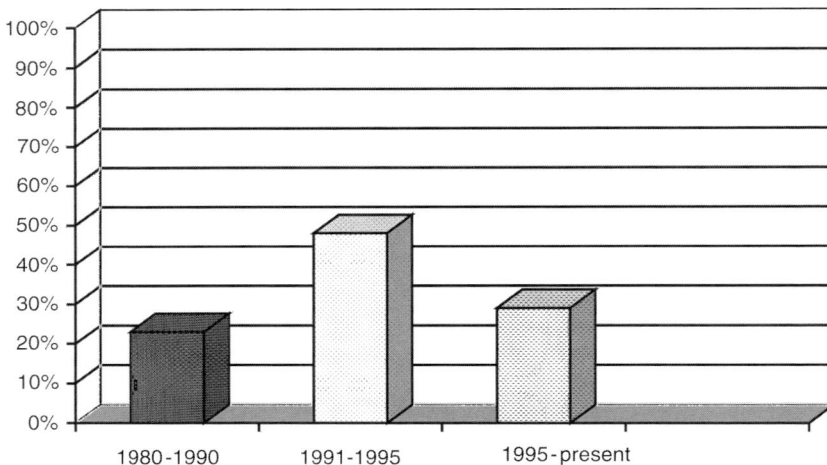

**Figure 1**  Eras of distribution of pancreas transplant recipients with posttransplant lymphoproliferative disease reported to the Israel Penn International Transplant Tumor Registry.

**Table 1**  Demographic Information and Lymphoma Subtype in Pancreas Transplant Recipients with PTLD

| | |
|---|---|
| Mean age of patients | 38.5 yr (range = 21–53 yr) |
| Transplant type | |
|   Solitary pancreas | 8 |
|   SPK | 44 |
| Median time from Tx to PTLD diagnosis | 7 mo (range = 0.9–91 mo) |
| B-cell positive | 89.3% (25 of 28 reported) |
| EBV positive | 92.3% (24 of 26 reported) |
| Monoclonal lymphoma | 92.9% (13 of 14 reported) |

*Abbreviations*: PTLD, posttransplant lymphoproliferative disease; EBV, Epstein-Barr virus; SPK, simultaneous pancreas/kidney.

Immunosuppression in pancreas transplant recipients favored the use of antibody induction therapy and maintenance immunosuppression with triple drug therapy (Table 2). Slightly more patients received OKT3 (63%) than antilymphocyte globulin (ALG) (56%) for induction or treatment of rejection, while 27% received both OKT3 and ALG posttransplant. Only 6% of patients received neither OKT3 nor ALG. Triple drug maintenance immunosuppression was primarily with corticosteroids, an antimetabolite, and a calcineurin inhibitor. All pancreas recipients with PTLD (100%) received prednisone as part of their baseline immunosuppression. Azathioprine was used more frequently than mycophenolate mofetil (MMF) (73% vs. 31%), and calcineurin inhibitor use favored cyclosporine (85%) over tacrolimus (29%).

PTLD presentation at multiple sites was slightly less common than at single sites (46% vs. 54%). Fifty-four percent of patients presented with disease at a single site, while 30% had disease at two sites, and 16% had disease at three or more sites. Of those with disease at a single site at presentation, disease in the LNs only was seen 37%, in the CNS 26%, in the kidney or pancreas allograft 18.5%, GI tract 11%, liver 7.4%, and spleen 0% (Fig. 2). In patients with multifocal disease at presentation, LN involvement was present in 63%, CNS in 14%, allograft in 36%, GI in 18%, liver in 41%, bone marrow in 32%, and spleen in 27% (Fig. 3). Overall, at the time of diagnosis, PTLD involved the LN in 40%, the allograft in 27%, liver in 20%, CNS in 20%, GI tract in 18%, and spleen in 12%. Two patients did not have data on sites of PTLD at diagnosis.

Treatment of PTLD consisted of combination therapy or monotherapy. Seventy percent of PTLD patients received combination therapy, while 30% received monotherapy. Monotherapy consisted of immunosuppression discontinuation or reduction (ISDR) (43%), chemotherapy (29%), radiation therapy (XRT) (21%), and surgery (7%) (Fig. 4). Combination therapy included ISDR + allograft removal (AR) (39%), ISDR + chemotherapy (21%), XRT + chemotherapy (11%), ISDR + XRT (4%), and ISDR + chemotherapy + XRT (4%) (Fig. 5). Four patients received no therapy because of refusal or advanced multisystem organ failure. Two patients were diagnosed postmortem and did not receive therapy prior to death. Therapeutic information was not available on four patients.

**Table 2**  Induction and Maintenance Immunosuppression in Pancreas Transplant Recipients with Posttransplant Lymphoproliferative Disease

| | Solitary pancreas | Simultaneous kidney–pancreas |
|---|---|---|
| OKT3 | 50% (4/8) | 66% (29/44) |
| ALG | 25% (2/8) | 61% (27/44) |
| OKT3 + ALG | 25% (2/8) | 27% (12/44) |
| OKT3 or ALG | 100% (8/8) | 93% (41/44) |
| No induction | 0% (0/8) | 7% (3/44) |
| Prednisone | 100% (8/8) | 100% (44/44) |
| Azathioprine | 75% (6/8) | 72% (32/44) |
| MMF | 38% (3/8) | 30% (13/44) |
| Cyclosporine | 75% (6/8) | 86% (38/44) |
| Prograf | 38% (3/8) | 27% (12/44) |
| Rapamycin | 0% (0/8) | 2% (1/44) |

*Abbreviations*: ALG, antilymphocyte globulin; MMF, mycophenolate mofetil.

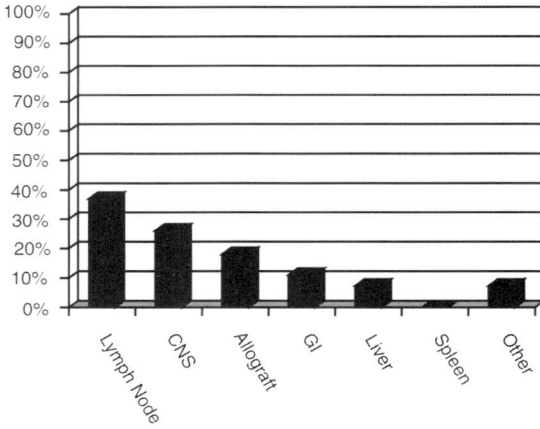

**Figure 2**  Frequency of unifocal sites of presentation of posttransplant lymphoproliferative disease in pancreas transplant recipients reported to the Israel Penn International Transplant Tumor Registry. *Abbreviations*: CNS, central nervous system; GI, gastrointestinal.

Involved sites, immunosuppression, and treatment were examined for effects on survival. Survival analysis according to involved sites did not show a survival benefit for single site versus multiple site presentation ($p = 0.2$) (data not shown). The effect of liver disease ($p = 0.07$), or of the absence of lymph node disease, approached significance ($p = 0.07$); however, the presence of splenic disease ($p = 0.12$), or gastrointestinal disease ($p = 0.2$), did not (data not shown). Pancreas recipients who had CNS involvement at diagnosis had a significantly shorter survival than those without CNS involvement ($p = 0.02$) (Fig. 6). The administration of chemotherapy did not improve survival ($p = 0.5$) (data not shown). Patients who had ISDR as a component of therapy had improved survival compared to those who did not have ISDR ($p = 0.03$) (Fig. 7). Removal of the kidney or pancreas allograft did not affect survival compared with retention of the allograft ($p = 0.07$) (data not shown).

## De Novo Solid Tumors

Data were collected on 61 pancreas transplant recipients with de novo solid tumors from 5/91 to 9/01. The distribution of times during which the patients were diagnosed is depicted in Figure 8. Skin cancer was the most common de novo solid tumor (69%), followed by vulvar/perineal Ca (10%), genitourinary cancer (8%), hepatobiliary (3%), cervical (3%), Kaposi's sarcoma (3%), lung cancer (1.5%), and thyroid cancer (1.5%) (Table 3). Age at diagnosis, time to diagnosis after transplant, and recurrence of cancer were similar between cutaneous cancers and noncutaneous cancers. However, time from initial diagnosis to recurrence of cancer was significantly shorter for cutaneous cancers (3.8 months) compared to noncutaneous cancers (15 months) ($p = 0.04$) (Table 4).

## Donor Associated Malignancy

Four cases of donor associated (potential or actual donor transmitted) malignancy have been reported to the IPITTR. These include two documented cases of donor-transmitted malignancy,

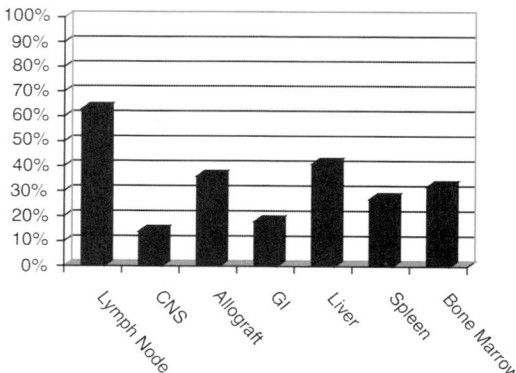

**Figure 3**  Multifocal posttransplant lymphoproliferative disease involved sites at the time of presentation in pancreas to recipients. *Abbreviations*: CNS, central nervous system; GI, gastrointestinal.

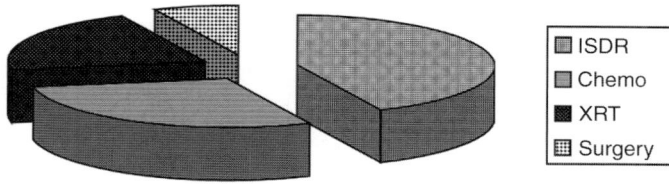

**Figure 4** Posttransplant lymphoproliferative disease monotherapy in pancreas transplant recipients. *Abbreviations*: ISDR, immunosuppression discontinuation or reduction; XRT, radiotherapy; Chemo, chemotherapy.

and two cases where the donor was found to have malignancy at the time of donation but did not transmit cancer to the recipient. The first case of documented transmission was a 36-year-old male who received an SPK transplant from a 24-year-old female who died secondary to intracerebral hemorrhage. The donor had had a prior history of malignant melanoma. The patient developed cutaneous melanoma eight months after transplantation. Karyotype analysis of the melanoma indicated both XX and XY cells present, consistent with donor transmission. At allograft removal, both kidney and pancreas were found to have extensive microscopic melanoma. The patient succumbed to widely metastatic melanoma two months after diagnosis. The second case of documented transmission was a 45-year-old male, who underwent simultaneous kidney–pancreas transplantation from a 55-year-old male donor, who died from intracranial hemorrhage. The donor had no history of malignancy. The patient had a spontaneous perforation of the pancreatic allograft duodenal segment 3 1/2 years posttransplant, which required allograft removal. The pathology showed a moderately differentiated adenocarcinoma consistent with pancreatic cancer infiltrating the recipient's ileal segment. Molecular typing of the tumor was consistent with donor origin. The patient died 11 months after diagnosis secondary to metastatic adenocarcinoma (10). The two cases of potential transmission involved patients who received organs from patients with a history of astrocytoma and colon cancer, but who did not develop a tumor after transplantation.

## DISCUSSION

While much has been published on cancer after kidney and liver transplantation, our understanding of the cancer risks after pancreas transplantation is limited. As Penn noticed different patterns of malignancies in liver and kidney transplant recipients (6,7), it therefore is reasonable to examine malignancies in pancreas transplant recipients. This reported experience shows a pattern of malignancy after pancreas transplantation, with some similarities to both kidney and liver transplant recipients (Table 5). Similar to liver transplant patients, PTLD was the most commonly reported tumor to the IPITTR in pancreas transplant recipients. However, the reported incidence of skin cancer was nearly identical for pancreas and kidney transplant patients (38% vs. 39%). Cutaneous cancers and PTLD comprised 84% of all de novo tumors in pancreas transplant patients.

The incidence of PTLD after transplantation is 28 to 49 times greater than in the general population (11). Moreover, the frequency varies depending on the type of transplant. The estimated incidence of PTLD is 1% to 4% in kidney transplant recipients and 2% in liver transplant recipients (12–14). Estimates of the incidence of PTLD after pancreas transplantation are based

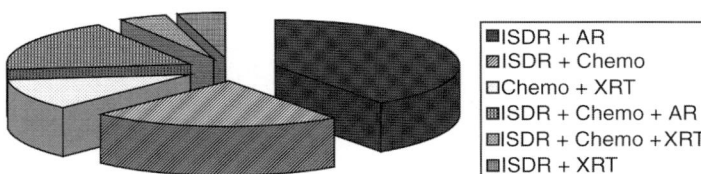

**Figure 5** Posttransplant lymphoproliferative disease combination therapy in pancreas transplant recipients. *Abbreviations*: ISDR, immunosuppression discontinuation or reduction with allograft removal; AR, allograft removal; Chemo, chemotherapy; XRT, radiotherapy.

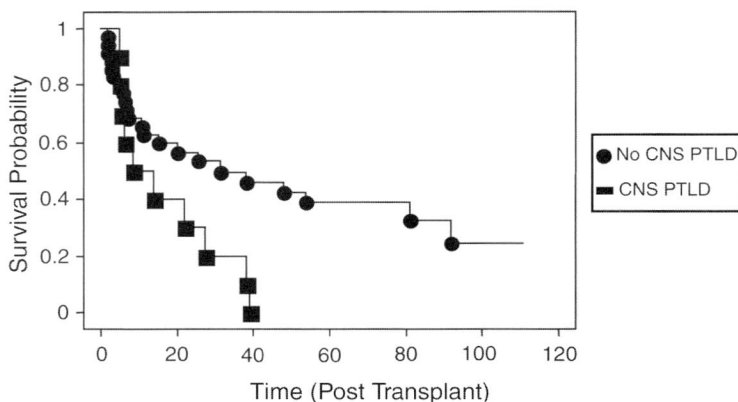

**Figure 6** Kaplan–Meier survival curves for pancreas transplant recipients with CNS involvement at time of PTLD presentation ($p = 0.03$). *Abbreviations*: CNS, central nervous system; PTLD, posttransplant lymphoproliferative disease.

on series of patients from single centers, with the estimated incidence varying from as low as 0.9% in larger single-center experiences to as high as 2.8% to 8.2% in some smaller series (8,9,15,16). It is not possible to determine incidence of PTLD in the IPITTR experience because of the inability to define the size of the total population at risk.

While the precise role of immunosuppression in the pathogenesis of PTLD has not been clearly defined, it has long been suspected that there is a direct correlation between the nature and magnitude of immunosuppression and the risk of PTLD. Since PTLD is most often related to a primary EBV infection or reactivation of a latent EBV infection, it is reasonable to expect that PTLD would be associated with intense immunosuppression. PTLD, however, has not been linked to any specific immunosuppressive regimen. PTLD was first described by Starzl and Penn in 1968, in five living-related kidney transplant recipients who received azathioprine and prednisone as maintenance therapy (2). Subsequently, PTLD has been seen with all types of immunosuppressive regimens. Multiple multicenter, randomized trials have failed to demonstrate an increased risk of PTLD in patients treated with cyclosporine, tacrolimus, or mycophenolate (17–24). A potential link between PTLD and OKT3 was made by Swinnen et al., who noted an increased rate of PTLD in cardiac transplant patients treated with OKT3 and particularly in those patients receiving over 75 mg as a cumulative dose (25). However, the total duration of anti-T-cell antibody therapy in these patients was excessive. OKT3

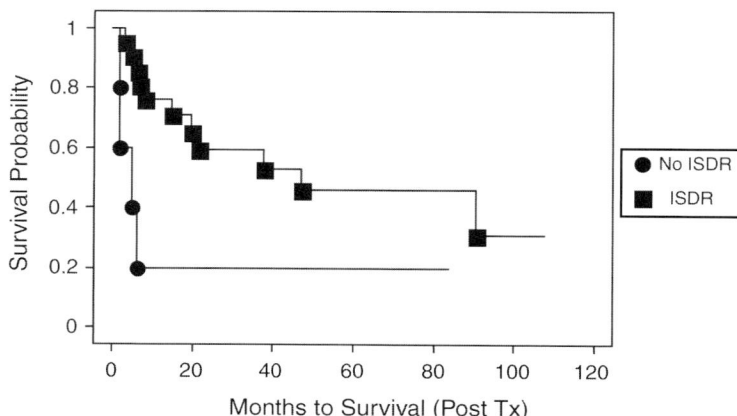

**Figure 7** Kaplan–Meier survival curves for pancreas transplant recipients who did or did not have ISDR as component of treatment of posttransplant lymphoproliferative disease ($p = 0.03$). *Abbreviation*: ISDR, immunosuppression discontinuation or reduction.

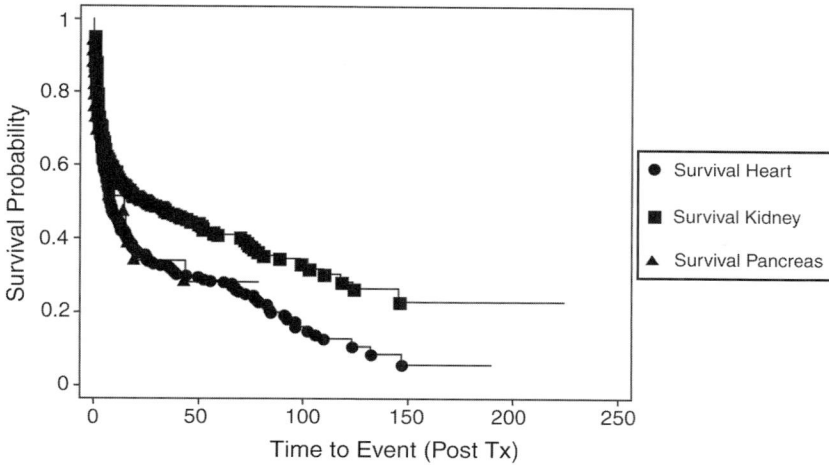

**Figure 8**  Kaplan–Meier survival curves for heart, kidney and pancreas transplant recipients diagnosed with post-transplant lymphoproliferative disease. Pancreas survival curve is partially obscured by heart survival.

use and cumulative OKT3 dose were not seen as primary risk factors for PTLD in a later study in cardiac transplants by Ratkovec et al (26). Thymoglobulin therapy, either for induction or for the treatment of rejection, has not been associated with a higher rate of PTLD, when compared with ATGAM (27,28). In the present study of cancer after pancreas transplantation, no clear correlation between type of immunosuppression and PTLD was found.

Triple immunosuppression, consisting of prednisone, azathioprine, and cyclosporine, was the most common maintenance immunosuppression in the present study, reflecting the period in which most of the patients were transplanted (i.e., prior to the availability of MMF and tacrolimus). Ninety-four percent of patients received some form of induction therapy, and 93% of patients were treated with OKT3, polyclonal antilymphocyte preparations, or both for induction or rejection. There was no clear correlation, however, between the use of OKT3 and PTLD in this patient population and no advantage or disadvantage in survival was seen in patients who received OKT3, polyclonal antilymphocyte preparations, or both.

The presentation of PTLD after pancreas transplantation was characterized by early onset, predominance of lymph node involvement, and poor survival in patients with CNS disease. The median time to presentation of PTLD after pancreas transplantation was seven months, compared to 18 months in renal transplant recipients (29). Similar to renal transplant

**Table 3**  Tumor Type and Reporting Incidence of Israel Penn International Transplant Tumor Registry for De Novo Solid (Non-Posttransplant Lymphoproliferative Disease) Tumors

| Type of tumor | No. of cases reported/ reporting incidence | (%) |
|---|---|---|
| Skin | 42/61 | (69%) |
| SCCa | 22/61 | |
| BCCa | 15/61 | |
| Melanoma | 2/61 | |
| SCCa + BCCa | 3/61 | |
| Vulvar/perineal | 6/61 | (10%) |
| Genitourinary | 5/61 | (8%) |
| Renal | 2/61 | |
| Bladder | 2/61 | |
| Prostate | 1/61 | |
| Hepatobiliary | 2/61 | (3%) |
| Cervical | 2/61 | (3%) |
| Kaposi's sarcoma | 2/61 | (3%) |
| Lung | 1/61 | (1.5%) |
| Thyroid | 1/61 | (1.5%) |

*Abbreviations*: SCCa, squamous cell cancer; BCCa, basal cell cancer.

**Table 4** Demographics and Recurrence Information on Pancreas Transplant Recipients with De Novo Solid Tumors (Non-Posttransplant Lymphoproliferative Disease)

|  | Skin cancer | Non-skin cancer | *p*-Value |
|---|---|---|---|
| Age at diagnosis | 43.5 yr (30.2–55.5 yr) | 44.6 yr (30.3–55.1 yr) | NS |
| Time from Dx to transplant | 56 mo (8.2–137 mo) | 56.4 mo (7.5–127.8 mo) | NS |
| Recurrence rate | Overall, 18%; BCCa, 6.7%; SCCa, 13.7%; melanoma, 50% | 7% | NS |
| Time from Dx to recurrence | 3.8 mo | 15 mo | *p* = 0.04 |

*Abbreviations*: SCCa, squamous cell cancer; BCCa, basal cell cancer; NS, not significant; Dx, detection.

patients, most PTLDs were EBV (+), B-cell (+), and monoclonal (29). Allograft involvement with PTLD was seen in 28% after pancreas/SPK transplantation compared to 20% in kidney transplant recipients (29). Involvement of lymph nodes at presentation was also common. Of patients with PTLD at a single site, lymph nodes were the site 37% of the time, while lymph nodes were involved in 63% of patients with disease at more than one site.

Patterns of presentation differed between those with single-site disease and those with multiple-site disease, as PTLD in the liver, spleen, and bone marrow was more likely in patients with disease at multiple sites. Survival of PTLD was not influenced by number of sites or the location of PTLD, with the exception of CNS disease. Patients with CNS involvement at the time of diagnosis had a significantly worse prognosis than those without CNS disease. This observation is consistent with the overall IPITTR experience, where CNS involvement with PTLD has been found to be associated with poor survival in a review of 910 kidney, heart, liver, and lung transplant recipients with PTLD (30).

Currently, there is no universally accepted treatment algorithm for PTLD. PTLD therapies have included antiviral therapy (acyclovir or gancyclovir) and intensive combination chemotherapy. In general, initial intervention is based on the location and severity of disease at presentation. The most immediate treatment option is ISDR. Previous reports have indicated that ISDR alone is sufficient treatment in 30% to 50% of cases (31–33). The potential consequence of significant rejection, and possible allograft failure, after ISDR, makes this a less attractive option in patients with PTLD after heart, liver, and pancreas transplantation. Which immuno-suppressive agent to reduce/discontinue, for how long, and how to predict efficacy are not known. While antiviral therapy may be used as a primary therapy for extensive nodal disease or as an adjunctive therapy, its efficacy has not been established. Radiation therapy has been used for CNS involvement and for localized disease. Chemotherapy is used primarily for those CNS tumors that are judged to be malignant. While earlier results with chemotherapy were poor, recent outcomes with CHOP-based chemotherapy have been more encouraging (34–38). The considerable variation in therapies for PTLD was likely related to the lack of consensus on an approach to treatment during the reporting time period. ISDR was the most frequently utilized monotherapy, and ISDR with allograft removal (concurrently or delayed) was the most common form of combination therapy. Failure to reduce or discontinue immunosuppression resulted in decreased overall survival. In spite of concerns of rejection of vital organs, ISDR has been shown to be a vital component of treatment of PTLD in this and other studies (39).

**Table 5** Israel Penn International Transplant Tumor Registry Reporting Frequency of De Novo Tumors in Renal, Liver, and Pancreas Transplant Recipients

|  | Renal (*n* = 7200) | Hepatic (*n* = 324) | Pancreas (*n* = 113) |
|---|---|---|---|
| Skin cancer | 2819 (39%) | 48 (15%) | 42 (38%) |
| PTLD | 828 (12%) | 189 (57%) | 52 (46%) |
| Kaposi's sarcoma | 314 (4%) | 10 (3%) | 2 (1.8%) |
| Cervical cancer | 278 (4%) | 4 (1%) | 2 (1.8%) |
| Renal cell cancer | 276 (4%) | 4 (1%) | 2 (1.8%) |
| Vulvar/perineal cancer | 207 (3%) | 2 (0.6%) | 6 (5.3%) |
| Colon cancer | 265 (4%) | 18 (5%) | 0 |

*Abbreviation*: PTLD, posttransplant lymphoproliferative disease.

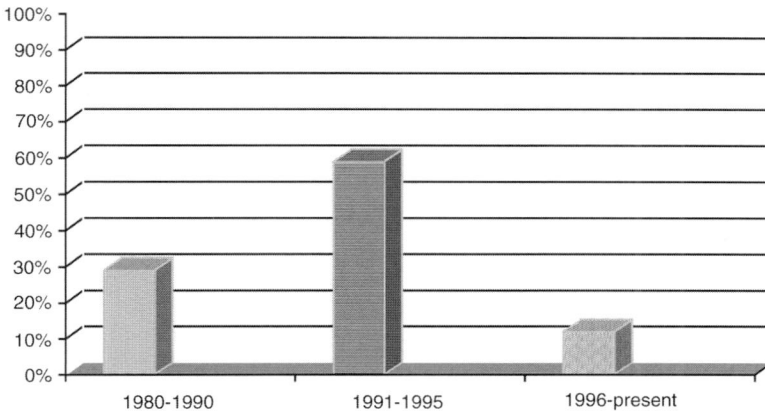

**Figure 9** Eras of distribution of pancreas transplant recipients with de novo solid tumors reported to the Israel Penn International Transplant Tumor Registry by ERA.

A consistent theme in the study of posttransplant malignancies is that tumors commonly seen in the general population are not seen with higher frequencies in the transplant population. The predominance of PTLD and skin cancer, seen in kidney and liver transplant recipients, is also observed in pancreas transplant patients (Table 5). These findings are consistent with those found in a smaller series of pancreas transplant recipients (8). The most frequent de novo solid (non-PTLD) tumors after pancreas transplantation were skin, vulvar/perineal, and genitourinary (Fig. 9).

The pattern of skin cancer in pancreas transplant patients differed in several ways from that seen in the general population. In the general population, BCCa outnumbers SCCa by a 5:1 ratio. In pancreas transplant patients, the reverse occurred, with SCCa outnumbering BCCa by a ratio of 1.2:1. In the general population, SCCa occurs most often in persons in their 60s and 70s, but the average age in pancreas transplant patients was 43. Recurrence of tumors after excision was not significantly different between skin Ca and non-skin Ca. However, the time to recurrence of cancers was significantly shorter for skin Ca than for non-skin Ca.

Donor-related transmission of malignancy has been reported sporadically over the past 30 years. Penn reported on 47 patients who received kidney transplants from 17 donors with known active malignancy at the time of donation (40). The two cases presented above raise several interesting points about donor-associated tumors. The first case involved a patient who developed metastatic melanoma of donor origin eight months after pancreas transplantation. Since this donor had a previous history of melanoma, the malignant cells very likely existed in the donor and were transferred to the recipient at the time of transplantation. Because of the high risk of transmission of melanoma, IPITTR recommends avoiding the use of donors with a history of this malignancy. The second case involved a patient who developed a pancreatic cancer in the transplanted pancreas 40 months posttransplantation. Given the age of the donor (55 years), the time from transplantation to tumor diagnosis, and lack of evidence of tumor at the time of transplantation, it is reasonable to conclude that the malignancy was not present at the time of transplantation but arose de novo from donor cells; alternatively, the malignancy was present but was too small to be appreciated. Understanding the potential for donor transmission and tumors at high risk for transmission (choriocarcinoma, melanoma, lymphoma, adenocarcinoma of lung, breast, colon, kidney) is critical for the prevention of such occurrences.

In summary, the present study indicates that cancer in pancreas transplant recipients demonstrates features similar to those in other solid organ transplant recipients.

Skin cancer and PTLD are the most frequently reported tumors in pancreas transplant recipients. Failure to reduce or discontinue immunosuppression after a diagnosis of PTLD also results in decreased survival, and CNS involvement of PTLD is associated with a poor prognosis. Finally, donor-transmitted tumors are uncommon but may be fatal when they do occur.

## ACKNOWLEDGMENTS

Thanks to the following for their contributions to this review: Dr. Dixon Kaufman, Dr. Alan Koffron, Dr. Ronald Pelletier, Dr. Ronald Ferguson, Dr. Robert Stratta, Dr. Ram Peddi. Thanks to Dr. Gopalan Sethuraman for his assistance with statistical analysis.

## REFERENCES

1. Penn I. De novo cancers in organ transplant recipients. Curr Opin Organ Transplant 1998; 3:188.
2. Penn I, Hammond W, Brettschneider L, Starzl TE. Malignant lymphomas in transplantation patients. Transplant Proc 1969; 1:106.
3. Penn I. Why do immunosuppressed patients develop cancer? CRC Crit Rev Oncogene 1989; 1:27.
4. Penn I. The problem of cancer in organ transplant recipients: an overview. Transplant Sci 1994; 4:23.
5. Penn I. Malignancy after immunosuppressive therapy: how can the risk be reduced? Clin Immunother 1995; 9:207–218.
6. Penn I. De novo cancers in organ allograft recipients. Curr Opin Organ Transplant 1998; 3:188.
7. Penn I. Posttransplantation de novo tumors in liver allograft recipients. Liver Transplant Surg 1996; 1:52.
8. Martinenghi S, DellAntonio G, Secchi A, DiCarlo V, Pozza G. Cancer arising after pancreas and/or kidney transplantation in a series of 99 consecutive diabetic patients. Diabet Care 1997; 20:272.
9. Keay S, Oldach D, Wiland A, et al. Posttransplant lymphoproliferative disorder associated with OKT3 and decreased antiviral prophylaxis in pancreas transplant recipients. Clin Infect Dis 1998; 26:596.
10. Roza A, Johnson C, Eckels D, et al. Adenocarcinoma arising in a transplanted pancreas. Transplantation 2001; 72:1156.
11. Boubenider S, Heisse C, Goupy C, et al. Incidence and consequences of post-transplant lymphoproliferative disorders. J Nephrol 1997; 10:136.
12. Firzzera G. Atypical lymphoproliferative disorders. In: Knowles DM, ed. Neoplastic Hematopathology. Baltimore, MD: Williams & Wilkins, 1992:459.
13. Le Meur Y, Poteleune N, Jaccard A, et al. Lymphoproliferative syndromes after renal transplantation. Nephrologie 1998; 19:255.
14. Raymond E, Tricottet V, Samuel D, Reynes M, Bismuth H, Misset JL. Epstein Barr virus-related localized hepatic lymphoproliferative disorders after liver transplantation. Cancer 1995; 76:1344.
15. Sutherland D, Gruessner R, Dunn D, et al. Lessons learned from more than 1,000 pancreas transplants at a single institution. Ann Surg 2001; 233:463.
16. Fernandez LA, Odorico JS, Sollinger HW, et al. The effect of mycophenylate mofetil on the incidence of PTLD compared to azathioprine in pancreas transplantation. International Islet and Pancreas Transplant Association Meeting, 2001. Abstract # 01–39.
17. The Canadian Multicenter Transplant Group. A randomized trial of cyclosporine in cadaveric renal transplantation. N Engl J Med 1983; 309:809.
18. European Multicenter Transplant Group. Cyclosporin in cadaveric renal transplantation: one year follow-up of a multicenter trial. Lancet 1983; 8357:986.
19. Legendre C, Kreis H. The effect of immunosuppression on the incidence of lymphoma formation. Clin Transplant 1992; 6:220.
20. Pirsch JD et al. CMV and PTLD in renal transplant recipients: results of the US Multicenter FK 506 Kidney Transplant Study Group. Transplantation 1999; 68:1203.
21. Pirsch JD, Miller J, Deierhoi M, et al. A comparison of FK 506 and cyclosporine for immunosuppression after cadaveric renal transplantation. Transplantation 1997; 63:977.
22. Weisner R. A long term comparison of FK 506 versus cyclosporine in liver transplantation: a report of the US FK 506 Study Group. Transplantation 1998; 66:493.
23. Sollinger HW et al. Mycophenolate mofetil for the prevention of acute allograft rejection in primary cadaveric renal allograft recipients. Transplantation 1995; 60:225.
24. Tricontinental Mycophenolate Mofetil Renal Transplantation Study Group. A blinded, randomized clinical trial of mycophenolate mofetil for the prevention of acute rejection in cadaveric renal transplantation. Transplantation 1996; 61:1029.
25. Swinnen L, Costanzo-Nordin M, Fischer SG, et al. Increased incidence of lymphoproliferative disorder after immunosuppression with the monoclonal antibody OKT3 in cardiac transplant recipients. N Engl J Med 1991; 323:1723.
26. Ratkovec RM, O Connell J, Bristow N, et al. Post-transplant lymphoproliferative disorder in cardiac transplant patients receiving OKT3 therapy. Clin Transplant 1992; 6:260.
27. Brennan D, Flavin K, Lowell J, et al. A randomized, double-blinded comparison of Thymoglobulin versus ATGAM for induction immunosuppression therapy in adult renal transplant recipients. Transplantation 1998; 67:1011.
28. Gaber AO, First M, Tessi R, et al. Results of a double blinded, randomized, multicenter phase III trial of Thymoglobulin versus ATGAM in the treatment of acute allograft rejection episodes after renal transplantation. Transplantation 1998; 66:29.

29. Trofe J, Sethuramam G, Buell J, et al. Renal allograft involvement by post transplant lymphoproliferative disorder: clinical implications. AJT 2002; 2:151.
30. Buell J, Gross T, Hanaway M, et al. Post transplant lymphoproliferative disorder: the significance of central nervous system involvement. AJT 2002; 2:373.
31. Starzl T, Penn I, Halgrimson CG. Immunosuppression and malignant neoplasms. N Engl J Med 1970; 283:934.
32. Benkerrou M, Durandy A, Fischer A. Therapy for transplant related lymphoproliferative diseases. Hematol Oncol Clin North Am 1993; 7:467.
33. Heslop HE, Brenner MK, Rooney C, et al. Clinical protocol: administration of neomycin gene marked EBV specific cytotoxic T lymphocytes to recipients of mismatched-related or phenotypically similar unrelated donor marrow grafts. Hum Gene Ther 1994.
34. Starzl T, Porter K, Iwatsuki S, et al. Reversibility of lymphomas and lymphoproliferative lesions developing under cyclosporine-steroid therapy. Lancet 1984; 1:583.
35. Hanto DW, Frizzera G, Galj-Peczalska, et al. Epstein-Barr virus, immunodeficiency and B-cell lymphoproliferation. Transplantation 1985; 39:461.
36. Raymond E, Tricottet V, Samuel D, et al. Epstein-Barr virus related lymphoproliferative disorders treated with cyclophosphamide–doxorubicin–vincristine–prednisone chemotherapy. Cancer 1995; 72:1344.
37. Garrett T, Chadburn A, Barr ML, et al. Post transplant lymphoproliferative disorders treated with cyclophosphamide–doxorubicin–vincristine–prednisone chemotherapy. Cancer 1993; 72:2782.
38. Swinnen L, Mullen G, Carr T, Costanzo M, Fischer R. Aggressive treatment for postcardiac transplant lymphoproliferation. Blood 1995; 86:3333.
39. Trofe J, Sethuraman G, Buell J, et al. Multivariate analysis of risk factors that influence survival in cardiac transplant recipients with PTLD. AJT 2002; 2:282.
40. Wilson RE, Penn I. Fate of tumors transplanted with a renal allograft. Trans Proc 1975; 7:327.

# 20 | Neurologic Complications of Pancreas Transplantation

**Benjamin H. Eidelman**

*Department of Neurology, Mayo Clinic, Jacksonville, Florida and Mayo Clinic College of Medicine, Rochester, Minnesota, U.S.A.*

The purpose of pancreas transplantation is to restore blood glucose homeostasis, improve the quality of life of the diabetic patient, and reverse the secondary complications of diabetes. Although refinements in surgical technique and improved methods of immunosuppression have resulted in decreased complication rates, pancreas transplantation may negatively affect the nervous system. The neurologic complications of pancreas transplantation may involve both the central and the peripheral nervous systems, and the pathologic changes may be localized or diffuse. The clinical disturbances are protean and may have a considerable effect on the recovery of the patient after transplantation. Much of the literature relating to the neurologic complications of pancreas transplantation reports on studies involving simultaneous kidney–pancreas transplantation (KPT). Although the present review focuses on complications that are largely attributed to transplantation of the pancreas, it also discusses certain complications common to all transplant recipients.

Disturbances in nervous system function in relation to transplantation have many causes. Diabetic patients are susceptible to various conditions that involve both the central and the peripheral nervous systems (1). Disorders in patients with diabetes may remain latent until the time of transplantation. Diabetic patients may also be predisposed to certain neurologic conditions. Neurologic complications may arise from the transplantation procedure itself or occur at various times after transplantation. Thus, an appreciation of the full extent of the neurologic events occurring in relation to pancreas transplantation requires review of the pretransplantation as well as the posttransplantation conditions that may affect the nervous system.

## PRETRANSPLANTATION CONDITIONS

Type 1 diabetes mellitus is the main indication for pancreas transplantation (2). In most pancreas transplant recipients, the disease has been present for a prolonged time, and the neuropathologic changes resulting from diabetes have been well entrenched. Pathologic processes present before transplantation may be overt or latent at the time of the operation. Recognition of these pathologic events is vital because they have important management implications.

Neurologic complications of diabetes are listed in Table 1, and are discussed below. Diabetic ketoacidosis is one of the most serious complications of diabetes (3,4), and often results in severe metabolic disturbances (5–7). These may have wide-ranging effects on the nervous system (8). Graft failure caused by conditions such as thrombosis of the pancreatic artery may result in acute hyperglycemia (9). Close postoperative monitoring and vigorous therapeutic measures, which have become standard practice in the management of the pancreas transplants, usually allow for rapid detection and correction of elevated blood glucose levels. Thus, diabetic ketoacidosis is unlikely to occur after transplantation. Diabetes increases the risk of stroke (10–12). In addition, comorbid conditions such as hypertension and hyperlipidemia further increase the stroke risk. Deficits from a pre-existing vascular event may become more obvious after transplantation and may be interpreted as a complication of the operation. Pretransplantation screening often identifies individuals who have had a stroke and have subtle or latent abnormalities that had been undetected. Review of the past history and the presence of clinical findings indicative of a chronic process may help in recognizing that strokes occurred previously. Imaging, particularly magnetic resonance studies, may help in determining the acuteness of an event.

**Table 1**  Neurologic Complications of Diabetes Mellitus

Metabolic disturbances
Cerebrovascular events
Seizures
Infections
Neuropathy

In general, diabetic patients are probably at higher risk of development of infection (13). Several infections involving the central nervous system (CNS) are also more likely to occur in diabetic patients (14). Rhinocerebral mucormycosis is an acute, potentially lethal, necrotizing infection of the nasopharnyx, with facial pain, swelling, proptosis, and ophthalmoplegia as prominent features (15). It requires prompt recognition and treatment. Malignant otitis media may be complicated by meningitis and venous sinus thrombosis (16). Spinal epidural abscess may manifest as back pain followed by radicular symptoms (17). Spinal cord compression may develop rapidly and, if not treated early, result in permanent paraplegia. Any of these infections may occur after transplantation, and awareness of the manifestations of each of them is important for their early detection and effective treatment.

## POSTTRANSPLANT CONDITIONS
### Early Posttransplantation Phase

Neurologic dysfunction manifesting during this critical phase, which may be defined arbitrarily as the first 30 days after transplantation, may originate from disease processes established before transplantation or from de novo events arising from the transplantation itself (Table 2).

### Late Posttransplantation Phase

The late posttransplantation phase may be defined as the period after the first month after transplantation. During the late phase, the transplanted organ is usually well established, but often immunosuppression is at a high level, creating favorable conditions for the development of certain types of pathologic processes (Table 3).

### THE EARLY POSTTRANSPLANTATION PHASE

The early posttransplantation phase may be particularly taxing because of the manifestation of pathologic conditions that developed before the transplantation, complications of the operation, or disease processes arising from the posttransplantation environment. Disease processes may include infection and the toxic effects of immunosuppressive agents. Several clinical entities may be encountered.

### Encephalopathy

Impaired consciousness is the primary feature of an encephalopathic state. In some instances, however, disturbances of concentration and lethargy may be the only signs of this condition (18). Some patients may appear confused and exhibit behavioral changes, including restlessness and agitation. Hallucinations may also be evident. Profound coma may ensue, with or without focal signs. The causes of encephalopathy in the immediate postoperative period include hypoxic ischemic states, lingering effects of pharmacologic agents, and nonconvulsive

**Table 2**  Neurologic Complications of Pancreas Transplant Patients in the Early Posttransplantation Phase (Within 30 Days After Transplantation)

Encephalopathy
Seizures
Cerebrovascular events
Metabolic disorders
Neuromuscular complications

**Table 3** Neurologic Complications of Pancreas Transplant Patients in the Late Posttransplantation Phase (After the First Month After Transplantation)

| |
|---|
| Infection |
| Posttransplantation lymphoproliferative disease |
| Seizures |
| Encephalopathy |
| Persistent weakness |

status epilepticus. Diabetic ketoacidosis and hypoglycemia are also important conditions to consider as causes of encephalopathy in diabetic patients. Diabetic ketoacidosis, however, is an unlikely occurrence because close postoperative monitoring allows for early detection and correction of elevated blood glucose levels. Hypoglycemia, however, may occur as a complication of pancreas transplantation (9,19). Although impaired consciousness is the most common feature, other neurologic manifestations include focal deficits and seizures (20). Generally, these disturbances are reversible with restoration of euglycemia. Permanent disturbances in neurologic function, however, may occur after prolonged hypoglycemia (21). In some instances, patients may recover consciousness postoperatively only to become encephalopathic in the days after the procedure. Toxic effects of immunosuppressive agents and infection are important to consider as causes of delayed-onset encephalopathy.

Acute pancreatitis may be a complication after pancreas transplantation (APT), and pancreatic encephalopathy is a rare complication of acute pancreatitis (22,23). Although pancreatic encephalopathy has not been reported specifically after pancreas transplantation, it is a potential complication, particularly if serum amylase and lipase concentrations are markedly elevated.

The investigation of encephalopathy requires careful clinical evaluation combined with laboratory and imaging studies directed at identifying possible metabolic disorders, infection, and structural brain conditions that may be causing the clinical disturbance.

## Seizures

Seizures occur frequently in transplant recipients (24), and seizures of various types may occur APT (25). These include generalized epilepsy, partial seizures, and partial complex seizures. The clinical presentation may be overt and readily diagnosed. In some instances, however, seizure manifestations may be subtle. Particularly, in the case of partial complex epilepsy, impaired consciousness may be the only feature. Seizures may be the manifestation of cerebral disease, they may be caused by metabolic disturbances, and frequently they may be induced by medications. Prominent causes of seizures in the immediate posttransplantation phase include drug toxicity, cessation of medical therapy, metabolic disturbances, and hypoxic-ischemic injury (26). Vascular events and infection may also cause seizures. The diagnostic approach requires clinical evaluation, laboratory tests directed at excluding metabolic disturbances and drug toxicity, and imaging studies, which are performed to exclude underlying structural disturbances. The electroencephalogram may be helpful in demonstrating paroxysmal activity, and, in some instances, it may yield information that directs attention to specific causes, particularly certain types of infection. Lumbar puncture is indicated when there is suspicion of a CNS infection, but further evaluation is required first. Specifically, imaging studies of the brain are necessary to exclude intracranial disease that may contraindicate a lumbar puncture, and the prothrombin time and a platelet count should be obtained before proceeding with a lumbar puncture.

## Cerebrovascular Events

As discussed in the "Pretransplantation Conditions" section, diabetes increases the risk of ischemic strokes (10–12). Indeed, they have been reported to occur with greater frequency in diabetic patients undergoing certain surgical procedures (27,28). Ischemic stroke has also been reported as a complication of pancreas transplantation (25). Strokes typically are a focal disturbance. The clinical features may include impaired consciousness, hemiparesis, language dysfunction, motor disturbances, and sensory abnormalities as well as involuntary movements. As already discussed, it is important to determine whether the deficits resulted from a previous stroke. When an acute process is suspected, further investigation is required, which may include brain imaging studies and, in certain instances such as when a cardioembolic stroke is suspected, carotid ultrasonography and echocardiography.

## Metabolic Disturbances

The early posttransplantation phase may be complicated by metabolic disorders, including metabolic acidosis (29), hyponatremia (30), and hypophosphatemia (31).

Metabolic disorders are reported to be more common with bladder drainage of exocrine secretions (32). Acidosis in itself is not associated with neurologic dysfunction. Coexistent disorders, however, may affect the nervous system. In particular, dehydration may increase the risk of thrombotic cerebrovascular complications. Hyponatremia, as with other metabolic derangements, is more likely to occur in patients who have undergone bladder drainage (32). Impaired renal function may also predispose patients to develop hyponatremia. The neurologic consequences of hyponatremia include seizures and encephalopathy (33). Prominent, but reversible focal deficits may also complicate the clinical picture (33). Appropriate treatment of hyopnatremia usually results in resolution of the neurologic deficits. Hypophosphatemia has been reported to be a complication of combined KPT (31). This disorder is characterized by ataxia, reduced muscle strength, absence of tendon reflexes, and distal sensory disturbances (34). The weakness associated with hypophosphatemia may be so profound that it mimics Guillain-Barre' syndrome (34). Neurologic function typically improves rapidly after recognition and treatment of hypophosphatemia.

## Neuromuscular Complications
### Persistent Weakness

Severe loss of strength may be encountered in the patient recovering from a transplantation procedure. Neuromuscular disturbances may occur in critically ill individuals regardless of pancreas transplantation. These well-documented complications include conditions such as polyneuropathy (35), acute myopathy, or a combination of both (36). These disorders should be considered in patients in whom weakness develops APT. The cause of these disorders has not been established, but many predisposing conditions have been incriminated singly or together (37). Weakness is the primary feature, and patients generally improve as the underlying processes are corrected.

### Carpal Tunnel Syndrome

Carpal tunnel syndrome has been reported as a peripheral nervous system complication developing soon after transplantation (38). Patients present with features typical of carpal tunnel syndrome usually within eight days postoperatively. Conservative treatment measures are typically effective, and spontaneous improvement is the rule. The pathogenesis is not well understood.

### Femoral Nerve Injury

This condition may develop after abdominal surgery (39) and is characterized by unilateral weakness of knee extension, depressed patellar tendon reflex, and impaired sensation over the anterior thigh. Compression of the femoral nerve along its intrapelvic course, by self-retaining retractor blades, and nerve ischemia have been postulated as mechanisms for the development of this neuropathy (40).

### Diabetic Peripheral Neuropathy

Diabetic peripheral neuropathy tends to stabilize APT, and improvement occurs in some patients (41,42). Progression of the neuropathy, however, has been described, despite adequate graft function and normal blood glucose levels (43). Although there is no clear explanation for the deterioration in peripheral nerve function that has been described, this neuropathy does not appear to be an entity specific to pancreas transplantation because there are many potential causes of neuropathy in solid organ transplant recipients.

### Muscle Disorders

Diabetic muscle infarction has been described after simultaneous KPT (44). This rare condition typically occurs in patients with long-standing type I diabetes mellitus. The clinical presentation is of an abrupt onset of focal muscle pain. Tenderness, local swelling, and weakness of the involved muscle are the hallmarks of the condition. Treatment is largely symptomatic, and the pain and swelling usually subside over time.

## THE LATE POSTTRANSPLANT PHASE

During the late posttransplantation phase, heavy early immunosuppression has been tapered, but long-term chronic immunosuppression is still required. Patients thus continue to be at risk of developing infections, such as opportunistic fungal or viral infections. However, during this phase several other entities may affect the nervous system. Neuropathologic changes, induced by immunosuppressive agents, neuromuscular conditions, and posttransplantation lymphoproliferative disease, are of particular importance.

### Infection

Information relating to the incidence of fungal infections in pancreas transplant recipients is lacking (45), but these patients have many risk factors predisposing them to fungal infection (45). In general, fungal and bacterial pathogens that may be encountered in transplant recipients include *Cryptococcus*, *Aspergillus*, *Listeria*, *Nocardia*, and *Toxoplasma* (46). The risk of infection is increased in patients who have received high doses of immunosuppressive agents to prevent or treat rejection. The clinical manifestation of CNS infection may take many forms, and may be quite subtle (47,48). Infection should thus be suspected in transplant recipients who present with combinations of headache, personality change, focal deficits, seizures, and disturbed consciousness.

There are more overt clinical syndromes. For instance, in some fungal infections, encephalopathy may be the main presenting feature. Patients with certain bacterial infections, particularly from *Listeria*, may present with encephalopathy, with signs of meningitis appearing only later. A meningitic syndrome with headache and neck rigidity may be the dominant clinical finding with particular infections, such as bacterial meningitis, but it can also occur with cryptococcal infections (49). Alternatively, prominent focal findings such as hemiplegia may occur with cerebral aspergillosis (49). Patients with brain abscess of bacterial origin may also present with these findings. Impairment of cognitive function may signal an infection. This can develop with any infection but is typical of progressive multifocal leukoencephalopathy, which is a subacute demyelinating condition that results from papovavirus (JC) infection (50).

It is important to emphasize that the typical manifestations of infection may be modified considerably or even absent if the patient is immunosuppressed. Thus, fever, neck rigidity, and elevated white blood cell count may not be present. However, even in the absence of the classic signs, infection should be suspected in patients presenting with headache, disturbed consciousness, and focal abnormalities.

The diagnosis of a CNS infection initially requires imaging studies to identify structural abnormalities. Ideally, the studies are magnetic resonance imaging examinations. Cerbrospinal fluid analysis is often indicated, but as previously discussed before carrying out a lumbar puncture, brain imaging is mandatory to exclude conditions that may contraindicate a lumbar puncture. In many instances, histologic confirmation of an infectious process is required, necessitating a brain or meningeal biopsy.

### Posttransplantation Lymphoproliferative Disorder

Lymphoproliferative disorders are a serious complication of chronic immunosuppression and may be encountered in any transplant recipient. The pathogenesis is related to B-cell proliferation induced by Epstein-Barr virus infection. Generally, the proliferating B-cells are of host origin (51). Three types of lymphoproliferative disease have been described (51,52). Extranodal disease occurs in the most malignant form and is characterized by monoclonal B-cell proliferation, cytogenetic abnormalities, and immunoglobulin gene rearrangements. This form may involve the CNS (53). Extranodal disease should be suspected when there are alterations in mental state and focal neurologic findings. Investigation requires imaging studies, which may show multifocal abnormalities (54). Diagnosis may be confirmed by the demonstration of malignant lymphocytes in the cerebrospinal fluid or by brain biopsy.

## Seizures

Seizures may occur at any time after transplantation, but seizure that occurs later in the post-transplantation course may be signs of infection or the toxic effects of immunosuppressive agents (55). Metabolic disturbances such as hypoglycemia, hyponatremia, and hypomagnesemia may also be complicated by seizures.

## Encephalopathy

The development of encephalopathy later in the posttransplantation phase in patients who were previously neurologically normal may indicate a systemic illness, CNS infection, toxic effect of an immunosuppressive agent, or other conditions. Clouding of consciousness and the accompanying array of clinical disturbances developing as components of an encephalopathy may be the first manifestations of systemic infections, metabolic disturbances, toxic states, and organ failure.

Many disorders must be considered, and the initial investigations should be clinically driven. Examination findings and medication history can yield important information and provide a focus for investigations. In many instances, laboratory study findings may be diagnostically useful. If focal neurologic signs are present, attention should be directed to the CNS. After appropriate testing, the absence of evidence of systemic illness may suggest that the encephalopathy is of CNS origin. Brain imaging studies, electroencephalographic examination, and cerebrospinal fluid analysis may be required as part of the investigation. Encephalopathy may develop as a complication of commonly used immunosuppressive agents, including tacrolimus (56), cyclosporine (57), and coricosteroids (58). The features may be nonspecific, but prominent movement disorders may be seen with toxicity induced by tacrolimus or cyclosporine. In some instances, the encephalopathy induced by these two agents may be accompanied by brain magnetic resonance signal abnormalities involving the white matter, often in a posterior distribution. Immunosuppression-induced neurotoxicity may not always be accompanied by elevated plasma concentrations of the therapeutic agent. The diagnosis should thus be considered when there has been a recent dose increase. Low levels of serum magnesium and cholesterol have also been implicated as risk factors for the development of immunosuppression-induced encephalopathy (59). This condition should be considered in the presence of an unexplained encephalopathy, but the diagnosis is one of exclusion and is arrived at only after completion of appropriate investigations.

## Weakness

Progressive loss of strength has been reported in the months after simultaneous KPT or pancreas after kidney transplantation (60). The weakness, which first appears several months after transplantation and may continue to progress for several more months, seems to be related to the development of a myopathy. Polyneuropathy that frequently occurs in diabetic patients does not seem to cause this particular syndrome. There is no clear understanding of the cause of the myopathy. Prolonged hospitalization, graft rejection, sepsis, intercurrent infections, and immunosuppressive agents may contribute to the development of this condition. Some patients show improvement in strength over time.

There are other causes of weakness. The peripheral nervous system is vulnerable to the toxic effects of agents that may be required to treat conditions arising APT. Use of corticosteroids or colchicines (61) may contribute to myopathy (58). Some findings suggest that cyclosporine may contribute to the development of myopathy (62), and focal weakness as a result of a demyelinating neuropathy has been ascribed to cyclosporine (63).

Weakness may be a vexing problem in the pancreas transplant recipient. In some instances, the cause may be apparent, but often it cannot be determined. Management then rests on identification and treatment of the conditions that may be contributing to the weakness. If the cause of the condition is unknown, symptomatic measures and clinical monitoring are indicated.

## REFERENCES

1. Watkins PJ, Thomas PK. Diabetes mellitus and the nervous system. J Neurol Neurosurg Psychiatry 1998; 65:620–632.
2. Steen DC. The current state of pancreas transplantation. AACN Clin Issues 1999; 10:164–175.
3. Umpierrez GE, Khajavi M, Kitabchi AE. Review: diabetic ketoacidosis and hyperglycemic hyperosmolar nonketotic syndrome. Am J Med Sci 1996; 311:225–233.
4. Chiasson JL, Aris-Jilwan N, Belanger R, et al. Diagnosis and treatment of diabetic ketoacidosis and the hyperglycemic hyperosmolar state. CMAJ 2003; 168:859–866.
5. Krentz AJ, Ryder RE. Hypokalemia-induced respiratory failure complicating treatment of diabetic ketoacidosis. J Diabet Complic 1994; 8:55–56.
6. Ionescu-Tirgoviste C, Bruckner I, Mihalache N, Ionescu C. Plasma phosphorus and magnesium values during treatment of severe diabetic ketoacidosis. Med Intern 1981; 19:63–68.
7. Bustamante EA, Levy H. Severe alkalemia, hyponatremia, and diabetic ketoacidosis in an alcoholic man. Chest 1996; 110:273–275.
8. Riggs JE. Neurologic manifestations of fluid and electrolyte disturbances. Neurol Clin 1989; 7:509–523.
9. Zaman F, Abreo KD, Levine S, Maley W, Zibari GB. Pancreatic transplantation: evaluation and management. J Intens Care Med 2004; 19:127–139.
10. Dalal PM, Parab PV. Cerebrovascular disease in type 2 diabetes mellitus. Neurol India 2002; 50:380–385.
11. Mankovsky BN, Metzger BE, Molitch ME, Biller J. Cerebrovascular disorders in patients with diabetes mellitus. J Diabet Complic 1996; 10:228–242.
12. Lukovits TG, Mazzone TM, Gorelick TM. Diabetes mellitus and cerebrovascular disease. Neuroepidemiology 1999; 18:1–14.
13. McMahon MM, Bistrian BR. Host defenses and susceptibility to infection in patients with diabetes mellitus. Infect Dis Clin North Am 1995; 9:1–9.
14. Smitherman KO, Peacock JE Jr. Infectious emergencies in patients with diabetes mellitus. Med Clin North Am 1995; 79:53–77.
15. Strasser MD, Kennedy RJ, Adam RD. Rhinocerebral mucormycosis. Therapy with amphotericin B lipid complex. Arch Intern Med 1996; 156:337–339.
16. Doroghazi RM, Nadol JB Jr., Hyslop NE Jr., Baker AS, Axelrod L. Invasive external otitis. Report of 21 cases and review of the literature. Am J Med 1981; 71:603–614.
17. Darouiche RO, Hamill RJ, Greenberg SB, Weathers SW, Musher DM. Bacterial spinal epidural abscess. Review of 43 cases and literature survey. Medicine (Baltimore) 1992; 71:369–385.
18. Johnson MH. Assessing confused patients. J Neurol Neurosurg Psychiatry 2001; 71(suppl 1):i7–i12.
19. Osei K. Post-transplantation hypoglycaemia in type 1 diabetic pancreas allograft recipients. Acta Diabetol 1998; 35:176–182.
20. Carter F, Taylor C. Transient hypoglycemic hemiparesis. J Natl Med Assoc 2002; 94:999–1001.
21. Gold AE, Marshall SM. Cortical blindness and cerebral infarction associated with severe hypoglycemia. Diabet Care 1996; 19:1001–1003.
22. Ruggieri RM, Lupo I, Piccoli F. Pancreatic encephalopathy: a 7-year follow-up case report and review of the literature. Neurol Sci 2002; 23:203–205.
23. Menza MA, Murray GB. Pancreatic encephalopathy. Biol Psychiatry 1989; 25:781–784.
24. Patchell RA. Neurological complications of organ transplantation. Ann Neurol 1994; 36:688–703.
25. Kiok MC. Neurologic complications of pancreas transplants. Neurol Clin 1988; 6:367–376.
26. Gilmore RL. Seizures and antiepileptic drug use in transplant patients. Neurol Clin 1988; 6:279–296.
27. Treiman GS, Treiman RL, Foran RF, et al. The influence of diabetes mellitus on the risk of abdominal aortic surgery. Am Surg 1994; 60:436–440.
28. Kaarisalo MM, Immonen-Raiha P, Marttila RJ, Salomaa V, Torppa J, Tuomilehto J. The risk of stroke following coronary revascularization—a population-based long-term follow-up study. Scand Cardiovasc J 2002; 36:231–236.
29. Ketel B, Henry ML, Elkhammas EA, Tesi RJ, Ferguson RM. Metabolic complications in combined kidney/pancreas transplantation. Transplant Proc 1992; 24:774–775.
30. Rabb HA, Niles JL, Cosimi AB, Tolkoff-Rubin NE. Severe hyponatremia associated with combined pancreatic and renal transplantation. Transplantation 1989; 48:157–159.
31. Tyden G, Fehrman I, Siden A, Persson A. Hypophosphataemia and reversible neurological dysfunction in a patient subjected to combined renal and pancreatic transplantation. Nephrol Dial Transplant 1988; 3:823–825.
32. Becker BN, Odorico JS, Becker YT, et al. Simultaneous pancreas–kidney and pancreas transplantation. J Am Soc Nephrol 2001; 12:2517–2527.
33. Arieff AI, Guisado R. Effects on the central nervous system of hypernatremic and hyponatremic states. Kidney Int 1976; 10:104–116.
34. Bugg NC, Jones JA. Hypophosphataemia. Pathophysiology, effects and management on the intensive care unit. Anaesthesia 1998; 53:895–902.

35. Jarrett SR, Mogelof JS. Critical illness neuropathy: diagnosis and management. Arch Phys Med Rehabil 1995; 76:688–691.
36. Gutmann L. Critical illness neuropathy and myopathy. Arch Neurol 1999; 56:527–528.
37. Garnacho-Montero J, Madrazo-Osuna J, Garcia-Garmendia JL, et al. Critical illness polyneuropathy: risk factors and clinical consequences. A cohort study in septic patients. Intens Care Med 2001; 27:1288–1296.
38. Wadstrom J, Gannedahl G, Claesson K, Wahlberg J. Acute carpal tunnel syndrome immediately after combined kidney and pancreas transplantation. Transplant Proc 1995; 27:3489–3490.
39. Ruston FG, Politi VL. Femoral nerve injury from abdominal retractors. Can Anaesth Soc J 1958; 5:428–437.
40. Jog MS, Turley JE, Berry H. Femoral neuropathy in renal transplantation. Can J Neurol Sci 1994; 21:38–42.
41. Kennedy WR, Navarro X, Goetz FC, Sutherland DE, Najarian JS. Effects of pancreatic transplantation on diabetic neuropathy. N Engl J Med 1990; 322:1031–1037.
42. Boucek P, Bartos V, Vanek I, Hyza Z, Skibova J. Diabetic autonomic neuropathy after pancreas and kidney transplantation. Diabetologia 1991; 34(suppl 1):S121–S124.
43. Norden G, Olausson M, Andersen O. A case of painful progressive peripheral neuropathy after successful pancreas transplantation. J Diabet Complic 1991; 5:249–251.
44. Delis S, Ciancio G, Casillas J, et al. Diabetic muscle infarction after simultaneous pancreas–kidney transplant. Clin Transplant 2002; 16:295–300.
45. Hagerty JA, Ortiz J, Reich D, Manzarbeitia C. Fungal infections in solid organ transplant patients. Surg Infect (Larchmt) 2003; 4:263–271.
46. Rubin RH. Infection in the organ transplant recipient. In: Rubin RH, Young LS, eds. Clinical Approach to Infection in the Compromised Host. 3rd ed. New York: Plenum Medical Book Co., 1994:629–705.
47. Conti DJ, Rubin RH. Infection of the central nervous system in organ transplant recipients. Neurol Clin 1988; 6:241–260.
48. Hooper DC, Pruitt AA, Rubin RH. Central nervous system infection in the chronically immunosuppressed. Medicine (Baltimore) 1982; 61:166–188.
49. Rubin RH, Hooper DC. Central nervous system infection in the compromised host. Med Clin North Am 1985; 69:281–296.
50. Weber T, Major EO. Progressive multifocal leukoencephalopathy: molecular biology, pathogenesis and clinical impact. Intervirology 1997; 40:98–111.
51. Liebowitz D. Epstein-Barr virus and a cellular signaling pathway in lymphomas from immunosuppressed patients. N Engl J Med 1998; 338:1413–1421.
52. Savage P, Waxman J. Post-transplantation lymphoproliferative disease. QJM 1997; 90:497–503.
53. Hanto DW. Classification of Epstein-Barr virus-associated posttransplant lymphoproliferative diseases: implications for understanding their pathogenesis and developing rational treatment strategies. Annu Rev Med 1995; 46:381–394.
54. Castellano-Sanchez AA, Li S, Qian J, Lagoo A, Weir E, Brat DJ. Primary central nervous system posttransplant lymphoproliferative disorders. Am J Clin Pathol 2004; 121:246–253.
55. Wijdicks EF, Plevak DJ, Wiesner RH, Steers JL. Causes and outcome of seizures in liver transplant recipients. Neurology 1996; 47:1523–1525.
56. Eidelman BH, Abu-Elmagd K, Wilson J, et al. Neurologic complications of FK 506. Transplant Proc 1991; 23:3175–3178.
57. Wijdicks EF, Wiesner RH, Krom RA. Neurotoxicity in liver transplant recipients with cyclosporine immunosuppression. Neurology 1995; 45:1962–1964.
58. Aita JA. Neurologic complications of corticosteroid therapy. Postgrad Med 1974; 55:111–115.
59. de Groen PC, Aksamit AJ, Rakela J, Forbes GS, Krom RA. Central nervous system toxicity after liver transplantation. The role of cyclosporine and cholesterol. N Engl J Med 1987; 317:861–866.
60. Dyck PJ, Velosa JA, Pach JM, et al. Increased weakness after pancreas and kidney transplantation. Transplantation 2001; 72:1403–1408.
61. Ducloux D, Schuller V, Bresson-Vautrin C, Chalopin JM. Colchicine myopathy in renal transplant recipients on cyclosporin. Nephrol Dial Transplant 1997; 12:2389–2392.
62. Breil M, Chariot P. Muscle disorders associated with cyclosporine treatment. Muscle Nerve 1999; 22:1631–1636.
63. Wilson JR, Conwit RA, Eidelman BH, Starzl T, Abu-Elmagd K. Sensorimotor neuropathy resembling CIDP in patients receiving FK506. Muscle Nerve 1994; 17:528–532.

# 21 | Radiology Aspects

**Michael P. Federle, Keyanoosh Hosseinzadeh, James V. Ferris, and Albert Zajko**
*Department of Radiology, University of Pittsburgh Medical Center, Pittsburgh, Pennsylvania, U.S.A.*

**Manuel Brown**
*Department of Radiology, Henry Ford Health System, Detroit, Michigan, U.S.A.*

## INTRODUCTION

Pancreatic transplantation is usually performed concomitantly with renal transplantation in patients with renal failure secondary to long-standing type I diabetes mellitus. In most cases, the pancreas and kidney are removed from the same deceased donor, along with the liver and other organs for other transplant recipients. The reluctance on the part of transplant surgeons to jeopardize the vascular supply of the donor liver has made the recovery and transplantation of the donor pancreas somewhat more difficult. While progress has been made in recent years, with success rates now matching those of other solid organs, pancreatic transplantation is still performed less often, and with a greater variety of surgical techniques than for other solid visceral transplants.

These, and other factors, pose opportunities and challenges for radiologic imaging and intervention for pancreatic graft dysfunction and complications. Close communication between the surgeons and imaging specialists is essential, including specific details of graft and vascular anastomosis, time interval since transplantation, and any clinical evidence of graft dysfunction, fever, etc. As an example, the imaging evaluation of a febrile patient ("R/O abscess or anastomotic leak") might be very different for a patient with a bladder-drained pancreas, compared to a patient with enteric drainage.

As a general principle, imaging tests are relatively sensitive in the detection of transplant dysfunction, but lack specificity for early or mild abnormalities of the pancreatic parenchyma. With increasing severity and duration of transplant damage, the potential contribution of the radiologist increases. In the immediate posttransplant setting, imaging studies are of enormous value, principally to verify vascular integrity and allograft viability.

Our approach in this chapter will be to present the technical aspects and "normal" posttransplant findings for the various imaging modalities, followed by a discussion of the evaluation and management of common complications and clinical problems.

## IMAGING TECHNIQUES
### Plain Radiography and Fluoroscopy

The role of conventional radiography is limited, beyond the usual assessment of complications following any major abdominal surgery, such as small bowel obstruction. The pancreatic and renal allografts may be evident on a supine abdominal radiograph as vague lower quadrant soft tissue masses, with the two rows of surgical staples marking the closed ends of the duodenal segment (DS).

For patients with bladder drainage, retrograde urethrography and cystography play a major role in the evaluation of urologic complications and anastomotic leaks (Fig. 1). Both the urinary bladder and the DS can be opacified under fluoroscopic control. Care should be taken not to overdistend the bladder, particularly in the early postoperative period, to avoid disruption of fragile suture lines. Cystitis and duodenitis may be evident by lack of distensibility and thickened mucosal folds. Urethral stricture and leak are best demonstrated by retrograde fluoroscopic studies.

### Nuclear Scintigraphy

Radionuclear scintigraphy has been utilized extensively since the earliest days of pancreatic transplantation. A variety of radiopharmaceuticals and techniques have been studied, including

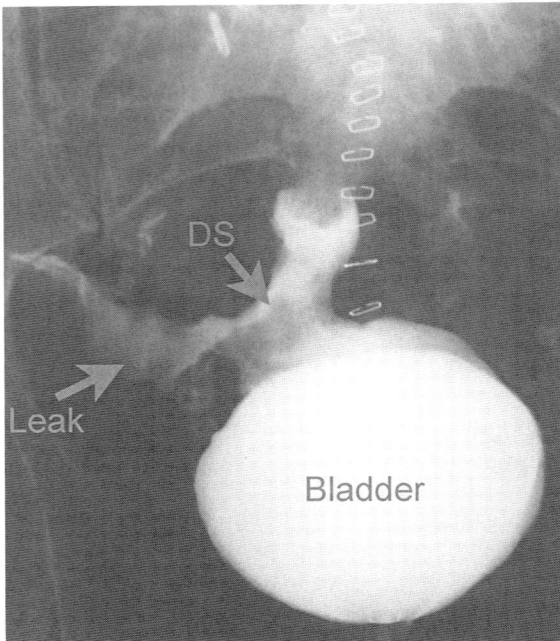

**Figure 1** Cystogram; anastomotic leak. Retrograde injection of contrast material through a Foley catheter demonstrates filling of the duodenal segment of the bladder-drained pancreatic transplant. An anastomotic leak is shown (*arrow*).

those that evaluate blood flow and perfusion ($^{99m}$Tc-DPTA or $^{99m}$TcMAG3); however, these agents only allow the evaluation of the flow phase and do not accumulate within the transplanted organ. Some investigators have used thallium-201 (1),$^{99m}$Tc Sestamibi (2), and $^{99m}$Tc-HMPAO (3), which allow for delayed static imaging. The third category of radiopharmaceuticals used for evaluating pancreatic transplants is $^{111}$In-labeled platelets to diagnose transplant rejection (4–6). The most common radiotracers are $^{99m}$Tc-DTPA or $^{99m}$MAG3. One hundred and twenty serial one-second perfusion images are obtained with a gamma camera placed over the lower abdomen and pelvis. These are often then summed to three to five seconds per image on the computer. These are followed immediately by a 500,000 count static image. Normal or well-functioning grafts show peak graft flow within three to six seconds of peak arterial flow and both will have equal intensity (Fig. 2). On sequential studies, the functioning graft will show very constant peak time, intensity, homogeneity, and size. Delay in time from peak iliac artery to peak graft activity, changes in the relative intensity, size, or homogeneity of the graft are nonspecific findings that may represent rejection or vascular complications.

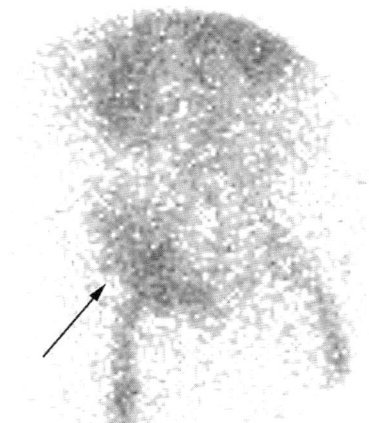

**Figure 2** Radionuclide flow scan; normal allograft. One of many sequential images following IV injection of Tc$^{99m}$-DTPA shows activity over the aorta and iliac vessels, and prompt uptake in the pancreatic allograft (*arrow*) indicating normal perfusion.

Using the agents that accumulate in the transplant (thallium-201, $^{99m}$Tc Sestamibi, or $^{99m}$Tc-HMPAO) may also reveal complications of transplantation by changes in graft size and/or change in homogeneity or uptake on sequential images (1–3).

$^{111}$In-labeled platelets have been shown to detect early pancreas allograft rejection and the effectiveness of anti-rejection therapy (4,5) in an animal model. Several reports have described diffuse increased uptake over the transplant in cases of rejection or diffuse increased uptake as focal accumulation in cases of venous thrombosis (6).

## Ultrasonography

Ultrasonography (US) plays an important role in the evaluation of the pancreatic allograft, but is technically very challenging and operator dependent (7–10). Sonographic technique includes oblique and transverse scan orientations parallel to the long and short axis of the graft, respectively, with typical abdominal 3.5–5 MHz curvilinear or sector probes used to delineate the morphology, echotexture, and vascularity of the gland (Figs. 3,4). For a bladder-drained allograft, moderate but incomplete distention of the urinary bladder facilitates localization of the pancreatic head along the superolateral margin of the bladder with the pancreatic tail oriented superolaterally from the head. For enteric drainage, US evaluation is more difficult, as the graft may be surrounded and obscured by bowel, with the head situated cranially. Additionally, absent in the transplant recipient is the overlying liver, which usually serves as a sonographic "window" and a reference for comparative echogenicity, with the normal pancreas being more echogenic than the normal liver. Since the pancreas lacks a firm capsule, it renders the borders indistinct, and differentiation of the gland from surrounding edematous and inflamed tissues is more difficult.

US is unable to distinguish between parenchymal abnormalities such as acute rejection or pancreatitis. In general, both of these acute processes result in an enlarged, hypoechoic, or heterogeneous gland, while chronic processes shrink the gland and increase its echogenicity (9). US has proven to be more reliable in screening for vascular complications and peripancreatic fluid collections. Color Doppler and power Doppler imaging enhance assessment of extraparenchymal and intraparenchymal vessels. Typically the "Y" graft anastomosis at the vascular pedicle and donor splenic artery and vein can be readily identified. However, the donor superior mesenteric artery and vein are often too small to be recognized, and thus indirect evidence of patency is provided by the presence of both arterial and venous Doppler waveforms within the head of the allograft (Fig. 5). "Normal" graft arterial waveforms show a low resistance, antegrade-only flow pattern. Venous flow is typically low velocity and mono- to minimally biphasic, similar to the signal from the portal vein.

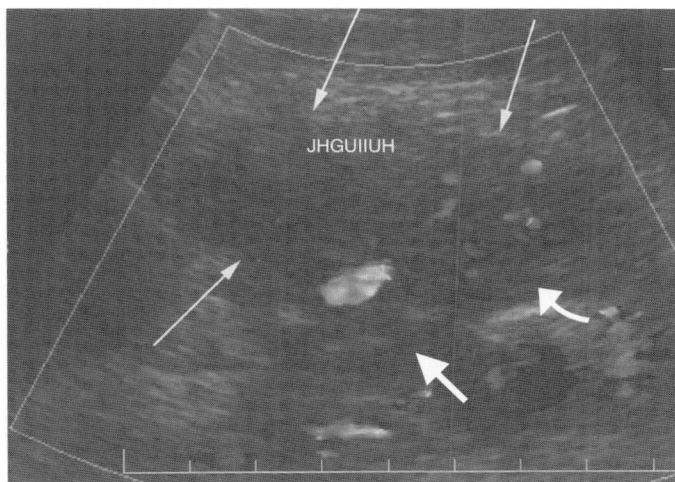

**Figure 3** Ultrasound; normal allograft. Color Doppler sonogram shows the normal homogeneous low-level echogenicity of the pancreatic allograft (*long arrows*) with arterial and venous flow indicated by short and curved arrows, respectively.

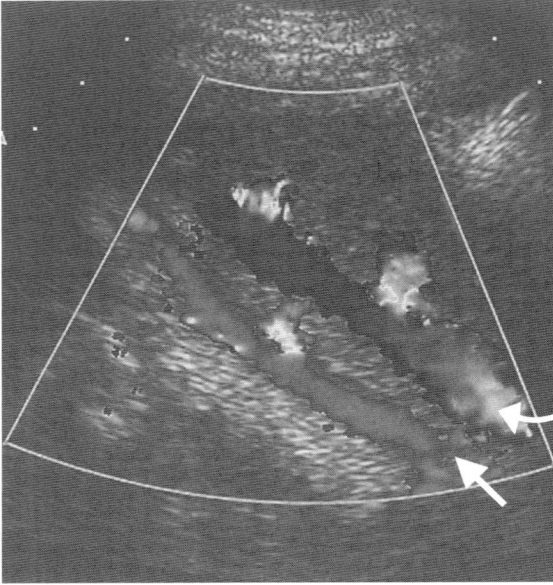

**Figure 4**  Ultrasound; normal allograft. Color Doppler sonogram along the long axis of the allograft shows normal artery (*straight arrow*) and vein (*curved arrow*) unusually well.

US is the optimal tool for guiding biopsy and drainage procedures, allowing one to avoid injury to the blood vessels, by providing real-time feedback for needle placement (Fig. 6) (11–15).

## Computed Tomography

Computed tomography (CT) plays a similarly important role, particularly in screening for severe pancreatic parenchymal damage and peripancreatic fluid collections (14,16,17). While intravenous contrast administration would be optimal, it is often not used because of the potential nephrotoxicity of iodinated contrast media. The use of oral contrast medium is mandatory in order to distinguish the graft or abnormal fluid collections from unopacified loops of bowel, and is especially useful in assessing the integrity of the enteric anastomosis for enteric-drained allografts. For bladder-drained allografts, we may obtain two series of CT sections through the lower abdomen and pelvis, one before and one following the catheter introduction of dilute (2%) contrast material in the urinary bladder. This "CT cystography" is especially useful in cases of suspected anastomotic leak.

The role of CT evaluation may have increased with the advent of multidetector CT scanners (14). These allow the rapid acquisition of thin (0.65–2.5 mm) sections through the abdomen within one breath hold, with decreased artifacts and increased resolution of small structures such as vessels, ducts, and small lesions. If the serum creatinine is normal or in the setting of pancreas transplantation alone, the use of a limited amount (usually 100 mL) of nonionic contrast material allows optimal demonstration of vascular anatomy and parenchymal enhancement. Multidetector CT enables high-quality two-dimensional or three-dimensional (3D) reconstructions of the vascular anatomy with respect to adjacent anatomic structures. Definition of blood vessels using this CT technique can rival the quality of conventional catheter angiography.

The "normal" pancreatic transplant is a vertically or horizontally oriented homogenous soft tissue structure (Figs. 7A,B). In patients with bladder drainage, the graft usually lies in the right iliac fossa and parallel to the ascending colon. The graft position may be more variable with enteric anastomosis, but is still usually vertical within the right side of the abdomen. Surgical staples placed along both ends of the duodenal stump may assist in localizing the transplant. In the early post-transplant period (less than four weeks), the graft may be enlarged and heterogeneous with surrounding fluid and hematoma, gradually becoming well defined and similar in density to the native pancreas, with little or no surrounding fluid or infiltration.

Conventional CT and CT fluoroscopy have been especially useful in guiding biopsy and drainage procedures, especially when US fails to demonstrate a safe pathway to the allograft (Figs. 8A,B).

**(A)**

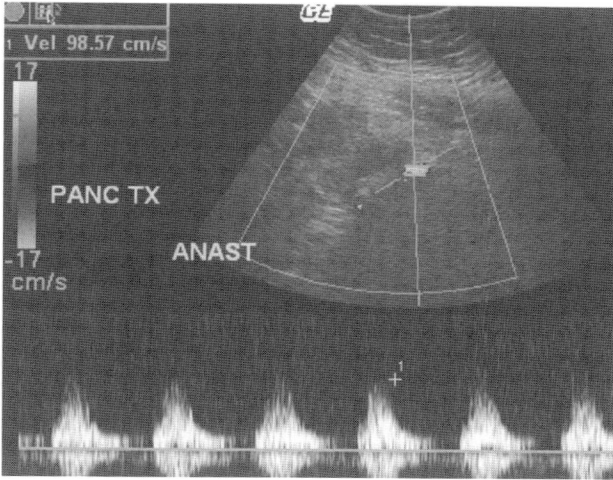

**(B)**

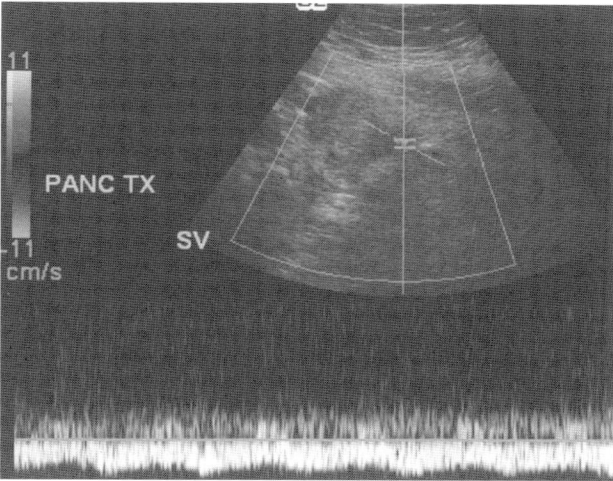

**Figure 5** Ultrasound; normal flow to allograft. (**A**) Doppler waveforms over the arterial anastomosis show low-resistance arterial flow with prompt "upstroke" and antegrade-only flow pattern. (**B**) Doppler waveforms over the venous anastomosis show normal low-velocity monophasic venous flow pattern.

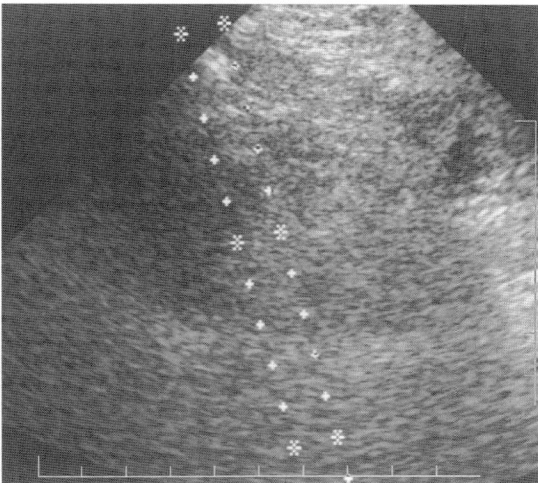

**Figure 6** Ultrasound-guided allograft biopsy. A guide mounted on the ultrasound transducer shows a needle biopsy path (*double row of cursors*) through the allograft, while avoiding major blood vessels or bowel.

**(A)**

**(B)**

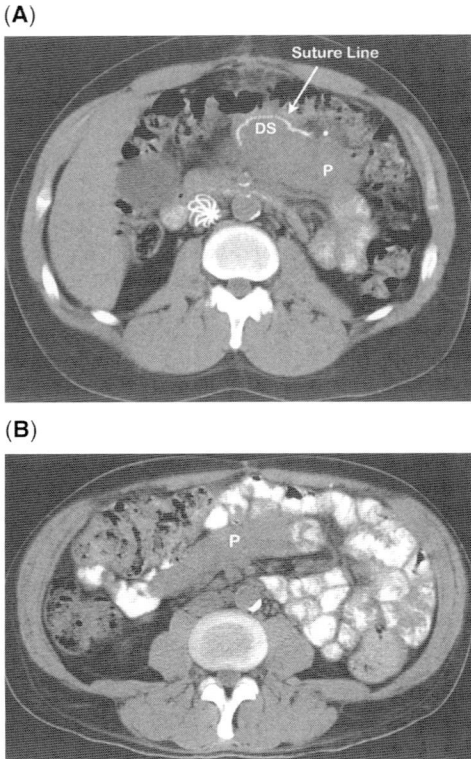

**Figure 7** Computed tomography; normal pancreatic allograft, enteric drainage. (**A** and **B**) A radiopaque row of sutures marks the anastomosis between the duodenal segment (DS) and bowel. The allograft (P) lies transversely and is distinct from the contrast-opacified small bowel.

## Magnetic Resonance Imaging

Ultrasound is typically the primary modality for assessment of the pancreas allograft. However, given the intraperitoneal location of the allograft, detailed assessment of the parenchyma and vasculature can be difficult with ultrasound in the presence of overlying bowel gas. While CT angiography (CTA) is technically less challenging, magnetic resonance angiography (MRA) offers similar noninvasive display of vascular anatomy and pathology without the use of potentially nephrotoxic contrast media (Figs. 9A,B). With improvements in technology and

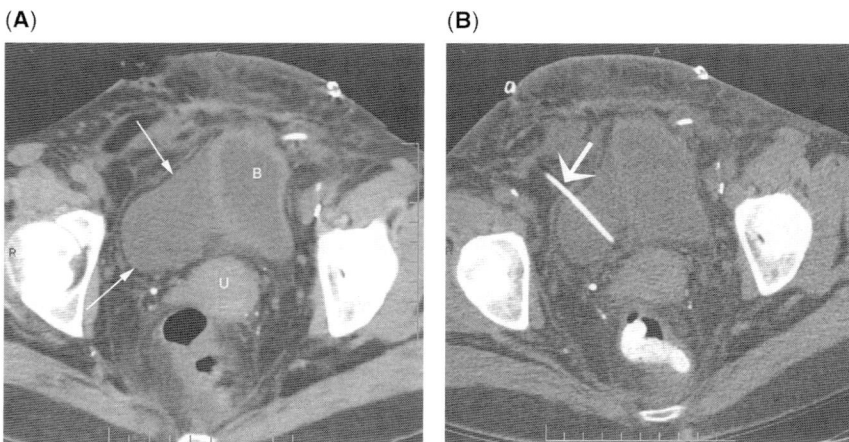

**(A)**

**(B)**

**Figure 8** Computed tomography (CT)-guided fluid drainage. (**A**) CT shows a loculated pelvic fluid collection (*arrows*) adjacent to the bladder (B) and uterus (U). (**B**) A pigtail catheter (*arrow*) was placed under CT guidance with successful drainage of the fluid.

**(A)**

**(B)**

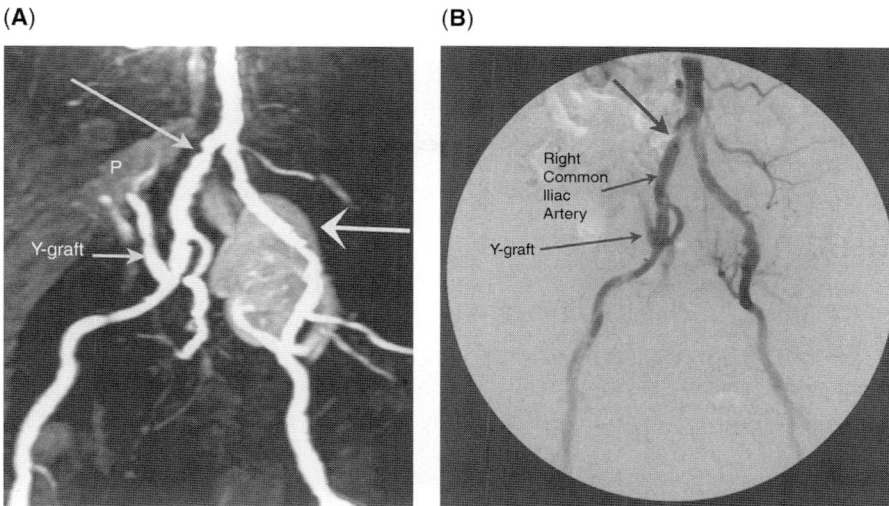

**Figure 9** Magnetic resonance (MRA) and catheter angiography (CA). (**A**) MRA shows normal flow to a left-lower quadrant renal allograft (*short, bold arrow*), and a patent "Y" graft to the right-side pancreatic allograft (P). Note atherosclerotic narrowing (*long arrow*) of the right common iliac artery. (**B**) CA shows similar vascular landmarks and narrowing (*arrow*) of the right common iliac artery.

increased availability of MR imaging (MRI), 3D MR angiography has been used occasionally for preoperative assessment of the recipient's pelvic vasculature and several studies have demonstrated the successful use of this technique in the evaluation of the pancreatic allograft and vasculature (18–21). In the evaluation of the allograft, MRA is as definitive as angiography, while MRA is superior in the evaluation of venous anatomy and parenchymal enhancement of the pancreas allograft. In the same MR examination, the renal allograft (if present) and its vascular supply are also displayed for evaluation (Fig. 10).

All pancreatic transplants preferably should be evaluated with a field strength of 1.5 T and higher, and a dedicated phased array coil. Both coronal and axial single shot fast spin echo T2-weighted sequences are performed to confirm the position of the pancreas allograft by identifying the duct and the duodenal stump, and to evaluate for peripancreatic fluid collections. A fat-suppressed, axial T1-weighted sequence is used to identify the normal high signal intensity of the pancreatic parenchyma and any peripancreatic hematoma or hemorrhagic necrosis. Fast spin echo T2-weighted imaging is most sensitive to abnormalities of the

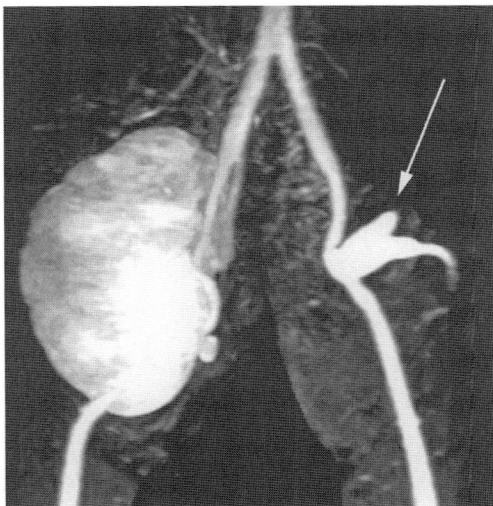

**Figure 10** Magnetic resonance angiogram (MRA); occluded arterial graft. MRA shows normal perfusion of the right lower quadrant renal allograft, but an occluded "Y" graft to the pancreatic allograft (*arrow*).

pancreas transplant, as the majority of pathologic processes increase glandular water content and these result in high-intensity (bright) lesions on T2-weighted MRI. The "normal" pancreas parenchyma is typically isointense to renal cortex on T1-weighted imaging and to muscle on T2-weighted imaging (Figs. 11A,B). Multiphase, breath-hold, pre- and post-contrast-enhanced, 3D fat-suppressed, T1-weighted MR angiography is performed in the coronal orientation to capture the arterial and venous phases of enhancement, followed by delayed axial, T1-weighted, fat-suppressed acquisition through the pancreas allograft. Postprocessing includes multiplanar reconstruction of the subtracted images, and 3D maximum intensity projections and volume rendering for vessel evaluation.

### Angiography and Other Interventional Modalities

Catheter angiography is largely limited to cases in which there is a high likelihood of a vascular complication, such as arterial or venous occlusion, pseudoaneurysm, or arteriovenous fistula (22–24). Proper performance and interpretation of angiography are impossible without detailed knowledge of the vascular anastomoses made in the patient to be studied. However, given advances in CT and MR angiography, catheter angiography is largely reserved for therapeutic intervention.

   Pancreatic transplant rejection is often monitored indirectly by assessing the urinary amylase (in bladder-drained cases) or by biopsying the coexisting renal transplant. Renal biopsy serves as a reasonable surrogate because rejection of the renal transplant generally coincides with pancreatic rejection, although "discordant" rejection may occur in a minority of cases. Direct confirmation or exclusion of pancreatic graft rejection by biopsy is sometimes necessary.

   Percutaneous needle biopsy is a standard means of evaluating possible rejection of the transplanted kidney or liver. Percutaneous biopsy of the transplanted pancreas, however, has been considered a high-risk procedure, with a relatively higher incidence of iatrogenic vascular injury, pancreatitis, or infection, either documented or feared. However, recent large clinical series (15,25) have documented a low incidence of significant complications (1.27–2.8%) and a high yield (89%) of diagnostic samples. Biopsies are best performed using real-time ultrasound guidance and an automated 18-gauge needle biopsy device. Alternatively, CT fluoroscopy can be used for biopsy guidance of the allograft.

   An alternative method for obtaining a pancreatic graft biopsy is to introduce a cystoscope through the bladder and into the pancreaticoduodenal segment in patients with bladder-drained grafts.

### COMPLICATIONS

The pancreas is a fragile organ and invariably suffers some damage during the transplantation process, usually attributed to preservation injury, ischemia, or simply the manual handling of the gland. Hyperamylasemia is common for the first five to seven days after transplantation.

(A)                                             (B)

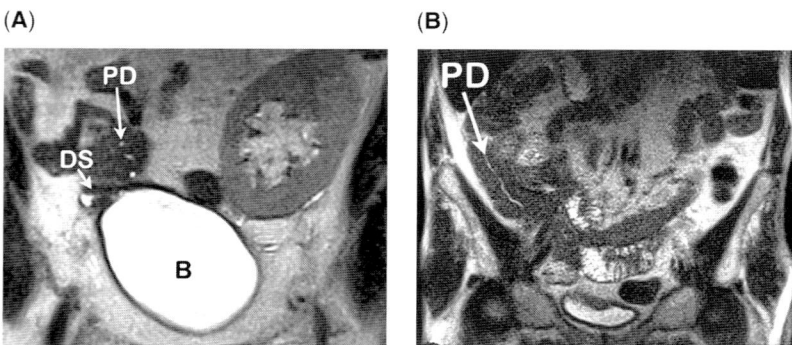

**Figure 11**   Magnetic resonance image; normal bladder-drained pancreatic allograft. (**A** and **B**) Coronal magnetic resonance sections show anastomosis between the bladder (B) and the duodenal segment (DS). Note the homogenous low intensity of the allograft and the normal pancreatic duct (PD).

Also occasionally seen is a transient leakage of fluid from the newly implanted graft. Some dismiss this as "pancreatic sweating" and attribute the fluid leak to disrupted lymphatics or exocrine secretions leaking through the thin pancreatic capsule (10). Drains placed at the time of transplantation may prevent the accumulation of these fluid collections (10).

## Rejection

Acute and chronic allograft rejection is common following pancreatic transplantation. The sonographic features of acute rejection are nonspecific and include allograft enlargement secondary to edema, which cannot be differentiated from acute pancreatitis. Elevated resistive indices within parenchymal arteries can be associated with chronic or severe acute rejection, although patients with no rejection or mild or moderate acute rejection may show no change in waveform (10,26). The hallmark of chronic rejection is an obliterative vasculopathy involving major pancreatic arteries and medium- and small-sized branches, which lead to parenchymal fibrosis (27). It is attributed to multiple episodes of undiagnosed or partially treated acute rejection. Chronic rejection is the leading cause of late allograft loss. Chronic rejection typically results in an atrophic and hyperechoic allograft (Fig. 12).

In acute rejection, T2-weighted images will show increased parenchymal signal intensity because of the presence of edema in an enlarged gland. In chronic rejection, the signal decreases because of parenchymal fibrosis and reduced extracellular fluid. Diffuse or patchy decreased glandular enhancement indicates some form of graft dysfunction (20,21), but does not reliably distinguish among various degrees of rejection, pancreatitis, or ischemia. The intravenous infusion of secretin in combination with dynamic contrast-enhanced MRI has been advocated by investigators as a measure of the ability of the pancreatic allograft to respond with increased output of pancreatic juice. This is an effective test to distinguish the healthy allograft from a dysfunctional allograft, but is not yet established as an accurate indicator of the etiology of the dysfunction (28).

Currently, the diagnosis of allograft rejection remains one of exclusion (e.g., imaging evidence of patent vasculature) and is confirmed by biopsy in most cases.

## Pancreatitis

Some degree of graft pancreatitis occurs commonly after pancreatic transplantation in the immediate postoperative period. Exocrine pancreatic effusions and hyperamylasemia usually decrease and stabilize within one week of surgery. The clinical diagnosis of transplant

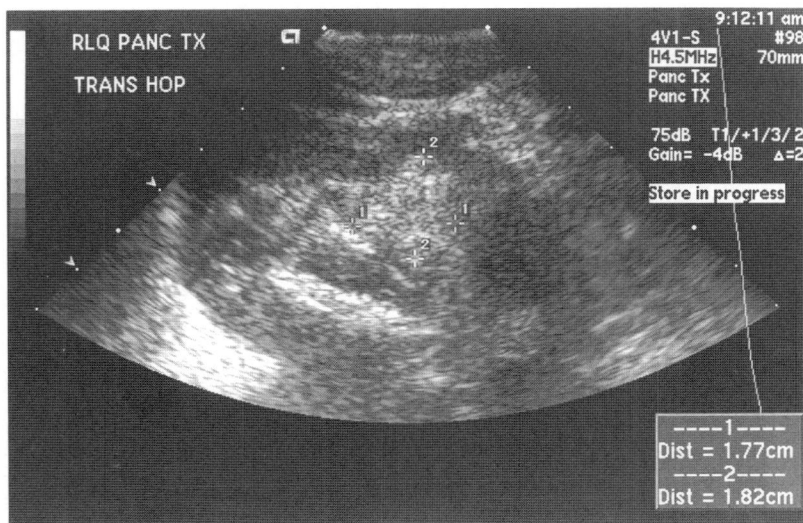

**Figure 12**  Ultrasound; chronic rejection. The pancreatic allograft (*between cursors*) is small and heterogeneously echogenic.

pancreatitis is usually suspected on the basis of right lower quadrant pain and tenderness and elevated serum amylase in the absence of demonstrable anastomotic leak. In cases of bladder drainage, severe pancreatitis may result from urinary reflux. Rarely, ampullary stenosis or a mucous plug may induce pancreatitis.

On radionuclide imaging, pancreatitis usually results in normal or increased flow on the dynamic images with patchy or poor uptake of tracer (Tc-DTPA or HMPAO) and prolongated washout of static images (2,3).

On CT and MR, pancreatitis is suggested by gland swelling, heterogeneity, and infiltration of peripancreatic fat planes (Figs. 13A–C). Non-loculated intraperitoneal fluid collections are common and are high in amylase content. Loculated fluid collections or pseudocysts may also develop a discrete wall evident on imaging (Figs. 14A,B). Bowel wall thickening of adjacent intestinal loops is a common secondary finding. Focal areas of ischemia or necrosis are sometimes seen, and in extreme cases, complete infarction of the graft may be found, with disorganized, liquefied parenchyma and gas bubbles present (Figs. 15A,B). In such cases, it is impossible to distinguish infarction from infected pancreatic necrosis, although graft pancreatectomy is usually required in either event.

By imaging criteria alone, it is difficult to judge the acuity or severity of pancreatitis in many cases. As previously noted, transient posttransplant pancreatitis is almost a constant, along with peripancreatic infiltration and fluid collections. In most cases, these resolve within a week, but the transplanted pancreas often appears enlarged and the fat planes somewhat blurred, in our experience, well after clinical signs of pancreatitis have resolved.

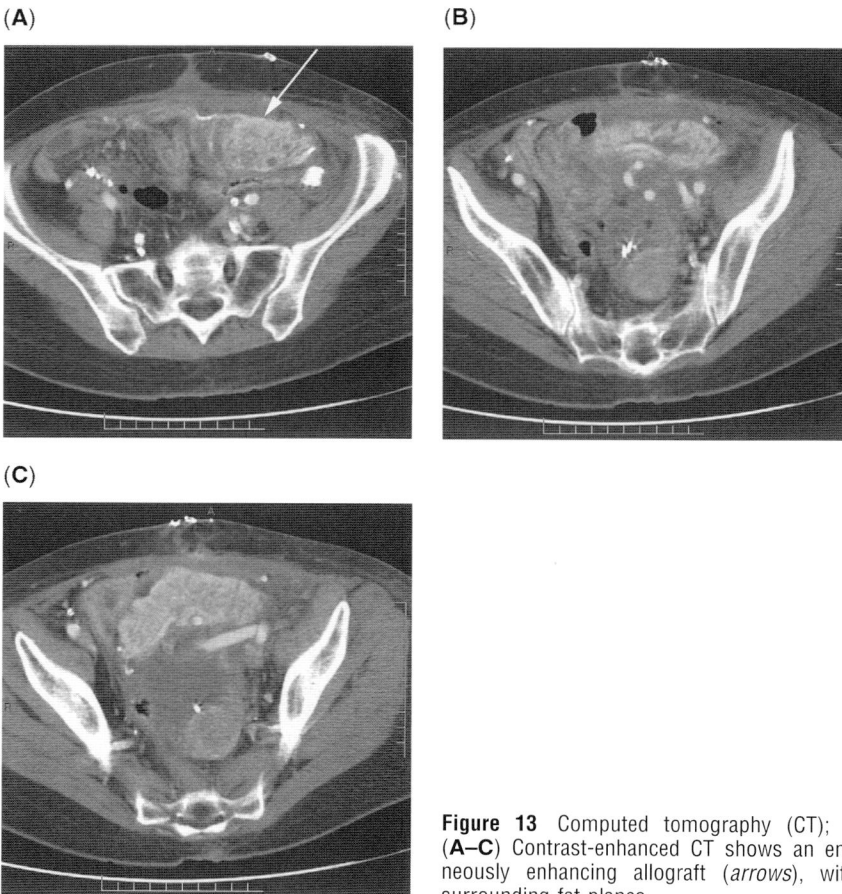

**(A)**

**(B)**

**(C)**

**Figure 13** Computed tomography (CT); allograft pancreatitis. (**A–C**) Contrast-enhanced CT shows an enlarged and heterogeneously enhancing allograft (*arrows*), with infiltration of the surrounding fat planes.

**(A)**            **(B)**

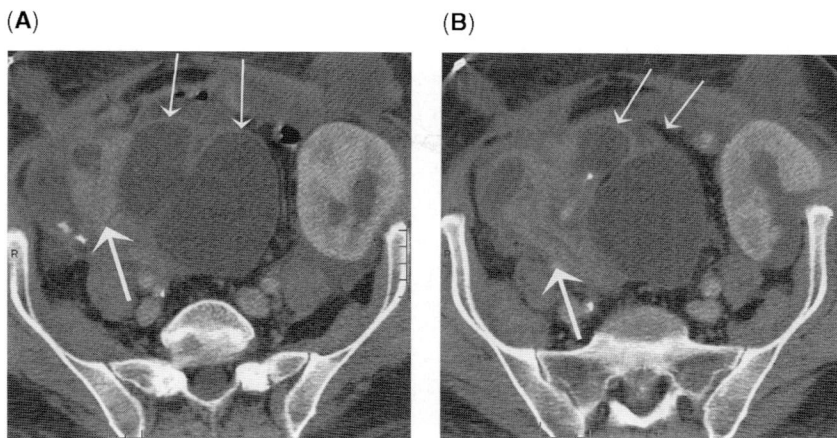

**Figure 14** Computed tomography (CT); allograft pseudocyst. (**A** and **B**) CT shows a multilobulated, encapsulated pelvic fluid collection (*thin arrows*) adjacent to the pancreatic allograft (*bold arrows*). Note left-sided renal allograft.

## Vascular Complications

A variety of vascular anastomoses are utilized, most involving the arterial anastomosis to the right external, common, or internal iliac artery. Venous drainage can be systemic (usually, the right external or common iliac vein) or portal (usually the superior mesenteric vein). Proper performance and interpretation of cross-sectional imaging or angiography are impossible without clear communication to the radiologists regarding the details of the vascular anastomoses.

    Vascular thrombosis is the second most common cause of pancreatic graft dysfunction after rejection, and, if not recognized early, will result in parenchymal infarction or necrosis, which would require pancreatectomy. Clinical signs of vessel thrombosis include sudden loss of graft function (e.g., hyperglycemia) with focal tenderness over a swollen gland. Vascular thrombosis is divided into acute and chronic graft thrombosis. Acute graft thrombosis usually occurs soon after transplantation, is more common in pancreatic than in other visceral transplants, and constitutes the most frequent cause of early graft failure. Among the reasons cited are the relatively small vessel size with reduced flow through the pancreas, the complex reconstruction of the vascular anastomoses, kinking or redundancy of the blood vessels, and injury caused by pancreatitis. Venous thrombosis is more common than arterial thrombosis, especially in the early postoperative period. Delayed graft thrombosis is an autoimmune phenomenon thought to be related to obliterative small vessel arteritis, which, in turn, leads to proximal vessel occlusion.

**(A)**            **(B)**

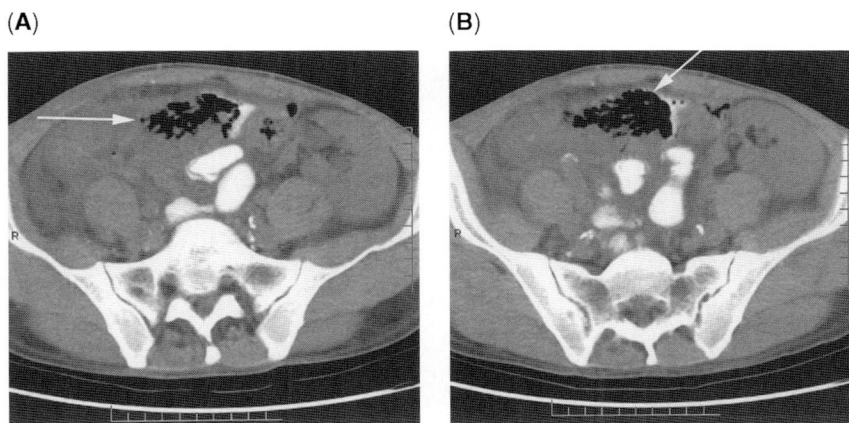

**Figure 15** Computed tomography; allograft necrosis. (**A** and **B**) The pancreatic graft is replaced with mottled gas (*arrows*) indicating infarction. There is little fluid evident to indicate pus.

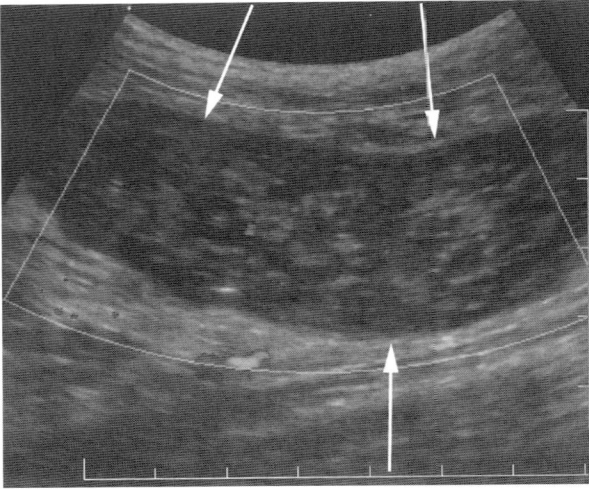

**Figure 16** Ultrasound; allograft necrosis. The allograft (*arrows*) is enlarged, hypoechoic, and shows no parenchymal vascularity.

The imaging modality of choice for vascular complications is sonography with color or spectral Doppler imaging. The infarcted pancreatic allograft is enlarged, hypoechoic, and heterogeneous (Fig. 16). Thrombosis must be demonstrated by both the absence of arterial or venous tracings in addition to the presence of intraluminal echogenic material occluding the vessel. Absence of color flow alone is insufficient to establish the diagnosis. However, if the donor graft or splenic veins are not visualized, the absence of venous tracings in the allograft parenchyma in combination with arterial resistive indices ≥1 has been shown to be highly suggestive of venous thrombosis in the first 12 days after transplantation (29). In bladder-drained cases, ultrasound is generally successful at detecting normal or abnormal flow within the anastomotic vessels. However, an experienced sonographer must optimize the scan parameters for small vessel flow, or a falsely positive diagnosis of vessel thrombosis is likely (13).

As stated earlier, MRI in combination with MRA can demonstrate the presence and extent of graft thrombosis and are increasingly being used over catheter angiography and CTA as a diagnostic modality (Fig. 17). MRA has the distinct advantage of mapping the entire arterial and venous anatomy, including the superior mesenteric artery and vein, and graft

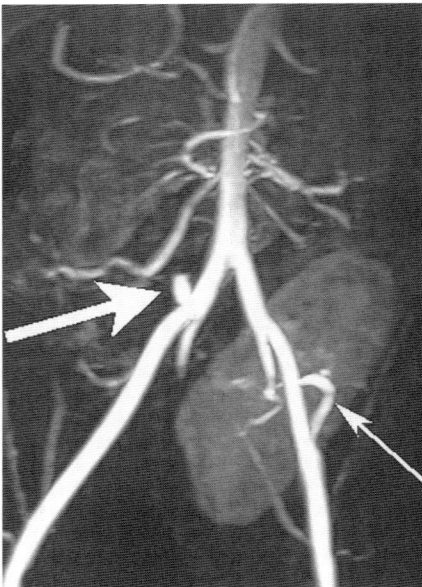

**Figure 17** Magnetic resonance angiogram (MRA); arterial graft occlusion. MRA shows occlusion of the arterial graft (*short arrow*) to the right side pancreatic allograft, and normal perfusion of the left renal graft (*long arrow*).

veins, which are infrequently seen on US. Graft viability is more accurately assessed by MRI. MRA is increasingly used to monitor anticoagulation therapy in patients with venous stump thrombosis, given the accurate delineation of the thrombus (19).

Catheter angiography is being used for embolotherapy (Figs. 18A,B). Radionuclide imaging may indirectly suggest vascular thrombosis by demonstrating decreased graft perfusion and uptake of the radiotracer and is used in the early posttransplantation period.

Doppler US is also useful in the diagnosis of anastomotic stenosis and pseudoaneurysm formation, which can further be evaluated by CTA or MRA. Arterial pseudoaneurysms at or near the anastomosis may occur, particularly as a result of adjacent infection or inflammation, made worse by the digestive action of exocrine secretions (17,18,22,23,28).

As the majority of recipients have peripheral vascular disease, vascular inflow to the allograft may be compromised by atherosclerotic plaques, which can be evaluated by MRA, and subsequently by diagnostic and therapeutic catheter angiography if needed.

## Bleeding

"Excessive" bleeding complicates about 1% of pancreatic transplantations. Clinical findings include pain and a falling hematocrit. Ultrasound would typically demonstrate nonspecific fluid collections, although low-level echoes or fluid–fluid levels may suggest a complex fluid collection. On a nonenhanced CT scan, the appearance of blood is quite specific, being higher than muscle density. Clotted blood or bleeding related to anticoagulation is easily diagnosed, the latter having a characteristic "hematocrit effect" (cellular fluid level).

Bleeding may also be intraluminal (enteric or bladder) and may be related to over anticoagulation, ischemia, or peptic ulceration. This is usually an endoscopic rather than radiologic diagnosis.

## Anastomotic Leak

The incidence, diagnostic evaluation, and sequelae of anastomotic leaks are related to the type of anastomosis constructed. Again, the complex surgical procedure and the presence of digestive enzymes make this complication uniquely common to pancreatic transplantation.

In bladder-drained cases, anastomotic leaks occur in as many as 14% of cases (30). Those that occur within the first few weeks after surgery usually involve some disruption of the pancreaticoduodenocystostomy anastomosis or disruption at the oversewn duodenal stump. These are often accompanied by significant local tissue necrosis and abscess, and patients have severe local pain but usually good graft function. Early leaks are attributed to surgical technical factors, whereas later leaks are felt to be due to infection, rejection, pancreatitis, or duodenitis. The diagnosis involves instillation of contrast medium into the bladder (Fig. 1). Small subacute

**(A)**                                              **(B)**

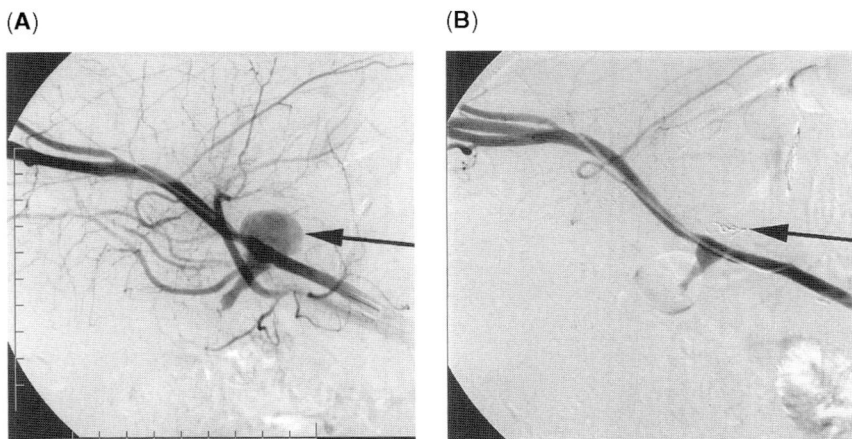

**Figure 18**   Angiography; pseudoaneurysm. (**A**) Catheter angiogram shows a pseudoaneurysm (*arrow*) arising from the pancreatic arterial graft. (**B**) An embolic coil (*arrow*) was placed into the aneurysm via the angiographic catheter, causing thrombosis.

leaks may be best diagnosed by a radionuclide voiding cystogram or a conventional fluoro-scopic cystogram with iodinated contrast medium. Our preferred method of evaluating anasto-motic leak (pancreatitis or abscess) is to obtain CT scans through the abdomen and pelvis both before and after the instillation of dilute contrast material into the bladder (30). The wall of the urinary bladder is usually evident, and the staple lines at the margins of the DS serve as useful anatomical landmarks. Extraluminal contrast media is diagnostic of a leak. Therapy for a sub-stantial leak is usually surgical, especially for an intraperitoneal leak, but a localized collection can usually be drained by closed drainage with ultrasound or CT guidance.

Leaks related to enteric drainage are more difficult to diagnose (17). Unless the surgeon has left a catheter from the skin to access the anastomosed bowel segment, it is very difficult to opacify or identifies a leak. The roux loop, if utilized, usually does not become opacified by orally administered contrast media. A loculated extraluminal fluid and/or gas may be present, and can be drained under ultrasound or CT guidance.

## Infection

Fever and sepsis are quite common in transplant recipients. The cause may be specific to the pancreatic transplantation (such as anastomotic leak or infected pancreatic necrosis), related to the immunocompromised state of the patient (e.g., opportunistic infection or posttransplant lymphoproliferative disorder), or simply related to the postoperative state of the patient [e.g., atelectasis, wound infection (Figs. 19A–C)]. CT is the most efficient means of evaluating such patients, and the entire abdomen from the lung bases to the symphysis pubis should be scanned.

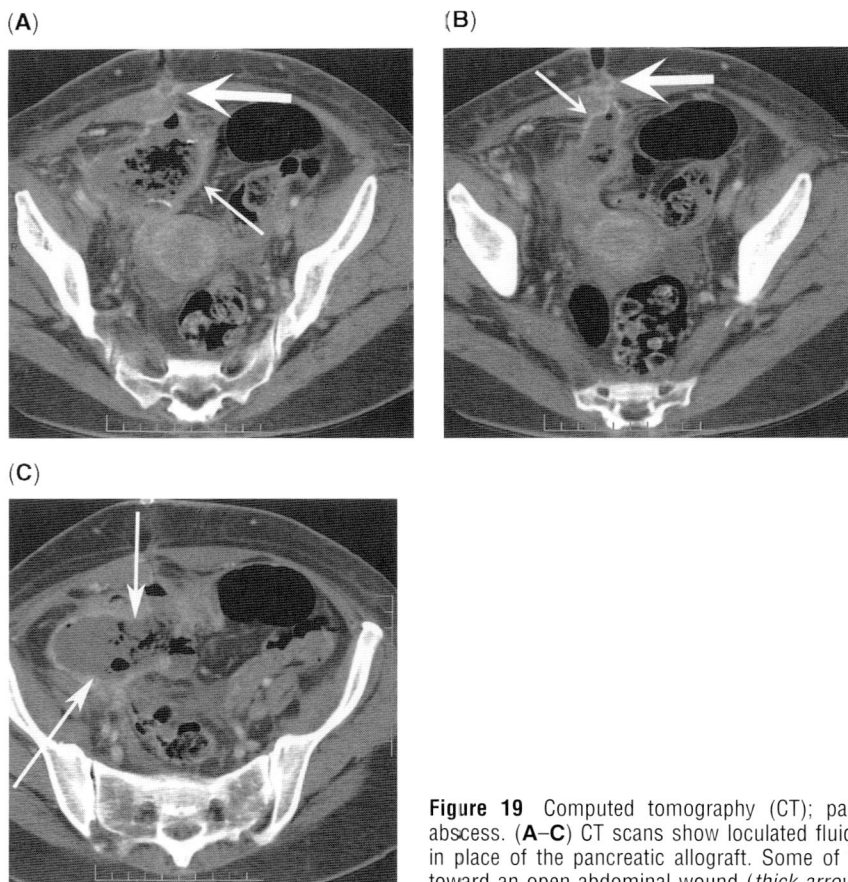

(A)

(B)

(C)

**Figure 19** Computed tomography (CT); pancreatic infarction and abscess. (**A–C**) CT scans show loculated fluid and gas (*thin arrows*) in place of the pancreatic allograft. Some of the gas and fluid track toward an open abdominal wound (*thick arrows*).

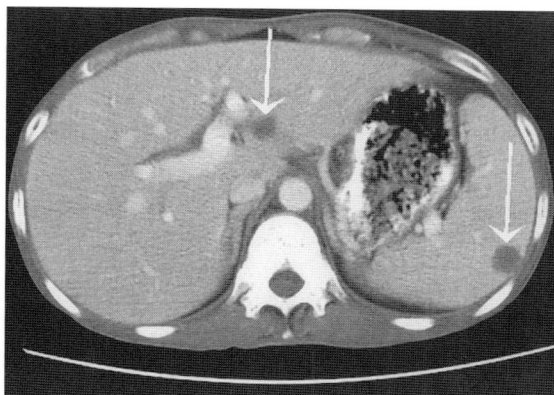

**Figure 20** Computed tomography (CT); posttransplant lymphoproliferative disorder. CT shows focal masses (*arrows*) within the liver and spleen, which were biopsied and proved to be posttransplant lymphoproliferative disorder.

An abscess is a loculated, encapsulated fluid collection, sometimes containing gas. Many abscesses can be treated effectively with CT or ultrasound-guided catheter drainage (Figs. 8A,B).

A common source of abdominal pain and fever in the posttransplant patient is enterocolitis. CT demonstrates a thick-walled bowel, often with a submucosal "halo" of edema or a "thumbprint" pattern of mucosal thickening. *C. difficile* is the most common specific causative organism for "pseudomembranous colitis."

## Urologic Complications

For patients with bladder drainage, urologic complications may occur, which has led to the development of the portal-enteric drainage as a primary procedure. Almost all patients develop at least transient hematuria, probably because of bladder manipulation. More severe or sustained hematuria, spasm, or frequency may be related to cystitis from pancreatic exocrine secretions. Cystitis and bladder infections are more frequent in bladder-drained pancreases. For patients who present with delayed onset of gross painless hematuria, ulceration of the DS may be the source. Evaluation of hematuria and cystitis is generally done by cystoscopy rather than by imaging.

The enzymatic assault on the urothelium may also result in urethral inflammation, stricture, or even disruption. In such cases, retrograde urethrography can be diagnostic.

## Posttransplantation Lymphoproliferative Disorder

Posttransplantation lymphoproliferative disorder (PTLD) is a rare complication of pancreas transplantation. PTLD has a spectrum of manifestations from benign lymphoid hyperplasia to aggressive malignant lymphoma. Extranodal involvement is the hallmark of PTLD, with the bowel and liver being common sites (Fig. 20). PTLD may involve the pancreatic allograft itself, usually manifested as a diffuse enlargement of the allograft, which is indistinguishable from rejection or pancreatitis by imaging techniques (31).

## SUMMARY

In the evaluation of pancreatic transplants, imaging should begin with US, which is best for assessing vascular integrity, especially in the early postoperative period. CT is useful in the evaluation for extra-allograft processes, especially sepsis, as it is often performed without intravenous contrast because of the nephrotoxic effects of iodinated contrast agent. MRI with 3D contrast-enhanced MRA is an accurate technique that is increasingly being used if sonography does not provide sufficient diagnostic information for vessel integrity and graft parenchyma viability. Imaging procedures are sensitive in the detection of graft dysfunction, but lack specificity in distinguishing among various parenchymal abnormalities, especially soon after transplantation. At this time, there is no reliable imaging modality to assess for acute rejection, although US- and CT-guided percutaneous biopsies are performed to diagnose and grade the severity of rejection. Percutaneous catheter drainage of certain fluid collections can be both diagnostic and curative. The optimal diagnosis and management of pancreatic transplant complications require close communication between radiologists and the surgeons caring for the patients.

## REFERENCES

1. Hirsch H, Fernandez-Ulloa M, Munda R, Fisher RA, Moulton JS, Hugh CJ. Diagnosis of segmental necrosis in a pancreas transplant by thallium-201 perfusion scintigraphy. J Nucl Med 1991; 32:1605–1607.
2. Elgazzar AH, Munda R, Fernandez-Ulloa M, Clark J, Ryan JR, Hughes JA. Scintigraphic evaluation of pancreatic transplants using technetium-99m Sestamibi. J Nucl Med 1995; 36:771–777.
3. van der Hern LG, van der Linder CJ, Ticheler CHJM, Hoitsma AJ, Corstens FHM. Early detection of post-transplant graft dysfunction with technetium-99m-HMPAO scintigraphy. J Nucl Med 1994; 35:1488–1490.
4. Kamps D, Cook K, Lieberman LM, Sollinger HW, Warner T. Early detection of pancreatic rejection with indium-labeled platelet scanning. Curr Surg 1984;29–32.
5. Sollinger HW, Lieberman LM, Kamps D, Warner T, Cook K. Diagnosis of early pancreas allograft rejection with indium-111-oxine-labeled platelets. Transplant Proc 1984; 3(XVI), pp 23–27.
6. Jurewicz WA, Buckels JAC, Dykes JGA, et al. 111-Indium platelets in monitoring pancreatic allografts in man. Br J Surg 1985; 72:228–231.
7. Letourneau JG, Maile CW, Sutherland DER, Feinberg SB. Ultrasound and computed tomography in the evaluation of pancreatic transplantation. Radiol Clin North Am 1987; 23:345–355.
8. Patel B, Markivee CR, Mahanta B, Vas W, George E, Garvin P. Pancreatic transplantation: scintigraphy, US, and CT. Radiology 1988; 167:685–687.
9. Nikolaides P, Amin RK, Hwang CM, et al. Role of sonography in pancreatic transplantation. Radiographics 2003; 23:939–949.
10. Wong JJ, Krebs TL, Klassen DK, et al. Sonographic evaluation of acute pancreatic transplant rejection: Doppler analysis versus guided percutaneous biopsy. AJR 1996; 166:803–807.
11. Kuhr CS, Davis CL, Barr D, et al. Use of ultrasound and cystoscopically guided pancreatic allograft biopsies and transabdominal renal allograft biopsies: safety and efficacy in kidney–pancreas transplant recipients. J Urol 1995; 153:316–321.
12. Nelson NL, Lowell JA, Taylor RJ, Stratta RJ. Pancreas transplants: efficacy of US guided cystoscopic biopsy. Radiology 1994; 191:283.
13. Pozniak MA, Propeck PA, Kelcz F, Sollinger J. Imaging of pancreas transplants. Radiol Clin North Am 1995; 33:581–594.
14. Freund MC, Steurer W, Gassner EM, et al. Spectrum of imaging findings after pancreas transplantation with enteric exocrine drainage. AJR 2004; 182:919–925.
15. Atwell RD, Gorman B, Larson TS, et al. Pancreas transplants: experience with 232 percutaneous US-guided biopsy procedures in 88 patients. Radiology 2004; 231:845–849.
16. Moulton JS, Mundra, Weiss MA, Lubbers DJ. Pancreatic transplants: CT with clinical and pathologic correlation. Radiology 1989; 172:21–26.
17. Dachman AH, Newmark GM, Thistlewaite JR Jr., et al. Imaging of pancreatic transplantation using portal venous and enteric exocrine drainage. AJR 1998; 171:157–163.
18. Hagspiel KD, Nandular K, Barkholder B, et al. Contrast-enhanced MR angiography after pancreatic transplantation: normal experience and vascular complications. AJR 2005; 184:465–473.
19. Dobos W, Roberts DA, Insko EK, et al. Contrast-enhanced MR angiography for evaluation of vascular complications of pancreas transplant. Radiographics 2005; 25:687–695.
20. Yuh WTC, Hunsicker LG, Nghiem DD. et al. Pancreatic transplants: evaluation with MR imaging. Radiology 1989; 170:171–177.
21. Krebs TL, Daly B, Wong-You-Cheong J, Carrol K, Bartlett ST. Acute pancreatic transplant rejection: evaluation with dynamic contrast-enhanced MR imaging compared with histopathologic analysis. Radiology 1999; 210:437–442.
22. Tobben PJ, Zajko AB, Sumkin JH, et al. Pseudoaneurysms complicating organ transplantation: roles of CT, duplex sonography and angiography. Radiology 1988; 169:65–70.
23. Snider JF, Hunter DW, Kuni CC, Castaneda-Zuniga WR, Letourneau JG. Pancreatic transplantation: radiologic evaluation of vascular complications. Radiology 1991; 178:749–753.
24. Rasmussen K, Burcharth F, Thomsen HS, Rygaard H. Monitoring of pancreas-graft perfusion by radionuclide and digital subtraction angiography. Diabetes 1989; 38:21–23.
25. Klassen DK, Weir MR, Cangro CB, et al. Pancreas allograft biopsy: safety of percutaneous biopsy—results of a large experience. Transplantation 2002; 73:553–555.
26. Aideyan DA, Foshager MC, Benedetti E, et al. Correlation of the arterial resistive index in pancreas transplants of patients with transplant rejection. AJR 1997; 168:1445–1447.
27. Papadimitriou JC, Drachenberg CB, Klassen DK, et al. Histologic grading of chronic pancreas allograft rejection/graft sclerosis. Am J transplant 2003; 5:599–605.
28. Heverhagen JT, Wagner H-J, Ebel H, et al. Pancreatic transplant: noninvasive evaluation with secretin-augmented MR pancreatography and MR perfusion measurements: preliminary results. Radiology 2004; 233:273–280.

29. Foshager MC, Hedlund LT, Troppmann C, et al. Venous thrombosis of pancreatic transplants: diagnosis by duplex sonography. AJR 1997; 169:11,269–11,273.
30. Bischof TP, Theoni RF, Melzer JS. Diagnosis of duodenal leaks from kidney–pancreas transplants in patients with duodenovesical anastomoses: value of CT cystography. AJR 1995; 165:349–354.
31. Meador TL, Krebs TL, Wong JJ, et al. Imaging features of post-transplantation lymphoproliferative disorder in pancreas transplant recipients. AJR 2000; 174:121–124.

# 22 | Islet Cell Transplantation

**Cynthia A. Smetanka**
*Thomas E. Starzl Transplantation Institute, University of Pittsburgh School of Medicine, Pittsburgh, Pennsylvania, U.S.A.*

**Rita Bottino**
*Islet Isolation Core, University of Pittsburgh, Pittsburgh, Pennsylvania, U.S.A.*

**Massimo Trucco**
*Division of Immunogenetics, Children's Hospital of Pittsburgh, Pittsburgh, Pennsylvania, U.S.A.*

## INTRODUCTION

Diabetes is one of the most devastating diseases known to mankind. Since it has the propensity to affect multiple organ systems, it is responsible for a tremendous amount of morbidity and mortality. Besides shortening life expectancy, it also seriously impairs the quality of life. It remains the most common cause of blindness and renal failure, and also causes impotence, neuropathy, various infections, vascular, and heart diseases. The cost of this disease is staggering and continues to climb. In 2002, the direct and indirect expenditures related to diabetes in the United States were estimated at $132 billion (1).

Because of the high impact this disease has on society, there is a tremendous amount of interest in exploring new treatment options. Despite the success of whole organ pancreas transplantation, an increasing interest has focused on cellular transplantation as a method to restore glucose homeostasis. Since only the insulin-secreting cells are ultimately required, islet cell transplantation and other cellular therapies have a great potential for the treatment of diabetes.

## HISTORY OF ISLET CELL TRANSPLANTATION

Islet cell transplantation is commonly described as a new treatment for diabetic patients. However, the history of its development dates back to the 1860s. Paul Langerhans first described the pancreatic islets in 1869, while working as a medical student (2). The first transplant using pancreatic fragments to reverse diabetes was done by Minkowski in 1892, but significant interest in the use of pancreatic tissue really began when Minkowski and Van Mering showed that the removal of the canine pancreas resulted in hyperglycemia in 1889 (3). Up until that time, the link between the pancreas and its role in disease was still very controversial.

In 1922, when insulin was discovered, it became possible to treat and save many lives that would have been lost to the severe consequences of insulin-dependent diabetes mellitus. Therefore, this early work on pancreatic fragments did not progress at this time because it was believed that insulin was the ultimate treatment. It was not known at that time that the chronic complications of diabetes could still develop despite intensive insulin therapy.

As clinicians and scientists learned more about diabetes and its complications, they became interested in separating the endocrine cells of the pancreas for possible treatment. In 1964, Hellerstrom used a microdissection technique to isolate islets from a rat pancreas (4). Moskalewski improved upon this technique by using collagenase to digest pig pancreata to improve the yield and function (5). An additional development was then made by Lacy and Kostianovsky, who introduced the idea of ductal distension of the pancreas, which they applied to the isolation of rat islets (6). The first successful islet transplant for the treatment of a diabetic animal was done by Ballinger and Lacy, who achieved euglycemia following the transplantation of 400 to 600 islets in diabetic Lewis rats (7). This demonstrated the feasibility of islet cell transplantation and paved the way for future clinical applications. The basic principles described by Lacy for the isolation of the islets are still used today, with some additional technical advances.

The most significant advance occurred in 1986, also at the Lacy laboratory. There, Camillo Ricordi et al. introduced the automated method for human islet isolation (8). In this method, the entire pancreas was loaded into a chamber, which became known as the Ricordi chamber. This automated method (described below) quickly became the standard method of islet isolation, and is still used today. Ricordi returned to Milan in 1988 to begin a clinical islet program, but just before starting, Ricordi was recruited by Dr. Thomas E. Starzl at the University of Pittsburgh. There Ricordi joined Daniel Mintz, Rodolfo Alejandro, and the Pittsburgh team to set up the human islet isolation lab. Just as the lab was completed, the St. Louis group reported the reversal of diabetes in a patient who had received a human islet transplant (9). Unfortunately, this patient was insulin independent for only 12 days (10).

It was at this time that the Pittsburgh trial began in January 1990. This trial represented the first unequivocal success of human islet allotransplantation, which resulted in the long-term reversal of diabetes (11). This initial study was a trial of nine patients who became diabetic after upper-abdominal exenteration, followed by liver transplantation and the infusion of allogeneic human islets. Early islet allograft function was seen in every recipient, which was sustained in five of these patients (11). Two of the best clinical results were seen in patients who received islets from a single donor (11). Some of these patients remained insulin free for up to six years. The islets were transplanted using a steroid-free protocol and the new drug FK-506 (tacrolimus—Prograf[®]) (11). The unprecedented success of this Pittsburgh trial was a major breakthrough in the field, which resulted in the initiation and resumption of clinical protocols for islet transplantation.

During the time period from 1990 to 1998, 267 islet allografts were transplanted; however, only 12.4% became insulin independent for more than a year (12). The reasons for these poor results included such factors as insufficient β-cell mass, the loss of β-cells during the isolation and transplantation process, and toxicity from the immunosuppressive regimen. In addition, these diabetic recipients also had the problem of autoimmunity, which might not have been fully appreciated at that time. With these poor results, the enthusiasm that occurred with the initial Pittsburgh trial was significantly dampened.

In 2000, a significant breakthrough occurred, with what became known as the Edmonton protocol. This protocol was used in a trial of seven patients with Type I diabetes (T1D), who all became insulin independent after islet transplantation using this new steroid-free protocol (13). This immunosuppressive regimen was initiated immediately prior to transplantation and consisted of the following drugs: sirolimus, low-dose tacrolimus, and daclizumab, a humanized monoclonal antibody against the interleukin-2 receptor (13). Besides the change in the immunosuppressive regimen, this trial also addressed other issues that were an impediment to successful transplantation. An increased number of islet cells were transplanted, which included more than one donor pancreas prepared in a xenoprotein-free medium (13). It is believed that the coating of the islets by a xenoprotein may target them for destruction. The Edmonton group also felt that their immunosuppressive regimen protected the islets not only from alloimmune reactivity but also from autoimmunity (13).

The news of this trial spread throughout the world. An unprecedented interest in islet cell transplantation blossomed, not only in the scientific and medical community, but also among the diabetic patient population. With the widespread use of the Internet, patients began contacting centers for information about clinical trials. New islet transplant centers began to spring up all over the world. Currently, there are 17 countries involved in human islet trials, with 19 centers in the United States. Numerous centers are actively collaborating, which will hopefully lead to a more rapid advancement of the field. Many improvements are being made in isolation techniques and in methods to minimize loss from thrombosis/inflammation; further improvements are being made in immunosuppressive regimens, and new technologies are being evolved to increase the supply of insulin-secreting cells. Overall, there have been a number of new developments that may result in a more durable survival of the islets. Ultimately, the development of an unlimited source of insulin-producing cells could significantly improve the life expectancy and quality of life for many diabetic patients.

## ISLET CELL BIOLOGY AND PHYSIOLOGY

The islets of Langerhans represent approximately 1% to 2% of the volume of the pancreas. They act as a single endocrine organ, which is comprised of several different cells. The insulin-producing β-cells represent approximately 50% to 70% of the endocrine cells. These cells are surrounded by several other endocrine cells. The majority of these cells are glucagon containing alpha cells (A cells). There are also a small number of D cells that secrete somatostatin, and PP cells that secrete pancreatic polypeptide. This cellular architecture results in autocrine effects that are mediated by the cell's own products, and also paracrine effects that influence other cells. The islets are highly vascular, with the arterioles penetrating the mantle, reaching the islet core, and then breaking up into capillaries (14). The blood flow within the islet then flows from the β-cell to the alpha and delta cells, carrying metabolic and hormonal information (14).

The vasculature of the islets exists in the form of a neurovascular stalk, which contains the parasympathetic and sympathetic nerves of the autonomic nervous system (15). These nerves allow the central nervous system to control the release of hormones from the islets using neurotransmitter receptors, such as muscarinic receptors from parasympathetic nerves for acetylcholine release and α- and β-adrenergic receptors for sympathetic release (15). These neurotransmitters are specifically involved in regulating insulin release. Acetylcholine can potentiate insulin release in response to glucose (15). Norepinephrine and epinephrine inhibit insulin secretion via the alpha-adrenergic receptors; however, activation via the β-adrenergic receptors stimulates insulin secretion (15).

Insulin secretion, which is exclusively limited to the beta cell, is controlled by glucose levels in the blood. This unique property is a combination of β-cell transcription, translation, and regulated secretory vesicle exocytosis. The insulin gene promoter is activated by a specific combination of transcription factors that are only found in the beta cell (16). This regulation is crucial. Although numerous other neuroendocrine cells have the ability to process and package exogenously expressed insulin via a different promoter into the secretory vesicles, insulin synthesis is restricted to the beta cell. This cell is the only one that has the ability to accurately sense changes in blood glucose levels and to respond in the acute setting and also on a long-term basis with appropriate insulin secretory rates. Insulin gene transcription occurs only in the beta cell, which is stimulated by increased glucose. The insulin promoter and transcription factors form a large transcription regulatory complex that involves a basic helix-loop-helix (neuro D) that combines with a specific protein, beta 2, and homeodomain factors, especially *PDX1*, along with many other factors, including the basal transcription machinery (16). The importance of these genes has been demonstrated in animal studies and also in humans (17–19). Inactivation of the beta 2/neuroD gene in mice has led to the development of severe diabetes resulting in death three to five days after birth (17). Mice that were homozygous for a targeted mutation in the *PDX1* gene were found to lack the pancreas (18). In a human report, a homozygous mutation of the *PDX1* gene resulted in the failure of pancreatic development (19).

With the necessary genetic machinery in place, the synthesis of insulin begins with the transcription of the DNA insulin gene to the messenger RNA in the cell nucleus. Then, in the ribosomes of the rough endoplasmic reticulum, the mRNA is translated to the peptide preproinsulin (15). The signal sequence is then cleaved and the proinsulin is transported to the Golgi apparatus via tiny membrane-bound vesicles (15). While the Golgi is packaging the proinsulin into secretory granules, the converting enzymes begin cleaving proinsulin to yield insulin and C-peptide (15). These secreting granules then enter a cytoplasmic storage pool, of which only 1% is available for immediate release due to its location near the plasma membrane (20). The release of these granules is thought to represent the first phase of insulin secretion, which occurs within minutes after glucose stimulation. Refilling then occurs from a larger reservoir, which is believed to represent the second phase of insulin secretion (21).

After the insulin has been synthesized and packaged into granules, there are complex signaling pathways, which result in the integration of metabolic and physiologic information so that an appropriate insulin release will occur. There are two major ion channels that are key to this signaling: the adenosine triphosphate (ATP)-sensitive potassium channel and the voltage gated calcium channel. Beta cell K-ATP channels maintain the membrane potential near the potassium equilibrium potential (22). These channels have two important receptors: the sulfonylurea receptor (SUR1) and the pore-forming (Kir6.2) subunit (23). The Kir6.2 subunit binds ATP and closes the channel, allowing the cell to depolarize. SUR1 binds nucleotide diphosphates in the presence of magnesium (such as Mg-ADP) and increases channel opening. Increasing glucose levels will convert more ADP to ATP through glycolytic and oxidative metabolism so that the opening effect of mg-adenosine diphosphate (ADP) is reduced, revealing the closing effect of free ATP. The depolarization due to the closing of K-ATP channels opens voltage-dependent calcium channels (22). At a glucose threshold level of near 5 mMol, the glucose-induced membrane depolarization is sufficient to trigger the opening of voltage-dependent calcium channels in the β-cell membrane (15). This admits the extracellular calcium into the pool of free calcium intracellularly, which then interacts with the exocytic components to fuse the granules to the plasma membrane, releasing insulin.

The calcium channels have an important, complex role in maintaining tight glucose control. The opening of these channels is precisely coordinated, resulting in the production of rhythmic oscillations of the membrane potential, which consists of trains of action potentials, which are superimposed on depolarized plateau potentials (24). At low glucose levels, the plateaus are brief and separated by silent phases. At half-maximal levels, the silent phases are brief and the plateaus are longer. At high glucose levels, the silent phases are gone and the cells remain depolarized, spiking persistently (24). The rhythmical pacing of the calcium uptake during the bursts of spikes is in parallel with the oscillation of the free calcium levels within the cells that are synchronized throughout the islets via electrical coupling (15). This modulation is due to the progressive closure of K-ATP channels, as the metabolic rate increases secondary to increased glucose stimulation.

In a simplistic analogy, the K-ATP channel acts as a control switch (22). When the switch is on, the potassium ions migrate out of the channel and hyperpolarize the beta cells, which puts a halt to the signal flow that controls insulin secretion. When the switch is off, the K-ATP channel removes the brake, which allows insulin release by the elevation of intracellular calcium, which then initiates the fusion of the insulin granules and the β-cell membrane. However, under normal conditions, the calcium signal is insufficient for the regulation of glucose-responsive insulin release (25). Pharmacological maneuvers have shown that elevating not only intracellular calcium but also glucose metabolism is necessary for dose-dependent, stimulated insulin release (22). K-ATP channels that are localized to the β-cell membrane couple glucose metabolism to the plasma membrane excitability, which switches on calcium influx for release. This triggers exocytosis of the primed insulin granules that are docked at the plasma membrane, which corresponds to the first phase release (20). K-ATP channels that are localized to the insulin granule membrane may have a role in coupling glucose metabolism to granule transport and exocytosis in a dose-dependent manner, which would represent the second phase response (22).

The study of these important channels, cellular signaling, and islet physiology are very clinically relevant. K-ATP channels are targets for antidiabetic drugs such as sulfonylureas, which close K-ATP channels by binding to the SUR1 receptor (15). Studies on calcium signaling are progressing to trying to develop better methods of viability testing for the islets so that in vivo results can be more accurately predicted. Increased knowledge of beta cell and islet physiology may enable us to establish improved methods to isolate and transplant these cells and also to develop new sources of insulin-producing cells. Understanding the precise mechanisms that the beta cell uses to sense and maintain normal glucose levels will ultimately be necessary.

## HUMAN ISLET ISOLATION—DONOR SELECTION, PROCEDURES, AND ASSESSMENT

Islet isolation is a highly specialized procedure. Generally, the pancreata that are not suitable for whole pancreas transplantation are allocated for use in islet transplantation and research. Pancreata that are used for islet transplantation are obtained from brain-dead, heart-beating multiorgan donors, who are usually between the ages of 15 and 50 (sometimes slightly older). Exclusion criteria include a history of diabetes, pancreatic trauma, any extracranial tumors, risk factors or positive testing for HIV, hepatitis B, or hepatitis C, and systemic infection (26). ABO compatibility and a negative cross-match are required. Human leukocyte antigen (HLA) matching is not routinely required (26). Additional criteria are also considered such as the cause of death, time in the ICU, overall hospital course, hemodynamic instability and the use of vasopressors, medications administered, such as steroids, and laboratory values, such as glucose and amylase. The pancreas harvesting procedure required for islet isolation use is virtually identical to the one required for whole organ transplantation. The organs are perfused in situ via the abdominal aorta with cold histidine tryptophan ketoglutarate or

University of Wisconsin solution. Cold ischemia time prior to islet isolation should be limited to 12 hours, since the islets are exquisitely sensitive to the ischemic damage that occurs during cold storage.

A major improvement in storage conditions of the pancreas for islets has been the introduction of the two-layer method (University of Wisconsin solution—perfluorocarbon plus $O_2$) that allows better preservation of the islets even over 12 hours of cold ischemia (27). The technique for human islet isolation has evolved from the classical methods mastered for animal islets. In the early 1920s, teleosts, insulin-producing cells, organized in clusters called Brockmann bodies (28), could be easily mechanically excised from the abdomen of the fish. Rodent islets were obtained only after the introduction of digestive solutions such as collagenases and the development of ductal distension of the pancreas (6), but large mammals and human islets remained difficult to isolate until the introduction of the semi-automated method developed by Camillo Ricordi et al. (8). Before the development of the semi-automated method, using the classic stationary digestion, which was used in the isolation of rodent islets, would have allowed the retrieval of only a minimal part of the human islet mass, making it impossible to even consider transplanting islets from deceased donors to human recipients. The semi-automated method, which implies the use of a digestion apparatus (the Ricordi chamber) (29), specifically designed to contain the human pancreas and maintain a flow of solution into and out of the system, has been modified over the years in an effort to further improve the isolation process and outcomes.

The isolation procedure involves several steps. First, organs are trimmed of as much surrounding fat and lymph nodes as possible. The main pancreatic duct is then cannulated according to size. Exogenous enzymes (collagenases, consisting of commercially available blends of purified collagenases and neutral proteases such as Liberase HI) (30) are reconstituted and dissolved in cold (4°C) Hank's balanced salt solution. The enzyme solution is then prewarmed to approximately 30°C before injection into the pancreas. Pancreata are intraductally injected with enzyme solution in either a recirculation system designed by Rajotte et al. (31), or manually via a syringe. Sufficient inflation of the pancreatic organ is an absolute necessity to obtain appropriate digestion of the tissue. Recently, a Swedish group has tested the use of metyltioninklorid and indermil (topical tissue adhesive) applied to the organ during distension to detect leakage of injected collagenase and to repair the damaged pancreatic glands (32). After inflation with warm enzyme solution, the pancreas is transferred to a Ricordi chamber, the apparatus designed to allow gentle disruption of the human pancreas. This chamber allows for chemical (enzymes) as well as mechanical (a chamber containing marbles) digestion of the pancreas. The chamber temperature is warmed to and maintained at 37°C and manually, mechanically shaken to allow for disruption of the pancreatic tissue. Chamber output is carefully monitored by taking regular samples that are then observed with a microscope after dithizone staining (dithizone is an organic chemical compound that binds to Zn+, which is abundant in the secretory granules of the islet cells), which allows for the identification of the islets. This helps to determine the condition of the islets, i.e., shape, size, architecture, condition, etc., and the degree of contamination with exocrine tissue. By monitoring the condition of the islets, it is possible to make informed judgments on when to stop the warm, enzymatic digestion and begin collecting the islets.

In the classical method, when large-sized, free islets are released with abundant digest, the digestion circuit is cooled by the addition of cold medium (containing serum or derived proteins) in order to abruptly reduce enzymatic activity. Cold dilution is then carried out for approximately 45 to 60 minutes (33). The switch from warm recirculation to cold collection is critical for allowing sufficient digestion of the pancreas while, at the same time, avoiding excess enzymatic activity on the cells that have already been released. In order to compensate for this problem, an additional collection can be added so that collection is started as soon as free, intact islets are seen in the digestion samples (34). For this collection, warm Hank's balanced salt solution is added into the circuit, while the digest is collected in 250 mL conical tubes. The cell suspension is immediately centrifuged and the supernatant containing the enzyme is again added to the digestion circuit. The cell pellet is then washed with fresh, serum-enriched, cold medium and maintained on ice. Centrifugation and refilling of the circuit is maintained continuously for approximately 10 to 15 minutes. After warm recirculation and collection, the circuit is filled with cold medium. The collection of the cells is continued using the previously described classical method. The cells are then washed and resuspended in University of Wisconsin solution and maintained on ice for about one hour. This allows for a reduction in dead cells and acinar tissue. The cells are then resuspended in polysucrose solution and purified with a COBE 2991 cell separator using discontinuous or continuous Euro-Ficoll gradients. The fractions of cells that are enriched in islets are either freshly infused into patients or subjected to culture. Islets are rarely obtained in highly purified fractions. Usually, exocrine tissue is always present in the preparation including the islet graft.

Islets represent approximately 1% to 2% of the pancreatic tissue. They are commonly quantified using an islet equivalent number, a parameter that expresses the volume of the islets in reference to an arbitrary islet of 150 μm diameter. Each islet is composed of a variable number of cells (500–2000), with sizes that range from 25 to 500 μm. The human pancreas contains approximately 700,000 to 1.5 millions islets, but only 50% can be retrieved consistently. Islet yield can be affected by a number of factors that include donor characteristics (age, body mass index, clinical history) or isolation-specific factors (reagent lots, time of digestion). Many groups have studied and reported on factors that can play a role in the isolation outcome.

Despite improvements in the isolation process, there are still many problems associated with islet isolation, particularly when it comes to using them for transplantation. The islet isolation process remains inefficient, often yielding an insufficient mass of functional islet cells needed to achieve adequate function in the recipient. The Edmonton study suggested that it was necessary to transplant each recipient with a minimal dose of 9000 IEQ/kg in order to achieve consistent insulin independence. Under current protocols, this would require obtaining islets from two to four different donor organs (35). Because of a limited and unpredictable supply of donor organs and the time and resources needed to isolate islets, this becomes a difficult task. Thus, efforts are being made to improve the yield of individual isolations. Many factors contribute to islet loss and insufficient metabolic function after transplantation (36–39). New data have shown that islet function is undermined by stressful events before transplantation (40,41). Improvements must be made in procurement procedures, storage, isolation and culture, as well as in immunosuppressive protocols, all of which contribute to islet loss and functional impairment. The field has to advance significantly if islet transplantation is to completely replace whole organ transplantation.

Clinical trials require quality control of the isolated islets. The release of islet batches for transplantation must meet protocol requirements for testing their function in vitro and in vivo in animal models. One of the requirements for appropriate function is the ability of islets to respond to ambient glucose variation with adequate and controlled insulin release. Islet samples can be loaded on a perifusion apparatus that allows the flow of a solution containing different glucose concentrations to stimulate the islets over time and determine their efficiency in stimulating release with increasing glucose concentration and reduction under nonstimulated conditions. Viability is also determined using confocal technology and viable fluorescent dye. Islet cell composition can be determined by immunostaining using anti-insulin (a marker of beta cells), anti-glucagon (alpha cells), anti-CK19 (ductal cells), and anti-amylase (exocrine) antibodies, which results in a more accurate estimate of the purity of the fraction compared to dithizone staining.

The most reliable assay for the assessment of islet function remains the in vivo study. There are several mouse models (nude mice, NODscid, Scid mice) that can accept implanted human tissue without unwanted rejection. These special recipients can be rendered diabetic by the injection of Streptozotocin or Alloxan, compounds that selectively destroy pancreatic beta cells and result in a diabetic state in the mouse. Diabetic animals can receive batches of human islets (500–1000 islets) under the kidney capsule as a cell pellet, which can reverse the diabetic state by the insulin released from the islet graft. Transplantation outcome is usually a good indicator of the quality of the islet preparation.

To date, however, there is no reliable and simple method that provides sufficient information in a short time on the quality of the islet preparation. A large effort is being made to find reliable and reproducible approaches that define islet potency. This is also required by the Food and Drug Administration (FDA), which regulates the process of isolation as well as clinical islet transplantation trials.

## INDICATIONS AND PATIENT SELECTION

Currently, there are three major indications for islet transplantation. The most common transplant performed is islets alone, in those patients with Type I diabetes with significant secondary complications but normal renal function. Islets can also be transplanted in patients who have received a kidney transplant, provided that it is possible to alter the immunosuppressive regimen to protect the islets. The third indication for islet transplantation is in the form of an autograft done in patients with severe chronic pancreatitis who require a pancreatectomy. In these patients, the islets are processed from their own pancreas to try to prevent the development of diabetes.

The indications for islets alone are the most extensive. There is a small amount of variability among centers; however, there are specific common indications. Candidates for islet alone transplantation are patients with Type I diabetes for greater than five years with frequent episodes of hypoglycemic unawareness, metabolic lability, and secondary complications. The most important indication is hypoglycemic unawareness. These episodes result in the need for assistance by others, frequent hospital visits, and a significant impairment in the quality of life. Metabolic lability should be persistent despite intensive insulin management efforts. This is usually defined as the monitoring of glucose levels at least three times a day with three or more insulin injections per day. An endocrinologist or a primary care physician with extensive diabetic experience should see these patients at least every three to four months. Despite this intensive insulin management, these patients usually have an HbA1C greater than 7 or 8. The C-peptide level should be $<0.5\,\text{ng/mL}$ ($<0.1\,\text{ng/mL}$ in some programs).

Potential candidates should have some evidence of progressive secondary complications, which are usually retinopathy, early nephropathy, and neuropathy. An ophthalmologist who is familiar with diabetic retinopathy must document this. Although progression is common in these patients, they must be stable at the time of transplantation. Nephropathy can be documented as a rising level of microalbuminurea, despite the use of angiotensin converting enzyme (ACE) inhibitors. However, for primary islet alone transplantation, a patient must not be in renal failure. Those patients who have end-stage renal disease can become candidates for islet after kidney transplantation or simultaneous islet/kidney transplantation. Neuropathy is also a fairly common finding which can affect many organ systems, resulting in gastroparesis, autonomic neuropathy, or a neurogenic bladder. Overall, patients who are candidates for islet alone transplantation should be those who are poorly controlled diabetics despite intensive insulin management, especially those with hypoglycemic unawareness and some evidence of secondary complications. This results in an appropriate risk–benefit profile for the transplantation of patients who will benefit most.

If a patient appears to meet the general indications for islet transplantation, then the evaluation process can begin. This evaluation process is very similar to protocols that are used for whole organ pancreas transplantation (42), but also includes some additional items related to the transplant procedure. A nurse coordinator will assist potential candidates in this evaluation process and coordinate all studies and physician consultations. An endocrinologist or medical physician who is experienced in the care of diabetic patients and a transplant surgeon will see these patients. These physicians will perform a history and physical examination and review all laboratory and medical records. A social worker will perform a psychosocial assessment to evaluate the appropriateness of candidacy and to investigate any compliance issues. Patients will see their own dentists and undergo a thorough dental exam to rule out any infectious or malignant conditions in the oral cavity. Female patients will be seen by a gynecologist for examination and Papanicolaou smear. Women who are 35 years and older will also undergo mammography. A pregnancy test will be done, as pregnancy is a definite contraindication to transplantation. (All candidates should be using appropriate contraceptive techniques.) Men over 40 years of age will obtain a prostate specific antigen (PSA level). If elevated, they will need a urological consultation and prostate biopsy. All patients 50 years and older will also be required to undergo colonoscopy. An ultrasound will also be done to assess portal vein patency and to rule out gallstones, hemangiomas, or any other liver lesion. A significant amount of blood work will be drawn, including hematological assessments, chemistries, serologies, etc. Additional studies will include chest X-ray, electrocardiogram (ECG), purified protein derivative (tuberculin skin test) (PPD), urine culture and 24-hour urine. The most important evaluation is the assessment of cardiac function. This can be done by a functional stress test; however, some programs are requiring cardiac catheterization. A summary of the required testing is given in Table 1.

The goal of this evaluation is to determine a patient's suitability for islet transplantation and to evaluate any conditions that would make the candidate ineligible. The most important

**Table 1**  Laboratory and Testing Requirements for Islet Cell Transplantation

History and physical examination, review of systems
CXR, ECG, PPD, functional stress test, ultrasound for portal vein patency and to assess for hemangiomas, gallstones, or any
    other lesions
Dental and psychosocial evaluation
Gynecological consultation for females, including PAP smear and mammography, if over 35.
PSA for men 40 years of age and older
Colonoscopy for patients older than 50
Hematology studies: CBC with differential, PT/PTT, INR, blood type (ABO, Rh), and cross-matching
Chemistries: electrolytes, BUN and creatinine, calcium, magnesium and phosphorus, complete liver panel, thyroid testing
    (thyroid stimulating hormone, T3 and T4), and amylase/lipase
Serologies: HIV, hepatitis panel, CMV, EBV, herpes zoster, herpes simplex, and varicella
Diabetes assessment: HbA1C, basal C-peptide (some programs also require stimulated C-peptide), a record of pre- and
    postprandial glucose levels (including any symptoms), fasting lipids (total cholesterol, HDL and LDL cholesterols,
    triglycerides)
Tissue typing: HLA, PRA
Autoimmune markers: GAD, insulin antibodies, islet cell antibodies
Urine tests: creatinine clearance, 24-hour protein, microalbumin, urine culture
Additional studies: Depending on the protocol, some programs will require additional diabetic studies such as various
    stimulated C-peptides, glucose tolerance testing, and possibly clamp studies

*Abbreviations*: ECG, electrocardiogram; PAP, papanicolaou; CBC, complete blood count; PT/PTT, prothrombin time/partial thromboplastin time; INR, international normalized ratio; BUN, blood-urea-nitrogen; CMV, cytomegalovirus; EBV, Epstein-Barr virus; HLA,
human leukocyte antigen.

consideration is the cardiac evaluation. Diabetic patients are well known to be at increased risk of accelerated atherosclerosis, and this needs to be evaluated carefully. Because of this risk, some programs routinely require cardiac catheterization in all patients. Others perform stress echocardiography with a minimal threshold for catheterization with any equivocal or positive finding. Other conditions such as hypertension, obesity and vascular disease, need to be carefully evaluated.

Risk factors that would adversely affect transplantation need to be evaluated and corrected, if possible. These include weight loss, possible coronary revascularization, and control of hypertension and hyperlipidemias. This evaluation should also identify any exclusion criteria so that the proper candidates will be transplanted, minimizing any potential risks. Exclusion criteria may vary among centers, although many are fairly standard. Although some patients may initially be ineligible because of cardiac issues, obesity, hypertension, etc., they may later become eligible after the appropriate treatment intervention has taken place. Table 2 lists a summary of some of the usual exclusion criteria.

Active infection and malignancy (with the exception of basal and in situ squamous skin cancers) are absolute contraindications to any cellular or organ transplant. However, once a patient is free of infection and also free of malignancy, they may become future candidates. The issue of malignancy is complex, requiring variable waiting times depending on the type

**Table 2**  Exclusion Criteria

Active infection or malignancy (except basal or in situ squamous skin cancers, which have been excised with a clear margin)
Severe cardiac disease: angiographic evidence of non-correctable coronary artery disease, recent myocardial infarction
    (within the last 6 mo), and ischemia on a functional stress test
Psychosocial issues: noncompliance, active substance abuse (which includes cigarette smoking in some programs),
    unstable psychiatric disorders such as uncontrolled psychosis or depression, inability to understand and provide informed
    consent, unwillingness or inability to take the appropriate medication, and comply with laboratory and physician visits
Abnormal liver function: elevated liver function studies, hepatitis, portal hypertension, gallstones, hemangiomas, or other
    liver lesions
Age: less than 18 or greater than 65 (some programs will transplant older individuals)
Body mass index: some programs exclude candidates with a body mass index $>26 \, kg/m^2$, while others are more liberal (up
    to $33 \, kg/m^2$)
Pregnancy: positive pregnancy test and also those who are unwilling to utilize effective contraceptive measures
Renal function: islet alone: creatinine $>1.5 \, mg/dL$, macroalbuminurea $>300 \, mg/24 \, hr$, creatinine clearance less than 60 mL/min
Other medical conditions: uncontrolled hypertension, hyperlipidemia, untreated proliferative retinopathy; use of Coumadin or
    other anticoagulants, except aspirin; medical conditions that require chronic steroid use (this is a relative exclusion
    depending on the condition and dosage)

of cancer (see Chapter 19). Severe cardiac disease is also one of the major exclusion criteria. However, some patients, with the exception of those with non-correctable disease, may also become candidates after appropriate intervention.

The evaluation of liver function is extremely important, as the islets will be placed intraportally. Patients with any abnormal lab values or lesions should not be transplanted. However, those who have gallstones can undergo cholecystectomy and become a candidate after an appropriate recovery time.

Psychosocial issues are extremely important. Patients need to be stable psychologically and compliant. They must be able to understand the risks involved and be willing to adhere to their medication schedules, lab requirements, and appointments.

The review and treatment of other medical conditions and secondary complications are extremely important. Patients with untreated proliferative retinopathy may not be transplanted; however, after appropriate ophthalmological treatment, they may become candidates. Hypertension and hyperlipidemia must be well controlled. Candidates for islets only must not be in renal failure. The creatinine should not exceed 1.5 mg/dL, with a clearance greater than or equal to 60 mL/min. Those in renal failure may possibly be candidates for islet/kidney or islet after kidney transplantation. Medical conditions requiring the use of anticoagulants (except aspirin) are contraindications because of the use of heparin in the procedure and the increased risk of bleeding. Patients with conditions requiring chronic steroid use may also be ineligible because of the adverse effect of steroids on the islets. This situation commonly comes up with patients who are on steroids for their kidney transplant. However, these patients may be weaned off steroids prior to islet transplantation. Some programs also have specific criteria regarding insulin requirements and HbA1C values. Although these are quite variable, all candidates need to be in the best metabolic control prior to transplantation.

## THE DAY OF THE TRANSPLANT: IMMEDIATE PRETRANSPLANT EVALUATION AND METHODS OF IMPLANTATION

On the day of the transplant, a brief workup is done to establish that no changes have occurred that would prohibit a successful transplant. The transplant surgeon will perform a brief history and physical examination while blood work is being drawn. This will include a complete blood count (CBC) with differential, prothrombin time/partial thromboplastin time (PT/PTT), international normalized ratio (INR), chemistries such as electrolytes, glucose, blood-urea-nitrogen (BUN), creatinine, calcium, magnesium and phosphorus, and a liver profile. Serologies for cytomegalovirus (CMV) and Epstein-Barr virus (EBV) will be repeated along with tissue typing, type and screen and cross-match. A chest X-ray, ECG, and urinalysis will also be done. If the results are satisfactory and the islet preparation is suitable for transplantation, the patient will be started on immunosuppression (see below.)

Prior to the release of the isolated islets for transplantation, a number of criteria must be met, which are mandated by the FDA [Code of Federal Regulations (CFR21)]. These criteria are essential to insure product safety and quality. Product safety involves the demonstration of sterility, with strict criteria for endotoxin and mycoplasma contamination. Quality is assessed by proper identification and quantification of the islets, purity of the preparation, and demonstrated potency. Some of the results will not be completed prior to transplantation, such as the culture results; however, there are specific criteria that must be met prior to transplantation. For product safety, samples of the islets and medium are analyzed for aerobic, anaerobic, mycoplasma, and endotoxin contamination. Strict requirements prior to islet release include a negative gram stain and an endotoxin load < 5 EU/kg body weight of the recipient. For islet quality, a sufficient mass must be available, which must be at least 5000 IE/kg but is usually higher (10,000–12,000 IE/kg). Viability of the islets must be at least 70%, and the purity of the preparation, which is expressed as the percentage of islets over the entire tissue preparation, must be at least 30%. Total volume of the preparation must not exceed 10 g of tissue. Islets that are cultured overnight should have a glucose-stimulated insulin release in vitro, which should show a stimulation index of greater than 1.

The most common method for islet cell transplantation is the percutaneous transhepatic intraportal technique, which is done in the interventional radiology suite. This has been the most effective site of implantation. Assess to the portal vein can also be accomplished via the transjugular approach. Prior to the procedure, all patients are given IV antibiotics (usually

Ancef or Levaquin). The patient is then sedated using a conscious sedation protocol with agents such as midazolam and fentanyl or propofol. An ultrasound of the liver is then done to again confirm the patency of the portal vein and to determine the optimal site into the portal system. The patient is then prepped and draped in the usual sterile fashion. After the infusion of a local anesthetic, a 22-gauge Chiba needle is advanced into the liver using a midaxillary approach at the level of the 9th or 10th intercostal space (43). Fluoroscopy and ultrasonography are both utilized to obtain safe portal vein access. Dilute contrast is injected as the needle is being withdrawn until a right tertiary portal vein branch is cannulated. A small guide wire (0.018 in) is then advanced into the main portal vein (43). Then, using the Seldinger technique, a six French vascular sheath is advanced over the guide wire into the main portal vein. Prior to infusion, catheter position is confirmed using portosplenography (43). Portal vein pressure is also measured.

Islet cell infusion is currently performed using a closed fed bag system (44). Using this method, the islets are infused by gravity; therefore, the infusion pressure can be minimized and controlled by adjusting the bag height in relationship to the portal vein. Besides controlling the infusion rate, this method also provides an additional safety measure because of the natural reduction of flow, which occurs with an increase in portal pressure (44). The bag method uses one or two sterile bags (depending on the pelleted volume of the final islet preparation) for the infusion of the islets and a sterile 150 mL bag for rinsing after the infusion. If two bags are used, it is preferable to fill the first bag with the purest islets (44). Each bag also holds a dose of 35 units/kg of heparin.

In the radiology suite, a sterile IV set is used as infusion tubing and is connected to the tip of the portal vein catheter using a wide bore three-way tap (44). The tubing is flushed retrograde. The 600 mL bag is then spiked and the infusion begun. During the infusion, under gravity, the bag is kept in motion, with the chamber filled with fluid at all times to avoid air moving into the infusion line and to maintain the islets in suspension (44). When the infusion is done, the bag is flushed with transplant medium to avoid the loss of the islets from the walls of the bag.

Throughout the procedure, portal pressure is carefully monitored. The first reading is taken before the procedure (43). Readings are also taken halfway through the completion of the 600 mL bag, at the end of the rinse, five minutes after completion of the infusion, and at any time when there are changes in vital signs or if the patient complains of any abdominal pain (44). These readings are repeated if a second bag is used.

Using portal pressures as a safety measure, there are specific indications for the termination of the infusion (44). If the opening portal pressure is greater than 20 mmHg, the infusion is not performed. If the portal pressure doubles during the infusion and is greater than 15 mmHg, the infusion is temporarily stopped until the pressure falls below 15 mmHg, and only then is the infusion restarted. If the portal pressure rises above 22 mmHg the infusion is stopped, but if it falls below 18 mmHg the infusion can be continued at a slower rate. If the pressure remains at 22 mmHg for more than 10 minutes, the infusion is terminated. This is also correlated with symptoms. Infusions may be stopped because of abdominal complaints by the patient at lower portal pressures. An immediate ultrasound is done at the end of the infusion (44). No post-infusion portogram is done to avoid exposure of the islets to the IV contrast. When the catheter tip is withdrawn into the liver parenchyma (about 3–4 cm from the liver edge), a small amount of contrast is injected to confirm the site.

A very important part of the procedure is the plugging of the catheter tract. This has been done using several techniques such as laser and gelfoam. However, the use of gelfoam alone sometimes failed, causing dislodgment or bleeding. Recently, a new technique has been introduced using D-Stat, a collagen/thrombin paste that is injected into the peripheral tract following the placement of a single gelfoam plug (44). This paste can be easily prepared by dissolving Thrombin in dilution fluid, which is then mixed with collagen. The dilution fluid can be replaced with contrast (up to a half) if needed (45).

In order to seal the tract, the catheter is retracted using fluoroscopy until the tip is in the parenchymal tract. A gelfoam plug is placed into the luer of a contrast-filled 1 cm$^3$ syringe (45). The syringe is attached to the catheter and the plug injected proximally. The plug is advanced further to the end of the catheter and then released by withdrawing the catheter over the pusher. The plug should be visible by fluoroscopy with no further blood return from the catheter (45). The syringe with the D-Stat is connected to the end of the catheter and slowly injected until it can be visualized at the end of the catheter. The injection is continued slowly, while withdrawing the catheter until it is removed so that the entire tract is filled.

This technique, along with the gravity bag described above, are recent advances that have shown that islet transplantation can be performed safely with minimal morbidity (43). Accessing the portal vein radiologically has some definite advantages and is attractive to the patient population. Patients can receive a transplant without having general anesthesia and an abdominal incision. The procedure is quick, less expensive, and requires only a brief hospital stay. Most transplants are currently performed in this manner.

Despite the attractiveness of the percutaneous approach, there are still some benefits and indications for performing an open procedure. Patients who cannot discontinue their aspirin or who may be on specific protocols requiring additional anticoagulants should have an open procedure. These patients would be at increased risk of bleeding, which would be more easily and safely identified and treated using an open approach. Patients with hemangiomas may need to have an open approach since it would be too risky to do percutaneously. There are some programs where an experienced interventional radiologist is not available, so the surgeons place the islets intraoperatively. Finally, there may be some patients who may feel more comfortable having an open procedure.

There are several ways to transplant the islets surgically. The least invasive method may be to cannulate a vein in the omentum, a tributary of the portal vein, with an 18-gauge IV catheter. It should be possible to measure portal pressure depending on the size of the vein. Portal angiography should be performed to confirm filling of the main portal vein. Alternatively, a small bowel venous tributary can be cannulated, also measuring portal pressure. Here the vein may be larger. An even larger vein such as the inferior mesenteric or middle colic could also be cannulated. This would allow a larger lumen catheter to be placed and threaded up to the portal vein, which could be confirmed fluoroscopically. Access using a dual lumen catheter would also allow continuous monitoring of portal pressures during the infusion.

Currently, the intraportal site (either open or percutaneous) is the standard method for clinical islet transplantation. Although there are risks associated with this site (see below), this has been the most effective site to date. The technical advances that have been described, such as the bag method and the use of gelfoam and D-Stat, have decreased the major risks of bleeding and thrombosis. However, there are additional studies to try to develop other techniques. The renal subcapsular site is quite interesting, since it is believed to represent an immunoprivileged site. However, despite its success in mouse models and some larger animals, there is concern about the ability of subcapsular islets to survive and function in humans. Another interesting procedure is the omental pouch method. This may allow better islet survival and function but would require an open operative procedure with the creation of multiple omental pouches. With continued research, it may be possible to transplant islets using these sites or another novel area; however, for the present, the intraportal route has been the most effective.

## PERITRANSPLANT MANAGEMENT AND MEDICATIONS

After the conclusion of the islet infusion, all patients are kept at bed rest, lying on their right side for four hours (43). Vital signs should be checked every 15 minutes for the first hour, every 30 minutes for the next hour, and then every four hours thereafter. When the patient returns from the interventional radiology suite, a CBC should be drawn.

Insulin regimens in the peritransplant period vary among different centers, and continue to evolve. Classically, there was a great effort to maintain tight euglycemic control to protect the newly transplanted islets from the increased physiological stress of elevated glucose levels. At the time of the transplant, patients were placed on intravenous insulin and a dextrose infusion to maintain euglycemia. Blood glucose levels were checked every one to two hours. As the glucose level fell, the insulin was appropriately decreased, and eventually replaced with subcutaneous injections. Currently, many programs do not use intravenous infusions and maintain glucose levels with subcutaneous injections as indicated. Post-transplantation, the glucose levels will vary from patient to patient depending on their previous insulin requirements and the function of the islets. The islets are not expected to be fully functional, since it may take up to 10 to 14 days for them to become fully vascularized.

A popular insulin regimen posttransplantation is the use of subcutaneous injections of Humalog (Lispro) insulin. This is a fairly new type of insulin, which has a very rapid effect. Its onset of action is within 15 minutes with a peak effect of 30 to 90 minutes and duration of three to five hours. Depending on the patient's insulin requirements and the function of the graft, neutral protamine hagedorn (NPH) insulin can also be added to the regimen. NPH is an intermediate acting insulin with an onset of four to six hours, peaking at 8 to 14 hours, and lasting for about 16 to 20 hours. While in the hospital, patients should have frequent blood glucose levels drawn, usually before and two hours after each meal, at bedtime, in the middle of the night, and early morning.

Patients are usually discharged from the hospital within 24 hours. Prior to discharge, their hemoglobin should be unchanged from admission, their liver function tests should be within acceptable levels, which is usually less than twice normal for the transaminases, and a repeat Doppler ultrasound should show a patent left, right, and main portal vein with no significant collections or hematomas. Following discharge, patients are followed closely in an outpatient unit with daily labs (CBC, PT/PTT, INR, liver function studies, BUN/creatinine, electrolytes, glucose and drug levels) for the first week after transplantation. Lovenox is given at a dose of 30 mg subcutaneously twice daily for seven days (43). Another ultrasound is done on day 7 to rule out any complications, such as a portal vein thrombus or perihepatic hematoma. Continued frequent blood glucose levels are done at least three to four times each day.

Metabolic monitoring can be done using various measures. The simplest indicator of graft function is the glucose levels and the dosage of exogenous insulin. Basal and stimulated C-peptide, and oral and intravenous glucose tolerance testing are also routinely done. In general, it is felt that intravenous glucose tolerance parameters may be a better measure of function. Intravenous glucose tolerance testing is used to assess acute insulin response ($AIR_g$), glucose disposal ($K_g$), and area under the curve for glucose, insulin, and C-peptide (46). This testing may be done on a specific schedule for clinical trials but may also be done based on clinical criteria. HbA1C is usually checked every month for the initial three months and then every three months thereafter. Various immunological assays are also measured post-transplantation, especially those that are related to autoimmunity, such as anti-GAD65 antibody, anti-ICA152, and anti-insulin antibody. Other immunological assays may also be done (which vary among different programs), such as proliferation assays, enzyme linked immunosorbent acid assays, and flow cytometry.

Immunosuppression is initiated immediately before islet transplantation. The original Edmonton protocol utilized three drugs: daclizumab (Zenapax), sirolimus (Rapamune), and tacrolimus (Prograf) (13). Sirolimus is given orally at a loading dose of 0.2 mg/kg/day, monitoring drug levels to maintain a trough level of 12 to 15 ng/mL for the first three months and 7 to 10 ng/mL thereafter. Low-dose tacrolimus is given orally at an initial dose of 1 mg twice daily to maintain a 12-hour trough level of 3 to 6 ng/mL. Daclizumab is given intravenously at a dose of 1 mg/kg every 14 days for a total of five doses. (There is a current trend to continue this treatment every two weeks.) For prophylaxis against *Pneumocystis carinii*, oral Bactrim is given three times a week. Valganciclovir is given daily (450 mg) for at least 12 weeks for prophylaxis against CMV. (The length of treatment is increasing due to the use of more potent antibody preparations.) Patients also receive oral supplementation of vitamin E (800 IU/day), vitamin $B_6$ (100 mg/day), vitamin A (30,000 IU/day), and vitamin C (1000 mg/day) (27) for antioxidant supplementation, which may help to protect the islets.

Most programs still follow the original Edmonton protocol; however, there are also new protocols using other agents. Some of the antibody preparations that are being introduced into these protocols include humanized OKT3, Campath-1H, and Thymoglobulin. There is a great deal of interest in agents that deplete T-cells, interfere with cellular signaling for lymphocyte activation, and alter lymphocyte trafficking and recruitment. Medications such as FTY 720, Everolimus, and CellCept are being used in various combinations in these new protocols. The current trend is to develop immunosuppressive protocols that are calcineurin-inhibitor free.

Besides the changes in immunosuppressive protocols, additional medications are also being investigated, such as infliximab and etanercept. Infliximab neutralizes the biological activity of tumor necrosis factor (TNF)-alpha and is commonly used in the treatment of Crohn's disease. Etanercept binds to TNF-alpha and blocks its interaction with cell surface TNF receptors. This drug has been used in rheumatoid arthritis and psoriasis patients. These drugs are being used in islet transplantation mainly as anti-inflammatory agents; however, they do have some immunomodulatory/immunosuppressive effects. The reason that there is an interest in using these agents is that there are a significant number of islets that are being destroyed possibly because of inflammatory events that occur during organ recovery, isolation, and transplantation. Reducing this inflammation may lead to improved long-term graft survival, using fewer islets.

In addition to these inflammatory and immunological events, there may be other reactions that may also destroy the islets. A unique thrombotic/inflammatory reaction has recently been described, which is believed to be elicited when isolated islets come in contact with ABO-compatible blood (47). This reaction, which is described as an immediate blood-mediated inflammatory reaction (IBMIR) may provide an explanation for early islet loss (see Chapter 23). This phenomenon is currently a very controversial topic. Some investigators deny its existence, while others feel it is a very important reaction, which must be treated. A confounding variable in the debate is that all centers use heparin, which is an antithrombotic agent. It may be possible that heparin mitigates this reaction, and it thus may not always be appreciated.

Because of this presumed reaction, several anticoagulant agents (melagatran and dextran sulfate) (47,48) are being studied to see if they can cause a reduction in IBMIR. Using an in vitro model with human islets, melagatran, a specific thrombin inhibitor, was found to reduce IBMIR (47). The authors suggested that the protective effect of melagatran indicated that thrombin plays an integral role in IBMIR and suggests that the inhibition of thrombin can improve clinical islet transplantation (47). Because of these studies and other ongoing work using dextran sulfate (48), it is likely that these agents will eventually be utilized in upcoming clinical trials, possibly replacing heparin. It is possible that these anti-inflammatory and anticoagulant medications may be just as necessary as immunosuppressive drugs and may even decrease the amount of immunosuppression needed to maintain long-term graft survival.

## COMPLICATIONS RELATED TO ISLET TRANSPLANTATION

The complications seen after islet transplantation are primarily related to the procedure and the immunosuppressive regimen. The most serious complications of the percutaneous hepatic approach are the risks of bleeding and thrombosis. Bleeding can be intrahepatic, perihepatic, or even intraperitoneal. Thrombosis can be partial, involving a branch of the portal vein or the main portal vein. In addition to these two major complications, others have been reported.

In a review of the clinical course of the initial 54 patients treated with the Edmonton protocol (35), these complications were discussed and quantified. At that time, there were five patients (9.2%) who had a post-procedure hemorrhage, four of whom required transfusion. There were also two cases (3.7%) of portal vein thrombosis, and two cases (3.7%) of gallbladder puncture. In one of the patients with a thrombus, anticoagulation was used, which led to bleeding, requiring the evacuation of the hematoma and a segmental hepatic resection. Two of the 54 patients experienced bradycardia. This may have been related to a rise in portal pressure or pain, or may have represented a vasovagal episode or a response to sedation.

A common side effect that has been reported is liver enzyme elevation. In a study of 84 consecutive islet transplant procedures, a significant increase in liver function tests was noted in more than 50% of the patients (49). The aspartate aminotransferase increased more than 2.5 times the normal value in 54% of the procedures, while a five-fold increase was noted in 27%. However, these levels normalized spontaneously in 90% of the recipients within four weeks. These findings have raised concerns about long-term sequelae that may occur in the liver following transplantation.

In a study that looked at the first 30 patients in a series of islet recipients, 20% were found to have periportal steatosis (50). However, diffuse fatty infiltration was not a common finding on ultrasound. The authors felt that the magnetic resonance imaging confirmed the benign nature of this finding by the normal T2 signal and by the lack of enhancement with gadolinium (50). The only clear difference in metabolic or any other clinical parameters between those with or without steatosis was that those with steatosis had a higher exogenous insulin requirement. Another interesting finding was that one subject with a complete loss of graft function had a complete resolution of the steatosis. The relationship between graft function and steatosis is currently unclear, as is the exact etiology (50). Although this phenomenon was originally thought to be solely related to the procedure and the islet infusion, it may be possible that immunosuppressive agents also play a role (50).

In general, the most serious complications remain those associated with bleeding or thrombosis. However, with improvements in techniques such as the bag method (44) (which decreases the risk of thrombosis) and the use of materials such as D-Stat (which decreases the risk of bleeding) (45), these complications have been rare or even nonexistent in recent studies (43). For example, in earlier procedures, the risk of serious complications including perihepatic bleeding and portal vein occlusion was 9% (51). However, in a recent study, none of the cases had any evidence of abdominal organ injury, bleeding, thrombosis, or any cardiac or pulmonary event (43). Only minimal complications were seen, such as nausea (59%), mild abdominal pain (71%), and elevated transaminases (2–3 times the normal value in 100%), which was self-limited (43).

Patients who may be at increased risk of bleeding may undergo an open procedure to infuse the islets. Although this may be safer for these patients, there are also some complications associated with this procedure. The severity of the complication is related to the size and location of the vessel that is used for the infusion. The least invasive method is to cannulate a vein in the omentum, a tributary of the portal vein, with an 18- or 20-gauge IV catheter. Because of the small size, it may be difficult to measure portal pressure because the catheter tip may be near the vein wall, dampening the signal. There may be the risk of a vein wall puncture or catheter dislodgement with spillage intraperitoneally. Therefore, the islets should not be infused under pressure. Alternatively, a small bowel venous tributary may be cannulated. Here, the vein is larger, which would make portal pressure monitoring easier; however, the catheter can still become dislodged. Ileus is more likely in this case because of bowel manipulation, and there is also a risk of devascularization of a segment of the bowel. Using a larger vein such as the inferior mesenteric or middle colic allows the use of a larger lumen catheter, which can be advanced up to the portal vein and confirmed fluoroscopically. Access using a dual lumen catheter would also allow continuous monitoring of portal pressure during the infusion. Surgical ligation of this vein could avoid the risk of postoperative bleeding, but this may compromise access for additional infusions. Although these risks are possible, only minimal complications have occurred using this technique.

Another major source of complications is the immunosuppressive agents. The standard Edmonton protocol consists of three immunosuppressive agents: daclizumab, tacrolimus, and sirolimus. Daclizumab binds specifically to the interleukin-2 receptor that is expressed on the surface of activated lymphocytes. It has been found to be well tolerated; however, it is occasionally associated with adverse events. These may include mild gastrointestinal symptoms, tremor, dizziness, headache, alterations in blood pressure and heart rate, pulmonary edema, musculoskeletal pain, and bleeding.

Tacrolimus inhibits T-lymphocyte activation by binding to an intracellular protein, FKBP-12. A complex is formed that inhibits calcineurin. This effect is thought to prevent the translocation of nuclear factor of activated T-cells, which is involved in the initiation of gene transcription for the formation of lymphokines (such as interleukin-2 and gamma interferon). It is fairly well tolerated at the low doses that are used in islet transplantation; however, it may act synergistically with sirolimus. Tacrolimus can cause neurotoxicity and nephrotoxicity. Hypertension can be fairly common; however, myocardial hypertrophy is rare. Hyperkalemia and hypomagnesemia are also fairly common but easily treated. Of additional concern is the diabetogenicity that may occur with the use of tacrolimus. Because of these side effects, new protocols are being developed which avoid calcineurin inhibitors.

Sirolimus binds to the immunophilin FK binding protein (FKBP-12) to generate an immunosuppressive complex that, has no effect on calcineurin activity. This complex binds to and inhibits the activation of the mammalian target of rapamycin, and this suppresses cytokine-driven T-cell proliferation. Some of the side effects associated with sirolimus include hypercholesterolemia, hyperlipidemia, hypertension, rash, diarrhea, anemia, thrombocytopenia, mouth ulcers, impaired wound healing, joint pain, and proteinuria. A significant number of these patients require treatment for their cholesterol and lipid levels. Because of these side effects, there have been cases where the dosage has been decreased or where mycophenolate mofetil has been substituted. Dosage reduction of tacrolimus has also been necessary in patients with rising creatinine levels and decreased creatinine clearance.

All immunosuppressive agents have the potential complications of infections, post-transplantation lymphoproliferative disorder (PTLD), and other malignancies (although sirolimus appears to be associated with a lower incidence of malignancy). Currently, in islet transplantation, there have been no cases of CMV, EBV, PTLD, or cancers. Newer protocols using calcineurin-inhibitor avoidance, antibody induction, and costimulatory blockade may reduce these side effects and may also increase graft survival.

## CURRENT OUTCOMES

After the introduction of the Edmonton protocol in 2000, replication of the outcomes has been confirmed in numerous centers. In North America, the Collaborative Islet Transplant Registry was established in 2001 to collect and analyze the data on islet transplantation (52). Currently, more than 300 recipients have received islet transplants since 1999 (53). Since this time, combined data from the three most experienced centers (Miami, Edmonton, and Minnesota) have revealed that 99% of the recipients had primary graft function, with 96% remaining C-peptide positive at one year (54). The one-year rate of insulin independence was 85%, with approximately 70% remaining insulin free at two years (54). These numbers illustrate the tremendous advances that have been made in the field since the 1990s, when only 8.2% of the patients remained insulin independent at one year post-transplant (12). Despite this significant achievement, the current hurdle is to increase the long-term survival of the islets. At three years post-transplantation, insulin independence drops to approximately 50% and, at five years, it decreases further, to approximately 24%. However, many of these patients still produce C-peptide, have lower insulin requirements, and also maintain an improved metabolic state. In a recent report of a five-year follow-up after islet transplantation, the majority of patients (approximately 80%) have C-peptide present; however, only a minority (about 10%) has maintained insulin independence (55).

In successful transplants, HbA1C has been maintained in the normal range (35). To date, there have been no mortalities and no cases of CMV, EBV, PTLD, or any other malignancies (54). In this recent combined experience, there have been no reports of portal vein thrombosis; however, in Edmonton (56), 4% of the patients had a segmental thrombosis of a branch of the portal vein believed to be associated with the infusion of a lower purity islet preparation.

The results of islet after kidney and simultaneous islet–kidney transplantation have also improved. Currently, the results of islet after kidney transplantation are similar to the results of islet alone transplantation after conversion to low-dose tacrolimus and sirolimus immunosuppression (57,58). Simultaneous islet–kidney transplantation has also been successfully performed using an open approach, by infusing the islets through a catheter placed in the mesenteric vein (59). In this series, five out of six patients became insulin independent (83%), with a follow-up of just over two years (59).

In addition to the benefit of insulin independence, islet transplantation is also associated with improvements in kidney graft survival and function in patients with Type I diabetes and kidney grafts (60). Specifically, islet transplantation reduces the fractional excretion of sodium, decreases the urinary excretion of albumin, and also reduces the 24-hour urinary sodium excretion rate (60). These clinical observations are associated with increases in Na+/K+-ATPase activity in the red blood cells and increased expression of Na+/K+-ATPase reactivity in the tubular cells of the kidney graft (60). Additional findings include a significant correlation between the Na+/K+-ATPase activity in the red blood cells and the C-peptide/creatinine ratio and also include a positive effect on systolic blood pressure. The restoration of C-peptide may have a protective role for the kidney (53), which may represent an important indication for performing islet transplantation in patients with kidney grafts (60).

In addition to these positive effects on renal function, islet transplantation has been found to improve vascular diabetic complications (61) and has also demonstrated a survival benefit for diabetics with functioning grafts (62). This may be due to the improvement in endothelial function and cardiovascular outcomes, as described by Fiorina et al. (62). Patients with functioning grafts demonstrated superior endothelial function compared with those without functioning grafts. Endothelial dysfunction, described by using von Willebrand factor and D-dimer fragment as markers, suggests an increased risk of accelerated atherosclerosis (62). Higher levels of these markers have been found in patients with nonfunctioning grafts. Cardiovascular death rates were also found to be significantly higher in this group of patients. Overall, this study showed that successful islet transplantation improves endothelial function, cardiovascular outcomes, and overall survival (62), which may be the result of improved blood glucose control and partial restoration of the islet endocrine function. Because of these positive findings, additional centers are investigating the possibility of setting up an islet program. Unfortunately, the maintenance of a sterile laboratory with trained professionals, and which meets FDA standards, requires a significant investment. A possible solution may be a collaborative effort between one center that has the complete facilities for islet transplantation and another program that may have the necessary clinical facilities and professionals but lacks an islet isolation laboratory. This type of collaborative effect is nicely illustrated in a paper that describes the first year review of patients transplanted at the Baylor program using islets isolated at the University of Miami (63). In this report, all patients produced C-peptide (basal and stimulated), with seven out of the 11 achieving insulin independence. There were no major complications related to the procedure. Only minor complications, such as abdominal pain, nausea, and transient elevations of serum transaminases were reported. This paper demonstrated that the use of a remote isolation center is safe and effective (63), something that has significant implications for the growth of this field. Since it takes an enormous amount of resources to maintain an islet isolation facility, having a smaller number of laboratories in strategic locations, which could ship islets to remote centers, could decrease the overall cost and also maintain a high-quality product. This would enable more centers to collaborate and facilitate patient access.

Despite this recent progress, one of the main criticisms remains the need for two or more donor pancreata to achieve insulin independence. This criticism is being addressed with data from the University of Minnesota (26). In a pilot study, six patients were transplanted with cultured islets using the two-layer perflurocarbon method. Four of the six patients became insulin independent and remained so throughout the one-year follow-up period. One recipient showed a transient 50% reduction in insulin requirements and another showed partial function with exogenous insulin doses of approximately 60% of pretransplant requirements (26). The immunosuppressive regimen that was used consisted of the humanized anti-CD3 monoclonal antibody hOKT3α1 (Ala-Ala), sirolimus, and low-dose tacrolimus. The success of this pilot trial was attributed to several factors: the quality of the islet preparation using the two-layer technique, careful donor and recipient selection, maintenance of adequate drug levels of the immunosuppressive agents, and the use of hOKT3α1 (Ala-Ala) antibody (54). The use of this antibody is associated with the emergence of CD4+CD25+ regulatory T-cell populations (26). Studies have shown that this antibody may regulate autoimmunity in Type I diabetes, which suggests that this may be a highly effective agent for islet transplantation (54).

## FUTURE PROSPECTS

There is an ongoing effort to improve upon these results and to develop additional methods to preserve islet mass. This includes improvements in the isolation methods through the use of antioxidants, gene therapy, and new culture media. Immunosuppressive regimens are being changed by the elimination of calcineurin inhibitors and the addition of anti-inflammatory and anticoagulant agents. Tolerance strategies are being tested to alter the immunological environment to decrease or eliminate autoimmunity and manipulate regulatory and effector T-cells. Preclinical studies are ongoing using various microencapsulation devices to protect the islets and to shield them from immune attack.

The predominant limiting factor remains the supply of insulin-secreting cells. There are over one million patients with Type I diabetes in the United States, but less than 1600 pancreata are recovered each year (based on OPTN data as of December 1, 2004). One method of increasing this supply is through the use of animal cells (xenotransplantation). The major barrier to the clinical application of xenotransplantation has been the innate immune response, which can result in hyperacute rejection. This is thought to be initiated by the binding of preformed host antibodies to specific α 1, 3 galactose epitopes on the recipients' vascular endothelium (64,65). This results in the activation of the complement cascade leading to rapid graft loss. This barrier was recently broken by cloning pigs with the inactivation of both of the α 1, 3 galactose gene alleles (66–68). Abrogation of these genes was proven to eliminate hyperacute rejection. These double knockout pigs are currently being tested in preclinical models. Additional transgenic pigs that express human decay activating factor and tissue factor inhibitors will also be tested.

Another promising technology to increase the supply of insulin producing cells is the use of stem cells. Many research efforts are ongoing, which are exploring this technology. One major issue is the type of cell that would be most efficacious. Some groups are studying tissue stem cells as potential progenitor cells, while others are investigating the use of embryonic stem cells. There are advantages and disadvantages to both (69). Some interesting and surprising findings have emerged from this work that challenge some of the common beliefs about β-cell development and function. Pluripotent stem cells were thought to be the source of new beta cells during adult life and after pancreatectomy (69), suggesting that they would be key cells to investigate. However, in a recent study, this notion has been challenged (70). These investigators have shown that pre-existing beta cells are the major source of new beta cells during adulthood and after pancreatectomy, suggesting that terminally differentiated beta cells maintain a significant proliferative capacity in vivo (70).

An important question relates to how pluripotent cell lines differentiate into specialized cell types, and whether this differentiation can be induced. To investigate these issues, mouse embryonic stem cells were studied in vitro, since their differentiation allows the observation of embryonic development and the specific differentiation of precursor cells to mature, specialized cells (69). This study illustrated key features in pancreatic development, including gene expression and regulation and the importance of *PDX1* expression in normal development. It also demonstrated the expression patterns of major islet hormones and the production of insulin-producing cells (69). A culture protocol was described, which supported the differentiation of embryonic stem cells throughout the early stages of pancreatic development, including the precursors of endocrine differentiation and the formation of all four of the major endocrine cell types (69).

Building on this work, additional culture modifications were made. In a study using human embryonic stem cells, and an improved protocol, these cells were modified to form insulin-producing cells (71). Using immunostaining and reverse transcriptase-polymerase chain reaction, the induced cells were found to be islet-like clusters similar to immature pancreatic beta cells, which secreted a substantial amount of insulin. Future studies are needed to develop methods to mature these cells, which may be a source for future cell therapy for the treatment of diabetes.

Additional efforts to discover cells that may be modified to produce insulin have revealed some surprising findings. In a study that looked at insulin gene expression and proinsulin production (72), the authors surprisingly found that hyperglycemia, with or without established diabetes, activated insulin gene transcription and proinsulin production, which resulted in the finding of insulin-positive cells in multiple tissues such as the liver, fat, spleen, thymus, and bone marrow (BM); these cells also produced glucagon, somatostatin, and pancreatic polypeptide (72). Bone marrow-derived cells appeared to be the major source of proinsulin expressing cells.

In a separate study, which specifically looked at bone marrow as a potential source of insulin-producing cells (73), stem cell lines were isolated from murine bone marrow and were found to express multiple genes that were related to β-cell development and function. Insulin and C-peptide production were identified. In vitro studies demonstrated glucose-stimulated insulin release. These cells were ultimately found to reverse diabetes and improve metabolic parameters in diabetic mice (73). The authors felt that their results indicated that the bone marrow contains cells that were capable of differentiation in vitro into insulin-producing cells (73). These cells could provide an unlimited source of insulin-producing cells. Because of the multiple influences on the differentiation of bone marrow-derived cells, there are additional studies that need to be carried out; however, this work appears to be quite promising.

The search for healthy, insulin-producing cells has resulted in numerous studies that are looking at methods to preserve and rescue β-cell mass as well as encouraging the differentiation of precursor cells. Rescue of β-cell mass may occur through increased β-cell replication, increased β-cell size, decreased β-cell death, and differentiation of possibly existing β-cell progenitors (74). It has been shown that occasional endocrine cells can be found embedded in normal pancreatic ducts. However, these cells are few and far between (75). The number of these duct-associated endocrine cells physiologically increases as a consequence of severe insulin resistance in obese individuals or during pregnancy (76,77). Similar histological changes are observed under conditions of tissue injury and repair after partial pancreatectomy, duct ligation, cellophane wrapping of the gland, or interferon-γ overexpression driven by the insulin promoter (78–81). Even then, within the ducts, only a small number of cells become insulin-positive. This suggests that, in the case in which some hypothetical precursors exist, the process of formation of endocrine cells (i.e., neogenesis) would not be a common property of the duct epithelium. On the other hand, the fact that α- and β-cells develop from a possibly common, non-hormone-expressing, yet *PDX1*-positive precursor (*PDX1* being a transcription factor required for pancreatic development) suggests that all cell types found within the islet may originate from a bona fide, common endocrine progenitor (82). These endocrine progenitors may be located close to the duct, but may not actually be components of the ductal epithelium (83). The progenitor cells could be mesenchymal in origin, or they could be cells differentiated from an unknown cell type. If the number of these progenitors is extremely small, lineage analysis becomes very difficult because of the lack of known appropriate markers. Moreover, if these cells are as rare as they appear to be, it becomes difficult to quantify their contribution to normal endocrine cell turnover. Seaberg et al. have shown that single murine adult pancreatic precursor cells can generate progeny with characteristics of pancreatic cells, including β-cells (84). These rare (one in 3000–9000 cells), pancreas-derived multipotent precursors (PMPs) do not seem to be conventional pluripotent embryonic stem cells, since they lack, for example, the Oct4 and Nanog markers that direct the propagation of undifferentiated embryonic stem cells, nor are these cells of clear ectodermal, mesodermal, or endodermal origin, since they failed to express other markers considered specific for precursors of each of the embryonic cell types (84,85). Since, surprisingly, these PMPs also lacked some β-cell markers (e.g., HNF3β) as well as ductal epithelium markers (e.g., cytokeratin), but were able to generate differentiation products with neural characteristics together with α, β, δ, and acinar pancreatic cells, the authors proposed the existence of a new and unique ectodermal/endodermal precursor cell present during embryonic development that could persist in adult tissues (84).

These results support the conclusions of another recent study in which multipotent pancreatic progenitors were prospectively isolated using flow-cytometric cell sorting (86). The marker used in this case was c-Met, the hepatocyte growth factor (HGF) receptor. The rationale for this choice was the known signal exchange between epithelial and mesenchymal cells, promoting the interaction between c-Met and HGF, which plays an important role in the development of the pancreas. The authors suggest that c-Met–HGF interaction is critically responsible for growth and differentiation of pancreatic stem and progenitor cells not only during development but also in the adult, where they maintain homeostasis and promote regeneration. Colonies derived from single c-Met–positive cells, sorted from neonatal and adult mouse pancreatic tissues, contained cells expressing several markers for endocrine, acinar, and ductal lineage cells. While neuroectodermal markers were not evaluated, the isolated pancreatic stem cells of Suzuki et al. (86) were also able to generate offspring cells expressing hepatocyte and gastrointestinal cell markers, possibly due to the selection marker used. Seaberg's PMP-derived cells were grown instead in the serum-free medium conditions normally used for neural stem cell culture (84).

All of these observations, even with their somewhat divergent outcomes, seem to support the conclusion that stem cells of some kind exist not only in the duct, but also within the islets themselves, since both subpopulations were independently used as the source of isolated single cell precursors (84,86). On the one hand, while this condition supports the working hypothesis of those who are proposing that pancreatic ductal cells can transdifferentiate into β-cells and that this is a physiologic process generally more efficiently activated by increased metabolic demand and tissue injuries (87), on the other hand, it may also accommodate the most recent results of Dor and colleagues (70), who propose instead that no β-cell can arise from non-β-cell progenitors, whether in the normal adult pancreas or after pancreatectomy. As a direct consequence, the number of β-cells should become virtually defined at a certain point of time and, afterwards, glycemia should be controlled only by that defined cellular pool. Dor et al.'s results were obtained by using a sophisticated Cre/lox system that, in transgenic mice, can be induced by Tamoxifen. This system labels fully differentiated β-cells (defined as postnatal cells transcribing the insulin gene) that express the human alkaline phosphatase protein, which is, in turn, revealed by a histochemical stain. In a defined period of time, the "chase," only the cells that are progeny of pre-existing and labeled β-cells are newly labeled. New β-cells derived from any non-β-cell source, including stem cells, are not labeled. The frequency and distribution of labeled β-cells within pancreatic islets, at the end of the chase period, should be inversely proportional to the number of new, non-labeled cells present in the same structures. If the frequency of labeled β-cells does not change as was observed, the number of cells derived from the differentiation of non-insulin-producing precursors must be minimal or null, while terminally differentiated insulin-producing β-cells themselves should be the cells that actually proliferate and give rise to other insulin-producing β-cells. While the results of Seaberg et al. (84) do not contest the proven, yet limited ability of a β-cell to divide, the failure of Dor et al. (70) to observe cells possibly differentiated from stem or precursor cells might actually be due to both their extremely limited number (84) and their technical issues. For example, the use of tamoxifen injected intraperitoneally or subcutaneously "twice a week for two and a half weeks" (70) might have blocked neogenesis from precursor cells "mainly in pancreatic ducts adjacent to involuted islets," as observed by Pelengaris et al. (88), and once the tamoxifen was withdrawn, these cells might not have had sufficient time to differentiate. At any rate, further studies are necessary to ultimately define the existence and significance of possible different sources of progenitor cells contributing to β-cell regeneration.

In the rat, experimental evidence supports the notion that precursor cells in both endocrine and exocrine tissue are not susceptible to damage by streptozotocin (STZ)—i.e., they are not Glut-2 positive since STZ, like alloxan, uses Glut-2 as the receptor to get into the target cells that it eventually kills (89,90)—and that local effects of residual β-cell mass are not important after 90% pancreatectomy (91). Also, even in neonatal STZ-treated rats, a combination of activin A and betacellulin, for example, promoted regeneration of pancreatic β-cells and improved glucose metabolism (92).

Experiments in monkeys indicate that, once the best immunosuppressive regimen is found, allo or even porcine islets can substitute for endogenous islets, producing enough insulin (monitored by porcine C-peptide) to maintain normal glycemia in the recipient animal. Pertinent to this discussion is, however, the observation that under a nondiabetogenic immunosuppressive protocol, and by adopting alternative means to correct hyperglycemia during the recovery process, the monkey's endocrine tissue is able to regenerate in a period of time similar to the one determined for the diabetic mouse. In the presence of calcineurin inhibitors in the immunosuppressive cocktail, regeneration was not seen. In our preliminary studies, all of the insulin+ and Glut-2+ cells disappeared in the pancreata of monkeys treated with one large (150 mg/kg) or two to three smaller (55 mg/kg) STZ dose infusions. Insulin+ and Glut-2 + cells reappeared after three to four months of treatment only when immunosuppressive protocols that did not contain calcineurin inhibitors were administered to the animal. This observation supports the conclusion that all the Glut-2 + β-cells of the recipient are ultimately killed by the STZ treatment when it is properly implemented. If regeneration is taking place, not only in rodents but also in the monkey, we can expect that the endocrine tissue regenerates in humans, once autoimmunity is properly and successfully abrogated. There is some evidence that supports these expectations.

One example is the case of a 13-year-old Caucasian boy. After suffering with a conventional T1D onset (i.e., after a history of polyuria, polydipsia, and weight loss), the boy presented with serum glucose levels up to approximately 500 mg/dL, glucosuria, and ketonuria. The boy initially required insulin; however, ultimately the insulin therapy was able to be completely stopped after 11 months of treatment. This case was recently published by the group from Ulm, Germany (93). The authors also reported that "Without further treatment, HbA1C and fasting glucose levels remained normal throughout the entire follow up of currently 4.5 years," and that serum autoantibodies to GAD65, IA-2 insulin, and ICA "were initially positive but showed a progressive decline or loss during follow up." A similar case was recently reported by David Harlan's group (94).

On this basis, we hypothesize that, not only in the rodents or in the monkey but also in humans, the abrogation of autoimmunity allows the physiological regeneration of the insulin-producing β-cells in the host endocrine pancreas even after the onset of the disease. These are the premises on which reliable and more clinically translatable alternatives than allogeneic bone marrow transplants or allogeneic or xenogeneic pancreatic islet transplants will be found to cure our young diabetic patients.

Precursors of a perhaps unconventional type (84,86) located both in close proximity and inside the endocrine tissue, which can be activated by increased metabolic demand or by various secreted factors, may be able, under normal conditions, to accelerate the process that guarantees islet of Langerhans cellular homeostasis. The physiologic equilibrium between lost and newly generated cells can be altered by the action of β-cell-specific, autoreactive T-cells, in instances in which autoimmunity develops (95). Once T-cell killing activity overcomes the regenerative compensatory activity of the organ, the number of functional β-cells progressively decreases until they become too few to maintain the glucose homeostasis of the entire body. The time of transition over this metabolic threshold becomes immediately evident with the presentation of the characteristic symptoms of the clinical onset of T1D. During the disease, even if the regenerative properties of the pancreas remain functional, the continued presence of diabetogenic, autoreactive T-cells consistently nullifies the reparative effort. The fact that these autoreactive T-cells remain present in the body of the diabetic patient for a long time is proven by experiments in which healthy islet cells transplanted into syngeneic, long-term diabetic mice or humans, are quickly killed by these same autoreactive T-cells (96).

The autoimmune response is successfully averted in the nonobese diabetic (NOD) mouse either by directly eliminating the majority of the autoreactive T-cells with anti-T-cell antibodies or by substituting all or part of the immunocompetent cell repertoire with BM cells obtained from diabetic-resistant donors. The treatment of overtly diabetic NOD mice with antilymphocyte serum (ALS) abrogates autoimmunity and achieves only partial clinical remission (97). Transient treatment of overtly diabetic NOD mice with ALS and exendin-4—a potent insulinotropic hormone that promotes replication and differentiation of β-cells in vitro and in vivo—achieved instead complete remission of 88% of the treated animals within 75 days, accompanied by progressive normalization of glucose tolerance, improved islet histology, increased insulin content in the pancreas, and almost normal insulin release in response to a glucose challenge. These results show that exendin-4 synergistically augments the remission-inducing effect of ALS, possibly by promoting differentiation of β-cell precursors (97).

We and others have shown that the successful induction of a mixed allogeneic chimerism obtained after transplanting BM from a diabetes-resistant donor into a diabetic animal following a sublethal dose of irradiation, is sufficient to block and eventually also revert the systematic invasion and inflammation of the islets by the autoreactive T-cells that results in insulitis (Fig. 1) (99–101).

Within the endocrine pancreas, once the insult of autoimmunity is abrogated, the physiologic process of regeneration can continue efficiently, eventually replenishing the population of insulin-producing cells to a number sufficient to maintain euglycemia, thus curing the diabetic recipient (Fig. 2) (98,103,104). While this process takes place, the recipient's glycemia must be controlled by additional, independent measures. The most commonly used technique is to transplant into the recipient islets from the same marrow donor. However, the successful engraftment of the transplanted bone marrow, or the establishment of a steady hematopoietic chimerism, would have to be maintained without the use of calcineurin inhibitors that will kill not only the autoreactive T-cells of the recipient but also the β-cells themselves, thereby defeating the purpose of the transplant (105–107).

The use of these diabetogenic immunosuppressive agents may also interfere with the observed rise of regulatory T-cells, a possible explanation for the long-lasting immunoregulatory cell-dominant condition observed in cured animals. Adoptive transfer experiments, in which both diabetogenic lymphocytes and splenocytes from ALS-treated, long-term diabetes-free NOD mice were transplanted in NODscid mice with no signs of diabetes induction, support this hypothesis (97).

A subject of ongoing debate is whether either or both the transplanted BM and the cotransplanted β-cells are necessary for promoting an efficient regenerative process, independent of their ability to block autoimmunity or preserve euglycemia, respectively. They may, for example, secrete factors such as glucagon-like peptides, which are useful in order to sustain an efficient regenerative process (97,108,109). Strong evidence suggests that the hematopoietic precursors present in the BM cell population do not directly participate in the reparative process of the insulin-producing cell population (Fig. 2) (98,104). In the cured recipient, insulin-producing cells that are genetically marked to indicate that they are of donor origin, are extremely rare, occurring in no more than two out of more than 100,000 β-cells. These cells may actually be the result of sporadic cell fusion processes (110). A different source of donor cells, from the spleen, for example, might be able to block autoimmunity and also provide mesenchymal β-cell precursors (111,112). However, the hypothesized presence in

Experimental Design

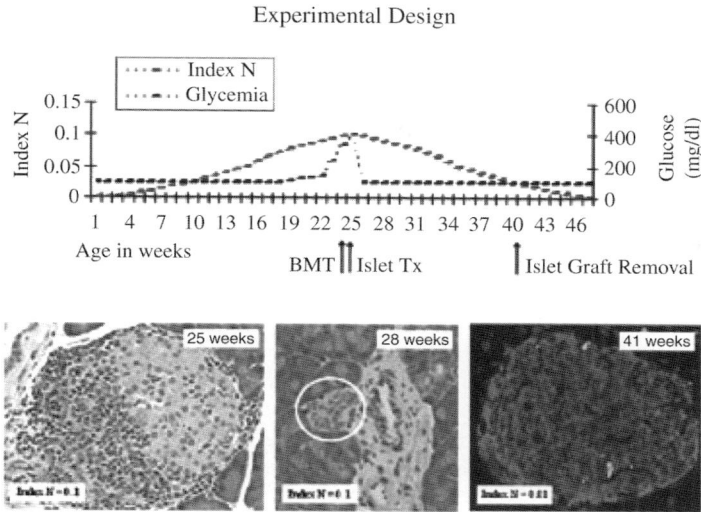

Figure 1  Schematic representation of the protocol used to test regeneration (or rescue) of the β-cell in diabetic non-obese diabetic (NOD) mice. In NOD mice, the infiltration of autoreactive T-cells into the islets of Langerhans (resulting in insulitis) begins at around four weeks of age. At 20 to 23 weeks, ~85% of female mice are diabetic, i.e., their glycemia is >300 mg/dL. When successfully transplanted with bone marrow from a nondiabetes prone donor and hematopoietic chimerism is established, the NOD mouse no longer shows signs of autoimmune activity. However, while there is no more evidence of insulitis in the endogenous pancreas, there is also no sign of insulin production. Three to four months after bone marrow transplantation, new insulin-positive cells are present throughout the endogenous pancreas. Thus, when the islets, transplanted under the kidney capsule in order to maintain euglycemia while regeneration takes place, are removed by nephrectomy, the mice remain nondiabetic. For "Index N" morphometric scoring system, see Ref. 99. *Abbreviation:* BMT, bone marrow transplantation. *Source:* From Refs. 98, 99.

the mouse spleen of embryonic mesenchymal cells that lack surface expression of CD45 and are able to differentiate into endothelial and endodermal cells remains to be confirmed by groups other than Faustman's.

As already stated, in humans, T1D most frequently presents with the clinical onset in children and adolescents who are genetically predisposed. In the late 1980s, in collaboration with Dr. Hugh McDevitt of Stanford University, we were able to map and identify the most influential single hereditary susceptibility factor in T1D: a single amino acid of the β-chain of the HLA-DQ histocompatibility molecule (113,114). Although T1D is recognized to be a multigenic disease (115), in humans the principal genetic susceptibility component was proposed to be any allelic form of the HLA-DQ molecule that lacks a charged amino acid at position 57 of its β-chain. Conversely, resistance to disease is associated with the inheritance

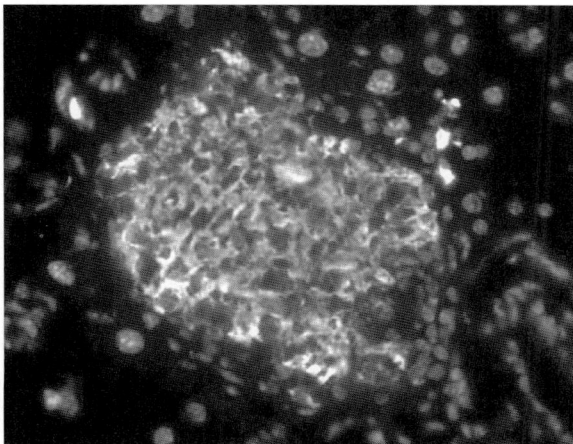

Figure 2  Using a GFP transgenic mouse as donor, it is possible to observe how the majority of the transplanted bone marrow cells do not directly participate in the regeneration of the endogenous pancreas. As shown here, there are no double-positive cells in the newly formed islets. The donor cells appear to be located close to possibly existing juxta-ductal precursor cells, which may be activated by marrow cell–secreted factors. Insulin-positive cells are shown. *Source:* From Ref. 102.

of HLA-DQ alleles containing a charged amino acid such as aspartic acid, at the same position (Asp-57). The physical explanation of the unusual importance of this particular single amino acid location for the development of the autoimmune characteristics of T1D came with the elucidation of the crystal structure of the HLA-DQ8 molecule, a non-Asp-57 molecule, which conferred the highest susceptibility to the disease (116). The most important feature of the susceptibility of HLA-DQ8 molecule relevant to diabetes immunology is that its crystal structure is identical to the homologous I-AG$^7$ molecule present in the NOD mouse (117). The peptide binding-site of the majority of human HLA-DQ and murine I-A molecules have an Asp-57 that points into the groove. In these allelic forms, Asp-57 forms an electrostatic salt bridge with the arginine in juxtaposition (i.e., in position 76) of the alpha chain of the molecule (Arg-76), which also points into the groove. HLA-DQ8 and I-Ag$^7$ lack Asp-57 and this variation disrupts the electrostatic interaction, leaving the Arg-76 free to interact with the aqueous environment and with any peptide able to lodge inside the binding groove of the molecule (118,119). The absence of Asp-57 allows the binding of peptides that may not find appropriate lodging inside other Asp-57+ molecule grooves, and may jeopardize an efficient presentation by the histocompatibility molecule to T-cells because of incorrectly positioned self-peptides. The susceptibility status can be correlated, in immunological terms, with impaired peptide lodging, impaired peptide presentation to T-cells with consequent reduction in positive selection of regulatory T-cells, or by the impaired negative selection of self-reactive T-cells (114–117). Indirect evidence supporting these hypotheses derives from transgenic NOD mice that express class II genes other than I-AG$^7$, which do not develop diabetes (120–123), and from the fact that transplantation of allogeneic BM from strains that do not spontaneously develop diabetes also prevents the occurrence of diabetes in NOD mice (98–100,104).

Recently, Tian and colleagues (124) demonstrated that T1D was prevented by transfecting the gene encoding a "diabetes-resistant" major histocompatibility complex class II β-chain into the hematopoietic stem cells of genetically susceptible (i.e., carrying a "diabetes-susceptible" allele) NOD mice. This strain of mice spontaneously develops T1D with pathogenetic characteristics very similar to the disease in humans. The expression of the newly formed diabetes-resistant molecule in the reinfused hematopoietic cells was sufficient to prevent T1D onset in the NOD mouse even in the presence of the native, diabetogenic molecule. Instead of approaching the problem using an alloreactive BM transplant, with all of its inherent severe contraindications (e.g., graft-versus-host disease), Tian et al. (124) transfected ex vivo the gene encoding a resistant, Asp-57 + β-chain into the BM cells isolated from the diabetes-prone NOD mouse. The expression of the newly formed diabetes-resistant molecule in the reinfused hematopoietic cells was sufficient to prevent T1D onset in the NOD recipient, even in the presence of the native, diabetogenic, non-Asp-57, Ag$^7$ molecule. Mechanistically, the authors suggested a model in which a subset of the engineered BM cells—i.e., hematopoietic precursor cells—migrate, populate the thymus, and become antigen-presenting cells involved in the negative selection of thymocytes that would otherwise mature into autoreactive T-cells. In fact, diabetes-free NOD mice exhibited neither the emergence into the blood stream of T-cells capable of responding to putative autoantigens nor the presence of β-cell–reactive T-cells in the pancreatic islets themselves (i.e., no insulitis).

If Tian's approach to obtain autoimmunity abrogation can facilitate a possible recovery of autologous insulin-producing cells also in the diabetic individual, safe induction of an auto-immunity-free status might become a new promising therapy for T1D (125), which would be a great benefit to patients. Figure 3 shows the theoretical basis of Tian's approach for autoimmunity abrogation in the nonobese diabetic mouse. In a healthy individual, the maturation of the T-cells, coming from precursors present in the bone marrow, takes place in the thymus, where they undergo a positive and a negative selection. In the thymus, peptides from antigens of self-tissues are presented to the various immature double positive, T-cells (A, B, and C) via the major histocompatibility complex (MHC) molecule. MHC class II molecules are heterodimers composed of an alpha and a beta chain that form their antigen-combining site. When, as in the A cell, the T-cell receptor (TCR) has a very low affinity for the MHC molecule/self-peptide complex (in the figure, contours of the MHC molecule/self-peptide complex do not fit with the contours of the TCR molecule), the developing T-cell does not receive the necessary positive signal to survive and exit the thymus for release into the periphery. However, if the affinity between the MHC molecule/self-peptide complex and the TCR is too high, as in the B-cell (in the figure, the contours of the MHC molecule/self-peptide complex fit

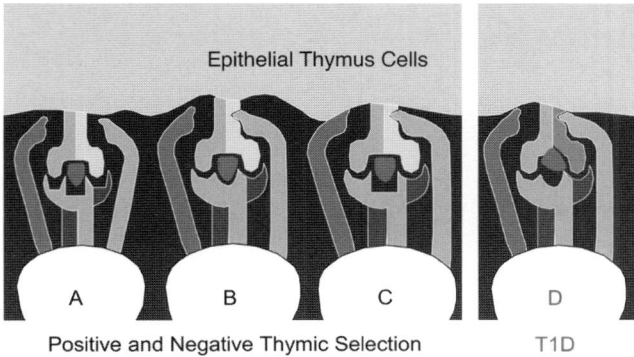

**Figure 3** Theoretical basis of Tian's approach for autoimmunity abrogation in the nonobese diabetic mouse. *Abbreviation:* T1D, Type I diabetes. *Source*: From Ref. 125.

precisely into the contours of the TCR molecule), the T-cell undergoes negative selection and dies inside the thymus. The T-cell shown in C, receives, instead, a positive survival signal because of the high-affinity interactions between its TCR with the MHC molecule, an affinity, however, that is not further enhanced by the presence of a self-peptide in its groove so that negative selection does not take place. This T-cell matures and goes into the circulation to protect the body from foreign (non-self) invaders, with which it is able to efficiently interact. The immunological basis of type 1 diabetes is schematically described in Type I diabetes. Here the D cell binds to an MHC molecule conferring susceptibility to diabetes (like the HLA-DQ8 in humans and the $I\text{-}Ag^7$ in the mouse), because it does not present the self-peptide properly. The T-cell, then, even if potentially autoreactive (D has the same TCR as B), is not subjected to negative selection and is free to leave the thymus to circulate in the blood. T-cells that are potentially reactive to self-antigens but fail to be deleted inside the thymus are able to attack tissues of the body expressing these same antigens, generating autoimmunity. The approach taken by Tian and colleagues (124) can be illustrated imagining that the diabetogenic $I\text{-}Ag^7$ molecule, carrying a non-Asp-57 beta chain, was supplemented in the hematopoietic cells of the nonobese diabetic mouse, with a nondiabetogenic MHC molecule, like the one interacting with A, B, or C. The ex vivo transfection of a gene encoding an $Asp\text{-}57^+$ beta chain, into the bone marrow stem cells, allowed the reconstruction of an efficient MHC molecule that, once the cells were returned into the donor, allowed the restoration of an efficient negative selection in the thymus (as in B), sufficient per se to delete autoreactive T-cells and consequently to prevent diabetes.

Our young diabetic patients must check their blood glucose levels and be injected with insulin multiple times each day. Concurrently, they live with the constant threat of unpredictable acute hypoglycemic episodes and the future concerns about chronic complications. Although human islet transplantation carries with it some potential for the treatment and possible cure of T1D, finding safe ways to block autoimmunity seems to be the first goal we should achieve in order to give our patients a reliable solution to their heavy, lifelong burden, since it is a prerequisite for the efficient use of the re-establishment of euglycemia, capitalizing on the pancreatic regenerative pathway.

# REFERENCES

1. American Diabetes Association. Economic costs of diabetes in the U.S. in 2002. Diabet Care 2003:917–932.
2. Langerhans P. Bertrage zur mikroskopischen anatomie der baushspeicheldruse. Inaugural dissertation, Medizinische Fakultat, Friedrich-Wilhelm-Universitat, Guston Lange, Berlin, 1869.
3. Minkowski O. Mitterlungen uber den diabetes mellitus nach extirpation des pankreas. Berl Klin Wochenschr 1892; 29:90.
4. Hellerstrom C. A method for the microdissection of intact pancreatic islets of mammals. Acta Endocrinol 1964; 45:122.

5.  Moskalewski S. Isolation and culture of the islets of Langerhans of the guinea pig. Gen Comp Endocrinol 1965; 5:342.
6.  Lacy PE, Kostianovsky M. Method for the isolation of intact islets of Langerhans from the rat pancreas. Diabetes 1967; 16(1):35–39.
7.  Ballinger WF, Lacy PE. Transplantation of intact pancreatic islets in rats. Surgery 1972; 72:175.
8.  Ricordi C, Lacy PE, Finke EH, et al. Automated method for isolation of human pancreatic islets. Diabetes 1988; 37:413.
9.  Ricordi, C. Lilly Lecture 2002. Islet transplantation: a brave new world. Diabetes 2003; 52:1595–1603.
10. Scharp DW, Lacy PE, Santiago JV, et al. Insulin independence after islet transplantation into Type I diabetic patient. Diabetes 1990; 39:515–518.
11. Tzakis AG, Ricordi C, Alejandro R, et al. Pancreatic islet transplantation after upper abdominal exenteration and liver replacement. Lancet 1990; 336:402–405.
12. Bretzel RG, Brendel MD, Hering BJ, et al. International Islet Transplant Registry Report. Vol. 8. Geissen: Justus-Liebis University of Geissen, 2001:1.
13. Shapiro AMJ, Lakey JRT, Ryan EA, et al. Islet cell transplantation in seven patients with Type I diabetes mellitus using a glucocorticoid-free immunosuppressive regimen. NEJM 2000; 343:230–238.
14. Bonner-Weir S. Anatomy of the islet of Langerhans. In: Samals E, ed. The Endocrine Pancreas. New York: Raven Press, 1991:15–27.
15. Ahren B, Taborsky GJ. Beta cell function and insulin secretion. In: Porte D, Sherwin RS, Baron A, eds. Ellenberg and Rifkin's Diabetes Mellitus. New York: The McGraw-Hill Companies, Inc., 2003:44–45.
16. Docherty K, Steiner DF. The molecular and cell biology of the beta cell. In: Porte D, Sherwin RS, Baron A, eds. Ellenberg and Rifkin's Diabetes Mellitus. New York: The McGraw-Hill Companies, Inc., 2003:29–32.
17. Naya FJ, Huang HP, Qiu Y, et al. Diabetes, defective pancreatic morphogenesis, and abnormal enteroendocrine differentiation in BETA2/Neuro D deficient mice. Genes Dev, 1997; 11:2323.
18. Jansson J, Carlsson L, Edlund T, et al. Insulin promoter factor 1 is required for pancreas development in mice. Nature 1994; 371:606.
19. Stoffers, DA, Zinkin NT, Stanojevic V, et al. Pancreatic agenesis attributable to a single nucleotide deletion in the human IPF1 gene coding sequence. Nat Genet 1997; 15:106.
20. Daniel S, Nada M, Straub SG, et al. Identification of the docked granule pool responsible for the first phase of glucose-stimulated insulin secretion. Diabetes 1999; 48:1686.
21. Rorsman P, Eliasson L, Renstrom E, et al. The cell physiology of biphasic insulin secretion. News Physiol Sci 2000; 15:72.
22. Geng X, Lehong L, Watkins S, Robbins PD, Drain P. The insulin secretory granule is the major site of K-ATP channels of the endocrine pancreas. Diabetes 2003; 52:767–776.
23. Li L, Wang J, Drain P. The I182 region of Kir 6.2 is closely associated with ligand binding in K-ATP channel inhibition by ATP. Biophys J 2000; 79:841–852.
24. Cook DL, Satin LS, Hopkins WF. Pancreatic beta cells are bursting, but how? Trends Neurosci 1991; 14:411.
25. Henquin JC. Triggering and amplifying pathways of regulation of insulin secretion by glucose. Diabetes 2000; 49:1751–1760.
26. Hering BJ, Kandaswamy J, Harmon JV, et al. Transplantation of cultured islets from two-layer preserved pancreases in Type I diabetes with anti-CD3 antibody. Am J Transplant 2004; 4:390–401.
27. Matsumoto S, Wualley SA, Goes S, et al. Effect of the two-layer (University of Wisconsin solution—perfluorochemical plus 0$_2$) method of pancreas preservation on human islet isolation, as assessed by the Edmonton isolation protocol. Transplantation 2002; 74(10):1414–1419.
28. Wright JR Jr. From ugly fish to conquer death: JJR Macleod's fish insulin research. Lancet 2002; 6359(9313):1238–1242. (http://www.ncbi.nlm.nhi.gov/entrez/query.)
29. Ricordi C, Lacy PE, Scharp DW. Automated islet isolation from human pancreas. Diabetes 1989; 38(suppl 1):140–142.
30. Linetsky E, Bottino R, Lehmann R, Alejandro R, Inverardi L, Ricordi C. Improved human islet isolation using a new enzyme blend, Liberase. Diabetes 1997; 46(7):1120–1123.
31. Lakey JR, Warnock GL, Shapiro AM, et al. Intraductal collagenase delivery into the human pancreas using syringe loading or controlled perifusion. Cell Transplant 1999; 8:285–292.
32. Goto M, Eich TM, Felldin M, et al. Refinement of the automated method for human islet isolation and preservation of a closed system for in vitro islet culture. Transplantation 2004; 78(9):1367–1375.
33. Ricordi C, Rastellini C. Automated method for pancreatic islet separation. In: Ricordi C, ed. Methods in Cell Transplantation. Austin: R.G. Landes Company, 1995:433–438.
34. Balamurugan AN, Chang Y, Fung JJ, Trucco M, Bottino R. Flexible management of enzymatic digestion improves human islet isolation outcome from sub-optimal donor pancreata. Am J Transplant 2003; 3:1135–1142.
35. Ryan EA, Lakey JR, Paty BW, et al. Successful islet transplantation: continued insulin reserve provides long-term glycemic control. Diabetes 2002; 51:2147–2148.
36. Linn T, Schneider K Hammes HP, et al. Angiogenic capacity of endothelial cells in islets of Langerhans. J FASEB 2003; 17:881–883.

37. Bottino R, Fernandez LA, Ricordi C, et al. Transplantation of allogeneic islets of Langerhans in the rat liver: effects of macrophage depletion on graft survival and micro-environment activation. Diabetes 1998; 47:316–323.
38. Gysemans C, Stoffels K, Giulietti A, et al. Prevention of primary non-function of islet xenografts in autoimmune diabetic NOD mice by anti-inflammatory agents. Diabetologia 2003; 46:1115–1123.
39. Wu Y, Han B, Luo H, et al. DCR3/TR6 effectively prevents islet primary non-function after transplantation. Diabetes 2003; 52:2279–2286.
40. Lakey JR, Burridge PW, Shapiro AM. Technical aspects of islet preparation and transplantation. Transplant Int 2003; 16:613–632.
41. Paraskevas S, Maysinger D, Wang R, et al. Cell loss in isolated human islets occurs by apoptosis. Pancreas 2000; 20:270–276.
42. McCauley J, Corry RJ. Pretransplant medical evaluation for pancreas transplant candidates. In: Hakim N, Stratta R, Gray D, eds. Pancreas and Islet Transplantation. New York: Oxford University Press, 2002:47–50.
43. Goss JA, Soltes G, Goodpastor SE, et al. Pancreatic islet transplantation: the radiographic approach. Transplantation 2003; 76:199–203.
44. Baidal DA, Froud T, Ferreira JV, Khan A, Alejandro R, Ricordi C. The bag method for islet cell infusion. Cell Transpl 2003; 12:809–813.
45. Froud T, Yrizarry JM, Alejandro R, Ricordi C. Use of D-Stat to prevent bleeding following percutaneous transhepatic intraportal islet transplantation. Cell Transplant 2004; 13:55–59.
46. Ryan EA, Lakey JRT, Rajotte RV, et al. Clinical outcomes and insulin secretion after islet transplantation with the Edmonton protocol. Diabetes 2001; 50:710–719.
47. Ozmen L, Ekdahl KN, Elgue G, Larsson R, Korsgren O, Nilsson B. Inhibition of thrombin abrogates the instant blood-mediated inflammatory reaction triggered by isolated human islets. Possible application of the thrombin inhibitor melagatran in clinical islet transplantation. Diabetes 2002; (51):1779–1784.
48. Goto M, Johansson H, Maeda A, Elgue G, Korsgren O, Nilsson B. Low-molecular weight dextran sulfate abrogates the instant blood-mediated inflammatory reaction induced by adult porcine islets both in vitro and vivo. Transplant Proc 2004; 36:1186–1187.
49. Rafael E, Ryan EA, Paty BW, et al. Changes in liver enzymes after clinical islet transplantation. Transplantation 2003; 76(9):1280–1284.
50. Bhargava R, Senis PA, Ackerman TE, et al. Prevalence of hepatic steatosis after islet transplantation and its relation to graft function. Diabetes 2004; 53:1311–1317.
51. Owen RJT, Ryan EA, O'Kelly K, Lakey JRT, et al. Percutaneous transhepatic pancreatic islet cell transplantation in Type I diabetes mellitus: radiological aspects. Radiology 2003:165–170.
52. Close NC, Hering BJ, Anand R, Eggerman T. Collaborative Islet Transplant Registry (CITR). In: Cecka M, Terasaki P, eds. Clinical Transplants. Los Angles, CA: UCLA, 2003.
53. Shapiro AMJ. Islet transplants and impact on secondary diabetic complications. Does C-peptide protect the kidney?. J Am Soc Nephrol 2003; 14:2214–2216.
54. Shapiro AMJ, Ricordi C. Unraveling the secrets of single donor success in islet transplantation. Am J Transplant 2004; 4:295–298.
55. Ryan EA, Paty BW, Senior PA, et al. Five-year follow up after clinical islet transplantation. Diabetes 2005; 54:2060–2069.
56. Casey JJ, Lakey JR, Ryan EA, et al. Portal venous pressure changes after sequential clinical islet transplantation. Transplantation 2002; 74:913–915.
57. Toso C, Morel P, Bucher P. et al. Insulin independence after conversion to tacrolimus and sirolimus based immunosuppression in islet–kidney recipients. Transplantation 2003; 76(7):1133–1134.
58. Kaufman DB, Barker MS, Chen X, et al. Sequential kidney/islet transplantation using prednisone-free immunosuppression. Am J Transplant 2002; 2:674–677.
59. Lehman R, Weber M, Berthold P, et al. Successful simultaneous islet–kidney transplantation using a steroid-free immunosuppression. Two-year follow-up. Am J Transplant 2004; 4:117–123.
60. Fiorina P, Folli F, Zerbini G, et al. Islet transplantation is associated with improvements of renal function among uremic patients with Type I diabetes mellitus and kidney transplants. J Am Soc Nephrol 2003; 14(8):2150–2158.
61. Fiorina P, Folli F, Moff P, et al. Islet transplantation improves vascular diabetic complications in patients with diabetes who underwent kidney transplantation: a comparison between kidney–pancreas and kidney-alone transplantation. Transplantation 2003; 75(8):1296–1301.
62. Fiorina P, Folli F, Bertuzzi, et al. Long-term beneficial effect of islet transplantation on diabetic macro/microangiopathy in Type I diabetic kidney transplanted patients. Diabet Care 2003; 26(4):1129–1136.
63. Barshes NR, Lee T, Goodpasture S, et al. Achievement of insulin independence via pancreatic islet transplantation using a remote isolation center: a first-year review. Transplant Proc 2004; 36:1127–1129.
64. Galili V. Evolution and pathophysiology of the human natural anti-alpha galactosyltransferase IgG (anti-Gal) antibody. Springer Semin Immunopathol 1993; 15:155.
65. Cooper DK, Koren E, Oriol R. Oligosaccharides and discordant xenotransplantation. Immunol Rev 1994; 141:31.

66. Phelps CJ, Koike C, Vaught TD, et al. Production of alpha 1,3-galactosyl-transferase-deficient pigs. Science 2003; 299(5605):411–414.
67. Koike C, Fung JJ, Geller DA, et al. Molecular basis of evolutionary loss of the alpha 1,3-galactosyl-transferase gene in higher primates. J Biol Chem 2002; 277(12):10,114–10,120.
68. Koike C, Friday RP, Nakashima I, et al. Isolation of the regulatory regions and genomic organization of the porcine alpha 1,3-galactowyltransferase gene. Transplantation 2000; 70(9):1275–1283.
69. Kahan BW, Jacobson LM, Hullett DA, et al. Pancreatic precursors and differentiated islet cell types from murine embryonic stem cells. An in vitro model to study islet differentiation. Diabetes 2003; 52:2016–2024.
70. Dor Y, Brown J, Martinez OI, Melton DA. Adult pancreatic beta-cells are formed by self-duplication rather than stem cell differentiation. Nature 2004; 429:41–46.
71. Segev H, Fishman B, Ziskind A, et al. Differentiation of human embryonic stem cells into insulin-producing clusters. Stem Cells 2004; 22:265–274.
72. Kojima H, Fugimiya M, Matsumura K, et al. Extrapancreatic insulin-producing cells in multiple organs in diabetes. PNAS 2004; 101(8):2458–2463.
73. Tang DQ, Cao LZ, Burhardt BR, et al. In vivo and in vitro characterization of insulin-producing cells obtained from murine bone marrow. Diabetes 2004; 53:1721–1732.
74. Lipsett M, Finegood DT. β-cell neogenesis during prolonged hyperglycemia in rats. Diabetes 2002; 51:1834–1841.
75. Gu D, Lee MS, Krahl T, Sarvetnick N. Transitional cells in the regenerating pancreas. Development 1994; 120:1873–1881.
76. Bernard-Karger C, Ktorza A. Endocrine pancreas plasticity under physiological and pathological conditions. Diabetes 2001; 50(suppl 1):S30–S35.
77. Brelje TC, Scharp DW, Lacy PE, et al. Effect of homologous placental lactogens, prolactins, and growth hormones in islet β-cell division and insulin secretion in rat, mouse, and human islets: implication for placental lactogen regulation of islet function during pregnancy. Endocrinology 1993; 132:879–887.
78. Rosenberg L. In vivo cell transformation: neogenesis of beta cells from pancreatic ductal cells. Cell Transplant 1995; 4:371–383.
79. Bouwens L. Transdifferentiation versus stem cell hypothesis for the regeneration of islet beta-cells in the pancreas. Microsc Res Tech 1998; 15:332–336.
80. Bonner-Weir S, Deery D, Leahy JL, Weir GC. Compensatory growth of pancreatic beta cells in adult rates after short-term glucose infusion. Diabetes 1989; 38:49–53.
81. Arnush M, Gu D, Baugh C, et al. Growth factors in the regenerating pancreas of gamma-interferon transgenic mice. Lab Invest 1996; 74(6):985–990.
82. Herrera PL. Adult insulin-and glucagon-producing cells differentiate from two independent cell lineages. Development 2000; 127:2317–2322.
83. Gu G, Dubauskaite J, Melton DA. Direct evidence for the pancreatic lineage: NGN3+ cells are islet progenitors and are distinct from duct progenitors. Development 2002; 129:244–2457.
84. Seaberg RM, Smukler SR, Kieffer TJ, et al. Clonal identification of multipotent precursors from adult mouse pancreas that generate neural and pancreatic lineages. Nat Biotechnol 2004; 22:1115–1124.
85. Weir GC, Bonner-Weir S. Beta-cell precursors—a work in progress. Nat Biotechnol 2004; 22:1–2.
86. Suzuki A, Nakauchi H, Taniguchi H. Prospective isolation of multipotent pancreatic progenitors using flow-cytometric cell sorting. Diabetes 2004; 53:2143–2152.
87. Bonner-Wier S, Sharma A. Pancreatic stem cells. J Pathol 2002; 197:519–526.
88. Pelengaris S, Khan M, Evan GI. Suppression of Myc-induced apoptosis in β cells exposes multiple oncogenic properties of Myc and triggers carcinogenic progression. Cell 2002; 109:321–334.
89. Szkudelski T. The mechanism of alloxan and streptozotocin action in B cells of the rat pancreas. Physiol Res 2001; 50:536–546.
90. Elsner M, Tiedge M, Guldbakke B, Lenzen S. Importance of the GLUT2 glucose transporter for pancreatic beta cell toxicity of alloxan. Diabetologia 2002; 45(11):1542–1549.
91. Finegood DT, Weir GC, Bonner-Wier S. Prior streptozotocin treatment does not inhibit pancreas regeneration after 90% pancreatectomy in rats. AJP-Endo 1999; 276:822–827.
92. Li L, Yi Z, Seno M, Kojima I. Activin A and Betacellulin. Effect on regeneration of pancreatic β-cells in neonatal streptozotocin-treated rats. Diabetes 2004; 53:608–615.
93. Karges B, Durinovic-Bello I, Heinze E, Boehm BO, Debatin K-M, Karges W. Complete long-term recovery of β-cell function in autoimmune type 1 diabetes after insulin treatment. Diabet Care 2004; 27:1207–1208.
94. Rother KI, Harlan DM. Challenges facing islet transplantation for the treatment of type 1 diabetes mellitus. J Clin Invest 2004; 114:877–883.
95. von Herrath M, Homann D. Islet regeneration needed for overcoming autoimmune destruction—considerations on the pathogenesis of type 1 diabetes. Pediatr Diabet 2004; 5:23–28.
96. Sutherland DE, Sibley R, Xu XZ, et al. Twin-to-twin pancreas transplantation: reversal and reenactment of the pathogenesis of type 1 diabetes. Trans Assoc Am Physicians 1984; 97:80–87.
97. Ogawa N, List JF, Habener JF, Maki T. Cure of overt diabetes in NOD mice by transient treatment with anti-lymphocyte serum and exendin-4. Diabetes 2004; 53:1700–1705.

98. Zorina TD, Subbotin VM, Bertera S, et al. Recovery of the endogenous beta cell function in auto-immune diabetes. Stem Cells 2003; 21:377–388.

99. Zorina TD, Subbotin VM, Bertera S, Alexander A, Styche AJ, Trucco M. Distinct characteristics and features of allogeneic chimerism in the NOD mouse model of autoimmune diabetes. Cell Transplant 2002; 11:113–123.

100. Li H, Kaufman CL, Boggs SS, Johnson PC, Patrene KD, Ildstad ST. Mixed allogeneic chimerism induced by a sublethal approach prevents autoimmune diabetes and reverses insulitis in nonobese diabetic (NOD) mice. J Immunol 1996; 156:380–388.

101. Ikehara S, Ohtsuki H, Good RA, et al. Prevention of type 1 diabetes in nonobese diabetic mice by allogeneic bone marrow transplantation. Proc Natl Acad Sci 1985; 82:7743–7747.

102. Trucco M. Regeneration of the β-cell. J Clin Invest 2005; 115:5–12.

103. Ryu S, Kodama S, Ryu K, Schoenfeld DA, Faustman DL. Reversal of established autoimmune diabetes by restoration of endogenous β-cell function. J Clin Invest 2001; 108:63–72.

104. Hess D, Li L, Martin M, et al. Bone marrow-derived stem cells initiate pancreatic regeneration. Nat Biotechnol 2003; 21:763–770.

105. Ricordi C, Zeng YJ, Alejandro R, et al. In vivo effect of FK506 on human pancreatic islets. Transplantation 1991; 52:519–526.

106. Tamura K, Fujimura T, Tsutsumi T, et al. Transcriptional inhibition of insulin by FK506 and possible involvement of FK506 binding protein-12 in pancreatic β-cell. Transplantation 1995; 59:1606–1615.

107. Bell E, Cao X, Moibi JA, et al. Rapamycin has a deleterious effect on MIN-6 cells in rat and human islets. Diabetes 2003; 52:2731–2739.

108. Paris M, Bernard-Kargar C, Berthault MF, Bouwens L, Ktorza A. Specific and combined effects of insulin and glucose on functional pancreatic β-cell mass in vivo and in adult rats. Endocrinology 2003; 144:2717–2727.

109. Farilla L, Hui H, Bertolotto C, et al. Glucagon-like peptide-1 promotes islet cell growth and inhibits apoptosis in Zucker diabetic rates. Endocrinology 2002; 143:4397–4408.

110. Lechner A, Yang YG, Blacken RA, Wang L, Nolan AL, Habener JF. No evidence for significant trans-differentiation of bone marrow into pancreatic β-cells in vivo. Diabetes 2004; 53:616–623.

111. Kodama S, Kühtreiber W, Fujimura S, Dale EA, Faustman DL. Islet regeneration during the reversal of autoimmune diabetes in NOD mice. Science 2003; 302:1223–1227.

112. Kodama S, Davis M, Faustman DL. Diabetes and stem cell researchers turn to the lowly spleen. Sci Aging Knowl Environ 2005; 3:pe2.

113. Todd JA, Bell JI, McDevitt HO. HLA-DQ beta gene contributes to susceptibility and resistance in insulin-dependent diabetes mellitus. Nature 1987; 329:599–604.

114. Morel P, Dorman J, Todd J, McDevitt H, Trucco M. Aspartic acid at position 57 of the HLA DQ-beta chain protects against type I diabetes: a family study. PNAS (USA) 1988; 85:8111–8115.

115. Davies JL, Kawaguchi Y, Bennett ST, et al. A genome-wide search for human type 1 diabetes susceptibility genes. Nature 2002; 371:130–136.

116. Lee KL, Wucherpfennig KW, Wiley DC. Structure of a human insulin peptide/HLA-DQ8 complex and susceptibility to type 1 diabetes. Nat Immunol 2001; 2:501–507.

117. Acha-Orbea H, McDevitt HO. The first external domain of the nonobese diabetic mouse class II I-A β-chain is unique. PNAS 1987; 84:2435–2439.

118. Trucco M. To be, or not to be Asp57, that is the question. Diabet Care 1992; 15:705–715.

119. McDevitt HO. Closing in on Type 1 diabetes. N Engl J Med 2001; 345:1060–1061.

120. Lund T, O'Reilly L, Hutchings P, et al. Prevention of insulin-dependent diabetes mellitus in non-obese diabetic mice by transgenes encoding modified I-A β-chain. Nature 1990; 345:727–729.

121. Bohme J, Shuhbaur B, Kanagawa O, Benoist C, Mathis D. MHC-linked protection from diabetes dissociated from clonal deletion of T cells. Science 1990; 249:293–295.

122. Parish N, Chandler P, Quartey-Papafio R, Simpson E, Cooke E. The effect of bone marrow and thymus chimerism between non-obese diabetic (NOD) and NOD-E transgenic mice, on the expression and prevention of diabetes. Eur J Immunol 1993; 23:2667–2675.

123. Pietropaolo M, Trucco M. Major histocompatibility locus and other genes that determine the risk of development of insulin-dependent diabetes mellitus. In: LeRoith D, Taylor S, Olefsky JM, eds. Diabetes Mellitus: a Fundamental and Clinical Text. 3rd. Philadelphia, PA: J. B. Lippincott Co, 2004:539–556.

124. Tian C, Bagley J, Cretin N, Seth N, Wucherpfennig KW, Iacomini J. Prevention of type 1 diabetes by gene therapy. J Clin Invest 2004; 114:969–978.

125. Trucco M, Giannoukakis N. MHC tailored for diabetes cell therapy. Gene Ther 2005; 12:553–554.

# 23 | New Approaches to Pig-to-Man Islet Transplantation

**W. Bennet and C. G. Groth**
*Karolinska Institute, Stockholm, Sweden*

Transplantation of the islets of Langerhans offers a logical means for treating insulin-dependent diabetes mellitus. However, if islet transplantation is to be widely applied, the supply of human islets will not suffice. An alternative would be the use of pig islets. Porcine islets are readily available, and porcine insulin has been used as a treatment for diabetes for several decades. In a pilot study in the early 1990s, 10 patients were transplanted with fetal porcine islets in Stockholm, Sweden (1). In eight patients, the islets were given by intraportal injection; four of these patients had evidence of islet survival, reflected in temporary excretion of small amounts of porcine C-peptide. Two of the patients had the islets placed under the kidney capsule; in one of these patients, a biopsy revealed surviving porcine islets three weeks after transplantation. No clinical benefit was, however, observed. Presumably, most of the transplanted porcine islets were destroyed early after transplantation.

The preferred route for islet transplantation is by intraportal injection. Thus far, little attention has been paid to the possibility that isolated islets, placed in the blood stream, may become the target of an injurious incompatibility reaction. We have recently developed an in vitro islet perfusion system that mimics the conditions encountered by intraportally transplanted islets. This system consists of plastic loops (polyvinylchloride), the inner surface of which has been coated with covalently bound heparin. A rocking device is used to generate flow in the loops (Fig. 1).

## ISLETS EXPOSED TO XENOGENEIC BLOOD UNDERGO INSTANT INJURY

When isolated adult porcine islets were perfused with fresh human blood for one hour in the loop system, an immediate, severe reaction was elicited (2). This reaction was characterized by a rapid activation and consumption of platelets, consumption of polymorphonuclear cells (PMNs) and monocytes, and activation of the coagulation and complement systems. Concomitantly, very high levels of porcine insulin appeared in the loops, presumably reflecting the "dumping" of insulin from damaged islets (Table 1). Morphological examination revealed damaged islets embedded in clots and infiltrated with leukocytes. C3a and C5b-9 was deposited on the islet surface, while human immunoglobulin was not (Fig. 2). Complement inhibition with soluble complement receptor 1 (sCR1) abrogated the complement activation and reduced the insulin release significantly; this implied that the islet injury was complement-mediated (Fig. 3).

To examine whether this reaction would occur also in vivo, adult pig islets were injected intraportally in cynomolgus monkeys (2). Immediately after transplantation, significant complement activation with generation of C3a and sC5b-9 occurred. Concomitantly, extremely high levels of porcine insulin were recorded in the recipients' plasma, indicating severe islet damage. Pretreatment of the monkeys with sCR1 resulted in suppression of complement activation and significantly less insulin release, compared to the findings in the untreated controls (Fig. 4). When the livers were examined 60 minutes post-transplantation, there was a difference in islet morphology. Islets from monkeys in the untreated group were to a large extent torn, small, and fragmented, whereas islets from the sCR1-treated monkeys showed significantly better morphology. There were complement C3 depositions around the islets in the untreated group, whereas very little complement was found in the treated monkeys.

Thus, xenogenic islets exposed to fresh blood in vitro, or injected into the portal vein in vivo, were found to elicit an instant reaction resulting in islet damage. This reaction has not

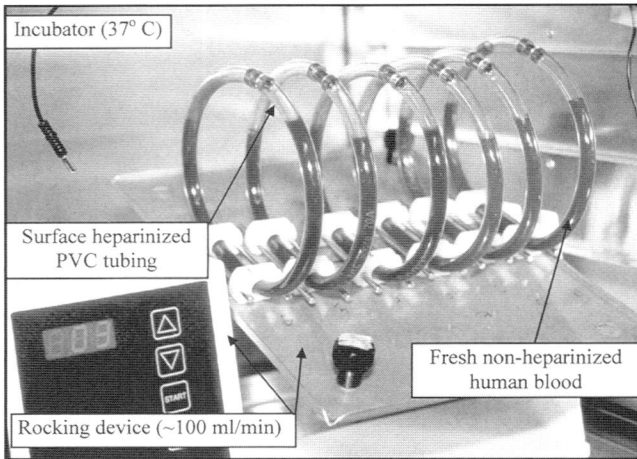

**Figure 1** The loop perfusion system (see text).

been described in detail previously and therefore lacks a descriptive name. We have chosen to name it an instant blood-mediated inflammatory reaction (IBMIR).

## THE ROLE OF PLATELETS IN IBMIR

Since islets are not damaged by fresh human serum during in vitro culture (3), cellular mechanisms or activation of complement or coagulation must be implicated in IBMIR. Recently, platelets have been found to be important mediators of inflammation; thus, platelets may play an important role in the protection against bacterial, parasitic, and foreign particle invasion (4).

Isolated islets of Langerhans consist of conglomerates of several kinds of endocrine cells bound together by fibroblasts and matrix proteins; the cellular conglomerate is surrounded by an incomplete collagen capsule. Thus, isolated islets have a heterogeneous surface, which exposes a variety of cells and matrix proteins. This surface could be expected to induce platelet activation similar to that occurring after vascular endothelial injury.

Indeed, when porcine islets were exposed to fresh human blood in vitro, a massive consumption of platelets and a marked reduction in PMNs occurred within minutes. The fact that the platelets were affected first, and that P-selectin–positive platelets were found to adhere to the islets, indicated that platelets were highly important for triggering the IBMIR. Moreover,

**Table 1** Blood Cell Counts, Coagulation, and Complement Parameters and Insulin Levels Before and After 60 Minutes of Perfusion of Pig Islets with Fresh Human Blood in the Loop

| | Before ($n = 19$) | Medium only added ($n = 19$) | Adult pig islets added ($n = 19$) | *p*-Value medium vs. pig islets added |
|---|---|---|---|---|
| Platelets ($\times 10^9$) | 241± 6.6 | 168± 8.3 | 4.6± 0.5 | < 0.001 |
| Neutrophils ($\times 10^9$) | 2.8± 0.2 | 2.6± 0.2 | 0.6± 0.1 | < 0.001 |
| Monocytes ($\times 10^9$) | 0.39± 0.03 | 0.39± 0.03 | 0.05± 0.01 | < 0.001 |
| Lymphocytes ($\times 10^9$) | 2.3± 0.1 | 2.0± 0.1 | 1.7± 0.1 | < 0.001 |
| C3a (ng/mL) | 83.6± 6.9 | 526± 54 | 1413± 156 | < 0.001 |
| C5b-9 (AU/mL) | 15.3± 1.5 | 63.3± 8.3 | 262.8± 33.4 | < 0.001 |
| FXIIa-AT (µmol/L) | 0.17± 0.07 | 0.16± 0.04 | 8.49± 1.28 | < 0.001 |
| FXI-AT (µmol/L) | 0.05± 0.001 | 0.18± 0.07 | 5.55± 1.57 | 0.003 |
| TAT (µg/mL) | 5.1± 1.3 | 123± 26 | 23,330± 3340 | < 0.001 |
| B-TG (U/mL) | 466± 74 | 1460± 114 | 7275± 538 | 0.025 |
| MPO (ng/mL) | 29.8± 12.4 | 33.7± 8.9 | 56.6± 18.7 | 0.006 |
| Insulin (pmol/L, $\times 10^3$) | 0.01± 0.001 | 0.1± 0.001 | 100.8± 26.2 | 0.001 |

Medium only was added in the control experiments.

**(A)**

**(B)**

**(C)**

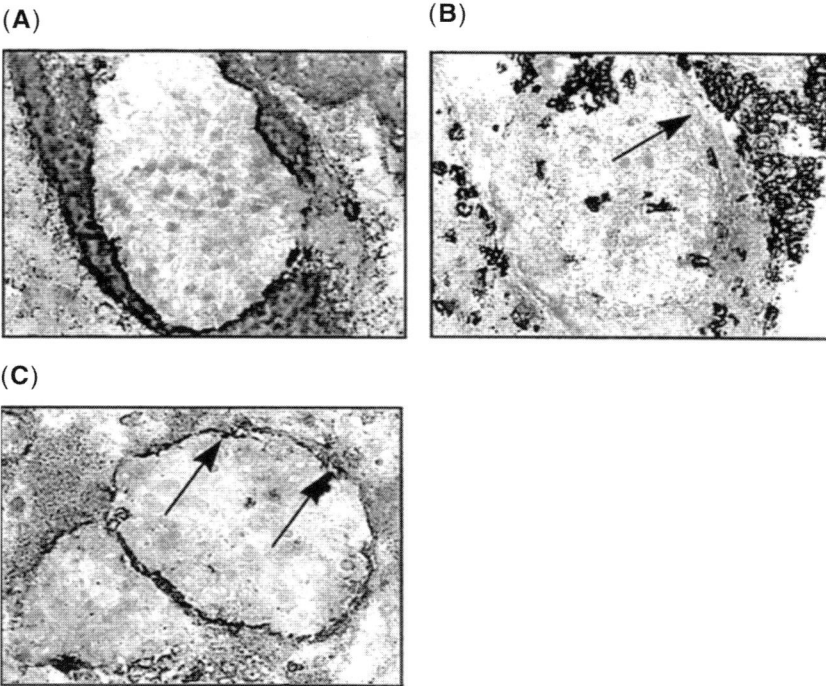

**Figure 2** Immunohistochemical staining of porcine islets after 60 minutes of islet perfusion with fresh nonheparinized human blood in the loop system. (**A**) There is adhesion of large numbers of platelets on the surface of the islets (*staining dark gray*). (**B**) Polymorphonuclear cells and monocytes were found accumulating in thrombi surrounding the islets (*arrow*). (**C**) C3c can be seen as a continuous layer surrounding the islets (*arrows*).

it was found that porcine islets exposed to platelet-rich plasma induced platelet aggregation. Scanning electron microscopic analysis of such islets revealed platelets adhering to the islet surface, with evidence of platelet activation as manifested by platelet spreading and "spiking."

Collagen and other matrix proteins, such as vitronectin and fibronectin, are exposed on the surface of isolated islets (5) and may presumably play a central role in triggering platelet aggregation. Secretion of clotting factors from the activated platelets, and upregulation of

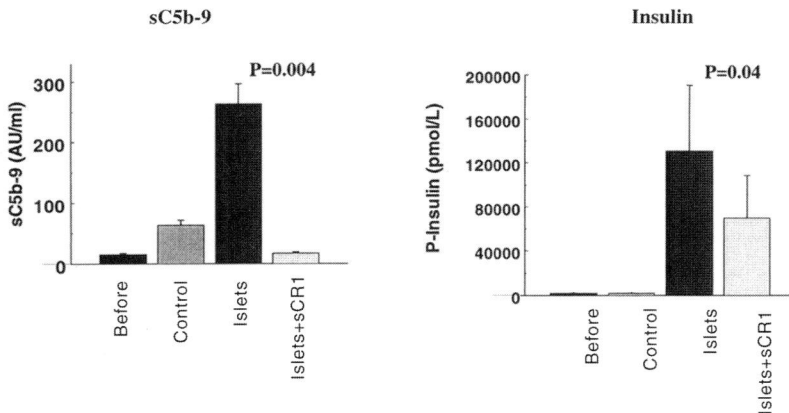

**Figure 3** Measures of complement activation, as reflected in sC5b-9 levels, and of pig islet injury, as reflected in insulin levels in the perifusate following loop perfusion with human blood. Findings in samples collected before and after 60 minutes of perfusion in loop to which saline (controls) or pig islets, or pig islets and soluble complement receptor 1 (sCR1) had been added. The pig islets elicited marked activation of complement and severe islet injury; sCR1 counteracted these changes.

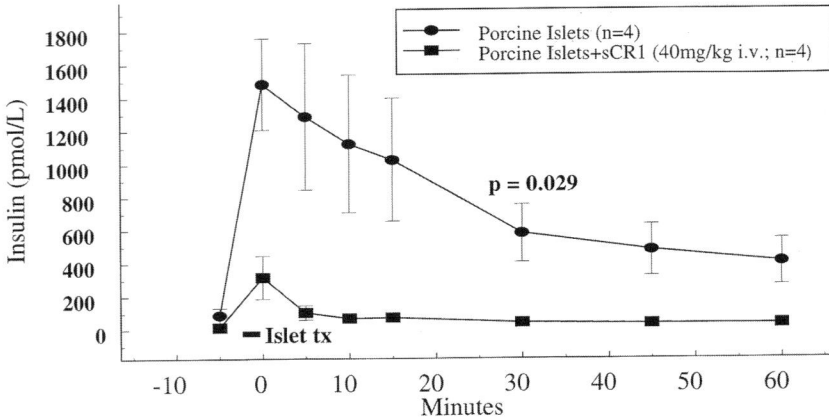

Mean sC5b-9 levels after porcine islet injection:

Control: 135 ± 6 (AU/ml)

sCR1:      54 ± 5 (AU/ml)

**Figure 4**  Levels of insulin and sCR5b-9 in the serum of cynomolgus monkeys measured after intraportal pig islet transplantation. In four animals that were given pig islets only, there were marked complement activation and a massive insulin release indicating severe islet injury. In four animals that were given soluble complement receptor 1 before the injection of the pig islets, complement activation was much diminished and so was insulin dumping.

P-selectin will further potentiate aggregation and clotting. The fibrinogen receptor, which is unique to platelets and plays a central role in platelet aggregation, can also bind to the PMNs (6). Upregulation of P-selectin on platelets will also mediate the binding of PMNs and monocytes to the developing blood clot. Other receptors, which mediate platelet binding to nonhematogenous cells, include the receptors for thrombospondin, vitronectin, and fibronectin. Thus, platelets are well equipped to recognize and to bind to the matrix and cell membrane proteins exposed on isolated islets.

In the intravascular compartment, platelet activation is strictly controlled by several regulatory mechanisms. These regulatory mechanisms are most likely absent on islet cells, and this may explain the extensive formation of thrombi around porcine islets in vitro and in vivo.

## THE ROLE OF COAGULATION IN IBMIR

Porcine islets generated extensive clotting during exposure to fresh human blood in the loop experiments. Clotting was apparent already at five minutes and the clots grew significantly larger during the remaining perfusion period. The findings indicated that coagulation was mainly a result of activation via the intrinsic pathway, possibly triggered by activated platelets (7). However, the extrinsic pathway may also have been triggered as a consequence of tissue factor upregulation on activated monocytes.

In the monkeys that had had porcine islets injected into the portal vein, macroscopic blood clots were detected in the portal branches of the sCR1-treated monkeys, whereas no clots were detectable in the nontreated control monkeys. It can be speculated that this difference was because IBMIR destroyed most of the islets in the untreated recipients, leaving little tissue on which to form clots. In the sCR1-treated recipients, more islets were preserved, improving the conditions for portal thrombosis.

Intraportal clotting in the context of intraportal islet transplantation has been observed previously in animal studies. Thus, rats that had syngeneic islets injected intraportally developed clots around the islets, with concomitant islet damage (8). We have previously observed intraportal clotting in an allogeneic model, in which pig islets were injected into pigs (9).

In clinical islet allo- and autotransplantation, intraportal clotting has also occurred. Portal hypertension, hepatic infarction, and even patient death have been described (10–12). In a liver biopsy obtained from a patient two days after islet allotransplantation, intraportal thrombi, composed of fibrin and leukocytes, clustering around islets were seen (13). This finding was referred to as an "islet cell thrombus" with portal inflammation. Furthermore, one of the patients receiving xenogeneic islets intraportally in Stockholm developed transient portal hypertension and significant platelet consumption (1). Thus, thrombotic complications may occur during intraportal islet transplantation, regardless of whether the islets are autologous, allogeneic, or xenogeneic.

The clots forming around the islets may be detrimental to the survival of the islets. In the early post-transplantation period, before revascularization occurs, islet metabolism depends on diffusion, and the entrapment of the islets in blood clots might hamper diffusion and contribute to islet ischemia (8,14).

## THE ROLE OF COMPLEMENT IN IBMIR

In addition to platelet activation and induction of coagulation, IBMIR was also characterized by complement activation both in vitro and in vivo. In the loop system, complement activation, measured as C3a and sC5b-9, was apparent after five minutes and continued to increase throughout the 60 minutes of study. The activation of complement appeared to occur somewhat more slowly than the very rapid onset of platelet activation. This may indicate that complement activation occurred secondarily to the activation of platelets and coagulation, or that the complement cascade system was triggered somewhat later. However, porcine islet histology did show human complement deposition on the islet surface already at five minutes, indicating that local activation on the islet surface did occur rapidly. Apparently, complement activation in the blood took somewhat longer. Notably, there was no binding of human Ig to the porcine islets, suggesting that complement activation through the classical pathway was unlikely. Intraportal injection of porcine islets into cynomolgus monkeys resulted in complement activation similar to what had been observed in the loops.

Apart from inflicting direct islet damage, the generation of complement factors will also promote activation of PMNs and monocytes, and also enhance platelet activation (15). C3a, C5a, and soluble C5b-9 are extremely potent proinflammatory agents and C5a also upregulates complement receptor 3 on PMNs and monocytes (16,17). In addition, C5a causes the release of toxic products from granulocytes and monocytes, which may inflict islet damage.

## COMPLEMENT INHIBITION AND HEPARIN ADMINISTRATION ABROGATE IBMIR

Since activation of the complement and coagulation systems was prominent feature of IBMIR, the effects of inhibiting these systems were investigated. Both in the loop perfusion experiments and in the monkey experiments, complement inhibition with sCR1 resulted in a nearly complete inhibition of complement activation. At the same time, the porcine insulin release was reduced to approximately half (2). However, consumption of blood cells and activation of coagulation remained unaffected. In addition, inflammatory cells still infiltrated the islets.

The addition of heparin to the loop system prior to porcine islet perfusion effectively inhibited coagulation and reduced consumption of blood elements and, to some degree, also complement activation. It did not, however, prevent platelet and fibrin binding, or leukocyte infiltration. Supplementing the blood with both sCR1 and heparin caused effective inhibition of both coagulation and complement activation. Furthermore, leukocyte infiltration was reduced, and islet morphology was improved (2). Thus, inhibiting IBMIR with combined treatment seemed to provide the most favorable conditions for islet survival.

## IBMIR IS AN INNATE INFLAMMATORY REACTION

In a previous study, we have shown that allogeneic islets also elicit IBMIR. Thus, when human islets were exposed to fresh human blood in the loop system, changes (9) were very similar to those seen when pig islets were used. Furthermore, when pig islets were injected into the portal vein in pigs, there was formation of intravascular clots surrounding the islets, presumably as a consequence of IBMIR.

Thus, IBMIR seems to be an innate response that occurs when nonhematological cells are exposed to fresh blood. In the context of intraportal allogeneic and xenogeneic islet transplantation, the islets will be exposed first to IBMIR, and then to the destructive mechanisms of allo- and xeno-rejection, respectively. The IBMIR will inflict damage to the islets by itself, but it will presumably also enhance the severity of the rejection process by augmenting antigen presentation (18,19). Autologous islets will presumably also elicit IBMIR, but since no immune rejection will follow enough islets may survive to allow for blood glucose control.

## FUTURE PROSPECTS

Counteracting IBMIR in the context of intraportal islet transplantation, either with xenogeneic or with allogeneic islets, should reduce early islet injury and improve subsequent islet function and survival. This may be achieved by inhibiting the activation of the platelets, or the coagulation or complement cascades, by some form of systemic treatment. Alternatively, the islet surface could be modified or covered, thereby reducing the exposure of collagen and other molecules, which might trigger the inflammatory response. Heparinization of the islet surface could offer a way to reduce activation of the coagulation cascade. The use of islets from transgenic pigs, which express human inhibitors of complement, would offer an alternative, attractive means to counteract complement activation.

The discovery that isolated porcine islets exposed to human blood elicit an IBMIR, that is injurious to the islets, and that there are means available to counteract this reaction, should have important implications for pig-to-man islet transplantation. Applying such measures in allogeneic human islet transplantation should also facilitate islet survival and function.

## REFERENCES

1. Groth CG, Korsgren O, Tibell A, et al. Transplantation of porcine fetal pancreas to diabetic patients. Lancet 1994; 344 (8934):1402.
2. Bennet W, Sundberg B, Lundgren T, et al. Damage to porcine islets of Langerhans after exposure to human blood in vitro, or after intraportal transplantation to cynomolgus monkey: protective effects of sCR1 and heparin. Transplantation 2000; 69:711–719.
3. Mirenda V, Le Mauff B, Cassard A, et al. Intact pig pancreatic islet function in the presence of human xenoreactive natural antibody binding and complement activation. Transplantation 1997; 63(10):1452.
4. Männel DN, Grau GE. Role of platelet adhesion in homeostasis and immunopathology. J Clin Pathol Mol Pathol 1997; 50:175.
5. van Suylichem PT, van Deijnen JE, Wolters GH, van Schilfgaarde R. Amount and distribution of collagen in pancreatic tissue of different species in the perspective of islet isolation procedures. Cell Transplant 1995; 4(6):609.
6. Sprangenberg P. Adhesion of activated platelets to polymorphonuclear leukocytes. Thromb Res 1994; 74:35.
7. Walsh PN, Sinha D, Koshy A. Functional characterization of platelet-bound factor XIa: retention of factor-XIa activity on the platelet surface. Blood 1986; 68:225.
8. Grotting JC, Rosai J, Matas AJ, et al. The fate of intraportally transplanted islets in diabetic rats. A morphologic and immunohistochemical study. Am J Pathol 1978; 92(3):653.
9. Bennet W, Sundberg B, Groth CG, et al. Incompatibility between human blood and isolated human islets of Langerhans: a finding with important implications for clinical intraportal islet transplantation. Diabetes 1999; 48:1907–1914.
10. Toledo-Pereyra LH, Rowlett AL, Cain W, Rosenberg JC, Gordon DA, MacKenzie GH. Hepatic infarction following intraportal islet cell autotransplantation after near-total pancreatectomy. Transplantation 1984; 38(1):88.
11. Shapiro J, Lakey J, Rajotte R, et al. Portal vein thrombosis after transplantation of partially purified pancreatic islets in a combined human liver/islet allograft. Transplantation 1995; 59:1060–1063.
12. Froberg MK, Leone JP, Jessurun J, Sutherland DR. Fatal disseminated intravascular coagulation after autologous islet transplantation. Hum Pathol 1997; 28:1295–1298.
13. Sever CE, Demetris AJ, Zeng Y, et al. Islet cell allotransplantation in diabetic patients. Histologic findings in four adults simultaneously receiving kidney or liver transplants. Am J Pathol 1992; 140(5):1255.
14. Cameron JL, Mehegan DG, Harrington DP, Zuidema GD. Metabolic studies following intrahepatic autotransplantation of pancreatic islet grafts. Surgery 1980; 87:397.
15. Sims PJ, Wiedmer T. The response of human platelets to activated components of the complement system. Immunol Today 1991; 12(9):338.
16. Fletcher MP, Stahl GL, Longhurst JC. C5a-induced myocardial ischemia: role for CD18-dependent PMN localization and PMN-platelet interactions. Am J Physiol 1993; 265(5 Pt 2):H1750.

17. Chenoweth DE, Hugli TE. Demonstration of specific C5a receptor on intact human polymorpho-nuclear leukocytes. Proc Natl Acad Sci USA 1978; 75(8):3943.
18. Carroll MC, Fischer MB. Complement and the immune response. Curr Opin Immunol 1997; 9(1):64–69.
19. Callucci S, Lolkema M, Matzinger P. Natural adjuvants: endogeneous activators of dendritic cells. Nat Med 1999; 5(11):1249–1255.

# 24 | Pregnancy After Pancreas Transplantation

**Velma P. Scantlebury**

*Department of Surgery, University of South Alabama, Mobile, Alabama, U.S.A.*

## INTRODUCTION

The success of combined pancreas–kidney transplantation has resulted in an improved quality of life, not only by restoring renal function, but also by stabilizing and/or eliminating some of the metabolic consequences of diabetes.

Diabetic patients with or without renal impairment often experience significant morbidity during pregnancy, resulting in neonates who are large for gestational age and are subject to an increased incidence of congenital abnormalities and respiratory distress syndrome. The restoration of renal function by kidney transplantation increases the chances of successful pregnancy. However, successful outcomes can still be compromised as a result of metabolic derangements associated with diabetes. Despite these increased risks, careful control of blood sugars and recent advances in neonatal care have resulted in improved fetal outcome.

It is well known that restoration of impaired renal function by kidney transplantation has resulted in increased numbers of successful pregnancies (1–4), primarily in nondiabetic patients. However, for diabetic renal transplant recipients in general, pregnancy has not been advised, primarily due to the increased maternal and perinatal mortality. Successful pregnancies have been reported in this group of patients (5–7), but with less frequency when compared with nondiabetic renal transplant recipients.

Many patients who undergo simultaneous pancreas–kidney (SPK) transplants are of childbearing age. With the improvements in the long-term results of SPK transplantation, many patients have an increasing desire to have children. The maternal risks of complications related to their original disease, such as retinopathy or arteriopathy, coupled with the risks of graft loss for those with an existing second organ, might be expected to be exponentially greater for these patients when compared to those with a kidney transplant alone.

In this chapter, we will outline the possible complications that can be encountered after pancreas transplantation for both the recipient and the fetus. A review of the literature and reported cases will be detailed. The need for a multidisciplinary approach in the management of these patients will be outlined and discussed, as well as recommendations for pre-pregnancy teaching pertinent to this patient population.

## BACKGROUND

The first reported successful pregnancy in an SPK recipient was published in 1986 (8). A juvenile diabetic since the age of nine years, this patient became pregnant 16 months after transplantation. Complications of renal graft dysfunction, proteinuria, and hypertension prompted a cesarean section at 35 weeks gestation. There were no perinatal complications, but the congenital abnormality of bilateral cataracts was noted in the baby. The number of reported pregnancies in SPK recipients has subsequently increased (Table 1). Despite the challenge placed on the endocrine function of the pancreas as a result of pregnancy, the overall outcome in these patients has been generally good (9–12).

Many of the earlier reports of pregnancies occurred in recipients who received segmental pancreas grafts (13,14); these outcomes were no different from those with whole pancreas grafts. Gunnar et al. reported that the risk of gestational diabetes in nondiabetic women (resulting from increased insulin resistance) seen in the third trimester of pregnancy was in the range of 0.15% to 12%. This being the case, patients with segmental pancreas grafts could conceivably be at greater risk as a result of the decreased islet cell mass and the diabetogenic effect of steroids and immunosuppressive drugs. The lack of data to substantiate this

**Table 1** Immunosuppressive Therapy and Outcome of Pregnancy in Combined Renal–Pancreas Transplantation Cases

| Author(s) | Live births | Time to conception (mean mo) | Complications | Gestational age (wk) | Fetal outcome |
|---|---|---|---|---|---|
| Skannal, et al. (9) | 1 | 21 | Early labor | 35 | Normal |
| McGrory, et al. (10) | 12 | 40.8 | Hypertension, pre-eclampsia, infections, graft dysfunction, hydronephrosis | <37 | Anemia, pneumonia (1 pt) |
| Midtvedt, et al. (11) | 2 | Unknown | Gram-negative septicemia and hyperemesis | 38 | Normal |
|  |  | 21 | Placental abruption | 36 | Normal |
| Barrou, et al. (12) (IPTR) | 19 | 32.6± 19 | Worsening retinopathy, graft dysfunction, septicaemia | 35.2± 2.2 | Double aortic arch (1 pt), bilateral cataracts (1 pt), DM at 3 yr (pt 1) |

*Abbreviations*: DM, Diabetes mellitus; IPTR, International Pancreas Transplant Registry; pt, patient.

theoretical risk has been encouraging and confirms the ability of the transplanted pancreas to handle the metabolic challenges of pregnancy.

The long-term consequences of diabetes, such as microvascular and neuropathic complications, can be stabilized or prevented by pancreas transplantation. For patients who undergo transplantation before the development of significant complications of long-term diabetes, such as renal disease, the improved patient and graft survival results in improved outcomes for both recipient and offspring. Thus, patients who have had successful solitary pancreas transplantation might be expected to have less morbidity and perinatal mortality when compared with patients who undergo renal transplantation alone. However, there are no data in the literature to confirm this hypothesis.

The overall risk of pregnancy after organ transplantation in this group of patients is influenced not only by the immunosuppressive therapy and the underlying renal and pancreatic graft function but also by the potential complications that could develop as a result of long-term diabetes (Table 2).

## IMMUNOSUPPRESSIVE DRUGS

The number of recipients who have undergone pancreas transplantation under cyclosporine (CyA)-based immunosuppression remains significantly greater than those treated with tacrolimus. The report from the International Pancreas Transplant Registry in 1998 by Barrou et al. (12) showed a total of 9012 pancreas transplants performed as of December 1996. All of these patients were treated with CyA-based therapy. Within this group, 19 pregnancies were reported, resulting in 19 live births in a total of 17 female recipients.

Maintenance immunosuppression consisted of various combinations of CyA, azathioprine, and prednisone. The management of CyA dosing in pregnancy after transplantation has been previously described by earlier experiences in liver and kidney transplant recipients (16–18).

The state of pregnancy is known to result in an overall increase in the glomerular filtration rate, which may explain the decrease in CyA levels especially seen in the third

**Table 2** Risks to Offspring of Allograft Recipients

Congenital abnormalities
   Related to immunosuppressive medication
Viral infections
   Cytomegalovirus
   Herpes simplex virus
   Infectious hepatitis
Possible long-term problems
   Fertility problems
   Chromosome breaks in offspring

*Source*: From Ref. 15.

trimester of pregnancy. Several other physiological changes that occur in pregnancy, such as the increase in body weight and fat content, could also alter the pharmacokinetics of CyA and its metabolism, as a result of the increase in the volume of drug distribution. While there is a tendency for trough levels to decrease, these changes are not consistent from patient to patient. One author reported an increase in the CyA requirement in three pregnancies of kidney transplant recipients (19), while other authors maintained the pre-pregnancy doses of CyA without any alterations during pregnancy (20). Armenti's review of patients on CyA therapy found that the data supported the concept that CyA bioavailability was altered during pregnancy. Decreasing CyA doses could perhaps contribute to adverse graft-related events, which, in turn, could affect neonatal outcome and graft survival. Although preventing rejection is the primary focus, the incidence of rejection during pregnancy has remained low, with few documented reports, especially in the third trimester. However, graft dysfunction during pregnancy or within two years after delivery (graft loss or rejection) was seen more in patients on lower CyA dosages (<3 mg/kg/day) with higher pre-pregnancy serum creatinines than in those whose pre-pregnancy CyA dosages were >4 mg/kg/day. In addition, those patients who experienced early graft dysfunction had neonates with lower birth weights and lower gestational age than those who experienced no graft dysfunction before or after delivery (21).

CyA is known to cross the placental barrier, but there have been no reports of direct harm to the fetus. Venkataraman et al. (22) documented the concentrations of CyA and its metabolites in the mother and the child, but these levels were essentially undetectable three to five days after birth in most cases (23). In the literature, there are no reports of CyA causing any mutagenic or carcinogenic changes.

Nausea and vomiting can be a factor in the patient's ability to tolerate the immunosuppressive drugs, and may necessitate hospitalization and intravenous fluid support to ensure appropriate dosing of medications and immunosuppressive drug levels. It is pertinent to monitor for changes in graft function during these episodes, in order to determine whether the fluctuations in CyA levels are affecting either the kidney or the pancreas graft function.

The use of azathioprine and prednisone during pregnancy is also well documented. Leukopenia and thrombocytopenia have been reported with the use of azathioprine, but at significantly higher doses than the standard 1–2 mg/kg/dose (24). While one study looking at the chromosomes of lymphocytes from an infant born to a mother on azathioprine showed some chromosomal abnormalities, these changes were said not to be evident at one year after birth (25). Similarly, studies on rats have shown normal first-generation offspring, but increased infertility in the second generation. Penn et al. reported two offspring of male recipients and four of female recipients who had congenital abnormalities present at birth. All six recipients were taking azathioprine prior to pregnancy. Data from Armenti's National Transplantation Pregnancy Registry (NTPR) (21) showed that neonates born to mothers on non-CyA regimens had more complications but were less likely to have low birth weights when compared to neonates born to patients on CyA. Five of six neonates who died were born to mothers on azathioprine and were conceived within two years after transplantation. However, the incidence remains small and can be multifactorial in origin. Analysis from all data sources is needed before specific conclusions can be drawn when comparing these patients to the general population.

Steroids have also been implicated in the increased incidence of premature rupture of membranes, as well as worsening hypertension. Adrenal insufficiency in an infant born to a mother on azathioprine and steroids has been reported by Penn et al. (3) in an earlier series of patients. With the introduction of newer immunosuppressive agents, current steroid requirements are lower, which is certainly more advantageous for patients.

Mycophenolate mofetil, a new purine antagonist, has been used more frequently in recent years as a third agent and is effective in reducing the incidence of acute rejection. Fetal abnormalities have occurred in animal studies, which has been seen as effects on organogenesis at lower dosages than those that result in maternal toxicity. However, there are no reports to date of such malformations in the offspring of female transplant recipients, despite the use of this drug in combination with Prograf and Neoral reported in data from the NTPR (26). With the increasing number of pregnancies that continue to be reported, more information will be needed before the actual risks can be determined (Table 2).

With the improved patient and graft survival under tacrolimus, reports of successful pregnancies in liver, kidney, and pancreas recipients have been increasing, as more and more patients achieve better long-term success and quality of life after transplantation (11,27). The earliest reports of live births from mothers receiving tacrolimus have been in liver transplant recipients (28,29). There were no reported birth defects or congenital abnormalities. Jain et al. reported one preterm fetal death that occurred at 22 weeks gestation born to a 20-year-old patient who conceived one month after liver transplantation. Twelve pregnancies reported by Armenti et al. (26) were all on tacrolimus at the time of conception. Despite the higher incidence of diabetes and infections seen during pregnancy, outcomes for both mother and child were comparable to those on CyA-based therapy.

The teratogenic effects of tacrolimus were studied by Farley et al. (30), who reported resorption of all fetuses in experiments using pregnant mice that were treated with high-dose tacrolimus. While there were no obvious detrimental effects on maternal health with either high- or low-dose tacrolimus, some resorptions of fetuses were seen at low doses. Those fetuses that did survive were without teratogenic changes and appeared the same as those born to the control animals. Farley concluded that the toxicity effects seen with tacrolimus are dose-dependent. Clinically, tacrolimus has been a safe and efficacious drug that can be used during pregnancy and has not been associated with any harmful effects to either mother or child.

## MATERNAL OUTCOME

For patients undergoing pancreas or kidney–pancreas transplantation for type I diabetes, the average duration of diabetes is about 20 years. The majority of pancreas–kidney recipients are of childbearing age, and, once beyond the perioperative period, generally are able to resume normal activities. These recipients have been cleared from a cardiac point of view by extensive preoperative workup. However, cardiac complications can also develop postoperatively, leading to significant morbidity and mortality despite good glycemic control. Barrou et al. (12) reported one death from a myocardial infarction, occurring five years after delivery despite normal pretransplant cardiac angiography and normal pancreas function. Long-term survival in this group is therefore dependent not only the complications of transplantation but also on the underlying disease process.

For most reports, the interval between transplantation and conception has ranged from one to three years. Many pregnancies were able to complete gestation to 35 weeks and even beyond. Elective cesarean sections occurred in nearly 80% of cases; these were often prompted by worsening hypertension, a decrease in fetal heart rate, and failure of labor to progress. Many cesareans were also performed as a result of concerns regarding the presence of the grafts within the iliac fossa and the desire to avoid potential injury by repeated uterine contractions.

Vaginal delivery has also been reported in pancreas–kidney transplant patients (31). This can be safe despite the presence of a pelvic pancreas transplant, if there is no extreme prolonged pelvic compression (32). The decision to proceed with vaginal delivery should be individualized and only undertaken with a combined multidisciplinary approach. McGrory et al. have also described maternal complications in their study of 15 pregnancies in 10 pancreas–kidney recipients (Table 3).

Pre-eclampsia is said to be more common in transplant recipients when compared to the general population. An incidence of 30% to 35% has been reported by a number of authors in renal transplant recipients (2,33). The onset of hypertension and proteinuria in the third trimester may be due to underlying renal dysfunction. Assessing the underlying pathology may be difficult, and some patients may experience a deterioration of renal function after delivery (Table 4). Often an early delivery can be prompted not only by pre-eclampsia but also by

**Table 3**  Percentage of Maternal Comorbid Conditions in Kidney–Pancreas Recipients (15 Pregnancies in 10 Recipients)

| Condition | No. of patients |
|---|---|
| Hypertension | 13 (87%) |
| Pre-eclampsia | 4 (32%) |
| Infections | 12 (73%) |
| Rejection | 2 (13%) |
| Graft dysfunction | 3 (20%) |

*Source*: From Ref. 10.

**Table 4** Outcomes of 12 Newborns of 10 Pancreas–Kidney Recipients (15 Pregnancies)

| | |
|---|---|
| Cesarean section | 8 (67%) |
| Mean gestational age at birth (±SD) | 38.7 (±2.1 wk) |
| Prematurity (<37 wk) | 9 (75%) |
| Mean birth weight (±SD) | 1873 (±468 g) |
| Low birth weight (<2500 g) | 10 (83%) |
| Complications of prematurity | 3 (25%) |
| Neonatal deaths | 0 |

*Source*: From Ref. 15.

ongoing hypertension. Van Winter et al. reported one patient with two pregnancies in whom severe labile hypertension precipitated early delivery despite good baseline renal and pancreatic function. An analysis of outcomes from the NTPR by McGrory et al. (10) reported the incidence of hypertension and urinary tract infections to be 87% and 73 %, respectively; these were the two highest comorbid conditions seen in the 10 transplant recipients with 12 live births. None of these infections were life threatening, and all were able to be resolved with appropriate treatment.

Transplant recipients are more susceptible not only to bacterial infections but also to viral infections. While reactivation of a maternal viral infection is a possibility, so far, there have been no reported cases of cytomegalovirus infections during pregnancy in pancreas transplant recipients. Whether such congenital viral infections may be asymptomatic or may result in congenital abnormalities such as hearing loss has yet to be determined.

Maternal complications related to the original disease are certainly risks that can complicate the pregnancy either during or after birth. Worsening retinopathy or arteriopathy are such concerns, but are not predictable. One such case of progressive retinopathy was reported by Barrou et al. (12), and occurred at the end of the pregnancy. Surgical complications have also been reported, such as roux-en-y loop obstruction requiring surgical correction. Both transverse and vertical hysterotomies have been used without any reported direct injuries to the nearby kidney and pancreas grafts.

However, in addition to the one case of a bladder injury reported, a tear to the duodenal segment of a pancreas graft was described as a complication of a cesarean section in the report by McGrory et al. (10). Whether this was directly related to the surgical procedure was not clear. This injury was successfully repaired.

## KIDNEY AND PANCREAS OUTCOME (FUNCTION)

The physiological changes of increasing renal blood flow and increase in glomerular filtration rate can lead to a rise in the creatinine clearance of nearly 50% in patients during early to mid-pregnancy (34). This elevation can continue throughout pregnancy. Hence, it is important to establish baseline function of the kidney by checking an initial 24-hour urine collection for creatinine clearance and protein excretion and then following serial 24-hour urines. An increase in protein excretion during pregnancy can be a sign of either pre-eclampsia or worsening renal function. However, many patients will have greater than 0.3 g/24 hours of proteinuria excreted after kidney transplantation. Thus, careful monitoring of kidney function is essential in order to assess potential complications.

Patients who have received segmental pancreas grafts have been able to meet the challenge of the increased need for insulin that occurs in the second and third trimester of pregnancy. There were no reported differences in the ability of the segmental grafts to function appropriately during pregnancy when compared to patients who received a whole graft. No reports of abnormal blood sugars have been documented.

Increased pelvic pressure from uterine growth can result in pancreatitis. Kairaitis et al. (35) reported such a case in a patient who had previously undergone enteric conversion of bladder-drained pancreatic graft to a loop of jejunum 18 months earlier. Graft pancreatitis occurred at 30 weeks gestation, caused either by direct graft compression or reflux into the pancreas. The patient was treated with total parenteral nutrition for two weeks, resulting in gradual but incomplete resolution of the patient's elevated enzymes.

The problems created by the enlarging uterus are a major concern not only for the pancreas but also for the kidney. Biesenbach et al. (19) reported two cases of mechanical obstruction of the transplant ureter in pancreas–kidney transplant recipients. Both required placement of a nephrostomy and underwent surgical revision four and eight weeks after delivery.

No pancreas rejections during pregnancy have been reported by any of the large series of cases. Tyden et al. (36) documented evidence of deteriorating kidney function at 33 and 34 weeks gestation in two of four patients reported in their early series. All four patients had received pancreas and kidney grafts. However, postpartum changes in graft function may be a late reflection of earlier graft dysfunction, such as that seen in the case reported by Barrou et al. (37). This report of acute rejection 2.5 months postpartum led to the need for allograft pancreatectomy. Such rejection might be the result of the termination of the natural immunosuppressive state of pregnancy.

The risks of acute rejection during or within three months of delivery are estimated to be 9% to 14.5%. McGrory et al. also reported three graft losses (two kidneys and one pancreas) within two years of delivery in two patients with elevated pre-pregnancy creatinine levels (1.9 and 2.3 mg/dL, respectively) (10). Worse baseline renal function pre-pregnancy has been determined to be a risk factor for complications during pregnancy and postpartum, and has been well documented in patients with renal transplants alone. The existence of pre-pregnancy hypertension, even if adequately treated, or hypertension occurring prior to 28 weeks' gestation may contribute to covert microvascular changes that could lead to the compromised development of uteroplacental circulation. A longer interval between transplantation and conception may increase the risk even in the absence of hypertension (38,39).

## FETAL OUTCOME

The most frequent fetal complications documented are prematurity, growth retardation, congenital anomalies, and occasional medical problems. Barrou et al. reported two cases of congenital malformations in their report of the International Pancreas Transplant Registry study (12). These were congenital bilateral cataracts and a double aortic arch, which required surgical correction three months later. Given that pancreas transplantation corrects the abnormal glucose metabolism, one would expect the rate of congenital abnormalities to be similar to that seen in the general population. This is perhaps borne out by the higher incidence of malformations in infants born to diabetic mothers who have not received transplants (5).

The incidence of prematurity is similar to that seen in kidney transplant recipients, ranging from 70% to 75%. The mean gestational age is in the range of 35 weeks. With the high rate of cesarean sections being performed, some of the main causes of early delivery are failure of labor to progress, decreased fetal heart rate, increasing maternal hypertension, and fear of harm to the pancreas graft by vaginal delivery. Mean birth weights are generally over 2000 g, averaging 2100 to 2300 g. McGrory et al. reported three of 12 newborns with birth weights less than 1500 g (10).

Cited medical complications include transfusion-required anemia, pneumonia, ventilatory support, and one case of candidiasis of the urinary tract. Follow-up of these infants has shown normal growth and development. No long-term sequelae from exposure to maternal immunosuppression have been recorded. However, the risk of diabetes in the offspring of diabetic mothers is 13% to 14%, if the maternal age of onset of diabetes is less than eight years. This compares to 2.5% if the maternal onset occurred after age 8 (40). In pancreas recipients, there is only one documented case of the development of type I diabetes, occurring in an infant at age 3 (12). Long-term follow-up of these children will be necessary to determine the actual rate of transmission in this group of diabetic mothers. It is unlikely that correction of the metabolic derangements by pancreatic transplantation will reduce the incidence of diabetes in the offspring. Such risks must be considered when considering the long-term consequences of pregnancy in these recipients.

## RECOMMENDATIONS

All potential pancreas–kidney recipients of childbearing age should be counseled regarding the resumption of sexual activity and the potential return of fertility after transplantation. The need for contraception should be stressed until their health is optimized in order to decrease the chances of complications. All potential problems should be discussed and the risks to both mother and child should be detailed. Barrier contraceptives are the preferred choice because of the risks of thrombosis associated with hormonal therapy. However, the recent development of low-dose estrogens can minimize the possible risks associated with oral contraceptives. They should only be used in consultation with a specialist.

The standard recommendation offered to kidney transplant recipients who desire to have children is an interval of at least two years of stable health between transplantation and conception (41). Analysis of data from the NTPR concluded that neonates conceived within two years of transplantation had significantly lower birth weights than those conceived greater than five years after transplantation (42). Information regarding the complications that can be encountered during and after pregnancy, as well as the chances for positive outcomes, should be discussed. Once pregnancy is established, a high-risk obstetrical evaluation should take place for early prenatal assessment, in collaboration with the transplant team. It is important to emphasize the following: (i) good physical health that would optimize the obstetrical outcome, (ii) minimal proteinuria, (iii) the absence of hypertension or well-controlled hypertension, (iv) no evidence of graft dysfunction, with a preferred base-line serum creatinine less than 1.5 to 2 mg/dL, (v) no evidence of mechanical obstruction of the kidney, and (vi) maintenance of low-dose immunosuppressive medications.

Early pregnancy may be complicated by emesis gravidarum, which may require hospitalization for fluid management to prevent dehydration. Renal dysfunction may also occur as a result of suboptimal immunosuppressive drug levels resulting from poor absorption related to continued emesis. It is important to rule out rejection at this stage. Continual evaluation of graft function by routine chemistries and 24-hour urine collections are important in detecting potential problems. These should be followed every four to six weeks for assessment of renal and pancreas function. Prenatal visits every two weeks until 30 weeks gestation are recommended, followed by weekly visits. Consideration should be given to the use of prophylactic antibiotics if there is history of bacteriuria to prevent infection. Ultrasound monitoring of the patient and the fetus from 20 weeks gestation is suggested, preferably every three to four weeks.

The most important factor for a successful delivery is the cooperation and communication between the transplant surgeon and the obstetrician. Once the delivery process is completed, continued monitoring of pancreatic and renal function is essential to diagnose any postpartum complications. The long-term graft survival after pregnancy in renal transplant recipients was compared with matched controls by Salmela et al. (43). They reported a 69% 10-year graft survival compared to 100% for control patients. It is known that a slow deterioration of the function of grafts occurs over time. Whether this deterioration is accelerated by pregnancy is certainly an issue to be considered.

While female pancreas–kidney transplant recipients generally can tolerate a pregnancy without significant detrimental effects to either mother or child, the increased risk of reduced long-term graft function should be considered and discussed in the counseling of these patients. As future analyses of data from pancreas transplant recipients are performed, the long-term outcomes in these patients will become more apparent.

# REFERENCES

1. Murray JE, Reid DE, Harrison JH, et al. Successful pregnancies after human renal transplantation. N Engl J Med 1963:269–346.
2. Davison JM. Pregnancy in renal allograft recipients: prognosis and management. Baillieres Clin Obstet Gynaecol 1987; 1:1027–1045.
3. Penn I, Makowski EL, Harris P. Parenthood following renal transplantation. Kidney Int 1980; 18:221–233.
4. Armenti VT, Ahlswede KM, Ahlswede A, et al. National Transplantation Pregnancy Registry—outcomes of 154 pregnancies in cyclosporine-treated female kidney transplant recipients. Transplantation 1994; 579(4):502–506.
5. Ogburn PL, Kitzmiller JL, Hare JW, Phillippe M, Gabbe SG, et al. Pregnancy following renal transplantation in class T diabetes mellitus. JAMA 1986; 255:911–915.
6. Levine MG, Miodovnik M, Siddigi TA, et al. A successful pregnancy in a juvenile diabetic with a renal transplant complicated by preeclampsia. Transplantation 1983; 35:498–499.

7.  Tagatz GE, Arnold NI, Goetz FC, Najarian JS, Simmons RL. Pregnancy in a juvenile diabetic after renal transplantation (Class T diabetes mellitus). Diabetes 1975; 24:497–501.
8.  Castro LA, Baltzer U, Hillebrand G, Landgraf R, Kuhlmann H, Land W. Pregnancy in juvenile diabetes mellitus under cyclosporine treatment after combined kidney and pancreas transplantation. Transplant Proc 1986; 28:1780–1781.
9.  Skannal DG, Miodovnik M, et al. Successful pregnancy after combined renal pancreas transplantation: a case report and literature review. Am J Perinatol 1996; 13(6):383–387.
10. McGrory CH, Radomski JS, Moritz MJ, Armenti VT. Pregnancy outcomes in 10 female pancreas recipients. J Transplant Coord 1998; 1:55–59.
11. Midtvedt K, Hartmann A, Brekke IB, Lyndgal PT, Bentdal O, Haugn G. Successful pregnancies in a combined pancreas and renal allograft recipient and in a renal graft recipient on tacrolimus treatment. Nephrol Dial Transplant 1997; 12:2764–2765.
12. Barrou BM, Gruessner AC, Sutherland DER, Gruessner RWG. Pregnancy after pancreas transplantation in the cyclosporine era. Transplantation 1998; 65:524–527.
13. Gunnar T, Brattstrom C, Bjorkman U, et al. Pregnancy after combined pancreas–kidney transplantation. Diabetes 1989; 38:43–45.
14. Calne RY, Brons IGM, Williams PF, Evans DB, Robinson RE, Dossa M. Successful pregnancy after paratopic segmental pancreas and kidney transplantation. BMJ 1988; 296:1709.
15. Armenti VT, Radomski JS, Moritz MJ, Branch KR, McGrory CH, Coscia LA. In: Cecka JM, Terasaki PI, eds. Clinical Transplants. Los Angeles, CA: UCLA, 1997:101–112.
16. Burrows L, Knight R, Thomas A, Panico M. Cyclosporine levels during pregnancy. Transplant Proc 1994; 26(5):2820–2821.
17. Thomas AG, Burrows L, Knight R, Panico M, Lapinski R, Lockwood CJ. The effect of pregnancy on cyclosporine levels in renal allograft patients. Obstet Gynecol 1997; 90:916–919.
18. Huynh, L, Min DI. Outcomes of pregnancy and the management of immunosuppressive agents to minimize fetal risks in organ transplant patients. Ann Pharmacother 1994; 28:1355–1356.
19. Biesenbach G, Zazgornik J, Kaiser W, et al. CyA requirements during pregnancy in renal transplant recipients. Nephrol Dial Transplant 1989; 4:667.
20. Bumgardner GL, Matas AJ. Transplantation and pregnancy. Transplant Rev 1992; 6:139–162.
21. Armenti V. Pregnancy in transplant recipients. Transplant Immunol Lett 1995; 11:4–6.
22. Venkataramanan R, Koneru B, Wang CC, et al. Cyclosporine and its metabolites in mother and baby. Transplantation 1988; 46(3):468–469.
23. Claris O, Picaud JC, Brazier JL, Salle BL. Pharmacokinetics of cyclosporine A in 16 newborn infants of renal or cardiac transplant mother. Dev Pharmacol Ther 1993; 20:180–185.
24. Davison JM, Dellagrammatikas H, Parkin JM. Maternal azathioprine therapy and depressed haemopoiesis in the babies of renal allograft patients. Br J Obstet Gynaecol 1985; 92:233–239.
25. Reimers TJ, Sluss PM. 6-Mercaptopurine treatment of pregnant mice: effects on second and third generations. Science 1978; 201:65–67.
26. Armenti V, Coscia L, McGrory H, Mortiz M. Update on pregnancy and renal transplantation. Nephrol News Issues 1998; August:19–22.
27. Jain A, Venkataramanan R, Fung JJ, et al. Pregnancy following liver transplantation under tacrolimus. Transplantation 1997; 64:559–565.
28. Jain A, Venkataramanan R, Lever J, et al. FK506 and pregnancy in liver transplant patients. Transplantation 1993; 56:1588–1589.
29. Winkler ME, Niesert S, Rege B, et al. Successful pregnancy in a patient after liver transplantation maintained on FK506. Transplantation 1993; 56:1589–1590.
30. Farley DE, Shelby J, Alexander D, Scott JR. The effect of two new immunosuppressive agents. FK506 and didemnin B, in murine pregnancy. Transplantation 1991; 52:106–110.
31. Armenti VT, McGrory CH, Cater J, Radomski JS, Jarrell BE, Moritz MJ. The National Transplantation Pregnancy Registry: comparison between pregnancy outcomes in diabetic cyclosporine-treated female kidney recipients and CyA-treated female pancreas–kidney recipients. Transplant Proc 1997; 29:669–670.
32. Allenby K, Campbell DJ, Lodge JPA. Vaginal delivery following combined pelvic renal and pancreatic transplant. Br J Obstet Gynaecol 1998; 105:1036–1038.
33. Van Winter JT, Ogburn PL, Ramin KD, Evans MP, Velosa JA. Pregnancy after pancreatic–renal transplantation because of diabetes. Mayo Clin Proc 1997; 72:1044–1047.
34. Kinkade-Smith PS, Fairley KF. Physiological adaptation in the kidney in pregnancy. In: Jones D, Theaker P, eds. The Kidney and Hypertension in Pregnancy. New York, NY: Churchill Livingstone, 1993:7–12.
35. Kairaitis LK, Nankivel BJ, Lawrence S, et al. Successful obstetric outcome after simultaneous pancreas and kidney transplantation. MJA 1999; 170:368–370.
36. Tyden G, Brattstrom C, Bjorkman U, et al. Pregnancy after pancreas–kidney transplantation. Diabetes 1989; 38(suppl 1):43.
37. Barrou B, Baldi A, Bitkerr MO, Squifflet JP, Gruessdner RW, Sutherland DER. Pregnancy after pancreas transplantation: report of four new cases and review of the literature. Trans Proc 1995; 27(6):3043.
38. Scantlebury VP. Pregnancy after kidney transplantation. In: Shapiro R, Simmons R, Starzl TE, eds. Renal Transplantation. Stamford: Appleton and Lange, 1997:503–551.

39. Sturgiss S, Davidson JM. Perinatal outcome in renal allograft recipients: ]prognostic significance of hypertension and renal function before and during pregnancy. Obstet Gynecol 1991; 78:573–577.
40. Bleich D, Polak M, Eisenbarth GS, Jackson RA. Decreased risk of type I diabetes in offspring of mothers who acquire diabetes during adrenarchy. Diabetes 1993; 42:1433.
41. Armenti VT, Ahlswede KM, Ahlswede BA, Cater JR, Moritz MJ, Burke. N.T.P.R: analysis of outcome/risks of 394 pregnancies in kidney transplant recipients. Transplant Proc 1994; 26:2535.
42. Ahlswede KM, Ahlswede BE, Jarrell BE, Moritz MJ, Armenti VT. Effect of transplant to conception interval on outcomes in pregnancies from 266 female renal transplant recipients. Surg Forum 1993; 44:535.
43. Salmela KT, Kyllönen LEJ, Holmberg C, Grönhagen-Riska C. Impaired renal function after pregnancy in renal transplant recipients. Transplantation 1993; 56:1372–1375.

# 25 | The Role of the Transplant Coordinator

**Deborah S. Good**
*Thomas E. Starzl Transplantation Institute, University of Pittsburgh School of Medicine, Pittsburgh, Pennsylvania, U.S.A.*

**Holly Woods**
*VA Pittsburgh Healthcare System, Pittsburgh, Pennsylvania, U.S.A.*

## INTRODUCTION

The increasing success of pancreatic transplantation has resulted from a number of factors, many of which have been discussed in some detail in other chapters in this book. Perhaps less well appreciated has been the critical role played by the transplant nurse coordinator. The transplant coordinator establishes the initial contact with a patient interested in transplantation and follows the patient through the entire transplant process. The coordinator maintains the lines of communication among patient, referring physician, and all members of the transplant team, in order to ensure proper care of the patient before and after transplantation.

This chapter will outline the role of the transplant coordinator, as it relates to pancreas transplantation. The referral and evaluation process, perioperative considerations, and postoperative care and management will all be described.

## REFERRAL

The patient's nephrologist, endocrinologist, primary care physician, or dialysis unit usually initiates the referral process. The patient or a family member may also contact the transplant center to begin the process. This is usually done either by a phone call or letter to the transplant physician or coordinator. It is the responsibility of the coordinator to obtain the patient's demographic and insurance information. At this time, the patient is given an appointment for evaluation clinic, and the insurance information is provided to the transplant credit department. Once insurance coverage for the evaluation is confirmed, the patient is sent a transplant teaching booklet and also given pertinent information regarding the appointment.

## THE EVALUATION

The potential transplant candidate ordinarily undergoes a one-day evaluation in an outpatient setting. The patient typically arrives at the transplant center in the morning and begins by having a chest X-ray and electrocardiogram. Following this, the patient is introduced to one of the transplant coordinators. The coordinator begins the nursing assessment; this includes a review of the patient history that usually has been completed by the patient or renal unit nurse prior to the day of the evaluation. The coordinator also completes an additional nursing history and physical examination, which includes vital signs, height and weight, allergies, social habits, previous transplant history, current medication regimen, and transfusion history. During this time, the coordinator also provides teaching regarding the evaluation process, activation on the transplant list, the surgery, inpatient care posttransplantation, and short- and long-term outpatient follow-up. The nurse also reviews the immunosuppressive medications and any other drugs that the patient will require after transplantation. Included in this discussion are the potential side effects of these drugs. The family members or significant others are strongly encouraged to participate in the entire evaluation process. Once the nursing assessment is completed, it is reviewed with the transplant surgeon and physician; they will then perform a more detailed history and physical examination, as described in Chapter 4. It is at this point that the need for specific additional testing is identified; this is subsequently coordinated through the referring physician's office.

A psychosocial evaluation is an essential part of the evaluation process. Every potential candidate is interviewed by a transplant social worker on the day of the evaluation. The social worker discusses family dynamics, work or school history, financial considerations, social habits, and insurance coverage for medications. The social worker from the patient's dialysis unit may also be contacted for additional information. If any problems are identified, the social worker may request further evaluation by a psychologist or psychiatrist. This evaluation is considered to be of critical importance prior to activation. In addition to these responsibilities, the social worker assists the potential recipients and family members with housing arrangements. Many of the transplant recipients do not live in the immediate area. It will, therefore, be necessary for them to stay locally during their recovery period and/or for return visits.

The patient's insurance coverage is reviewed by a credit analyst from the transplant credit department. At this time, insurance benefits are reviewed with the patient in an attempt to identify potential problems with coverage, not only for the surgery and hospitalization but also for long-term follow-up care.

The remainder of the evaluation consists of laboratory studies, which include human leukocyte antigen typing, DR typing, quick panel reactive antibody, circulating antibodies, viral serologies, RPR, and blood type. A punfred protein duodenum (PPD) and an anergy panel are also administered by the nurse coordinator. The patient is provided with instructions regarding the reading of the TB test, which is usually done by a nurse or physician at the dialysis unit.

## FURTHER STUDIES

After the evaluation, the nurse coordinator will send a letter to each of the referring physician, dialysis unit, and the patient. This letter includes a list of additional studies that will need to be completed prior to the presentation of the patient to the transplant evaluation committee (see Chapter 4). Specific additional studies are based on the history and physical examination performed on the day of the evaluation. The length of time needed for completion of these studies is dependent upon both the number of studies requested and the motivation of the patient to complete these tasks. A quarterly letter is generated to keep the patient informed of outstanding studies.

Once all the testing has been completed, the results are forwarded to the transplant coordinator. The coordinator is responsible for the collection of all patient data and prepares the patient's medical record for presentation to the transplantation evaluation committee. In our institution, it is the task of the transplant fellow to review the chart and present the patient to the committee. At this time, the patient may be medically cleared for transplantation, or additional testing may be required. If further testing is requested, another letter is generated to the patient and the patient's physician requesting these studies. After completion of this additional testing, the patient is then re-presented to the committee, and a decision is made. Occasionally, a patient may be found unsuitable for pancreas transplantation, and may be rejected by the committee. In some cases, this patient may be able to be listed for a kidney transplant alone if the patient has concurrent renal failure.

The next step in the activation process involves obtaining fiscal clearance for the transplant surgery and hospitalization. This is the responsibility of the credit analyst.

Once fiscal approval is obtained, the patient is activated on the United Network for Organ Sharing (UNOS) waiting list. The patient, referring physician, and, if applicable, the dialysis unit will receive an activation letter, which will provide information regarding the need for monthly blood samples. The patient is requested to call the transplant coordinator with any change in physician, renal unit, type of dialysis, phone numbers, and/or home address. While the patient is active on the transplant list, a quarterly letter is sent to the renal unit or physician to request information regarding any change in the patient's medical condition.

### Transplantation

When a donor is available, the transplant coordinator on call is involved in the process of recipient selection. Initially, the pancreas transplant surgeon contacts the coordinator. The surgeon selects several candidates, and the immunopathology laboratory initiates the cross-match procedure. Recipient selection is based on cross-match results, the waiting time of the recipient, and antigen matching. Once a recipient is selected, the ABO of the recipient is confirmed with the blood bank. Prior to contacting the recipient, the coordinator obtains medical clearance from the referring physician. The recipient is subsequently notified that a donor is available. The potential recipient is questioned regarding transfusion history, dialysis schedule, and any changes in medical condition, including recent fever or infections. Recipient and donor information is conveyed to the transplant fellow on call. The procurement agency and tissue typing laboratory are notified of the recipient selection.

After transplantation, the recipient is removed from the UNOS waiting list, and the transplant center's database is updated with donor and recipient information. The transplant surgeon will contact the referring physician by phone regarding the recipient's medical condition and function of the transplanted organs. A follow-up letter is sent by the transplant coordinator after this initial contact. It is equally important that follow-up be made available to the donor family. This is done by the procurement agency, with input from the transplant coordinator, within 48 hours of surgery. Recipient follow-up is also sent to the donor family on a yearly basis.

## INPATIENT FOLLOW-UP

The role of the transplant coordinator is not limited to the outpatient setting. Therefore, it is vital that the lines of communication between the inpatient and outpatient nursing staff are maintained. This is accomplished in various ways, such as rounding with the transplant physicians, participating in the weekly discharge planning meeting, attending a weekly morbidity and mortality conference, and communicating with the nursing staff, case manager, and transplant social worker. At our transplant center, a postoperative teaching book is provided to the patient by the transplant coordinators. A prerecorded audiotape is provided to patients who are visually impaired or illiterate. During their hospital stay, information provided in the teaching book is reviewed by the inpatient nursing staff, the transplant pharmacist, and the transplant social worker. After discharge, the patient is followed on a daily basis in the outpatient unit, which is located within the hospital close to the inpatient unit. Seeing the patient on a daily basis not only provides the physicians with the ability to monitor closely the patient's graft function and overall medical condition but also allows for ongoing patient education.

## OUTPATIENT FOLLOW-UP

After discharge from the outpatient unit, the patient is followed in the transplant clinic. Initially, this may occur twice a week. Laboratory studies may be drawn in the clinic on the morning of the visit or at a local laboratory near the patient's home on the day prior to the appointment. The transplant coordinator is responsible for the initial assessment of the patient. This assessment includes a brief summary of the patient's overall status, vital signs, weight, glucose readings, and medication regimen. The coordinator is present during the physician's visit to assist with wound care, review changes made in the medication regimen, and provide instructions regarding future clinic visits and laboratory studies.

Another responsibility of the transplant coordinator is to conduct the postoperative teaching class. This class is scheduled during the clinic, and it is recommended that every recipient and the recipient's family members attend. It is during this class that the postoperative teaching book is reviewed. A test is provided at the end of the class to assess the patient's understanding of the information reviewed.

Once the transplant physicians feel that the patient is stable, a letter to the referring physician is sent by the coordinator and a copy of all pertinent information is forwarded. Each patient is encouraged to return to the referring physician for medical follow-up. The patient is expected to continue with routine laboratory studies as requested by the transplant team, with periodic return visits to the transplant clinic. It is the responsibility of the coordinator to review the results of all laboratory studies with the transplant physician and notify both the patient and the referring physician of any changes made in the medication regimen. The coordinator maintains communication among the patient, transplant team, and referring doctor on an ongoing basis. Similarly, the referring physician maintains contact with the coordinators through office notes or phone calls.

## POSTTRANSPLANT ON-CALL RESPONSIBILITY

The transplant coordinator is available for consultation on a 24-hour/day basis. After office hours, the coordinator answers patient phone calls through an answering service. These calls may include sick calls, abnormal laboratory results, questions regarding a patient's medication regimen, local emergency room calls, or calls from referring physicians. The coordinator has access to the attending physician on call. The nurse once again acts as a liaison among the transplant surgeon/physician, referring physician, and the patient. If further intervention is needed, the transplant coordinator will make the necessary arrangements. In order to maintain continuity of care, all activity is documented on the patient's chart. As previously discussed in this chapter, the coordinator is also responsible for donor calls.

## ADDITIONAL RESPONSIBILITIES

The transplant coordinator has additional responsibilities outside of the office, clinics, and call. These include in-services at dialysis units regarding all aspects of transplantation, participating at school for career days or educational lectures, and other speaking engagements. The nurses are actively involved in Donor Awareness Week, The International Transplant Nursing Society, The North American Transplant Coordinator Organization, The Transplant Recipient International Organization, and The National Kidney Foundation. When physicians are involved in research projects, the coordinators may assist in gathering information or may actively participate as the research nurse for a specific project.

## SUMMARY

It is the responsibility of the transplant coordinator to ensure that the transplant patient is followed from the time of referral through the transplant process and for the remainder of the time the recipient has a functioning graft. Although the transplant recipient also returns to the care of the recipient's referring physician, posttransplant follow-up, especially regarding the management of immunosuppression, has been the responsibility of the transplant center. It has been the practice of our center to maintain close contact not only with the patient but also with the referring physician. In today's health care environment, this approach can be problematic, but can be accomplished by the cooperation and dedication of all caregivers. In this way, the patient receives the best possible care before, during, and after transplantation.

# 26 | Pancreas Transplantation at the University of Minnesota: 1966–2005

**David E. R. Sutherland, Rainer W. G. Gruessner, David L. Dunn, Arthur J. Matas, Abhinav Humar, Raja Kandaswamy, Angelika C. Gruessner, and John S. Najarian**
*Department of Surgery, University of Minnesota, Minneapolis, Minnesota, U.S.A.*

**S. Michael Mauer**
*Department of Pediatrics, University of Minnesota, Minneapolis, Minnesota, U.S.A.*

**William R. Kennedy**
*Department of Neurology, University of Minnesota, Minneapolis, Minnesota, U.S.A.*

**Frederick C. Goetz and R. Paul Robertson[a]**
*Department of Medicine, University of Minnesota, Minneapolis, Minnesota, U.S.A.*

## INTRODUCTION

The world's first clinical pancreas transplant was done simultaneously with a kidney graft on December 16, 1966 to treat a uremic diabetic patient at the University of Minnesota Hospital (1). From then through 2005, more than 24,000 pancreases have been transplanted (2); of these, nearly 8% have been done at the University of Minnesota (Fig. 1).

In addition to reports on the variety of specific aspects of pancreas transplantation, the cumulative experience with pancreas transplantation through the first thousand cases at the University of Minnesota as of 2000 has been published in a series of periodic overviews (3–8). This chapter resummarizes our early experience and gives an update to include our total experience with more than 1800 pancreas transplants through 2005.

For diabetic patients dependent on exogenous insulin for survival, the objectives of pancreas transplantation are to make them insulin-independent and normoglycemic, improve day-to-day quality of life (QOL), and ameliorate secondary complications. That the first objective could be achieved was obvious from the first case (1); the others had to be proven, and that is part of the multidecade story told here.

The evolution of pancreas transplantation at the University of Minnesota is closely intertwined with the advances in surgical techniques, (9–14) organ preservation technology (15), and immunosuppressive modalities (16–20) that have occurred in other pioneering programs, but some aspects of the Minnesota program have been decidedly different (6,8). An analysis of outcome over such a long time span in a constantly changing field can only be done by eras. Although each era has distinctive features, there is much overlap between, as well as heterogeneity within, eras. The similarities and differences with other programs are indicated in the following description of the Minnesota pancreas transplant program by six eras, the first, led by Lilleihei, being labeled 0, and the next five, initiated five years after the Lilleihei, divided according to changes in protocols, and particularly according to the dominant immunosuppression regimen in the various recipient categories (Table 1).

## ERA 0

From 1966 to 1973, 14 pancreas transplants were done from deceased donors (DDs), the first, a duct-ligated segmental graft in which William Kelly and Richard Lillehei collaborated (1). The next 13 were whole pancreas grafts (the first five with a cutaneous graft duodenostomy; the

---

[a] Dr. Robertson is currently with the Department of Medicine, University of Washington, Seattle, Washington, U.S.A.

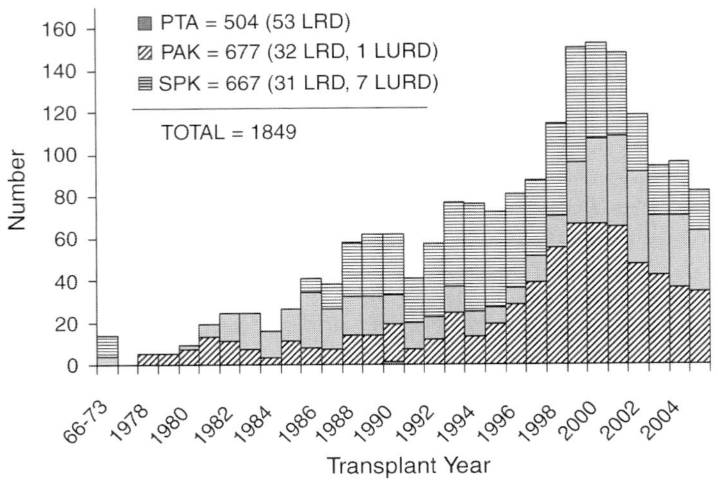


**Figure 1** Number of pancreas transplants at the University of Minnesota according to recipient category. SPK, PTA, PAK, and SPL from LRD and LURD. Inclusive dates are December 16, 1966 to December 31, 2005. *Abbreviations:* SPK, simultaneous pancreas-kidney; PTA, pancreas transplant alone; PAK, pancreas after kidney; SPL, simultaneous pancreas-liver; LRD, living related donors; LURD, living unrelated donors.

next seven with internal exocrine drainage via a Roux-en-Y duodenojejunostomy; and the last with only the graft papilla of Vater retained for anastomosis to recipient bowel), in a personal series by Lillehei (7). Era 0 will not be included in the detailed analyses to come; this era and its influence will be simply summarized in this introduction.

In brief, the first 11 cases were done in uremic diabetic patients, 10 as simultaneous pancreas-kidney (SPK) transplants and 1 as a pancreas transplant alone (PTA) in a patient who remained on dialysis. At the outset, it was thought that to do kidney transplants successfully in uremic patients would require correction of the diabetic state (3). However, because of the initially high complication rate with pancreaticoduodenal transplants, this concept was challenged internally (21). A series of kidney transplants alone (KTA) from living donors (LDs) or DDs was initiated in uremic diabetic patients (22,23), ultimately producing a large number of candidates (24) for pancreas after kidney (PAK) transplants in Era 1 (4). Lillehei switched to doing PTA in nonuremic diabetic patients, but had only three cases, and all grafts were rejected within three months (7,25). Interestingly, none of the pancreas allografts were rejected in the uremic diabetic patients (all SPK transplants except one), all losses due to technical complications (thrombosis, infection, anastomotic leak) or death with a functioning graft (DWFG) (7).

**Table 1** Dates of Eras for Analyses and Dominant Immunosuppression Protocol Within Eras for University of Minnesota Pancreas Transplant Program

| | | Dominant immunosuppression | | |
|---|---|---|---|---|
| Era | Dates | Induction | Maintenance | Recipient category |
| 0 | 12/16/1966–1973 | None | Aza/Pred | SPK, PTA |
| 1 | 7/25/1978–6/30/1985 | MALG | Aza/Pred | PAK, PTA |
| 2 | 7/1/1985–6/24/1994 | MALG | Csa/Aza/Pred | SPK, PAK, PTA |
| 3A | 6/25/1994–3/171998 | ATGAM | Tac/MMF/Pred | SPK, PAK |
| 3B | 6/25/1994–12/9/1998 | ATGAM | Tac/MMF/Pred | PTA |
| 4A | 3/18/1998–2/18/2003 | TMG/Zen[a] | Tac/MMF | SPK, PAK |
| 4B | 12/10/1998–2/18/2003 | Tac, MMF, TMG, Zen | Tac/MMF | PTA[b] |
| 5 | 2/19/2003–12/31/2005 | Campath[c] | Campath/MMF | SPK, PAK, PTA[d] |

[a]Anti–T-cell agent(s) given prevascularization of the graft(s).
[b]PTA candidates given TAC and MMF while on waiting list.
[c]Campath used for induction and maintenance immunosuppression.
[d]PTA candidates given MMF while on the waiting list.
*Abbreviations*: Aza, azathioprine; Pred, prednisone; Csa, cyclosporine; Tac, tacrolimus; MMF, mycophenolate mofetil; MALG, Minnesota anti-lymphocyte globulin; ATGAM, antithymocyte globulin; SPK, simultaneous pancreas-kidney; PAK, pancreas after kidney; PTA, pancreas transplant alone; TMG, thymoglobulin; Zen, Zenopax (daclizumab).

One SPK recipient (case number 6, or number 5 as tabulated by Lillehei (7); he called the first case done with Kelly number 0), however, was insulin independent for more than one year (3), until dying with a functioning pancreas graft, after losing the kidney to renal artery stenosis and returning to dialysis (7). This was the longest functioning pancreas graft in the world until a series of SPK segmental transplants drained into the ureter by Gliedman et al., beginning in the early 1970s, produced a recipient whose new pancreas functioned (insulin-independent) for five years (26).

The Lillehei series ended in 1973 with the hope that islet transplantation would quickly be developed for clinical application and succeed pancreas transplantation as total endocrine replacement therapy for diabetes (27). Islet transplantation research had begun at Minnesota in the late 1960s (28) and has continued to this day (6,29), but it was apparent by the late 1970s that clinical application (30), at least for islet allografts (islet autografts were successful (31,32), even the first case (30), would require many more years of research (33,34)—research that finally did come to fruition (35–37). Thus, after further laboratory experiments designed to refine surgical techniques (6,38), a new series of clinical pancreas transplants was begun in 1978 (Era 1) (4,39).

We took with us several lessons from the Lillehei series (25). In Era 0, only azathioprine (Aza) and prednisone (Pred) were used for immunosuppression; although adequate to prevent at least early rejection of SPK grafts, such a regimen was inadequate for PTA cases. The Lillihei series was the first to make a distinction in immunological risk for PTA versus SPK transplants (7,25), a distinction that has persisted even though the gap between the groups clearly narrowed over time (40). Conversely, in the Lillehei series, PTA recipients had much less morbidity than SPK recipients (7). Thus, in Era 1, we were swayed to reduce the magnitude of the operative procedures for uremic diabetic patients by doing a KTA with a PAK after an interval of recovery (4). We were also impressed by the high complication rate in the Lillehei series, seemingly associated with the duodenal portion of the whole pancreas graft (7). So, like others (9–11), we initially believed that it was better to do a segmental graft and avoid the duodenum (39,41). These concepts changed as Era 1 progressed (4,5), but early on, much of what we did was related to what we perceived as good or bad from Era 0. We continue to expound Lillehei's belief that PTA should be the norm and not simply the future of pancreas transplantation (42). Lillehei deserves the credit for being the first proponent (7).

## ERA 1

Era 1 began in July 25, 1978 with a DD segmental pancreas transplant (39). Based on animal experiments (38,43), the graft duct was left open, allowing the exocrine secretions to drain freely into the peritoneal cavity of a diabetic woman who had received a successful kidney transplant from her mother six years earlier. The recipient was insulin independent for $17\frac{1}{2}$ years when she died with a functioning graft after being thrown off a horse. At the time she died, she had the world's longest functioning graft, though ultimately six patients from Era 1 achieved over 20 years of pancreas graft function, five of whom are still insulin independent, two LD enteric drained (ED) segmental PTAs, one LD ED segmental PAK, one DD duct-injected PTA, and one DD ED PAK), while one (an LD duct-injected segmental PAK) finally failed at over 23 years. Thus, Era 1 initiated the first series of pancreas transplants where truly long-term graft function was destined to occur (44), even though our initial success rate was low and we had not yet developed a good method for monitoring solitary pancreas transplants for rejection.

Era 1 ended on June 30, 1986 when we resumed SPK transplants, giving us the maximal flexibility to manage uremic diabetics. In the eight-year period of Era 1 (July 1978–June 1986), we only did solitary (65 PAK and 83 PTA) pancreas transplants ($n = 148$). In contrast, every other program in the world did only or predominantly SPK transplants during this period (45).

Initially, we did not have a good marker to monitor for solitary pancreas graft rejection episodes, because an elevation in plasma glucose is a very late manifestation (as opposed to elevation of serum creatinine in kidney graft recipients, which is a relative early marker of renal allograft rejection, and one that gives an immunological advantage to SPK recipients because serum creatinine can be used as a surrogate marker to detect rejection that usually affects both organs from the same donor (SD). Duct management techniques later solved the problem, but initially we used other tactics. One was to administer Minnesota antilymphocyte globulin (MALG), which we had already showed, reduced the rejection response in renal allograft recipients (46). The other was to use LDs for segmental grafts (47) as we knew that the rejection episode rate was much less for kidney grafts from LD than from DD (48,49). Although the technical failure (TF) rate of LD segmental pancreas transplants was initially high, the tactic was an immunologic success; particularly when the LD had previously given a kidney to the recipient, the rejection rate was low (50).

For DD solitary pancreas transplants, the rejection rate remained high with immunosuppression available at the time (MALG, Aza, and Pred). Although International Pancreas Transplant Registry data (45) showed that SPK transplants gave an advantage in terms of pancreas graft survival, we believed that the immunologic problems of solitary pancreas transplants could be overcome. We persisted with the philosophy that PTA was the most logical application (why wait for secondary complications?) (51).

In Era 1, emphasis was on developing the best surgical technique, particularly for duct management. We sequentially used every duct management technique devised [open duct (OD), 1978; duct injection (DI), 1980; enteric drainage (ED), 1981; urinary drainage via the bladder, bladder drained (BD), 1983], with overlap in application (52). The OD technique was used in our first few cases (41). We then compared (4) OD to the polymer DI technique developed by Dubernard et al. (10) in France and to a variant of the ED technique for segmental grafts popularized by Groth et al. (11) in Sweden. By mid-1983, we stopped doing DD segmental grafts routinely (4) and returned to the whole pancreas technique (with papilla of Vater) used by Lillihei in his last case (7). We did only a few cases by this technique before following the lead of Starzl et al. (13) at Pittsburgh to include the entire duodenum (53), as originally described by Lillihei (3). Urinary drainage, initially introduced by Gliedman et al. (9) in the early 1970s by anastomosing the pancreatic duct of a segmental graft to the recipient ureter, was modified by Sollinger et al. (12) in the early 1980s by directly anastomosing a whole pancreatic graft to the bladder. Once we learned how useful a decline in urine amylase (UA) activity was as a marker for rejection episodes (54,55), we used BD almost exclusively for solitary pancreas transplants (53).

In the beginning, however, we used the OD technique clinically because of its uniformly successful application in dogs that were controls for an experiment testing the DI technique (56). Half of the human recipients of OD segmental grafts did very well surgically, presumably because the enzymes remained inactive and the peritoneal cavity absorbed the pancreatic secretions, but the other half developed chemical peritonitis and the grafts had to be removed (41). For this reason, we switched to the DI and ED techniques until these were superseded by BD near the end of Era 1 (53,55).

Other technical aspects of Era 1 included portal venous drainage of segmental pancreas grafts via the interior mesenteric vessels in a few cases (57); routine procurement of whole pancreas grafts from liver donors (58) with reconstruction of the graft arterial system via a Y graft of donor iliac artery (59); and development of a reliable method of cold storage of pancreas grafts for over 24 hours in silica gel filtered plasma (SGFP) (60,61), the latter superseded in Era 2 by the nonbiologic (eliminating the risk of disease transmission) University of Wisconsin (UW) solution developed by Belzer (15). We also began to do pancreas graft biopsies (62) to help diagnose the cause of graft dysfunction (63).

During Era 1, immunosuppression evolved (64), from Aza/Pred to cyclosporine (Csa)/Pred to Csa/Aza/Pred (triple therapy), using MALG for induction in nearly all cases (65). Uniquely, we performed segmental pancreas transplants from nondiabetic identical twin LDs to their diabetic twin counterparts under the mistaken impression that we could do so without immunosuppression (66); we observed recurrence of autoimmune isletitis (67) and diabetes (66), a definite confirmation of the autoimmune etiology of Type-I diabetes (68), and a hard lesson (69).

In Era 1, nearly all pancreas candidates and recipients participated in baseline and serial follow-up studies of metabolism (70) and secondary diabetic complications of the eyes (71), nerves (72), and kidneys (73) to determine whether their lesions progressed, stabilized, or regressed (74). The studies have been continued longitudinally across all subsequent eras.

Era 1 was an exciting period of development, with numerous international conferences bringing together individuals from the few institutions applying pancreas transplantation as a treatment for diabetes (75–77). The lessons from our own experience and that of others during Era 1 were undoubtedly responsible for the improved results in Era 2.

## ERA 2

Era 2 began on July 1, 1986 when we resumed SPK transplants (78). From then on, we offered pancreas transplants liberally in all three recipient categories (79,80). Our basic immunosuppressive regimen (quadruple therapy) at that time consisted of MALG for induction and the combination of Csa/Aza/Pred for maintenance (65). We conducted a randomized study of MALG versus OKT3 (Ortho) for induction therapy in KTA and SPK recipients (81); substituted antithymocyte globulin (ATGAM, Upjohn) for MALG, when the latter became unavailable at the end of 1993 (82); and instituted anti-T cell agents as the first line of therapy for all first rejection episodes in pancreas recipients (83). We found that aggressive treatment of rejection episodes could preserve long-term endocrine function even when exocrine function was lost (84,85). However, the pancreas graft failure rate was high enough (86) for us to accumulate a large series of pancreas retransplants (87,88). Era 2 ended in June 1994 when new agents for maintenance of immunosuppression became available (17,89).

During the eight-year interval of Era 2, we did 462 pancreas transplants, of which slightly more than half were SPK, the others being nearly equally divided between the solitary PAK (24%) and PTA (26%) categories [with one simultaneous pancreas-liver (SPL) transplant]. LDs were used for 6% of transplants in Era 2, predominantly in recipients of solitary pancreas transplants (12% of the cases, equally distributed in the PAK and PTA categories) (90). The incentive for solitary pancreas transplants with LDs lessened as the results of DD pancreas transplants improved and waiting times became short by use of outside donors (91). Thus, near the end of Era 2 (91), we expanded our LD program to include SPK transplants for uremic diabetics who wanted one operation to become insulin independent as well as dialysis free without a long wait (92). The goal of one operation to receive both a kidney and a pancreas was also achieved in a few Era 2 patients (four), who received a DD pancreas simultaneously with an LD kidney (6). Interestingly, for logistical and allocation reasons, three SPK recipients in this era received both organs from different DDs.

BD predominated as the duct management technique, with ED done in only 5% of our cases, most early in Era 2 to complete a study initiated with the 101st case in Era 1 of ED versus BD for solitary pancreas transplants (53). This study showed that the solitary pancreas rejection loss rate (RLR) was significantly lower in BD recipients treated for rejection based on a decline in UA activity (units per hour) (53). Thus, we began to use BD for almost all solitary pancreas transplants (79). A decrease in exocrine function, as detected by UA monitoring, always preceded hyperglycemia as a manifestation of rejection in pancreas grafts (55), and the incidence of rejection episodes was high with the immunosuppressants available during this era (93). In special cases such as with patients who had both pancreatic exocrine and endocrine deficiency as a result of pancreatectomy-induced diabetes, we would do ED to correct both (94).

For SPK BD transplants, monitoring of UA was less important to detect rejection because a serum creatinine elevation usually preceded a UA decline when the rejection episode affected both organs (95). However, experimental studies showed that the incidence of discordant rejection (one organ involved when the other was not) was on the order of 10% (96), and clinical observations (97) corroborated the experimental ones (98). Thus, we continued to do BD with UA monitoring even for SPK transplants in Era 2, because it allowed the salvage of the occasional pancreas affected by a discordant rejection, as documented by transcystoscopic biopsies (99–101). We managed the chronic bladder-related complications (primarily recurrent urinary tract infections and metabolic acidosis from bicarbonate loss) by converting to ED (102,103); during Era 2 our conversion rate was 9% to 19% by two years, depending on the recipient category (104).

We made some modifications in surgical technique during Era 2, such as using a stapler for the duodenocystostomy of BD grafts (105); using every donor for both liver and pancreas procurement (106,107); and splitting the DD pancreases into two segments for transplantation to two recipients (108) (especially useful when two patients with a high panel-reactive antibody level to human leukocyte antigens (HLA) have a negative crossmatch to the SD). We began using pancreas grafts procured by surgeons outside our region (91), leading to an increase in our pancreas transplant volume with no detrimental affect on outcome. We converted from using SGFP to UW for pancreas organ preservation with no difference in results (109). Long-term endocrine function was similar for grafts preserved with either solution for up to 30 hours (109).

Donor (110) and recipient risk factors were redefined in this era (111). We accepted all referrals (6,111), but initiated measures to treat risk factors such as coronary artery disease, pretransplant (112).

The observations and studies we initiated in Era 1 on the pathogenesis of diabetes and the course of its complications continued in Era 2. We added to our series of identical twin donor segmental pancreas transplants, but with prophylactic immunosuppression (113). Of the three twin transplants done in Era 2, only one recipient has manifested disease recurrence; on immunosuppression, it progressed slowly and graft function was maintained for eight years. The other two recipients had no evidence of disease recurrence in follow-up graft biopsies (6), and are currently insulin independent at 10 and 13 years, respectively.

Studies of metabolism (84,114–118) and secondary diabetic complications (6) in pancreas recipients continued in Era 2. Pancreas transplantation did not alter the immediate course of advanced eye disease, but by three years, stabilization occurred (71). Neuropathy improved (119) and neuropathic patients with successful pancreas transplants had a survival advantage (120). Recurrence of diabetic nephropathy in renal allografts was also ameliorated by a successful pancreas transplant (121).

Although the results of solitary pancreas transplants improved in Era 2, we were not satisfied (6). The success rate was still higher in SPK recipients, particularly in the subgroup of young patients without vasculopathy, but we wanted to continue to offer pancreas transplants for all categories and stages of diabetic complications. Although rejection episodes were usually readily reversed in SPK recipients, the incidence of rejection episodes was high in all categories. Rejection episodes were harder to reverse or had a higher recurrence rate, for solitary pancreas transplant recipients. We knew that new immunosuppressive approaches were needed.

## ERA 3

Era 3 began on June 25, 1994 when tacrolimus (Tac) was approved for clinical use by the U.S. Food and Drug Administration (FDA). We immediately used it for clinical pancreas transplants (122). A year later, mycophenolate mofetil (MMF) was also approved by the FDA, and again, we immediately used it for pancreas transplants (123), including in combination with Tac (124). We continued to use anti-T cell agents, ATGAM for induction immunosuppression Orthoclone (OKT3, Ortho) for treatment of rejection episodes. BD predominated for pancreas graft duct management in all recipient categories in Era 3.

Era 3 ended on March 17, 1998 for the SPK and PAK categories and on December 9, 1998 for the PTA category. In this Era 3, with Tac initially and then with Tac-MMF as the principal maintenance immunosuppressants, we did 297 pancreas transplants. As in Era 2, about half of Era 3 transplants were in the SPK category (49%) and half in the solitary pancreas transplant category. However, the proportion of PAK transplants was higher (35%) in Era 3 than in Era 2.

The rate of surgical complications declined in all categories in Era 3 (125). The incidence of rejection episodes declined more in SPK and PAK than in PTA (126), and percutaneous pancreas graft biopsies were used routinely to confirm the diagnosis (127).

The metabolic studies initiated in the previous eras continued in Era 3 (128). The durability of pancreas graft insulin secretory reserve for more than one, or nearly two decades, was documented (129). Likewise, the studies on diabetic secondary complications in pancreas graft recipients continued (130,131). Nerve regeneration following successful pancreas transplantation in patients with diabetic neuropathy was clearly shown (132), and the survival advantage of a successful pancreas transplant in neuropathic patients was confirmed (133). With regard to diabetic nephropathy in native kidneys, surprisingly over a 10-year period, even structural glomerular lesions could regress (134).

Era 3 ended on these optimistic notes. The main remaining challenges were to further reduce the rate of surgical complications and to refine immunosuppression to improve PTA results, both early and late.

## ERA 4

Era 4 began for SPK and PAK recipients on March 18, 1998, and for PTA recipients on December 10, 1998, when we added daclizumab (Zenopex, Roche Laboratories), alone or in combination with polyclonal anti-T cell antibody (ATGAM, initially; Thymoglobulin when it was FDA approved in 1999) to our induction immunosuppressive regimen. We also began to give anti-T cell agents before graft revascularization, following the lead of others (135). In the PTA category, we also began to give Tac and MMF to the candidates while waiting (136,137). Concomitantly, we began to use ED as our principal exocrine drainage technique in SPK recipients of CAD grafts (exceptions were some high-risk elderly or obese patients or patients with chronic peritonitis from peritoneal dialysis). BD remained the preferred drainage technique for DD solitary and all LD segmental pancreas transplants.

Through February 18, 2003, we did 666 pancreas transplants in Era 4. Even though the absolute annual number was greater (42/yr vs. 26/yr and 40/yr, respectively), the proportion of pancreas transplants that were in the SPK category in Era 4 (32%) was less than in Eras 2 (50%) and 3 (49%), while the proportion of PAKs increased (43% vs. 24% and 35%, respectively). In Era 4, ED was used in 68% of SPK transplants, but in only 9% of PAK and PTA transplants. The overall outcomes for the first half of Era 4 have been published previously (8), and analyses on several topics relevant to our experience during this era have also been published (as cited below), but the outcomes for the entire era are presented here for the first time.

In Era 4, we found that steroids could be safely withdrawn with no added risk of rejection in our pancreas transplant recipients (138,139), and we initiated steroid-free immunosuppression beginning at the time of transplantation (Table 1). Elimination of steroids was not seen as a reduction in overall immunosuppression because we used anti-T-cell agents so liberally for induction, both depleting and nondepleting (8). If anything, our immunosuppressive regimen was more potent without steroids, made possible by the fact that we could give effective prophylaxis (gancycolivr) against cytomegalovirus (CMV) infections (140).

The need to continuously refine immunosuppression was apparent from our observations on chronic rejection in pancreas transplants, particularly in recipients of solitary grafts (141). Fortunately, chronic rejection of the exocrine pancreas does not inevitably lead to loss of endocrine graft function and a relatively high proportion of recipients remain insulin independent after loss of all exocrine function.

Besides trying to improve our results by changes in immunosuppression, we also reevaluated the technical aspects of pancreas transplantation and donor and recipient risk factors (142) such as obesity (143). The risk of TF decreased in Era 4 for both primary (125) and retransplant (144) cases for a variety of reasons. For example, even though DD pancreas transplants with preservation times over 30 hours have been done successfully (145), the risk of TF increased with increasing preservation time (146). Thus, during Era 4, we tested a new preservation technique, the two-layer method in which the pancreas is suspended between UW solution and perflorechemical with oxygen bubbled through and originally designed to improve yield and viability of islets following isolation (147), and found it allowed preservation of pancreas for clinical transplantation at least as long as required with a low TF rate (148).

Nevertheless, in order to shorten pancreas preservation times as much as possible, in Era 4, we proceeded to transplantation without waiting for a final crossmatch in unsensitized patients whenever logistically advantageous (149,150). We also did some pancreas transplants with past positive T-cell and/or current B-cell positive crossmatches in patients whose high panel reactivity on the relevant samples was a limiting factor in finding a donor in a reasonable time to whom all testing was negative (151). There were more early and late rejections in this group than in those without positive crossmatches, but the graft survival rate was acceptable and without taking the risk, some patients would never get transplanted (152).

We continued to do LD segmental pancreas transplants in Era 4 (153), primarily in patients who were sensitized but with a negative crossmatch to a living volunteer. We also initiated LD laparoscopic distal pancreastectomy, with or without simultaneous donor nephroctomy (154). We also continued to emphasize performing a LD kidney transplant to preempt dialysis in nephropathic diabetic patients, followed by a DD pancreas transplant (PAK) (155). Such an approach lowered the overall mortality that would occur if the patients had to wait for an SPK, and our analyses showed superior patient and kidney graft survival compared to diabetic recipients of a KTA (156).

The proportion of our pancreas transplant recipients over 45 years of age, as well as the proportion with vascular disease (VD) more than doubled in Era 4 (see Table 8). Thus, coronary artery intervention pretransplant became common, particularly in our SPK population (157).

Finally, in Era 4, we were able to do metabolic studies in a large number of pancreas transplant recipients (158,159) and LDs (159,160) accumulated from previous eras, showing remarkable stability of endocrine function for nearly two decades in some patients.

What did concern us as Era 4 came to an end were the pancreas transplant recipients in all categories who developed native or chronic allograft nephropathy with superimposed or etiologic calcineurin-inhibitor (CI) nephrotoxicity, and thus Era 5 began with an attempt to eliminate CIs from our immunosuppressive regimen while still keeping it steroid free (161).

## ERA 5

Era 5 began on February 19, 2003, when we began a novel CI- and steroid-free protocol using parenteral Campath for both induction and maintenance immunosuppression, the latter combined with an oral antimetabolite (MMF if tolerated, otherwise Rapamycin) for the first year posttransplant and thereafter, oral antimetabolite monotherapy in patients with lower than two rejection episodes (161). The objective was to improve recipient renal function (compared to historical controls) without compromising patient and graft survival rates. The preliminary results with this protocol have been published (162), showing that slightly better renal function was achieved in all three categories of recipients, even though there was a higher incidence of rejection episodes in SPK recipients compared to historical controls. Late follow-up also showed a higher incidence of rejection graft losses in the PTA recipients (163), and PAK recipients had the best outcome with this protocol. Late follow-up also showed some unique complications with the protocol in a few patients, particularly red cell aplasia or autoimmune hemolytic anemia, both of which responded to conversion from MMF to Rapamycin (163). However, there were no cases of posttransplant lymphoproliferative disorder (PTLD), consistent with our long-term observations published in Era 5 that PTLD has a low incidence in pancreas recipients (164).

Through December 31, 2005 we performed 262 pancreas transplants in Era 5. The proportion of pancreas transplants that were in the SPK category continued to decline (25%), the proportion of PAKs was stable (42%), while the proportion of PTAs increased (34%) compared to the previous era, what we consider a natural evolution in the quest to perform pancreas transplants earlier rather than later in the course of the disease (165). In Era 5, ED was used less often than in Era 4 in primary DD SPK transplants (57%), but the proportion of DD PAK and PTA transplants done with ED increased substantially, to 45% and 42%, respectively. The outcomes for the first part of Era 5 have been published previously (162), but are given here for the entire era.

Besides the use of a CI, steroid-free regimen with anti-T-cell agents (mainly Campath, or altuzemab) for both induction and maintenance immunosuppression (162,163), we published about several other aspects of our pancreas transplant program, including our outcomes in recipients with Type-II diabetes mellitus (166), the factors that predispose to late surgical complications (167), an update on our use of LDs for segmental grafts procured laparoscopically (168) and an update on the remodeling that occurs in native kidneys of PTA recipients with pretransplant lesions of diabetic nephropathy (169).

## SUMMARY OF PROCEDURES

Between December 16, 1966 and December 31, 2005 (Fig. 1), we performed 1849 pancreas transplants at the University of Minnesota (667 SPK, 677 PAK, 504 PTA, and 1 SPL). Of these, 1528 were primary and 321 were retransplants (265 second, 51 third, and 5 fourth). We retransplanted 31 second and 3 third pancreas allografts in 32 patients who received first or first and second transplants elsewhere and a second only ($n = 29$) or both a second and third ($n = 2$) or third only ($n = 1$) at the University of Minnesota, so the total number of patients enrolled in our program as of December 31, 2005 was 1561.

We did 1718 DD (1390 primary, 318 retransplants) and 124 LD (121 primary, 3 retransplants) pancreas transplants. Of the SPK transplants, the pancreas graft came from an LD in 38 (kidney from SD) and a DD in 623 cases (in 36, the kidney was from a different donor than the pancreas, 4 from a DD and 32 from an LD); of the PAK, from an LD in 33, a DD in 644; of the PTA, from an LD in 53, a DD in 451. Of the retransplants, 54 were SPK

(39 second, 13 third, and 2 fourth), 165 PAK (137 second, 25 third, and 3 fourth), and 102 PTA (89 second and 13 third).

Pancreas graft duct management or exocrine drainage technique was via a cutaneous graft duodenostomy in 5 (all Era 0); OD-free intraperitoneal drainage in 15 (all Era 1); duct occlusion (4 simply ligated, 46 polymer injected) in 50 (Eras 0, 1, 2, 3, and 5); enteric drainage (ED) in 411 (all Eras); and urinary drainage (4 ureter; 1353 bladder, BD) in 1357 cases (all Eras). The recipient portal venous system was used for the pancreas graft venous effluent in 14 cases (3 ED SPK, 7 ED and 1 duct-occluded PAK, 3 ED PTA; Eras 1, 2, 4, and 5).

## STATISTICAL ANALYSES

Analyses were done on all pancreas ($n = 1835$) transplants performed at the University of Minnesota from July 25, 1978 through December 31, 2005 [the 14 from Era 0 (10 SPK, 4 PTA)] were not included. Patient survival rates, pancreas and kidney graft survival rates (GSRs), RLRs, and reversible rejection episodes (RRE) rates, were calculated by the Kaplan–Meier method using SAS 6.12 software.

Pancreas grafts were considered functioning as long as the recipients were insulin independent. DWFG was considered a graft failure in our analyses of all cases. In our analyses of immunologic events (rejection), we excluded TFs and pancreas graft primary nonfunction cases (the remaining cases were considered technically successful (TS). In all analyses of TS cases, those with DWFG were censored at the time of death. TFs included primary graft thrombosis or removal of functioning grafts for complications such as anastomotic leak, perigraft infection, or bleeding. Kidney grafts were considered functioning as long as the graft was still in place and the patients on dialysis pretransplantation were dialysis free posttransplant or the posttransplant serum creatinine was below the pretransplant level in recipients who were never dialyzed.

In univariate actuarial analyses, $p$-values were calculated by the Wilcoxon (WC) and logrank (LR) tests and refer to the significance of the differences between the overall survival curves. The WC test primarily reflects the probability that early differences are significant; the L-R is weighted to detect late differences. $p$-Values below 0.2 are indicated numerically; all others are designated nonsignificant (NS). We also performed logistic and Cox multivariate regression analyses using multiple variables in the models to ascertain the relative risks for patient death, graft failure in general, TF, and rejection loss. The significance of differences in proportions of events comparing categorical variables of one group with another was determined by the Chi-square or Fisher's exact test. Continuous variables were analyzed parametrically using the T test. Means are given with 1 standard deviation.

## RECIPIENT CATEGORIES AND DUCT MANAGEMENT OVERALL AND BY ERA

The total number of pancreas transplants done from 1978 through 2005 (Eras 1–5 combined) is shown in Table 2 according to recipient category, donor source for primary or retransplants, recipient gender and dominant duct management technique. Of the 1835 pancreas transplants, more than a quarter were PTAs, while the rest were nearly equally divided among SPK and PAK recipients; of the primary transplants, overall lesser than 1/12 were LD, but the percentage

**Table 2**  University of Minnesota Pancreas Transplant Recipient Demographics for Eras 1 to 5 (1978–2005)

| Category | 1°DD | 1°LD[b] | 2°DD[c] | 2°LD | Total | Female | BD |
|---|---|---|---|---|---|---|---|
| SPK [36%] | 565 | 38 (6%) | 54 | 0 | 657 | 295 (45%) | 467 (71%) |
| PAK [37%] | 480 | 32 (6%) | 163 | 1 | 676 | 314 (46%) | 523 (77%) |
| PTA [27%] | 347 | 53 (13%) | 101 | 2 | 501 | 336 (67%) | 360 (72%) |
| Total [100%] | 1393[a] | 123 (8%) | 318 | 3 | 1835 | 945 (51%) | 1351 (74%) |

*Note*: [ ], vertical percentage, ( ), horizontal percentage.
[a]Includes one primary DD BD SPL.
[b]Percentage of primary (1°) transplants that were from LDs.
[c]2°, retransplantation, second, third, or fourth.
*Abbreviations*: DD, deceased donor; LD, living donor; BD, bladder drainage; SPK, simultaneous pancreas and kidney transplant; PAK, pancreas after kidney transplant; PTA, pancreas transplant alone.

was highest in the PTA category (more than double that of the others, primarily due to liberal application in the early ears). Very few pancreas retransplants were done with LDs. Overall, pancreas transplants were equally divided among males and females, but in the SPK PAK categories, there were more males, while in the PTA category, there were more females. BD drainage predominated overall and was done in approximately three-fourths of the recipients in each category, though again the proportion varied considerably by era (Table 3).

In Era 1 ($n = 148$), we did only PAK (44%) and PTA (56%) cases (15 OD, 41 DI, 3 ligation, 77 ED and 12 BD). In Era 2 ($n = 462$), we did all categories: SPK (51%), PAK (23%), PTA (26%), and 1 SPL (431 BD, 3 ureter, 24 ED, and 3 DI). In Era 3 ($n = 297$), 49% were SPK, 35% PAK, and 16% PTA (286 BD, 6 ED, and 5 DI).

In Era 4 ($n = 666$), 32% were SPK, 43% PAK, and 25% PTA (488 BD and 178 ED). (One PTA retransplant was with ED to provide intestinal exocrine function in a native pancreatectomized recipient with a functioning primary BD pancreas transplant). In Era 5 ($n = 262$), 25% was SPK, 42% PAK, and 33% were PTA (135 BD and 122 ED).

The specifics of the surgical techniques we have used for pancreas transplants over the years have been described in detail (165).

With regard to the SPK category, 36 of the recipients had the pancreas and kidney from different donors (Table 4), including 7 in Era 2, 14 in Era 4, and 15 in Era 5. Of these, 89% had the pancreas from a DD and the kidney from a LD, but 11% had both from different DDs.

With regard to the PAK category (Table 5), more than one-quarter had their kidney transplant elsewhere and the pancreas transplant at the University of Minnesota. The proportions

**Table 3** Number of Pancreas Transplants in Analysis by Recipient Category, Duct Management, Donor Source, and Era

| Category | Era 1 ($n = 148$) 1978–86 | Era 2 ($n = 462$)[a] 1986–94 | Era 3 ($n = 297$) 1994–98 | Era 4 ($n = 666$) 1998–03 | Era 5 ($n = 262$)[b] 2003–05[b] | Total ($n = 1835$) |
|---|---|---|---|---|---|---|
| *Simultaneous pancreas-kidney* | | 233 (19Re) | 146 (9Re) | 213 (19Re) | 65 (7Re) | 657 (54Re)[c] |
| Deceased donor | | 231 | 125 (9Re) | 200 (19Re) | 63 (7Re) | 619 (54Re) |
| ED | | 8 | – | 136 | 36 | 180 |
| BD | | 222 | 123 | 64 | 26 | 435 |
| Other | | 1 | 2 | – | 1 | 4 |
| Living donor | | 2 (0Re) | 21 | 13 | 2 | 38 (0Re) |
| ED | | – | – | 1 | 1 | 2 |
| BD | | – | 20 | 12 | – | 32 |
| Other | | 2 | 1 | – | 1 | 4 |
| *Pancreas after kidney* | 65 (12Re) | 109 (35Re) | 104 (18Re) | 288 (72Re) | 111 (28Re) | 677 (165Re) |
| Deceased donor | 47 (11Re) | 96 (35Re) | 103 (18Re) | 288 (72Re) | 110 (28Re) | 644 (164Re) |
| ED | 7 | – | 6 | 26 | 49 | 88 |
| BD | 3 | 96 | 97 | 262 | 59 | 517 |
| Other | 37 | – | – | – | 2 | 39 |
| Living donor | 18 (1Re) | 13 (0Re) | 1 (0Re) | – | 1 (0Re) | 33 (1Re) |
| ED | 12 | 3 | – | – | – | 15 |
| BD | – | 6 | – | – | – | 6 |
| Other | 6 | 4 | 1 | – | 1 | 12 |
| *Pancreas transplant alone* | 83 (15Re) | 119 (32Re) | 47 (6Re) | 165 (23Re) | 86 (26Re) | 500 (102Re) |
| Deceased donor | 49 (13Re) | 104 (32Re) | 46 (6Re) | 162 (23Re) | 86 (26Re) | 447 (100Re) |
| ED | 29 | 2 | – | 15 | 36 | 82 |
| BD | 9 | 102 | 45 | 147 | 50 | 353 |
| Other | 11 | – | 1 | – | – | 12 |
| Living Donor | 34 (2Re) | 15 (0Re) | 1 (0Re) | 3 (0Re) | 0 (0Re) | 53 (2Re) |
| ED | 29 | 11 | – | – | – | 40 |
| BD | – | 4 | 1 | 3 | – | 8 |
| Other | 5 | – | – | – | – | 5 |

[a]In Era 2 there was one DD/BD simultaneous pancreas liver transplant.
[b]As of December 31, 2005.
[c]Two simultaneous pancreas kidney transplants were done after previous liver transplants, one in Era 3 and one in Era 4.
*Abbreviations*: ED, enteric drained; BD, bladder drained.

**Table 4** Simultaneous Pancreas-Kidney Transplants According to Donor Source (Same or Different; LD or DD) of Each Organ

| Era (N) | Same (619) | | Different (36) | |
|---|---|---|---|---|
| | **DD** | **LD** | **DDPx/DDKd** | **DDPx/LDKd** |
| 2 (233) | 224 (96%) | 2 (1%) | 3 (4%) | 4 (2%) |
| 3 (146) | 125 (86%) | 21 (14%) | 0 (0%) | 0 (0%) |
| 4 (213) | 186 (87%) | 13 (6%) | 1 ($<$1%) | 13 (6%) |
| 5 (65) | 48 (74%) | 2 (3%) | 0 (0%) | 15 (23%) |
| Total (657) | 583 (89%) | 38 (6%) | 4 (1%) | 32 (5%) |

*Abbreviations*: LD, living donor; DD, deceased donor; Px, pancreas; Kd, kidney.

of PAK recipients who had the kidney outside the University of Minnesota remained relatively constant from era to era (Table 5).

## Recipient Demographics
### Age of Recipients
The age range of the recipients was extreme (11–67 years) in all categories and in all eras, 12 to 62 years in the SPK, 20 to 65 years in the PAK, and 11 to 62 years in the PTA category. Only seven pancreas transplants, however, were in children ($<$18 years): four PTA, (15 to 17 years), one SPL, (16 years), and two SPK, (11 and 12 years) (170).

The mean age tended to increase in successive eras in each category. In SPK recipients, from Eras 2 through 5, it went from 38 to 40 to 43 to 44 years; in PAK recipients, from Eras 1 through 5, it went from 33 to 36 to 40 to 42 to 45 years; and in PTA recipients, from 31 to 34 to 36 to 41 and 41 years (medians differed from means by no more than one year). The proportion of DD primary pancreas transplant recipients above 45 years approximately doubled in each category in Eras 4 and 5 compared to Era 3, in SPK going from 28% to 45%, in PAK from 14% to 47%, and in PTA from 16% to 39% (see Table 8).

Analyses of outcome according to recipient age were done for primary DD pancreas transplant cases in Eras 3 to 5 combined, with the demographics in each category for this period given in Table 6. The mean and median ages were identical within each category, 43 years for SPK, 43 years for PTA, and 40 years for PTA, with half of the recipients being between 36 and 49 years of age for SPK, 37 and 48 years for PAK and 33 and 48 years for PAK cases, with a quarter being younger and a quarter older in each category. Patient and pancreas GSRs within each category were calculated for recipients below 30 versus 30–to 45 versus. above 45 years of age. The proportion below 30 years of age was very small in the SPK (less than 1:30) and PAK (1:20) categories, but was above 1:8 in the PTA category.

### Gender
Overall (1978 to 2005), the proportion of male and female pancreas recipients was nearly equal (49% and 51%, respectively), but there were fewer female recipients in the SPK (45%) and PAK (46%) categories, while substantially more females in the PTA category (67%). The female:male ratio in each category was constant across eras (Table 2).

The slightly higher proportion of males in the SPK and PAK categories can be explained by the fact that diabetic males are more likely to be afflicted by endstage renal disease than diabetic females (171). However, this fact does not explain why females comprise such a high

**Table 5** Pancreas After Kidney Transplants by Era and Site of Kidney Transplant

| Era (N) | University of Minnesota Medical Center | Other |
|---|---|---|
| 1 (65) | 46 | 19 (29%) |
| 2 (109) | 77 | 32 (30%) |
| 3 (104) | 82 | 22 (21%) |
| 4 (288) | 212 | 76 (26%) |
| 5 (111) | 71 | 40 (36%) |
| Total 677 | 488 | 189 (28%) |

**Table 6**  Age (Years) Distribution of Recipients Primary Deceased Donor Pancreas Transplants Eras 3 to 5 Combined

| Category (N) | SPK (353) | PAK (383) | PTA (239) |
|---|---|---|---|
| Mean± SD | 43± 8 | 43± 8 | 40± 10 |
| Youngest | 12 | 20 | 15 |
| Q1 (yrs) | 36 | 37 | 33 |
| Median (yrs) | 43 | 43 | 40 |
| Q3 (yrs) | 49 | 48 | 48 |
| Oldest (yrs) | 62 | 65 | 65 |
| 12–29 (yrs) | 3% | 5% | 13% |
| 30–44 (yrs) | 54% | 52% | 51% |
| > 45 (yrs) | 43% | 43% | 37% |

*Note*: Q1, oldest in 2nd quartile; Q3, oldest in 3rd quartile.

proportion of PTA recipients, because the incidence of Type-I diabetes is equal in males and females (171). It appears that nonuremic diabetic females are more likely to seek pancreas transplantation as an alternative to treatment with exogenous insulin.

### General Vascular Disease

The proportion of recipients with preexisting VD, cardiovascular (CVD), cerebral, or peripheral vascular disease (PVD), as indicated by events or the need for therapeutic intervention pretransplant, was determined by entry of patients in Eras 3, 4, and 5 into a formal study (Table 7). CVD was defined as a documented myocardial infarction (MI), or the need for pretransplant coronary artery bypass (CAB) or coronary artery angioplasty (CAA); cerebral VD as a documented stroke or transient ischemia attack (TIA); and PVD as a history of claudication with documented arterial lesions, previous arterial bypass, or a major (extremity) or minor (digit) amputation.

In Era 3, approximately half the SPK and PAK recipients had at least one manifestation of VD, but in Eras 4 and 5, more than two-thirds in both categories manifested VD and the differences by era were significant (Table 7); for Era 5, in the SPK category, a recipient without VD was a rarity. For PTA recipients, the incidence of VD of any kind was relatively low in Era 3 (less than one-fifth), but in Eras 4 and 5, more than half had preexisiting VD, again a significant change by era (Table 7).

In a separate analysis, we had done for two periods (1995–1998 vs. 1999–2005 or nearly corresponding to Era 3 vs. Eras 4 and 5 combined) on the presence of CVD, with our without assessment of or other manifestations of VD, again there was a significant change of prevalence in our pancreas transplant recipients by period (Table 8). Of the patients studied, at least one of the criteria for CVD (MI or need for CAB or CAA) was present pretransplant in 22% of 1995–1998 SPK recipients ($n = 102$) versus 75% of 1999–2005 combined recipients ($n = 220$), with 18% versus 65%, respectively, needing pretransplant coronary artery revascularization ($p < 0.0001$ for both comparisons); in 22 % of 1995–1998 ($n = 92$) versus 74% of 1999–2005 ($n = 333$) PAK recipients, with 18% versus 66% needing revascularization ($p < 0.0001$ for both); and in 13% of 1995–1998 ($n = 38$) vs 54% of Eras 1999–2005 ($n = 235$) PTA recipients, with 13% versus 50% requiring revascularization ($p < 0.001$ for both).

Thus, not only did the prevalence of general vascular disease (GVD) increase significantly from Era 3 to Eras 4 and 5, but also the prevalence of CVD by itself more than tripled ($p < 0.001$) in each category. The increase, in part, may be because of the increase in the proportion of recipients of each category that were elderly (over 45 years), going from 28% in

**Table 7**  Pretransplant Vascular Disease (Cardiovascular or Peripheral Vascular Disease) Incidence in Pancreas Transplant Recipients by Era and Category

| Category (N) | Era 3 (n) | Era 4 (n) | Era 5 (n) | p |
|---|---|---|---|---|
| Simultaneous pancreas-kidney (334) | 51% (97) | 67% (181) | 84% (56) | < 0.0001 |
| Pancreas after kidney (375) | 47% (81) | 72% (213) | 69% (81) | < 0.0002 |
| Pancreas transplant alone (232) | 18% (40) | 55% (135) | 51% (57) | 0.0002 |

**Table 8**  Incidence of Pretransplant Vascular Disease and of Elderly Patients in the University of Minnesota Pancreas Recipient Vascular Disease Study by Period and Category

| Category | 1995–1998 | 1999–2005 | p |
|---|---|---|---|
| Simultaneous pancreas kidney transplant (n) | 102 | 220 | |
| > 45 y/o % | 28 | 45 | 0.004 |
| With VD % | 22 | 75 | < 0.0001 |
| Coronary revascular (%) | 18 | 65 | < 0.0001 |
| Pancreas after kidney (n) | 92 | 333 | |
| > 45 y/o % | 14 | 47 | < 0.0001 |
| With VD % | 22 | 74 | < 0.0001 |
| Coronary revascular (%) | 18 | 66 | < 0.0001 |
| Pancreas transplant alone (n) | 38 | 235 | |
| > 45 y/o % | 16 | 39 | 0.005 |
| With VD % | 13 | 54 | 0.0002 |
| Coronary revascular (%) | 13 | 50 | < 0.0001 |

*Abbreviations*: y/o, years old; VD, vascular disease.

1995–1998 to 45% in 1999–2005 combined for SPK, from 14% to 47% for PAK and from 16% to 39% for PTA recipients ($p < 0.01$ for each comparison).

The incidence of GVD as well as CVD was lower in PTA than in SPK and PAK recipients in all eras ($p < 0.05$), but nevertheless, in Eras 4 and 5, more than half were affected. The increased incidence of GVD in Eras 4 and 5 versus Era 3 correlated with the increase in mean age of recipients, as well as in the proportion over 45 years old (nearly doubled in the SPK and more than doubled in PAK and PTA categories).

## Donor Demographics
### Deceased Donor Age
DD age was available only for Eras 2 to 5. In Eras 1 to 5, all categories combined, the age range of our DDs was 4 to 69 years. The means of the ages of DDs for SPK transplants in the successive Eras 2 to 5 were 35, 32, 35, and 32 years (medians 33, 31, 36, and 26 years, respectively). DDs for solitary pancreas transplants tended to be younger, the means of the ages in the successive Eras 1 to 5 being 34, 31, 25, 30, and 27 years in the PAK (medians 27, 29, 21, 28, and 24 years, respectively) and 35, 31, 27, 30, and 25 years in the PTA (medians 35, 30, 25, 28, and 22 years, respectively) category.

### Deceased Donor Organ Preservation Time
All eras included, our DD pancreas allograft preservation times ranged from 1 to 33 hours, from 3 to 34 hours for SPK, 5 to 38 for PAK, and 1 to 33 for PTA transplants. During Era 1, we made a transition from Collins solution to SGFP for cold storage preservation, and during Era 2, from SGFP to UW solution. The preservation times tended to be shorter during Era 1, when we only did solitary transplants and started out using Collin's solution, with a mean of 12 hours in the PAK and 10 hours in the PTA category, than during Eras 2 to 5. Preservation times varied little during Eras 2 to 5, regardless of recipient category, the mean times in the successive eras being 16, 18, 19, and 17 hours for SPK transplants; 15, 17, 18, and 17 hours for PAK transplants; and 16, 17, 18, and 17 hours for PTA transplants (the median preservation times differed from the means by no more than one hour in each category and era).

### Deceased Donor Human Leukocyte Antigen Mismatches
Beginning in Era 2, we deliberately attempted to minimize pancreas donor HLA mismatches (MMs) with PTA, and to some extent with PAK, but not SPK recipients. Thus, with few exceptions the average HLA-A, B, DR mismatch in each era was greater for SPK than for PAK recipients and the latter in turn was greater than for PTA recipients. In successive Eras 2 to 5, the mean total HLA MMs (range 0–6) were 3.34 ($n = 228$), 3.30 ($n = 146$), 3.03 ($n = 213$), and 4.03 ($n = 59$) in the SPK category ($p = 0.004$); 3.04 ($n = 109$), 2.97 ($n = 104$), 3.35 ($n = 288$), and 3.47 ($n = 97$) in the PAK category ($p = 0.006$); and 3.05 ($n = 116$), 2.23 ($n = 47$), 2.67 ($n = 165$), and 2.84 ($n = 70$) in the PTA category ($p = 0.002$). The differences in average mismatch between eras

**Table 9**  Relationship of Living Segmental Pancreas Donors to the Recipients in Eras 1 to 5 Combined

|  | Simultaneous pancreas-kidney (38) | Pancreas after kidney (33) | Pancreas transplant alone (58) | Total |
|---|---|---|---|---|
| HLA-identical sibling | 6 | 13 | 20 | 39 |
| Identical twin | 0 | 1 | 9 | 10 |
| HLA-MM related | 25 | 18 | 24 | 67 |
| Unrelated | 7 | 1 | 0 | 8 |
| Total | 38 (31%) | 33 (27%) | 53 (43%) | 124 (100%) |

*Abbreviations*: HLA, human leukocyte antigens; MM, mismatches.

were statistically significant in each category. In both the PAK and PTA categories, the average mismatch was least in Era 3, but even in Eras 4 and 5 we have continued to try to minimize MMs for solitary pancreas transplants, especially in PTA recipients where even in Era 5, the average mismatch is well below that of the other categories.

In the analyses presented here, DWFG censored GSRs, and RRE rates, according to total number of HLA MMs, or by the number of MMs at just Class I or Class II loci, or for 0 versus 1 or above MMs at each locus, were calculated for recipients in each category of TS primary DD BD pancreas transplants in Eras 3 and 4 combined.

### *Living Donors*

The relation of the 124 living segmental pancreas donors to the recipients in each category for Eras 1 to 5 combined are shown in Table 9. There were 80 siblings (51 sisters, 29 brothers), 28 parents (19 mothers, 9 fathers), 2 offsprings (both daughters), 3 distant related, 8 unrelated, and 3 unclassified donors. Of the siblings, 49 (61%) were HLA identical [including the 10 identical twins of the 33 PAK and 53 PTA donors, all but 6 (2 PAK, 4 PTA)] were done in Era 1 and 2. Of the 38 SPK donors, 36 were done in Eras 3 to 5. The age range of the donors was 20 to 59 years.

The first donor (1979) remains normoglycemic, as do nearly all the others. However, six have developed diabetes treated with insulin, all with a body mass index (BMI) above 28 kg/m$^2$. The donors have been studied extensively by metabolic testing (160,172,173). Donors who had a 300% increase in plasma insulin levels from baseline during the first 1 to 3 minutes after a predonation intravenous glucose or arginine challenge have remained with normal glucose tolerance. Our current criteria to be a pancreas LD includes a BMI below 28 kg/m$^2$, a normal glucose tolerance test (GTT), and a threefold increase in plasma insulin concentration after both glucose and arginine stimulation.

### OUTCOME ANALYSIS

Patient and graft (DWFG counted as a failure) survival rates, TF rates, immunologic or rejection loss rates (RLR) (TS grafts analyzed with DWFG censored), and RRE rates for our pancreas and diabetic kidney recipients are given according to eras, recipient category, pancreas graft duct management, primary or retransplant status, donor source, and recipient and donor demographic features. The outcomes (patient and graft survival and RLRs) by era for primary, DD transplants are shown for each category in Figures 2–4 with each category discussed in detail following a general overview.

In general, our pancreas GSRs improved from era to era (Fig. 2B, 3B, and 4B), particularly for PAK and PTA recipients in whom the early era GSRs were relatively low because of the high RLR versus the SPK category, but reduction of the TF rates contributed to the improvement of GSR in all categories.

For all primary DD pancreas transplants from 1978 through 2005, the collective TF rate was 10% (135/1393), with minimal or no differences between categories, being 11% in SPK (62/565) and 9% in both PAK (42/480) and PTA (31/347) recipients. The TF rates for all categories combined in the successive eras went from 18% in Era 1 (13/72) to 14% in Era 2 (48/345) to 7% in Era 3 (16/241) and 9% in Era 4 (49/536) to only 4% in Era 5 (9/198). The reduction in TF rates over time occurred with both ED and BD, though in both Eras (4 and 5) where both techniques of exocrine drainage were frequently used, the TF rate was lower with BD; the TF

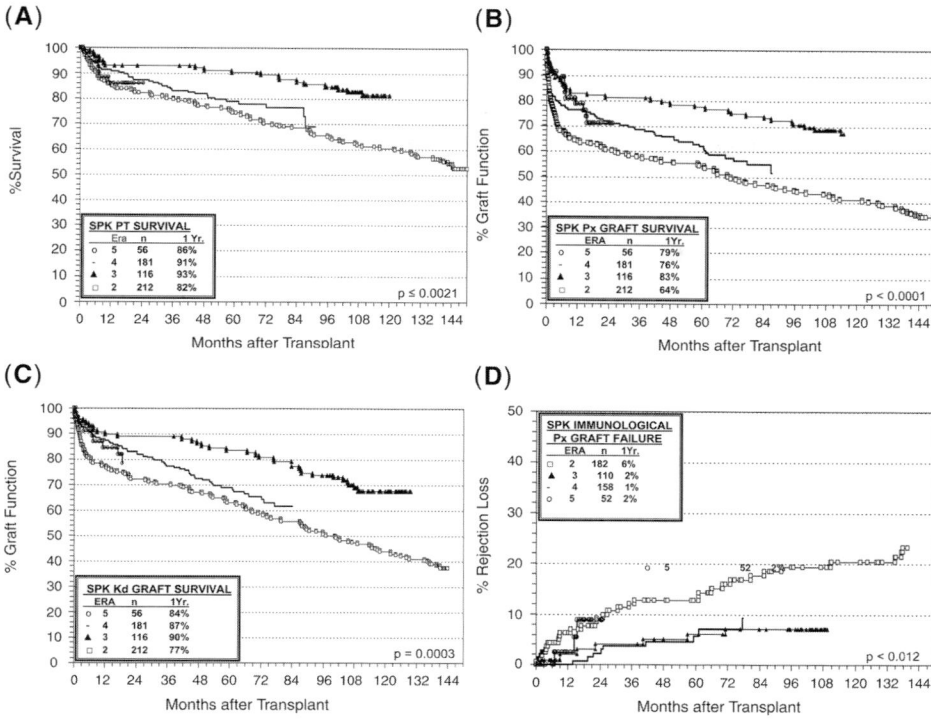

**Figure 2** Primary deceased donor simultaneous pancreas kidney (**A**) patient, (**B**) pancreas graft, (**C**) kidney graft functional survival rates, and (**D**) pancreas graft immunological failure rates by eras.

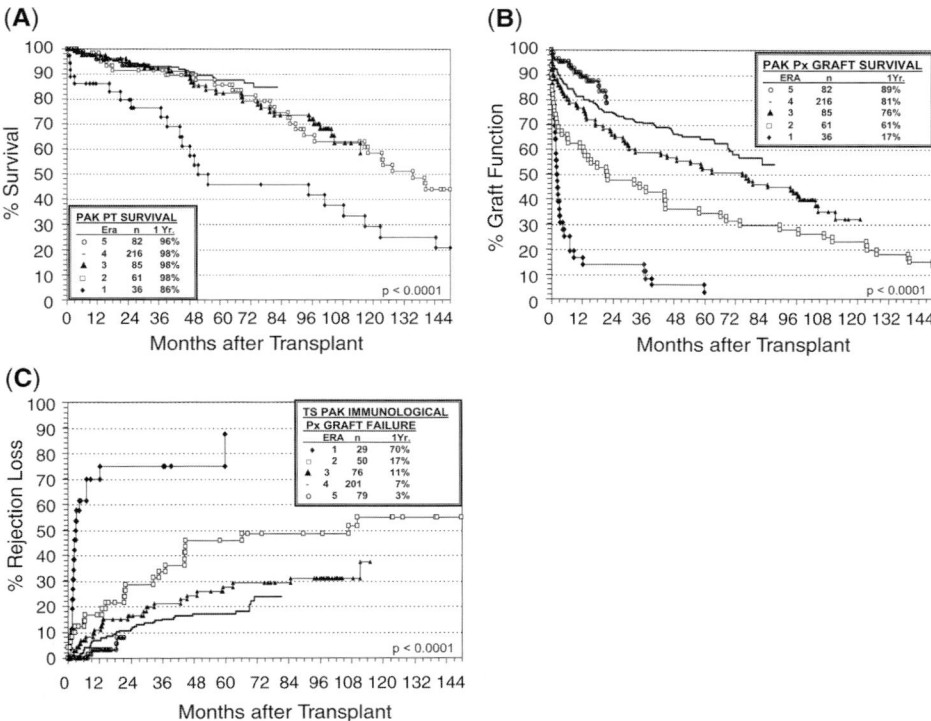

**Figure 3** Primary deceased donor pancreas after kidney (**A**) patient and (**B**) pancreas graft functional survival rates and (**C**) pancreas graft immunological failure rates by eras.

**(A)**

**(B)**

**(C)**

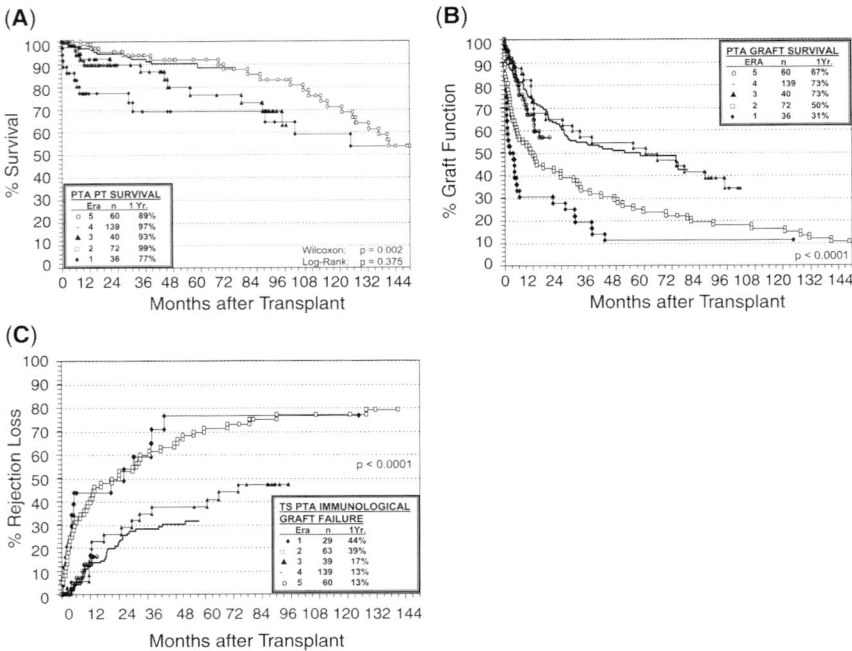

**Figure 4** Primary deceased donor pancreas transplant alone (**A**) patient, (**B**) pancreas graft functional survival rates, and (**C**) pancreas graft immunological failure rates by eras.

rate for primary DD went from 12% for ED transplants in Era 4 (18/151) to 7% in Era 5 (7/96), and for BD from 8% (31/385) to 2% (2/101) in the respective eras.

The reduction in TF rates impacts the early GSRs. The reduction in RLR (DWFG censored) is best measured long term. As expected, the five-year RLR for DD primary pancreas transplants decreased in all categories from the early to latest eras (Fig. 2C, 3C, and 4C), but was less dramatic in SPK recipients because it was low from the beginning. Indeed, in spite of the very large reduction in RLR in the PAK and PTA categories, in the most recent era (Era 4) where five-year outcomes can be calculated, the RLRs are higher in PAK and PTA recipients than for SPK recipients in the earliest era (Era 2) in which we did pancreas transplants in all three categories. Progressively, from Eras 2 to 4, the five-year RLR went from 13% to 6% to 6% in the SPK category, from 46% to 27% to 17% in the PAK category, and from 71% to 38% to 32% in the PTA category. It is too early to assess the five-year RLR in Era 5, but at least for PTA recipients, it is likely to remain relatively high because at one year it is 13% (Fig. 4C), versus. 2% in both the SPK (Fig. 2C) and PAK (Fig. 2C) recipients of this era.

The best estimate of current long-term pancreas GSRs comes from Era 4, at five years 62% for SPK (69% for the kidney grafts), 64% for PAK, and only 48% for PTA recipients (Figs. 2B, 3B, and 4B). The corresponding five-year patient survival rates for Era 4 SPK, PAK, and PTA recipients of primary DD transplants are 79%, 88%, and 88%, respectively (Figs. 2A, 3A, and 4A).

## Era Analysis of Outcome for Primary Deceased Donor Transplants by Recipient Category
### Simultaneous Pancreas Kidney Transplants
We did no SPK transplants in Era 1. The primary DD SPK patient survival rates (Fig. 2A), pancreas (Fig. 2B) and kidney (Fig. 2C) GSRs, and pancreas immunological loss rates (Fig. 2D) are shown by era. Although the immunological loss rates were highest in Era 2 and equally low in Eras 3, 4, and 5, the overall results (patient and nondeath censored GSRs) were superior in Era 3, an era where the vascular risk factors were half as prevalent as in the subsequent two eras (Table 7).

The principal difference between Era 2 versus 3 and 4 was the use of Csa-Aza in the former and Tac-Aza or Tac-MMF in the latter for maintenance immunosuppression (8). The principal difference in Era 5 was the use of Campath for both induction and maintenance immunosuppression for one year with oral monotherapy with MMF or, if MMF was not tolerated, Rapamycin (163). BD predominated for duct management of SPK transplants in Eras 2 and 3, and ED predominated in Eras 4 and 5. SPK patient (Fig. 2A) and non-DWFG censored GSRs [Fig. 2A (pancreas) and 2B (kidney)] were highest in Era 3, an Era with a relatively low incidence of GVD and CVD, but pancreas RLR were relatively low and equal in Eras 3 to 5 versus Era 2 (Fig. 2D). In Era 3, five year SPK patient, pancreas and kidney survival rates were 90%, 77%, and 83%, with a pancreas RLR of 6%. The principal cause of early pancreas graft loss in SPK recipients of each era was TF, but was lower in Era 3 (5%) than in Eras 2 (14%), 4 (12%), and 5 (7%) ($p = 0.06$).

### Pancreas After Kidney Transplants
Primary DD PAK patient (Fig. 3A) survival rates improved significantly from Era 1 to Era 2 and stayed high thereafter (>96% at one year in each of the Eras 2–5 and >82% at five years in each of the Eras 2–4). PAK pancreas GSRs (Fig. 3B) improved significantly in each successive Era from 1 to 5, reaching 89% at one year in Era 5 and 64% at five years in Era 4. The improvement in PAK GSRs was due both to sequential reduction in TF rates from Eras 1 to 5 [successively 17%, 16%, 11%, 6%, and 4% ($p = 0.02$)]; and to reduction in RLRs (Fig. 3C), at five years in successive Eras 1 to 4, 88%, 46%, 27%, and 17% ($p < 0.0001$).

The principal differences between Era 1 versus 2 for PAK recipients was the consistent use of Csa-Aza for immunosuppression and BD for pancreas graft duct management in Era 2, allowing early diagnosis and treatment of rejection episodes. The principal change in Eras 3 and 4 was the use of Tac-/MMF and, in Era 5, the use of Campath-MMF for maintenance immunosuppression.

### Pancreas Transplant Alone
Primary DD PTA patient (Fig. 4A) survival rates also improved dramatically from Era 1 to Era 2 and stayed high through Era 4; in Era 5 the PTA patient survival rate declined, perhaps due to the increased incidence of GVD and CVD in the recipient population (Table 4). PTA pancreas GSRs (Fig. 4B) also dramatically increased from Era 1 to 2, and improved again as much in Era 3, remained stable in Era 4 (50% functioning at five years), and then slightly declined in Era 5. Both the TF (19%) and rejection loss (77% at five years) rates were high for PTA recipients in Era 1, but thereafter both declined, the TF rate in successive Eras 2 to 5 being 11%, 2%, 9%, and 3% ($p < 0.5$) and the RLRs at five years in successive Eras 2 to 5 being 71%, 38%, and 32%, the latter being much higher than in both the SPK (especially) and the PAK categories.

## Influence of Duct Management on Outcome
### Era 1
All duct management techniques were used in Era 1. The TF rate was high except with DI (7%), but each technique was compatible with long-term success. The first OD graft (segmental DD PTA) functioned for 17 years, until DWFG occurred. A DI graft (segmental LD PAK) functioned for 25 years. The longest functioning DD donor DI graft (PTA) is 23 years. The longest functioning ED graft (LD PTA) is 24 years; the longest functioning DD graft (PAK) is 22 years. The longest functioning BD graft, also from Era 1 (DD PTA), is now 20 years.

In Era 1, we did only solitary pancreas transplants. The OD technique was used in 12 primary PAK (TFs in 3/9 DD, 2/3 LD); and in three primary PTA (all TFs, 1 CAD, 2 LD). The DI technique was used in 28 PAK (TF in 1/25 DD, 1/3 LD), 23 primary (TF in 1/20 DD, 1/3 LD), and 5 retransplants (all DD, no TF); and in 12 PTA (TF in 1/9 DD, 0/3 LD), 10 primary (TF in 1/7 DD, 0/3 LD) and 2 retransplants (both TS DD). Overall, the TF rate was 53% with OD ($n = 15$) and 7% with DI ($n = 40$) in Era 1.

ED was also used in Era 1: in 19 PAK (TFs in 3/7 DD, 5/12 LD), 15 primary (TFs in 3/4 DD, 4/11 LD) and 4 retransplants (TFs in 0/3 DD, 1/1 LD); and in 58 PTA (TFs in 10/29 DD, 9/29 LD), 50 primary (TFs in 9/23 DD, 8/27 LD) and 9 retransplants (TFs in 1/7 DD, 2/2 LD).

We began to use BD near the end of Era 1: in three DD PAK (all TFs), two primary and one retransplant; and in nine DD PTA (2 TF), five primary (1 TF) and four retransplants (1 TF). The overall TF rate for BD in Era 1 ($n = 12$) was 42%. However, the RLR in the TS BD cases in Era 1 was low; of the TS PTA transplants ($n = 7$), only one was rejected at below one year, with a two-year GSR of 86%. After Era 1, we rarely used any technique other than BD or ED, and predominantly BD until Era 4.

## Era 2

Of the 24 ED transplants done in Era 2, eight were in DD SPK recipients (TFs in 3/7 primary, 0/1 retransplant); three in primary LD PAK (2 TFs); and 13 in PTA recipients, two DD retransplants (no TF) and 11 primary LD (3 TFs). The one TS ED PAK retransplant in Era 2 was rejected at below one year.

In Era 2, the one-year GSRs were 50% for all ED DD SPK ($n = 8$) and 64% for all ED LD PTA ($n = 11$) transplants. The one- and five-year GSRs for the corresponding TS transplants were 80% and 40% in the ED DD SPK ($n = 5$) and 88% and 75% in the ED LD PTA ($n = 8$) recipients.

Of the primary DD BD grafts in Era 2, the TF rate was 23% in PAK ($n = 61$) and 15% in PTA ($n = 72$) recipients. For DD BD retransplants in Era 2, the TF rate was 29% in PAK ($n = 35$) and 10% in PTA ($n = 30$) recipients.

The one-year GSRs in all BD DD PAK ($n = 95$) and PTA ($n = 102$) recipients in Era 2 were 47% and 51%, respectively; for the corresponding TS cases, 72% ($n = 69$) and 64% ($n = 85$).

For primary BD DD PAK ($n = 51$) and PTA ($n = 64$) TS transplants the one-year GSR was 82% and 60%, respectively. BD was used in four LD PTA recipients in Era 2 [1 TF; 2/3 TS grafts functioned >one year (67%) and one is still functioning at >16 years]. Urinary drainage was used in 10 LD PAK recipients in Era 2, via the bladder in six [2 TF; 5/6 TS grafts (83%) are still functioning at 12 to 21 years] and via the ureter in four (two TFs; the two TS grafts are still functioning >12 years).

## Era 3

With very rare exceptions, we continued to use BD in DD PTA recipients in Era 3 ($n = 45$), with no TFs in 39 primary cases and one TF in six retransplants (17%). For the primary DD BD PTA cases ($n = 39$) in Era 3, the one-year GSR was 82%. Most DD PAK transplants were also done with BD in Era 3 (n=97), with a TF rate of 10% for primary ($n = 81$) cases and 42% for the retransplants ($n = 16$). However, six PAK transplants (4 primary, 2 retransplants) in Era 3 were done with ED (1 TF, a primary graft).

In Era 3, the one-year GSR for primary DD BD PAK transplants ($n = 81$) was 78% with a rejection graft loss rate at one year of 11%. We did not do an ED SPK transplant in Era 3, but did 123 BD SPK transplants with an overall TF rate of 6%, 4% for primary grafts ($n = 114$) and 22% for retransplants ($n = 9$).

## Eras 4 and 5

In Eras 4 ($n = 666$) and 5 ($n = 262$) we used ED or BD in large proportions of the recipients in all categories. The number of pancreas transplants in both eras combined was 928, of which 32% were ED and 67% BD, 27% versus 73% in Era 4 and 47% versus 52% in Era 5.

In the SPK category, in both eras combined ($n = 278$), 63% were ED, 64% in Era 4 ($n = 213$), and 58% in Era 5 ($n = 65$); in the PAK category, both eras combined ($n = 399$), 19% were ED, 9% in Era 4 ($n = 288$) and 44% in Era 5 ($n = 111$); in the PTA category, both eras combined ($n = 251$), 20% were ED, 9% in Era 4 ($n = 165$), and 42% in Era 5 ($n = 86$).

The TF rates for primary DD ED ($n = 159$) versus BD ($n = 77$) SPK transplants in Eras 4 and 5 combined were 13% versus 8%, 13% ($n = 127$) versus 9% ($n = 54$) in Era 4 and 9% ($n = 32$) versus 4% ($n = 23$) in Era 5; for primary DD ED ($n = 53$) versus BD ($n = 245$) PAK transplants in the combined eras, 8% versus 5%, 7% ($n = 15$) versus 6% (n=201) in Era 4 and 8% ($n = 38$) versus 0% ($n = 44$) in Era 5; for primary DD ED ($n = 35$) versus BD ($n = 164$) PTA transplants in the combined eras, 3% versus 9%, 0% ($n = 9$) versus 10% ($n = 130$) in Era 4 and 4% ($n = 26$) versus 3% ($n = 34$) in Era 5.

GSRs for ED versus BD transplants were calculated within each Era (4 and 5) and for the combined eras for each category. For Era 4, GSRs at one year for ED versus BD transplants in the SPK category were 77% ($n = 127$) versus 74% ($n = 54$); in the PAK category, 73% ($n = 15$) versus 82% ($n = 201$); and in the PTA category, 78% ($n = 9$) versus 73% ($n = 30$). For Era 5, GSRs at one year for ED versus BD in the SPK category were 76% ($n = 32$) versus 81% ($n = 23$); in the PAK category, 92% ($n = 38$) versus 88% ($n = 44$); and in the PTA category, 65% ($n = 26$) versus 69% ($n = 34$). The GSRs for ED versus BD cases by category for the combined eras (4 and 5) are

**Table 10** Deceased Donor Primary Pancreas Transplant Graft Survival Rates by Duct Management and Recipient Category for Eras 4 and 5 Combined

|  | SPK | | PAK | | PTA | |
|---|---|---|---|---|---|---|
|  | ED | BD | ED | BD | ED | BD |
| (N) | 159 | 77 | 53 | 245 | 35 | 164 |
| GSR | 13% | 8% | 8% | 5% | 3% | 9% |
| 1 yr | 77% | 77% | 83% | 83% | 69% | 73% |
| 3 yr | 68% | 66% | 57% | 72% | 48% | 53% |
| 5 yr | 64% | 57% | 53% | 67% | 32% | 44% |
| p values (WC/LR) | N | S | 0.15/0.08 | | N | S |

Abbreviations: WC, Wilcoxin Test; LR, Log-Rank Test; NS, not significant ($p > 0.2$).

shown in Table 10: for ED ($n = 159$) versus BD ($n = 77$) SPK cases, one- and five-year GSRs were 77% versus 76% and 64% versus 57%; for PAK cases, 87% ($n = 53$) versus 82% ($n = 245$) and 53% versus 67%; and for PTA cases, 68% ($n = 35$) versus 71% ($n = 164$) and 45% versus 45%.

Overall, there was a slightly higher TF rate for ED versus BD during Eras 4 and 5, but there were no significant differences in GSRs in any category according to duct-management. ED avoids the chronic complications of BD (urinary infections, hematuria, metabolic acidosis, dysuria) that may lead to the need to convert to ED (174). In Eras 4 and 5 combined, the actuarial incidence of conversion of TS primary DD BD grafts to ED by three years post transplant was 24% for SPK ($n = 71$), 25% for PAK ($n = 232$), and 24% for PTA ($n = 150$) cases. Thus, the higher early TF rate for SPK ED transplants is offset by the higher, chronic complication rate with BD, but the latter does not lead to graft loss, and thus for solitary pancreas transplants or for high risk SPK transplants, we continue to use BD.

The main difference for Era 4 as opposed to Era 3 (when our results were the best) was the much higher incidence of VD risk factors in all categories, and the high incidence of VD, and particularly CVD, continued in Era 5. The main difference for Era 5 as opposed to Era 4 was the change in immunosuppression protocol from CI maintenance to anti-T-cell maintenance for one year with Campath. In the SPK and PAK categories, GSRs were similar in the two eras, but in the PTA category, the GSRs were better in Era 4 than in Era 5. In Era 5, GSRs were highest in the PAK category, further justifying our preferred approach to preempt dialysis in nephropathic diabetes with a LD kidney with either a simultaneous LD or DD pancreas or a subsequent DD pancreas (PAK) with either ED or BD.

## Outcome by Recipient Risk Factors
### *Recipient Age*
The age range of the pancreas recipient population expanded in each successive era, mainly in the direction of older population. Across all Eras, only seven recipients were below 18 years (four PTA, two SPK, one SPL). One pediatric LD PTA graft functioned for four years, while the other PTA grafts failed between two and six months. The two pediatric SPK recipients (170) currently have functioning pancreas grafts at nearly 10 years, though one needed a kidney retransplant at nine years because of renal insufficiency from CI-induced nephropathy.

At the other extreme, for primary DD pancreas transplants in Eras 4 and 5 combined, 45% of SPK, 47% of PAK, and 39% of PTA recipients were 45 years or older, as compared to 28%, 22%, and 16%, respectively, in Era 3. For assessment of pancreas transplant outcomes (patient and GSRs, uncensored, and TF rates) according to recipient age, we analyzed DD primary pancreas transplant cases in Eras 3 to 5 combined (June, 1994 to December, 2005), for age groups below 30 versus 30 to 45 versus above 45 years old in each category (Tables 11–13).

The TF rates for pancreas transplants did not differ significantly according to recipient age in any category (Table 11). In recipients below 30, 30 to 44, and above 44 years, the pancreas graft TF rates were 17%, 13%, and 10%, respectively, in the SPK ($p = 0.6$); 15%, 8%, and 8% in the PAK ($p = 0.5$); and 10%, 10%, and 8% in the PTA ($p = 0.9$) category.

Although patient survival rates, at least long term, might be expected to be lower in the older recipients, statistically significant differences according to age were only seen in the SPK category (Table 12), and were both early ($p = 0.15$ WC) and late ($p = 0.18$ LR). SPK patient

**Table 11**  Technical Failure Rates for Primary Deceased Donor Pancreas Transplants According to Recipient Category and Age in Eras 3 to 5 Combined

| Category (N) | < 30 (n) | 30–45 (n) | > 45 (n) | p Value $\chi c^2$ |
|---|---|---|---|---|
| Simultaneous pancreas-kidney (353) | 17% (12) | 13% (190) | 10% (151) | 0.58 |
| Pancreas after kidney (383) | 15% (20) | 8% (200) | 8% (163) | 0.52 |
| Pancreas transplant alone (239) | 10% (30) | 10% (121) | 8% (88) | 0.88 |

survival rates in recipients <30 vs 30 to 45 vs >45 years were 100% vs 93% vs 88% at one year and 86% vs 84% vs 73 at seven years posttransplant.

For PAK recipients <30, 30 to 45, and >45 years old, the patient survival rates at one year were 100%, 96%, and 98%, respectively, at seven years 83%, 80%, and 77%. For PTA recipients in the respective age groups, the patient survival rates at one year were 93%, 96%, and 93% ($p = 0.11$ WC), at seven years 59%, 84%, and 87% ($p = 0.08$ LR).

GSRs, uncensored, according to age in each recipient category are shown in Table 13. In the SPK category, neither pancreas nor kidney GSRs differed significantly early or late according to recipient age. At one year, the pancreas GSRs were 83%, 79%, and 79% and the kidney GSRs 92%, 89%, and 85% in those <30, 30 to 44, and >45 years old; at seven years, for the pancreas 60%, 61%, and 60% respectively, for the kidney, 63%, 69%, and 65%.

Likewise, in the PAK category, pancreas GSRs did not differ significantly by recipient age. GSRs at one year for PAK recipients <30, 30 to 44, and >44 years old were 75%, 80%, and 84%, at seven years, 43%, 49%, and 58%, respectively.

However, in the PTA category, GSRs differed significantly by age, both early ($p = 0.04$ WC) and late ($p = 0.03$ LR), being highest in the oldest and lowest in the youngest recipients. GSRs at one year for PTA recipients <30, 30 to 44, and >44 years old were 60%, 71%, and 78%; at seven years 22%, 38%, and 55%, respectively.

Thus, the older PTA recipients (>45 years old) did surprisingly well, with significantly higher GSRs, both early and late, than their younger counterparts, particularly those <30 years old. Of the > 45-year old PTA recipients, more than half were still insulin-independent at 10 years and with a survival rate at least as high, if not higher than their younger counterparts who reject more, perhaps showing the benefit on survival of persistent graft function a diabetic category (PTA), where the main indication for the pancreas transplant was hypoglycemic unawareness.

### *Vascular Disease*
A comparison of outcome was done for the study cohort recipients of primary DD pancreas allografts with ≥1 vascular risk factor (MI, CAB, CAA, stroke, TIA, arterial bypass, amputation)

**Table 12**  Patient Survival Rates for Primary Deceased Donor Pancreas Transplant According to Recipient Category and Age in Eras 3 to 5 Combined

| Category and age (N) | Years posttransplant | | | | | p Values (WC/LR) |
|---|---|---|---|---|---|---|
| | 1 yr | 3 yr | 5 yr | 7 yr | 10 yr | |
| *SPK (353)* | | | | | | |
| 12–29 (12) | 100% | 100% | 100% | 86% | 86% | 0.015/0.018 |
| 30–44 (190) | 93% | 90% | 88% | 84% | 78% | |
| > 45 (151) | 88% | 82% | 76% | 73% | 65% | |
| *PAK (383)* | | | | | | |
| 12–29 (20) | 100% | 100% | 100% | 83% | 42% | 0.27/0.55 |
| 30–44 (200) | 96% | 94% | 86% | 80% | 65% | |
| > 45 (163) | 98% | 90% | 84% | 77% | 65% | |
| *PTA (239)* | | | | | | |
| 12–29 (30) | 93% | 84% | 67% | 59% | 59% | 0.11/0.08 |
| 30–44 (121) | 96% | 92% | 89% | 84% | 84% | |
| > 45 (88) | 93% | 90% | 87% | 87% | 56% | |

*Abbreviations*: WC, Wilcoxin Test; LR, Log-Rank Test; SPK, simultaneous pancreas-kidney; PAK, pancreas after kidney; PTA, pancreas transplant alone.

**Table 13**  Pancreas (and Kidney in SPK) Graft Survival Rates for Primary Deceased Donor Transplants According to Recipient Category and Age in Eras 3 to 5 Combined

| Category and age (N) | Years posttransplant | | | | | p Value (WC/LR) |
|---|---|---|---|---|---|---|
| | 1 yr | 3 yr | 5 yr | 7 yr | 10 yr | |
| SPK (353) | Pancreas (Kd) | Pancreas (Kd) | Pancreas (Kd) | Pancreas (Kd) | Pancreas (Kd) | |
| 12–29 (12) | 83 (92) | 83 (92) | 75 (83) | 60 (63) | 30 (31) | 0.92/0.88 |
| 30–44 (190) | 79 (89) | 72 (83) | 69 (78) | 61 (69) | 57 (62) | (0.27/0.22) |
| >45 (151) | 79 (85) | 72 (76) | 65 (67) | 60 (65) | 51 (55) | |
| PAK (383) | Pancreas | Pancreas | Pancreas | Pancreas | Pancreas | |
| 12–29 (20) | 75 | 55 | 50 | 43 | 16 | 0.33/0.21 |
| 30–44 (200) | 80 | 68 | 60 | 49 | 45 | |
| >45 (163) | 84 | 68 | 65 | 58 | 34 | |
| PTA (239) | Pancreas | Pancreas | Pancreas | Pancreas | Pancreas | |
| 12–29 (30) | 60 | 38 | 34 | 22 | 22 | 0.04/0.03 |
| 30–44 (121) | 71 | 51 | 45 | 38 | 38 | |
| >45 (88) | 78 | 63 | 59 | 55 | 35 | |

*Abbreviations*: WC, Wilcoxin Test; LR, Log-Rank Test; Kd, kidney.

versus those without a vascular risk factor in combined Eras 3 to 5. Even though the incidence of VD in all recipient categories was higher in Eras 4 and 5 than in 3 (Table 7), we combined all three eras for analsysis of the VD impact on outcome because within each group, patients with and patients without VD, they were similar across eras. In other words, eras differed only in the frequency distribution of the subgroup types, not in the types themselves.

Of the 1025 recipients of primary DD pancreas allografts in Eras 3 to 5, we had information in our database on their VD status in all but 25, giving 369 SPK, 381 PAK, and 242 PTA cases for anlaysis. Of these, 64% of SPK, 65 % of PAK, and 47% of PTA recipients had VD. Patient and GSRs for those with and without VD in each category are shown in Table 14.

Patient survival rates were statistically significantly lower in those with vs those without VD both early ($p = 0.02$ WC), 89% vs 95% at one year, and late ($p = 0.003$ LR), 73% vs 92% at

**Table 14**  Outcome by Vascular Disease in Recipients of Primary Deceased Donor in Eras 3 to 5 Combined

| Category (N) p-values years | SPK p = 0.0003/ < 0.001 | | PAK p = 0.10/0.04 | | PTA p = 0.25/0.35 | |
|---|---|---|---|---|---|---|
| Patient survival (%) | Yes (235) | No (134) | Yes (381) | No (249) | Yes (113) | No (129) |
| 1 | 89 | 95 | 97 | 98 | 95 | 95 |
| 3 | 84 | 94 | 91 | 95 | 92 | 89 |
| 5 | 80 | 93 | 83 | 89 | 90 | 82 |
| 7 | 73 | 92 | 72 | 88 | 90 | 76 |
| 10 | 61 | 87 | 57 | 77 | – | – |
| | SPK p = 0.02/0.003 | | PAK p = 0.29/0.13 | | PTA P = 0.34/0.32 | |
| Pancreas GSR (%) | Yes | No | Yes | No | Yes | No |
| 1 | 77 | 83 | 80 | 84 | 76 | 71 |
| 3 | 70 | 77 | 66 | 69 | 58 | 60 |
| 5 | 62 | 76 | 60 | 63 | 52 | 46 |
| 7 | 55 | 69 | 46 | 56 | 47 | 38 |
| 10 | 44 | 66 | 26 | 48 | – | – |
| | SPK p = 0.009/0.003 | | | | | |
| Kidney GSR (%) | Yes | No | | | | |
| 1 | 88 | 90 | | | | |
| 3 | 77 | 88 | | | | |
| 5 | 70 | 82 | | | | |
| 7 | 62 | 77 | | | | |
| 10 | 48 | 68 | | | | |

seven years, in SPK recipients; and at least late ($p = 0.04$), 72% vs 88% at seven years, in PAK recipients (Table 14). However, in the PTA category the patient survival rates did not differ significantly according to the presence or absence of VD.

In the SPK category, uncensored pancreas and kidney GSRs were also significantly lower, both early ($p < 0.02$ WC) and late ($p = 0.003$ LR), in recipients with vs without VD (Table 14), for pancreas 77% vs 83% at one year and 55% vs 69% at seven years, and for kidney 88% vs 90% at one year and 62% vs 77% at seven years. However, in the PAK and PTA categories, pancreas GSRs did not differ significantly between those with and without VD (Table 14). For PAK recipients with and without VD, one-year GSRs were 80% and 84%; at seven years, 46%, and 56% respectively. For PTA recipients with and without VD, the GSRs were 76% and 71%, at one year and 47% and 38% at seven years, respectively.

In general, the pancreas transplant outcomes for diabetic recipients without VD are good in all categories, but satisfactory outcomes are also achieved in most recipients with VD, especially considering the poor prognosis of uremic diabetic patients without a transplant (175,176).

## Outcome by Donor Risk Factors
### *Human Leukocyte Antigen Matching*

We analyzed TS primary DD **BD** GSRs and RRE rates by the overall number of donor HLA Class I (A and B loci) and II (DR locus) matches or MMs, or at individual loci, within each recipient category for combined Eras 3 and 4 both early (one year) and late (>five years) effects, if any, could be discerned (Tables 15–23).

The first analysis was of pancreas GSRs according to total number of MMs at HLA Class I and II loci combined (seven groups, sequentially 0 to 6 MMs Table 15). Only in the PTA category were there differences in outcomes according to combined number of HLA-A, B, and DR MMS that approached or were statistical significance ($p = 0.10$ by WC test for early and 0,05 by LR for late differences). However, in each category (SPK, PAK, and PTA), the seven-year pancreas GSRs were 100% for recipients of BD transplants from DDs with zero MMs at all HLA loci.

**Table 15**  Graft Survival Rates (DWFG Censored) for TS Primary DD BD Pancreas Transplants According to Number of HLA MMs (All Loci, A, B, and DR) for Eras 3 and 4 Combined

| Category (*N*) and HLA MMs (*N*) | Years posttransplant | | | | *p* Value (WC/LR) |
|---|---|---|---|---|---|
| | 1 yr | 3 yr | 5 yr | 7 yr | |
| *SPK (158)* | | | | | 0.64/0.71 |
| 0 (10) | 100 | 100 | 100 | 100 | |
| 1 (6) | 100 | 100 | 100 | 100 | |
| 2 (17) | 100 | 94 | 88 | 88 | |
| 3 (44) | 98 | 98 | 95 | 95 | |
| 4 (43) | 98 | 92 | 86 | 86 | |
| 5 (28) | 100 | 100 | 100 | 95 | |
| 6 (101) | 100 | 88 | 88 | 88 | |
| *PAK (260)* | | | | | 0.68/0.84 |
| 0 (1) | 100 | 100 | 100 | 100 | |
| 1 (20) | 84 | 79 | 79 | 79 | |
| 2 (46) | 98 | 92 | 92 | 80 | |
| 3 (71) | 93 | 84 | 79 | 76 | |
| 4 (82) | 90 | 82 | 77 | 74 | |
| 5 (36) | 91 | 79 | 76 | 76 | |
| 6 (4) | 100 | 100 | 100 | – | |
| *PTA (155)* | | | | | 0.10/0.05 |
| 0 (8) | 100 | 100 | 100 | 100 | |
| 1 (20) | 89 | 63 | 63 | 63 | |
| 2 (47) | 84 | 96 | 74 | 66 | |
| 3 (51) | 89 | 66 | 66 | 66 | |
| 4 (24) | 83 | 78 | 66 | 57 | |
| 5 (5) | 80 | 20 | – | – | |

*Abbreviations*: DWFG, death with functioning graft censored; TS, technically successful; DD, deceased donor; BD, bladder drainage; MM, mismatches; WC, Wilcoxin test; LR, log-rank test; HLA MMS, human leukocyte antigens; SPK, simultaneous pancreas-kidney; PAK, pancreas after kidney; PTA, pancreas transplant alone.

**Table 16**   Graft Survival Rates (DWFG Censored) for TS Primary DD BD Pancreas Transplants According to Number of HLA MMs at the *A Locus* for Eras 3 and 4 Combined

| Category (N) and MMs (N) | Years posttransplant | | | | p Value (WC/LR) |
|---|---|---|---|---|---|
| | 1 yr | 3 yr | 5 yr | 7 yr | |
| *SPK (158)* | | | | | |
| 0 (30) | 97 | 88 | 88 | 88 | 0.61/0.82 |
| 1 (73) | 98 | 98 | 93 | 89 | |
| 2 (55) | 100 | 96 | 94 | 94 | |
| *PAK (260)* | | | | | |
| 0 (53) | 92 | 87 | 57 | 78 | 0.70/0.68 |
| 1 (157) | 93 | 82 | 79 | 77 | |
| 2 (50) | 90 | 86 | 79 | 74 | |
| *PTA (155)* | | | | | |
| 0 (55) | 83 | 69 | 69 | 66 | 0.72/0.77 |
| 1 (90) | 88 | 71 | 66 | 60 | |
| 2 (10) | 100 | 76 | 76 | 73 | |

*Abbreviations*: DWFG, death with functioning graft censored; TS, technically successful, DD, deceased donor; BD, bladder drainage; MM, mismatches; WC, Wilcoxin Test; LR, Log-Rank Test.

We next calculated GSRs separately according to number of MMs at either the HLA-A or -B loci or -DR loci (Tables 16–18). There were no significant differences in pancreas GSRs according to number of MMs by themselves at the A locus in any category (Table 16), but at the B locus (Table 17) GSRs differed significantly in the PAK category ($p = 0.016$ WC and 0.019 LR) and highly significantly in the PTA category ($p < 0.001$ both WC and LR): seven-year GSRs for 0, 1, and 2 HLA-B MM recipients were 80% vs 81% vs 67%, respectively, in the PAK; and 71% vs 66% vs 22%, respectively, in the PTA category (Of note, the 0 MM B locus PAK and PTA recipients still had lower GSRs than the SPK recipients regardless of the number of B locus MMs.) At the DR locus, like the A locus, there were no differences in GSRs according to number of MMs that were statistically significant, though the $p$-values approached significance in the SPK category where GSRs were progressively higher with decreasing number of MMs (Table 18).

In the analyses of incidence of RREs according to HLA MMs at the individual loci (Tables 19–21), no differences were found at the A locus in any recipient category (Table 19). At the B locus (Table 20), however, the incidence of RERs—both early and late—increased with increasing number of MMs in the SPK category. In the PTA category, the incidence of RERs was very high with 2 MMs at the B locus, approaching statistical significance especially for the late follow up ($p = 0.12$ LR). At the DR locus (Table 21), only in the SPK category was there a effect of the number of MMs on the incidence of RREs with significantly fewer, both

**Table 17**   Graft Survival Rates (DWFG Censored) for TS Primary DD BD Pancreas Transplants According to Number of HLA MMs at the *B Locus* for Eras 3 and 4 Combined

| Category (N) and MMs (N) | Years posttransplant | | | | p Value (WC/LR) |
|---|---|---|---|---|---|
| | 1 yr | 3 yr | 5 yr | 7 yr | |
| *SPK (158)* | | | | | |
| 0 (30) | 100 | 93 | 93 | 93 | 0.86/0.69 |
| 1 (73) | 99 | 97 | 91 | 91 | |
| 2 (55) | 98 | 94 | 94 | 89 | |
| *PAK (260)* | | | | | |
| 0 (53) | 91 | 85 | 85 | 80 | 0.016/0.019 |
| 1 (157) | 96 | 90 | 85 | 81 | |
| 2 (50) | 85 | 72 | 90 | 67 | |
| *PTA (155)* | | | | | |
| 0 (55) | 97 | 85 | 82 | 71 | < 0.001/0.001 |
| 1 (90) | 87 | 69 | 66 | 66 | |
| 2 (10) | 50 | 33 | 33 | 22 | |

*Abbreviations*: DWFG, death with functioning graft censored; TS, technically successful; DD, deceased donor; BD, bladder drainage; MM, mismatches; WC, Wilcoxin Test; LR, Log-Rank Test.

**Table 18** Graft Survival Rates (DWFG Censored) for TS Primary DD BD Pancreas Transplants According to Number of HLA MMs at the *A Locus* for Eras 3 and 4 Combined

| Category and MMs (N) | Years posttransplant | | | | p Value (WC/LR) |
|---|---|---|---|---|---|
| | 1 yr | 3 yr | 5 yr | 7 yr | |
| *SPK (158)* | | | | | |
| 0 (36) | 100 | 100 | 97 | 97 | 0.15/0.13 |
| 1 (80) | 99 | 97 | 94 | 92 | |
| 2 (42) | 98 | 89 | 86 | 82 | |
| *PAK (260)* | | | | | |
| 0 (41) | 83 | 77 | 77 | 73 | 0.41/0.36 |
| 1 (146) | 94 | 84 | 79 | 73 | |
| 2 (73) | 94 | 87 | 85 | 85 | |
| *PTA (155)* | | | | | |
| 0 (31) | 86 | 72 | 72 | 72 | 0.80/0.57 |
| 1 (94) | 86 | 71 | 70 | 64 | |
| 2 (30) | 90 | 69 | 60 | 52 | |

*Abbreviations*: DWFG, death with functioning graft censored; TS, technically successful; DD, deceased donor; BD, bladder drainage; MM, mismatches; WC, Wilcoxin Test; LR, Log-Rank Test.

**Table 19** Reversible Rejection Episode Rates for TS Primary DD BD Pancreas Transplants According to Number of HLA MMs at the *A Locus* for Eras 3 and 4 Combined

| Category and MMs (N) | Months and years posttransplant | | | | | | p Value (WC/LR) |
|---|---|---|---|---|---|---|---|
| | 6 mo | 1 yr | 2 yr | 3 yr | 5 yr | 7 yr | |
| *SPK (155)* | | | | | | | |
| 0 (30) | 24 | 33 | 33 | 33 | 42 | 42 | 0.38/0.46 |
| 1 (73) | 31 | 38 | 43 | 43 | 44 | 47 | |
| 2 (85) | 22 | 26 | 28 | 28 | 36 | 36 | |
| *PAK (260)* | | | | | | | |
| 0 (53) | 24 | 38 | 42 | 45 | 47 | 63 | 0.33/0.39 |
| 1 (157) | 28 | 36 | 40 | 44 | 46 | 52 | |
| 2 (50) | 22 | 26 | 28 | 28 | 36 | 36 | |
| *PTA (155)* | | | | | | | |
| 0 (55) | 36 | 44 | 48 | 52 | 55 | 59 | 0.98/0.98 |
| 1 (90) | 32 | 50 | 52 | 56 | 59 | 59 | |
| 2 (10) | 30 | 30 | 50 | 50 | 60 | 60 | |

*Abbreviations*: DWFG, death with functioning graft censored; TS, technically successful; DD, deceased donor; BD, bladder drainage; MM, mismatches; WC, Wilcoxin Test; LR, Log-Rank Test.

**Table 20** Reversible Rejection Episode Rates for TS Primary DD BD Pancreas Transplants According to Number of HLA MMs at the *B Locus* for Eras 3 and 4 Combined

| Category and MMs (N) | Months and years posttransplant | | | | | | p Value (WC/LR) |
|---|---|---|---|---|---|---|---|
| | 6 mo | 1 yr | 2 yr | 3 yr | 5 yr | 7 yr | |
| *SPK (158)* | | | | | | | |
| 0 (19) | 22 | 22 | 22 | 22 | 30 | 30 | 0.08/0.04 |
| 1 (81) | 22 | 28 | 32 | 32 | 36 | 36 | |
| 2 (58) | 36 | 42 | 46 | 46 | 51 | 54 | |
| *PAK (260)* | | | | | | | |
| 0 (34) | 32 | 44 | 44 | 50 | 54 | 54 | 0.046/0.165 |
| 1 (144) | 25 | 33 | 37 | 40 | 43 | 54 | |
| 2 (82) | 32 | 45 | 51 | 56 | 56 | 56 | |
| *PTA (155)* | | | | | | | |
| 0 (43) | 36 | 43 | 49 | 51 | 54 | 40 | 0.22/0.12 |
| 1 (100) | 29 | 44 | 48 | 53 | 55 | 55 | |
| 2 (12) | 58 | 75 | 75 | 75 | 83 | 83 | |

*Abbreviations*: DWFG, death with functioning graft censored; TS, technically successful; DD, deceased donor; BD, bladder drainage; MM, mismatches; WC, Wilcoxin Test; LR, Log-Rank Test.

**Table 21** Reversible Rejection Episode Rates for TS Primary DD BD Pancreas Transplants According to Number of HLA MMs at the *DR Locus* for Eras 3 and 4 Combined

| Category and MMs (N) | Months and years posttransplant | | | | | | *p* Value (WC/LR) |
|---|---|---|---|---|---|---|---|
| | 6 mo | 1 yr | 2 yr | 3 yr | 5 yr | 7 yr | |
| *SPK (158)* | | | | | | | |
| 0 (36) | 15 | 18 | 22 | 22 | 29 | 29 | 0.0003/0.00022 |
| 1 (80) | 21 | 29 | 33 | 33 | 36 | 36 | |
| 2 (42) | 49 | 51 | 54 | 54 | 57 | 64 | |
| *PAK (260)* | | | | | | | |
| 0 (41) | 42 | 51 | 51 | 54 | 59 | 59 | 0.30/0.40 |
| 1 (146) | 26 | 36 | 41 | 44 | 47 | 55 | |
| 2 (73) | 24 | 34 | 40 | 46 | 46 | 58 | |
| *PTA (155)* | | | | | | | |
| 0 (31) | 35 | 52 | 52 | 59 | 59 | 59 | 0.46/0.86 |
| 1 (94) | 36 | 46 | 50 | 54 | 56 | 56 | |
| 2 (30) | 21 | 41 | 48 | 52 | 62 | 71 | |

*Abbreviations*: DWFG, death with functioning graft censored; TS, technically successful; DD, deceased donor; BD, bladder drainage; MM, mismatches; WC, Wilcoxin Test; LR, Log-Rank Test.

early and late [$p < 0.0003$ both WC and LR as the number of MMs decreased (incidence more than doubled at all time points for 2 vs 0 DR MMs)].

Thus, as far as HLA MMs are concerned, we can show in impact of the B locus on GSRs in solitary (PAK, PTA) pancreas transplant recipients, of both the B and DR loci on RERs in the SPK category.

We also did an analysis of GSRs and RRE rates according to HLA matching (as opposed to mismatching) at the Class II (A and B) loci combined, comparing those matched for no antigens with those matched for at least one antigen (Tables 22,23). In the SPK category, there were no differences in GSRs or RRE rates for 0 vs >1 antigen matched recipients (Table 22). However, in the PAK and PTA categories, GSR rates were significantly higher both early and late ($p < 0.05$ both WC and LR), in recipients who were matched for at least one antigen versus those who were not matched at all. The differences in RRE rates for matched vs unmatched solitary pancreas recipients did not reach statistical significance (Table 23), though it was very close, at least in the PAK recipients early on ($p = 0.06$ WC and 0.11 LR).

Previous Cox regression analyses have shown that minimizing MMs at the HLA B locus had a significant impact on pancreas graft survival, especially for PTAs (8). Currently, for solitary pancreas transplants, HLA matching does not carry a penalty in terms of waiting time because the ratio of number of pancreas transplant candidates on the waiting list to the number of DDs with suitable pancreases is low, so with a measurable effect there is no good reason not to apply a matching strategy.

**Table 22** Graft Survival Rates (DWFG Censored) for TS Primary DD BD Pancreas Transplants According to Number of HLA Matches (0 vs. ≥1) at the *A,B Loci* for Eras 3 and 4 Combined

| Category and matches (N) | Years posttransplant | | | | *p* Value (WC/LR) |
|---|---|---|---|---|---|
| | 1 yr | 3 yr | 5 yr | 7 yr | |
| *SPK (158)* | | | | | |
| 0 (89) | 99 | 95 | 94 | 90 | 0.47/0.84 |
| ≥1 (69) | 99 | 97 | 91 | 91 | |
| *PAK (260)* | | | | | |
| 0 (110) | 88 | 79 | 74 | 70 | 0.048/0.034 |
| ≥1 (150) | 94 | 88 | 85 | 81 | |
| *PTA (155)* | | | | | |
| 0 (21) | 71 | 56 | 56 | 47 | 0.028/0.039 |
| ≥1 (134) | 90 | 73 | 70 | 66 | |

*Abbreviations*: DWFG, death with functioning graft censored; TS, technically successful; DD, deceased donor; BD, bladder drainage; WC, Wilcoxin Test; LR, Log-Rank Test.

**Table 23** Reversible Rejection Episode Rates for TS Primary DD BD Pancreas Transplants According to Number of HLA Matches (0 vs. ≥1) at the *A,B Loci* for Eras 3 and 4 Combined

| Category and matches (N) | Months and years posttransplant | | | | | | p Value (WC/LR) |
|---|---|---|---|---|---|---|---|
| | 6 mo | 1 yr | 2 yr | 3 yr | 5 yr | 7 yr | |
| *SPK (158)* | | | | | | | |
| 0 (89) | 29 | 34 | 36 | 36 | 42 | 43 | 0.52/0.51 |
| ≥1 (69) | 24 | 31 | 37 | 37 | 40 | 40 | |
| *PAK (260)* | | | | | | | |
| 0 (110) | 32 | 43 | 49 | 54 | 54 | 60 | 0.06/0.11 |
| ≥1 (150) | 25 | 34 | 38 | 41 | 44 | 53 | |
| *PTA (155)* | | | | | | | |
| 0 (21) | 43 | 52 | 62 | 62 | 75 | 75 | 0.28/0.18 |
| ≥1 (134) | 31 | 46 | 48 | 53 | 55 | 57 | |

*Abbreviations*: DWFG, death with functioning graft censored; TS, technically successful; DD, deceased donor; BD, bladder drainage; MM, mismatches; WC, Wilcoxin Test; LR, Log-Rank Test.

## Kidney Transplant Outcomes for PAK and KAP Recipients

Virtually all uremic diabetic patients referred to our program since Era 1 were offered the option of an LD or DD KTA, with the possibility of a subsequent PAK transplant, or an SPK transplant (in Era 2 from a DD) donor, in Eras 3 to 5 from either an LD or DD donor). We strongly encourage LD kidney transplants (177), and a high proportion of our uremic diabetic pancreas transplant candidates underwent an LD KTA. For those without an LD, a DD SPK transplant was possible only in those with adequate financial coverage: This proportion increased from Era 2 to Era 3 and 4. The proportion of LD and DD KTA recipients who went on to get a PAK transplant also depended on their financial coverage; again, this proportion increased from era to era. However, a substantial number of LD and DD KTA recipients were not able to, or chose not to, have a subsequent pancreas transplant. Thus, we are able to compare both patient and kidney GSRs both in Era 2 and Era 3,and 4 combined for DD SPK versus LD or DD KTA recipients as well as for DD PAK (with the previous kidney from either an LD or DD donor) versus LD or DD KTA recipients.

Our PTA recipients were nonuremic at the time of transplant, but some with moderate nephropathy pretransplant developed progressive renal insufficiency after the pancreas transplant and went on to have a kidney after pancreas (KAP) transplant (178). The outcome in this group is also described.

### *Living Donor and Deceased Donor Kidney Graft Survival Rates in Pancreas After Kidney Recipients*

Kidney GSRs in PAK recipients can be calculated from the time of the kidney or the time of the pancreas transplant. All PAK recipients have a functioning kidney graft at the time of the pancreas transplant, so it is a select group of KTA recipients who have a PAK transplant. In previous publications we compared kidney GSRs for PAK vs KTA recipients from the time of the kidney transplant and found those in PAK recipients to be significantly higher (179).

Our PAK kidney GSRs from the time of the pancreas transplant in all cases (primary and retransplant, DD and LD pancreas transplants) in each era are shown in Table 24A and for primary DD PAK cases only in Table 24B. The differences by era are statistically significant $p < 0.035$ for both WC and LR), but in each of Eras 2 to 5 the primary DD PAK one-year post–pancreas transplant kidney allograft GSRs were >94%. For Eras 1 to 4, where long-term GSRs can be calculated, at seven years postpancreas transplant in primary DD PAK recipients, >50% of the previously placed renal allografts were still functioning, including 75% in Era 4.

The excellent kidney GSRs following a PAK occurred, whether the kidney came from a LD or DD, as shown in an analysis of primary DD PAK cases in Eras 3 and 4 combined (Table 25). At one-year post–pancreas transplant, 95% of LD and 97% of DD kidney were functioning in the PAK recipients, at seven years at least two-thirds of either LD or DD kidneys were still functioning, and at 10 years half were functioning. The fact that there was no difference in LD vs DD kidney GSRs after a PAK transplant may reflect that to get a PAK transplant, the recipient has to have stable renal allograft function and once stability is achieved, it is independent of the original source of the kidney.

**Table 24** Kidney Graft Survival Rates (%) from the Time of the Pancreas Transplant in Recipients of Deceased Donor PAK Allografts for All (A) or Primary (B) Cases by Era

| | Years posttransplant | | | | | | | |
|---|---|---|---|---|---|---|---|---|
| **ERA (N)** | **1** | **2** | **3** | **5** | **7** | **10** | **15** | **20** |
| *(A) All cases (672)* | | | | | | | | |
| 1 (65) | 88 | 81 | 78 | 59 | 48 | 30 | 27 | 21 |
| 2 (107) | 92 | 84 | 81 | 69 | 58 | 47 | 26 | 24 |
| 3 (104) | 94 | 89 | 83 | 70 | 61 | 49 | – | – |
| 4 (287) | 94 | 89 | 85 | 73 | 69 | – | – | – |
| 5 (109) | 93 | 79 | 76 | – | – | – | – | – |
| $p = 0.030/0.035$ | | | | | | | | |
| *(B) Primary PAK (510)* | | | | | | | | |
| 1 (53) | 87 | 81 | 77 | 56 | 50 | 29 | 75 | 21 |
| 2 (73) | 97 | 90 | 89 | 79 | 64 | 53 | 28 | 28 |
| 3 (86) | 94 | 91 | 83 | 72 | 60 | 45 | – | – |
| 4 (216) | 96 | 91 | 88 | 79 | 75 | – | – | – |
| 5 (82) | 94 | 81 | 78 | – | – | – | – | – |
| $p = 0.003/0.012$ | | | | | | | | |

*Note*: $p =$ Wilcoxin/Log-Rank Tests.

### Kidney After Pancreas Transplants in Pancreas Transplant Alone Recipients

In the entire cohort of primary PTA recipients in all eras ($n = 398$), 62 went on to have at least one subsequent kidney transplant (of which 6 had subsequent kidney retransplants). Of the primary KAP transplants, 29 were from LDs (with no other concomitant transplant) and 33 were from DDs; of the latter (DD KAP) 14 were done simultaneously with a pancreas (re-)transplant from the SD DD S (re-P) K, and one was done simultaneously with a heart transplant (SHK) from the SD, while 17 had a simple DD KAP with no concomitant transplants. The cumulative incidence of KAP after primary PTAs in the entire series (Eras 1–5 combined) was 3% by one year and 18% by seven years, and is shown for each era in Table 26. The incidence of KAP transplants, both early ($p = 0.12$) and late ($p = 0.11$) after a PTA, has varied only slightly in successive Eras 1 to 5 (Table 26), at three years 16%, 9%, 6%, 5%, and 2%; at seven years (Eras 1–4), 31%, 15%, 18%, and 16%, respectively.

The KAP GSRs in each Era 1 to 5, and for all five eras combined, whether done as a solitary kidney or as part of an SPK (pancreas retransplant) case, is shown in Tables 27 and 28. The differences in KAP GSRs by era are not significant (Table 27). For the 62 primary KAP transplants (including those done as a SPK transplant) done in all five eras combined, the one-year kidney GSR was 85% and 61% in the five-year, less in those done as a DD SPK ($n = 14$, 50% of kidneys functioning at one-year and $-21\%$ at five years) vs those done as a solitary kidney, ($n = 46$, 98% functioning at one year, 76% at five years $p < 0.001$). The one DD SHK done as a KAP died 10 months later with both the kidney and the pancreas (seven years) functioning.

For the nephropathic PTA recipients whose pancreas graft is functioning, the advantage of an LD over a DD KAP is mainly one of timing (Table 28). The KAP GSR was 100% in LD and 94% in DD recipients of a solitary kidney only, but at five years the GSR was 76% in both groups. What is clear is that in PTA recipients whose pancreas has failed, an S (re-P) K has a lower kidney graft GSR than the solitary kidney KAP recipients, whether LD or DD ($p < 0.001$ WC and LR).

**Table 25** Kidney Graft Survival Rates from Time of Pancreas Transplant in Recipients of Primary Deceased Donor PAK Allografts According to the Source of the Kidney (LD or DD) in Eras 3 and 4 Combined

| Donor source (302) | 1 | 2 | 3 | 5 | 7 | 10 | 15 | 20 |
|---|---|---|---|---|---|---|---|---|
| LD (238) | 95 | 91 | 86 | 77 | 69 | 52 | ? | ? |
| DD (64) | 97 | 92 | 87 | 73 | 66 | 49 | – | – |
| $p = 0.84/0.61$ | | | | | | | | |

*Note*: $p =$ Wilcoxin/Log-Rank Tests.
*Abbreviations*: LD, living donor; DD, deceased donor.

**Table 26** Cumulative Incidence of Primary Kidney Transplants (KAP) in Recipients Originally Given a Pancreas Transplant Alone (PTA): Years Post-PTA (Percent Given Kidney Transplant)

| Era (N) | 1 yr | 2 yr | 3 yr | 5 yr | 7 yr | 10 yr |
|---|---|---|---|---|---|---|
| 1 (68) | 5 | 10 | 16 | 18 | 31 | 35 |
| 2 (87) | 5 | 7 | 9 | 13 | 15 | 23 |
| 3 (41) | 0 | 0 | 6 | 15 | 18 | 38 |
| 4 (142) | 1 | 3 | 5 | 7 | 16 | – |
| 5 (60) | 2 | 2 | 2 | – | – | – |
| Total (398) | 3 | 5 | 7 | 13 | 18 | 30 |
| $p = 0.12/0.11$ | | | | | | |

*Note*: $p =$ Wilcoxin/Log-Rank Tests for comparison of eras.

With these results, our approach for PTA recipients with declining renal function is to add a kidney transplant early, rather than risk pancreas graft rejection by lowering the dose of CI to suboptimal immunosuppression levels in an attempt to lessen nephrotoxicity and put the patient in need of both organs.

## Pancreas Retransplants

In our series (Eras 1 to 5) of pancreas transplants from 1978 to 2005 ($n = 1,835$), 321 (17%) were retransplants (14% second transplants, 2.5% third, 0.5% fourth); all but 3 were from DD donors. The category of the second pancreas transplant according to the category of the first transplant is shown in Table 29. Of the 265 second pancreas transplants [39 SPK (15%), 137 PAK (52%), and 89 PTA (34%)], the primary was an SPK in 86 (32%), the second a SPK in 23 (27%) and a PAK in 63 (73%); a PAK in 81 (31%) [the second an SPK in 8 (10%), and a PAK in 73 (90%); and a PTA in 98 (37%) [the second an SPK in 8 (8%), a PAK in 1 (1%), and a PTA in 89 (91%)]. Of the 39 SPK second transplants, the first was an SPK in 23 (59%), a PAK in 8 (21%), and a PTA in 8 (21%); of the 137 PAK second transpants, the first was an SPK in 63 (46%), a PAK in 73 (53%), and a PTA in 1 (1%); of the 89 PTA second transplants, all the first, of course, were PTAs (100%). Of the second pancreas transplants done at the University of Minnesota, 31 (12%) had their first transplant elsewhere, as shown by category and era in Table 30.

Analyses of DD retransplant outcomes were done by era and recipient category, one analysis for second transplants only (Table 31) and one for all retransplants (second, third, and fourth combined, Table 32). As for primary pancreas transplants, the PAK and PTA retransplant GSRs significantly improved in successive eras, while for SPK retranspants, the GSRs were relatively high to begin with and thus the differences between eras were not significant.

### Simultaneous Pancreas Kidney Retransplants

In Eras 2 to 5 combined, we did 53 DD SPK retransplants (38 seconds), with no significant differences in pancreas GSRs between eras (Tables 31,32). The overall (Eras 2–5 combined) one-year pancreas GSR was 62% for all SPK retransplants together and 66% for second SPK transplants only, at three years 45% for all and 52% for second transplants only.

**Table 27** KAP kidney Graft Survival Rates (GSRs) by Era Years Post-Kidney Transplant (Percent Functioning)

| Era (N) | 1 yr | 2 yr | 3 yr | 5 yr | 7 yr | 10 yr |
|---|---|---|---|---|---|---|
| 1 (27) | 77 | 59 | 54 | 54 | 54 | 49 |
| 2 (18) | 83 | 78 | 72 | 60 | 33 | 27 |
| 3 (10) | 90 | 80 | 80 | 40 | – | – |
| 4 (11) | 100 | 83 | 83 | 83 | – | – |
| 5 (1) | 100 | 100 | – | – | – | – |
| All eras (62) | 85 | 73 | 69 | 61 | 49 | 43 |
| $p = 0.58/0.70$ | | | | | | |

*Note*: $p =$ Wilcoxin/Log-Rank Tests comparing GSRs by eras.
*Abbreviations*: KAP, Kidney after pancreas (PTA) transplant; PTA, pancreas transplant alone.

**Table 28** KAP Graft Survival Rates[a]

| Donor category | 1 yr | 2 yr | 3 yr | 5 yr | 7 yr |
|---|---|---|---|---|---|
| All eras (62) | 85 | 73 | 69 | 49 | 43 |
| LD (29) | 100 | 88 | 82 | 69 | 60 |
| DD Kd (17) | 94 | 82 | 76 | 57 | 47 |
| DD S (Re-P) K (14) | 50 | 36 | 36 | 14 | 14 |
| p = 0.007/0.002 | | | | | |

[a]All eras combined by donor category.

### Pancreas After Kidney Retransplants

In Eras 1 to 5 combined, we did 163 DD PAK retransplants (135 seconds). DD PAK retransplant GSRs differed significantly by era ($p = 0.001$ WC and LR), with the improvement over time greatest from Eras 1 to 2 to 3 (Tables 31,32). For Eras 3 to 5 combined, the one-year GSR for DD PAK retransplants with second, third, and fourth included ($n = 117$) was 67% and for second transplants only ($n = 99$) was 65%, at three years 51% for all, and 50% for second transplants only.

### Pancreas Transplant Alone Retransplants

In Eras 1 to 5 combined, we did 99 DD PTA retransplants (86 second transplants). DD PTA retransplant GSRs also differed significantly by era ($p \leq 0.08$ WC, $\leq 0.05$ LR), with the improvement over time greatest from Eras 1 to 3 to 4 to 5 (Tables 31,32). For Eras 4 and 5 combined, the one-year GSR for DD PAK retransplants with 2nd, 3rd, and 4th included ($n = 49$) was 67% and for second transplants only ($n = 43$) was 66%, and at three years 50% for all and 48% for second transplants only.

### Living Donor Pancreas Transplants

Nearly all of the LD solitary (PAK and PTA) pancreas transplants were done in Era 1 and 2 (Table 3). All but two of the LD SPK transplants ($n = 38$) were done in Eras 3 to 5 combined (Table 3). The results in the early eras have been illustrated in detail in a previous publication (8). The relation of the living segmental pancreas donor to the recipients is shown in Table 9.

In Era 1, we primarily used LDs because the rejection rate for solitary DD pancreas transplants was very high with the immunosuppressive regimens we then used. The TF rate was high for both DD and LD PAK transplants in this era (23% and 33%, respectively), so the main gain of using LDs was immunologic, as reflected by the GSRs for TS PAK transplants. For TS PAK transplants from LD ($n = 10$) versus DD ($n = 37$) donors, the pancreas GSRs were 90% versus 22% at one year ($p = 0.004$) and 70% versus 9% at five years ($p = 0.002$).

Also in Era 1, the improvement in pancreas GSRs with LDs was much higher for PAK than for PTA transplants. It may be that the chronic immunosuppression, which the PAK recipients were already on, contributed to this difference, but it should also be noted that most (84% of TS cases) of the LD PAK recipients had previously received a kidney from the SD and, thus, had been selected as having an immunologically favorable state with their particular donor. That situation was not the case with DD PAK transplants, where the pancreas always came from a different donor than the kidney, or with PTA transplants, where donor selection based on a previously favorable outcome was not possible.

**Table 29** Second Pancreas Transplants Eras 1 to 5 According to Category of Original Transplant

| Second transplant category | First transplant category | | |
|---|---|---|---|
| | SPK | PAK | PTA |
| SPK (39) | 23 (59%) | 8 (21%) | 8 (21%) |
| [15%] | [27%] | [10%] | [15%] |
| PAK (137) | 63 (46%) | 73 (53%) | 1 (1%) |
| [52%] | [73%] | [90%] | [1%] |
| PTA (89) | 0 (0%) | 0 (0%) | 89 (100%) |
| [34%] | [0%] | [0%] | [91%] |
| Total (265) | 86 (32%) | 81 (31%) | 98 (37%) |

**Table 30**  Pancreas Retransplants by Site of First Transplant

| Type/Era | UMMC | Other |
|---|---|---|
| *SPK (39)* | 28 | 11 (28%) |
| 2 (11) | 8 | 3 (27%) |
| 3 (9) | 5 | 4 (44%) |
| 4 (13) | 12 | 1 (8%) |
| 5 (6) | 3 | 3 (50%) |
| *PAK (137)* | 119 | 18 (13%) |
| 1 (9) | 9 | 0 (0%) |
| 2 (28) | 27 | 1 (4%) |
| 3 (16) | 12 | 4 (25%) |
| 4 (62) | 54 | 8 (13%) |
| 5 (22) | 17 | 5 (23%) |
| *PTA (89)* | 87 | 2 (2%) |
| 1 (13) | 13 | 0 (0%) |
| 2 (28) | 27 | 1 (4%) |
| 3 (5) | 5 | 0 (0%) |
| 4 (21) | 21 | 0 (0%) |
| 5 (22) | 21 | 1 (5%) |
| *Total (265)* | 234 | 31 (12%) |
| 1 (22) | 22 | 0 (0%) |
| 2 (67) | 62 | 5 (7%) |
| 3 (30) | 22 | 8 (3%) |
| 4 (96) | 87 | 9 (9%) |
| 5 (50) | 41 | 9 (18%) |

## Living Donor Pancreas After Kidney

Of 10 TS LD PAK recipients in Era 1, 9 had the SD for the kidney and pancreas (sequential operations). The only early failure (<one year) was part of the identical twin series [the only one with a kidney transplant (66)]; the recipient was not immunosuppressed for either organ (inconsequential for the kidney), and the pancreas graft developed recurrent autoimmune isletitis (67). The immunological privilege in this case did not extend to the beta cells. The other nine TS LD PAK grafts in Era 1 (including the one from a different donor, who was HLA ident-

**Table 31**  Graft Survival Rates for Deceased Donor Second Pancreas Transplants by Recipient Category and Era Years Posttransplant (Percent Functioning)

| Era (*N*) | 1 | 3 | 5 | 10 |
|---|---|---|---|---|
| *SPK (38)* | | | | |
| 1 (0) | — | — | — | — |
| 2 (11) | 73 | 45 | 45 | 27 |
| 3 (8) | 63 | 38 | 38 | 25 |
| 4 (13) | 54 | 54 | 11 | — |
| 5 (6) | 80 | 80 | — | — |
| *p* = 0.54/0.36 | | | | |
| *PAK (135)* | | | | |
| 1 (8) | 12 | 12 | 12 | 12 |
| 2 (28) | 32 | 18 | 11 | 7 |
| 3 (16) | 81 | 62 | 56 | 50 |
| 4 (61) | 61 | 47 | 44 | — |
| 5 (22) | 66 | 44 | — | — |
| *p* = < 0.001 | | | | |
| *PTA (86)* | | | | |
| 1 (11) | 36 | 9 | 9 | 0 |
| 2 (27) | 48 | 37 | 30 | 15 |
| 3 (5) | 40 | 40 | 20 | 20 |
| 4 (21) | 71 | 52 | 52 | — |
| 5 (22) | 61 | 45 | — | — |
| *p*=0.08/0.05 | | | | |

*Note*: *p* values = Wilcoxin/Log-Rank Tests.

**Table 32** Graft Survival Rates for All Deceased Donor Pancreas Re-Transplants (2nd, 3rd, and 4th Combined) by Recipient Category and Era Year Posttransplant (Percent Functioning)

| Era (N) | 1 | 3 | 5 | 10 |
|---|---|---|---|---|
| SPK (53) | | | | |
| 1 (0) | – | – | – | – |
| 2 (19) | 58 | 37 | 37 | 26 |
| 3 (8) | 63 | 38 | 38 | 25 |
| 4 (19) | 63 | 47 | 18 | – |
| 5 (67) | 69 | 69 | – | – |
| $p = 0.8/0.8$ | | | | |
| PAK (163) | | | | |
| 1 (11) | 27 | 27 | 18 | 9 |
| 2 (35) | 29 | 14 | 9 | 6 |
| 3 (18) | 83 | 61 | 56 | 44 |
| 4 (71) | 62 | 51 | 44 | – |
| 5 (28) | 68 | 42 | – | – |
| $p = <0.001$ | | | | |
| PTA (99) | | | | |
| 1 (13) | 38 | 15 | 8 | 0 |
| 2 (31) | 52 | 35 | 29 | 16 |
| 3 (6) | 50 | 50 | 33 | 17 |
| 4 (23) | 74 | 52 | 52 | – |
| 5 (26) | 61 | 49 | – | – |
| $p = 0.08/0.04$ | | | | |

Note: p values = Wilcoxin/Log-Rank Tests

ical with both the kidney donor and the recipient) all have functioned for more than one year, the longest for >24 years (a DI segmental graft done in 1980, a year after a kidney transplant from the SD) before finally failing, presumably from duct-injected graft sclerosis over time, though possibly from recurrence of disease, certainly not from rejection because the kidney from the SD continues to function (serum creatinine <1 mg/dL in 2006 at >27 years post-transplant).

In Era 2, the rejection rate of TS CAD PAK transplants ($n = 46$) was much lower than in Era 1; thus the advantage of a TS LD PAK ($n = 7$) was less in Era 2, at least early on (functional survival rates for LD versus CAD grafts were 71% versus 82% at 1 year; and 71% versus 53% at 10 years ($p = $ NS). Of the seven TS LD PAK transplants in Era 2, the only two graft losses occurred when the pancreas came from a different donor than the kidney. In the other five, the kidney and pancreas grafts came from the SD in sequential operations, and all are functioning between 11 and 18 years.

The LD PAK transplant outcomes in Era 1 and 2 demonstrate the potential for lifelong function of a pancreas graft. Of the 30 primary LD PAK transplants done in the combined eras, patient survival rates at 1, 5, and 10 years were 100%, 91%, and 75%. With TFs included in the calculations and DWFG counted as a graft failure, 14 LD PTA grafts (47%) were functioning at 1 year, 11 (37%) and 7 (23%) at 10 years. Of the two LD PAK transplants done in Eras 3 to 5, both are currently functioning, the longest for nearly >nine years. The RLR for LD PAK transplants has been low, particularly when from the SD at the kidney. However, because of the immunologically privileged nature of LD PAK transplants, the immunologic advantage, or lack thereof, of a LD pancreas transplant over a DD transplant is more easily discerned in the PTA category.

### Living Donor Pancreas Transplant Alone

In Era 1, the TF rates for primary LD PTA ($n = 33$) and DD PTA ($n = 36$) were both 33%. Our hope that the rejection rate would be less for TS LD PTA ($n = 22$) than for TS CAD PTA ($n = 24$) grafts turned out not to be the case for Era 1: primary GSRs at 1 year were 53% versus 52%; at 10 years, 24% versus 22% ($p = $ NS).

Also in Era 1, we were making the transition from Aza-Pred to Csa-Pred for maintenance immunosuppression. It was not until Era 2, when we went to Csa-Aza-Pred (triple therapy) for maintenance, which we saw an improvement in TS PTA GSRs, but with LD only. In Era 2,

GSRs for TS LD PTA ($n = 11$) versus TS CAD PTA ($n = 60$) were 82% versus 60% at 1 year ($p = 0.05$) and 64% versus 23% at 10 years ($p = 0.04$), respectively.

Of the 47 primary LD PTA cases in Eras 1 and 2 combined, patient survival rates at 1, 5, and 10 years were 91%, 91%, and 82%, respectively. With TFs included in the calculations, DWFG counted as a graft failure, 21 LD PTA grafts (45%) were functioning at 1 year, 14 (30%) at 5 years, and 12 (26%) at 10 years. Of the four LD PAK transplants done in Eras 3 to 5, all functioned >one year and three are currently functioning for >four years.

With triple therapy (Csa-Aza-Pred) in Era 2, LDs definitely gave an advantage for PTA. (Introduction of triple therapy had much more of an impact on DD PAK than on DD PTA results.) It was not until Era 3 (FK/MMF) that DD PTA one-year GSRs (40) equaled those of LD PTA in Era 2.

Thus, in Era 3 we placed less emphasis on LDs for PTA transplants because DD pancreas grafts were readily available in the United States for the small number of PTA candidates listed, and the success rate with DD grafts had improved (91).

The potential for PTA grafts to function for a lifetime was shown in the Era 1 series. Eight of the grafts (five from LDs and three from DD donors) are currently functioning 20 to 24 years posttransplant.

### Living Donor Simultaneous Pancreas Kidney

We initiated LD SPK transplants in March 1994, just before Era 3 began (92). Of the 38 donors, 6 were HLA identical siblings, 25 were HLA-mismatched relatives, and 7 were unrelated (Table 9). Two donors were ABO-blood type-incompatible and antibody reduction was successfully accomplished with plasmapherisis (148) and both grafts are currently functioning at >six years. In the overall series of 38 LD SPK transplants, the one-, five-, and one-year patient survival rates are 100%, 100%, and 84%, respectively; the segmental pancreas GSRs (TFs included, DWFG counted as a graft failure) are 84%, 70%, and 60%, respectively; and the kidney GSRs are 100%, 86%, and 67%, respectively.

We used DI in four LD SPK transplants, the first two SPK segmental pancreas grafts (one still functioning at >12 years; one failed at >10 years), and as well as in two later cases (one pancreas failed at 4 months, the kidney is still functioning at >10 years; in the other both grafts are functioning at >one year).We used ED in two cases (both organs are functioning at >two and >seven years) and BD in the other 32.

A comparison of outcomes in Eras 3 to 5 combined was made for primary LD SPK ($n = 36$) versus primary DD SPK ($n = 324$) transplants (Table 33). The patient survival rates were significantly higher ($p = 0.01$ WC and 0.03 LR) in the LD vs DD cases, at one, three, and seven years post-transplant, 100%, 100%, and 95% in LD versus 90%, 86%, and 79% in DD recipients. Pancreas GSRs were not significantly different between the LD and DD SPK recipients, at one, three, and seven years posttransplant, 86%, 78%, and 67% in the LD, and 78%, 74%, and 62% in the DD cases. Kidney GSRs were marginally significantly higher ($p = 0,09$ WC, 0.19 LR) in LD vs DD SPK recipients, at one, three, and seven years posttransplant, 100%, 91%, and 79% in the LD versus 87%, 86%, and 67% in the DD cases.

### Quality of Life Study

In Eras 2, 3, and 4 combined, 316 SPK, 204 PAK, and 98 PTA recipients enrolled in a prospective study of QOL changes after pancreas transplantation (8). For QOL assessment, we used

**Table 33**   Primary SPK Living Donor (LD) vs. Deceased Donor (DD) Outcomes for Eras 3–5 Combined

| Years posttransplant | Patient survival | | Pancreas | | Kidney GSR | |
|---|---|---|---|---|---|---|
| | LD | DD | LD | DD | LD | DD |
| 1 | 100% | 90% | 86% | 78% | 100% | 87% |
| 3 | 100% | 86% | 78% | 74% | 91% | 86% |
| 5 | 100% | 85% | 74% | 69% | 86% | 73% |
| 7 | 95% | 79% | 67% | 62% | 79% | 67% |
| 10 | 79% | 72% | 67% | 55% | 65% | 57% |
| | $p = 0.01/0.03$ | | $p = 0.03/0.41$ | | $p = 0.09/0.19$ | |

*Note*: $p$ = Wilcoxin/Log-Rank tests

**Table 34**  Pretransplant Baseline Quality of Life (QOL) Scores in Eras 2 to 4[a]

| Category (N) | Q1 | Median | Q2 |
|---|---|---|---|
| SPK (316) | 8.4 | 11.3 | 14.6 |
| PAK (204) | 11.7 | 13.3 | 15.9 |
| PTA (98) | 8.1 | 10.9 | 13.4 |

[a]Pancreas Transplant Recipient Study patients (range of middle two quartiles).

four dimensions of the Karnofsky Index: status of health, management of life, life satisfaction, and health satisfaction. Each recipient's response was recorded on a 1 (low) to 5 (high) scale for each parameter. A total score was calculated from the sum of the four parameters (maximum score possible, 20). The impact of a successful or failed transplant was assessed by the changes in scores from baseline in annual follow-up evaluations.

The baseline (prepancreas transplant) median total scores (Eras 2–4 combined) were significantly higher ($p < 0.0001$) in the PAK than in the SPK and PTA candidates. The ranges of baseline scores for the two midquarters in each recipient category are given in Table 34. Interestingly, pretransplant (baseline) QOL scores became successively higher in Era 2 versus 3 versus 4. The mean baseline scores in these eras were $9.5 \pm 2.6$ ($n = 109$), $12.3 \pm 3.9$ ($n = 131$), and $13.0 \pm 3.7$ ($n = 62$) for SPK ($p = 0.0001$); $10.9 \pm 2.6$ ($n = 32$), $13.9 \pm 3.3$ ($n = 82$), and $15.2 \pm 2.8$ ($n = 46$) for PAK ($p = 0.0001$); and $9.9 \pm 2.9$ ($n = 26$), $10.3 \pm 3.6$ ($n = 30$), and $12.7 \pm 3.3$ ($n = 24$) for PTA ($p = 0.009$) candidates. Possibly diabetic patients are coming to pancreas transplantation in better health condition than in the past.

It is not the absolute QOL score that is telling, but rather the change (delta) in score from the pretransplant baseline to the posttransplant evaluation that is important. The total score deltas for each recipient category according to graft function at one year are shown in Tables 35,36.

### Simultaneous Pancreas Kidney

SPK recipients were divided into four groups by graft status: (i) both grafts had sustained function ($n = 130$); (ii) the pancreas had sustained function, but the kidney graft failed ($n = 5$); (iii) the kidney graft had sustained function, but the pancreas graft failed ($n = 24$); or (iv) both grafts failed ($n = 2$).

At one-year posttransplant, the mean increase from baseline in total QOL scores was highly significant ($p = 0.0001$) in the SPK recipients with both grafts functioning but not in those with a functioning pancreas but a failed kidney (Table 35). In those with a functioning kidney but a failed pancreas graft, there was virtually no change from baseline. Only two recipients in whom both grafts failed completed the follow-up evaluation at one year: the total score did not change in one; it was lower, compared with pretransplant baseline in the other. The results in the SPK recipients in whom only one graft failed suggest that achieving insulin independence improves QOL more than becoming dialysis free.

### Pancreas After Kidney

At one year, the mean total QOL score increased significantly ($p = 0.0001$) from baseline in PAK recipients with sustained graft function ($n = 55$)(but not in those with failed grafts ($n = 16$)) (Table 36).

### Pancreas Transplant Alone

At one year, the mean total QOL score increased significantly ($p = 0.0001$) from baseline in PTA recipients with sustained graft function ($n = 25$) but not in those with failed grafts ($n = 12$) (Table 36).

**Table 35**  One Year Posttransplant Change in Quality of Life Score from Pretransplant Baseline in SPK Recipients According to Graft Function (Fxn) or Failure (Fld)

| Graft status (N) | Pancreas Fxn kidney Fxn (130) | Pancreas Fxn kidney Fld (5) | Pancreas Fld kidney Fxn (24) | Pancreas Fld kidney Fld (2) |
|---|---|---|---|---|
| QOL score change | $5.2 \pm 4.0$ | $2.4 \pm 1.5$ | $0.2 \pm 3.7$ | $\leq 0$ |
| p Value | 0.0001 | 0.12 | $> 0.5$ | NA |

**Table 36** One Year Posttransplant Change in Quality of Life Score from Pretransplant Baseline in Solitary Pancreas Transplant Recipients with Functioning or Failed Grafts

| Graft status | Functioning | Failed |
|---|:---:|:---:|
| PAK (N) | 3.7± 4.1 (55) | 0.9± 2.5 (16) |
| p value | 0.0001 | 0.009 |
| PTA (N) | 5.9± 4.2 (25) | 2.8± 4.8 (12) |
| p value | 0.0001 | 0.07 |

### Long-Term Quality of Life

The increase in mean total points from pretransplant baseline was sustained in succeeding years in patients with functioning grafts. At two years, the mean increases were 4.3 + 0.8 points for SPK ($n = 100$), 3.7 + 5.6 for PAK ($n = 32$), and 6.4 + 4.3 for PTA ($n = 8$)($p = 0.0001$). ). For 50 SPK study patients who completed the evaluation at four years, the mean increase in total points from baseline was 6.2 + 4.6 ($n = 50$) ($p = 0.0001$).

Overall, our study showed that diabetic patients, who become insulin independent, perceive their QOL as having improved in spite of immunosuppression. The data presented here is original and complements past QOL studies, done by independent investigators (180–186), of the Minnesota pancreas recipients.

## Metabolic Studies

Formal metabolic studies of the Minnesota pancreas recipients and LDs have been conducted since the inception of our program (70) and are still ongoing (160).

In Era 1, the studies were initiated by coauthor Goetz and were very basic: 24 metabolic profiles (MPs) of glucose and insulin values before and after meals, and standard oral or intravenous GTTs in pancreas recipients who were insulin-independent as a result of a functioning graft (70). The profiles usually resembled those of nondiabetic individuals, or at least those of nondiabetic kidney allograft recipients, with or without portal drainage of the graft venous effluent (57).

The MP and GTT studies were used in Era 2 to compare posttransplant endocrine function by duration of pancreas graft preservation (109) and to compare function in recipients who did or did not have RREs (84). MP and GTT results were similar regardless of preservation time or occurrence of rejection episodes in recipients with sustained insulin independence; glycosolated hemoglobulin levels (115), both short-term (187) and long-term (117), were normal.

Era 2 saw the introduction of more sophisticated metabolic studies using new methods initiated by coauthor Robertson (188) and carried out by a series of fellows and associate faculty members in the Division of Endocrinology (114,116,172,173,189–194). Parallel studies of our islet auto- and allograft recipients were also done (195–199). These studies not only examined pancreatic graft beta cell function, but also alpha cell function, glucose counter-regulatory mechanisms, and the impact of the site of venous drainage (systemic or portal) of a pancreas graft.

Diem et al. (114) were the first to establish systemic venous drainage as the principal cause of systemic venous hyperinsulinemia after pancreas transplantation. A smaller portion of the hyperinsulinemia could be attributed to recipients' glucocortocoid use. In spite of this metabolic abnormality, virtually all measures of carbohydrate metabolism in the fasting state and after a mixed meal remained normal (189).

Possible adverse effects of immunosuppressive drugs on beta cell function and glucose tolerance were also studied. Many of the drugs are known to interfere with insulin synthesis or secretion, or action. Teuscher et al. (194) assessed insulin secretory reserve in pancreas transplant recipients by measuring glucose potentiation of arginine-induced insulin secretion and observed abnormally low insulin responses. Because diminished insulin secretory reserve was also observed in nondiabetic kidney recipients, the immunosuppressive drugs were the likely causes of this metabolic abnormality. A similar defect was observed in psoriasis patients treated with Csa, but not in arthritis patients treated with glucocorticoids; thus, Csa was the likely cause of diminished insulin secretory reserve (194). However, despite the hyperinsulinemia consequent to systemic drainage and glucocorticoids, and despite the diminished insulin secretory reserve attributable to Csa, we (RPR, DERS) have recently reported normal levels of fasting plasma glucose and hemoglobin A1C in a group of pancreas recipients followed for 10 to 18 years (129).

Defective glucagon and epinephrine counter-regulatory responses to hypoglycemia are very serious consequences of Type 1 diabetes. These abnormalities can lead to dangerous levels of hypoglycemia that incapacitate patients and seriously compromise their QOL. This scenario is made all the worse because such patients lose normal symptom recognition of hypoglycemia, which prevents them from taking early corrective measures. Studies by Diem et al. (116) demonstrated that a successful pancreas transplant restores normal glucagon responses. Later studies by Kendall et al. (197) concluded that the transplanted pancreas, rather than the alpha cells in the native pancreas, provided the restored glucagon response. Barrou et al. (192) utilized isotopic infusions and hypoglycemic clamp methodology to demonstrate that the restored glucagon response normalized hepatic glucose production during hypoglycemia. Kendall et al. (193) demonstrated that a successful pancreas transplant partially restored epinephrine response during hypoglycemia. More important, these studies also documented that recipients of a successful pancreas transplant reestablish normal symptom recognition.

More recently, coauthor Robertson and his fellow, BW Paty, have shown that restored hypoglycemic counterregulation is stable in pancreas recipients with functioning grafts for at least two decades after transplantation (158). RPR has also studied the effect of the occurrence of posttransplant obesity in pancreas recipients and saw a detrimental effect on metabolism similar to that in the general population (159).

Although most of our pancreas transplants were from DD donors, nearly 10% were segmental grafts from LDs. The metabolic responsivity of the transplanted hemipancreas is generally indistinguishable from that of the whole pancreas grafts. Donors of the pancreatic segments generally maintain normal glucose levels, but follow-up studies of the donors of Era 1 and the early part of Era 2 (before we established out current criteria to be an LD) show that about 25% had metabolic evidence of acquired glucose intolerance several years after donation (172). Studies by Seaquist et al. (190) established that both beta cell and alpha cell responses were compromised in hemipancreatectomized donors during measurements of insulin secretory reserve. Later studies by Seaquist et al. (173) showed that hemipancreatectomy was also associated with elevated circulating levels of proinsulin, presumably due to release of immature insulin granules in which cleavage of C-peptide from proinsulin was not yet complete.

The results of these studies prompted us to modify our criteria to be an LD. Now, all LDs must have a BMI $<28 kg/m^2$, in addition to having a normal GTT results, and plasma insulin levels must increase by 300% within 1 to 2 minutes after intravenous stimulation with glucose or arginine. LDs who meet these criteria have so far remained euglycemic and insulin independent, but they need to be carefully studied over time. Recent studies by RPR of living hemipancreatectomized donor and their recipients during the second decade postsurgery has shown a relationship between the development of obesity and occurrence of diabetes (159), and thus the potential for weight gain in both must be taken into account when selecting LD donors and recipients for hemipancreatecomy and segmental pancreas transplantation, respectively. However, the vast majority of LD segmental pancreas donors retain normal hormonal responses to metabolic challenges (160).

## Studies of Diabetic Secondary Complications

Formal studies on the course of preexisting diabetic secondary complications after pancreas transplantation were initiated at the beginning of Era 1 (74,200). The multicenter Diabetes Control and Complications Trial (DCCT) (of which the University of Minnesota was a part) was just beginning (201). Until it was completed in 1993 (near the end of Era 2), the best evidence that a constant euglycemic state mitigated the progression of secondary complications was from our studies [by us (71,72,119–121) and those of others (202)] of (203) pancreas recipients. These studies were carried out by members of our faculty from ophthalmology (71), pediatric nephrology (121,134), and neurology (119,120,132,133). The failure rate of pancreas transplants was relatively high in Era 1 and 2, generating a control group for these studies. Recipients were studied at baseline, and subsequently divided into 2 groups: (i) those with early pancreas graft failure (<three months) and (ii) those with sustained graft function for more than one year.

## *Retinopathy*

Ramsay et al. (71) studied solitary pancreas recipients in Era 1 and 2. Retinopathy and visual acuity were quantitated before and serially after transplantation. Most candidates had advanced, proliferative retinopathy. At two years posttransplant, the incidence of progression to a higher grade of retinopathy was the same (~30%) in the eyes of recipients with versus without graft function. After three years, however, no further progression occurred in the recipients with functioning grafts. However, 70% with failed transplants advanced to a higher grade by five years. Only a few recipients had no retinopathy at the pretransplant baseline examination, but disease has not emerged in the subgroup with continuously functioning pancreas grafts.

## *Nephropathy*

Studies of diabetic nephropathy focused on disease recurrence or on preventing it in the kidney grafts of diabetic KTA, SPK, or PAK recipients (121,204,205), as well as on disease progression, stabilization, or regression of disease in the native kidneys of PTA recipients (134,169).

Mauer et al. documented the recurrence of diabetic nephropathy [vascular lesions (206) and an increase in glomerular (G) and tubular (T) basement membrane (BM) and mesengial matrix (204)] in nearly half of kidneys transplanted without a pancreas in uremic diabetic recipients (207).

Initial evidence that a successful pancreas transplant can influence the course of diabetic nephropathy came from kidney allograft biopsy studies in PAK recipients by Bilous et al. (121). At the time of the pancreas transplant one to seven years (mean, four years) after the kidney transplant, the graft glomerular mesengial volume was moderately increased and glomerular basement membrane (GBM) moderately thickened. There was no progression; indeed there was regression of glomerular lesions, in follow-up biopsies taken 2 to 10 years later (mean, 4.5 years). These findings contrasted to those in the KTA recipients, where progressive diabetic glomerulopathy occurred (207), leading to kidney graft failure and the need for a kidney retransplant in some recipients (208).

The most dramatic and surprising findings came from studies by Fioretto et al. (134,169) of native kidneys in our PTA recipients. We obtained baseline biopsies of native kidneys in most of the PTA recipients (209). Follow-up biopsies in some have shown Csa-induced lesions that were associated with a progressive decline in kidney function, independent of the diabetic lesions already present (131,205,210). The diabetic kidney lesions were distinct. In eight PTA recipients, who were nonuremic at the time of the pancreas transplant but who had mild to moderately advanced lesions of diabetic nephropathy at baseline, 10-year follow-up biopsies showed that GBM and tubular basement membrane (TBM) thickness and mesangial fractional volume of the glomerulus had decreased and, indeed, returned to normal (134). In follow-up studies, Fioretta et al. also demonstrated remodeling of renal interstitial and tubular lesions in the kidneys of the pancreas transplant recipients (169). Although these studies were in patients with diabetic nephropathy, the fact that structural lesions could be reversed shows in principle that the kidney has the capacity for remodeling if the environmental perturbations responsible for the lesions originally are removed, having implications for renal disease in general, and not just that secondary to diabetes.

Thus, although it takes at least five years of normoglycemia, a pancreas transplant can reverse the lesions of diabetic nephropathy. Such reversal does not guarantee normal function because independent damage to the kidney may occur from the CIs needed to prevent pancreas rejection (131). Hence the need for attempts to develop effective non-nephrotoxic immunosuppressive regimens (162). If successful, nearly all patients with early diabetic nephropathy would benefit from a pancreas transplant.

## *Neuropathy*

As with the eye and kidney, our pancreas recipients had baseline neurological studies with serial follow up (71,119,132). More than 80 of our recipients had symptomatic neuropathy and more than 90% had an abnormal neurologic exam at baseline (130). Kennedy et al. (119) showed significant improvement in motor and sensory indices as well as autonomic function between one and four years posttransplant; we concluded that progression of diabetic neuropathy is halted and that an improvement is possible with sustained normoglycemia.

Navarro et al. (120) found higher mortality rates were higher in patients with autonomic dysfunction or abnormal nerve conduction studies, compared with that in those with minimal disease. The mortality rate was also high in nontransplanted diabetic patients with neuropathy. However, in neuropathic patients with a successful pancreas transplant, the mortality rate was significantly lower even if in neuropathy improved only minimally (133). The combination of diabetes and severe neuropathy is lethal; correction of diabetes improves survival even if neuropathy persists.

Navarro et al. (132) did follow-up studies at 10 years of diabetic pancreas recipients. In control patients (those with a failed transplant), neuropathy progressively worsened, while in recipients with sustained graft function, the improvement in neuropathy seen early on was sustained.

### General

The most remarkable feature of the studies on diabetic secondary complications in our pancreas recipients was the positive impact on advanced disease. In the DCCT (201), at entry, diabetic patients had either no or minimal manifestation of secondary complications. Even with intensive insulin treatment, new lesions emerged, and lesions already present progressed in some patients (211). The secondary diabetic lesions at baseline were much more advanced in our patients than in the DCCT. The regression of neuropathic and nephropathic lesions seen after a successful pancreas transplant did not occur with intensified insulin treatment (212). Other groups have now also shown that a successful pancreas transplant can ameliorate microvascular complications (213,214), including retinopathy (215), nephropathy (203), and neuropathy (202,216).

Although a main objective of pancreas transplantation is to improve day-to-day QOL by omitting the need for insulin injections and glucose monitoring, the fact that secondary complications are also favorably influenced gives even greater impetus to apply this treatment modality.

### GENERAL DISCUSSION

Clinical pancreas transplantation, begun at Minnesota in 1966, now encompasses a period of nearly 40 years. Transplantation of endocrine tissue (pancreatic islet beta cells) is the only treatment that can induce insulin independence for Type 1 diabetic patients. As predicted (217), the results of islet transplantation have improved in recent years (218–223), but transplantation of islets within an immediately vascularized graft (pancreas) remains more successful and efficient (2,224) than as a free cellular graft (225).

Nevertheless, recent successes with clinical islet allotransplantation at our own (36,37) and other institutions (226–229), including one from a LD with alloislets from half a pancreas being sufficient to reverse pancreatic diabetes (230), suggest that eventually beta-cell replacement will be done routinely as a minimally invasive procedure rather than by the major surgery of pancreas transplantation, especially if our outcomes using single islet donors to achieve insulin-independence (36,37) can be universally replicated.

Meanwhile, pancreas transplantation continues to be done, and the lessons learned over many years at our own and other centers (only a few examples are referenced) (231–243), including recent advances such as steroid-free immunosuppression (244–247), use of cardiac death donors (248), and an intraretroperitoneal approach for portal-enteric drainage (249) rather than the anterior approach in general use elsewhere (250), some of which have contributed to the high success rate now achieved in both uremic and nonuremic diabetic recipients (2). Indeed, there is good evidence that a pancreas transplant prolongs survival of both nephropathic (251–254), neuropathic (133), and vasculopoathic (255) diabetic patients.

A recent concern that solitary pancreas transplants may slightly increase the mortality risk over that of pancreas transplant candidates on the waiting list (175) was not substantiated on more detailed analysis, indeed just the opposite effect was found, survival was slightly better in PTA and PAK recipients than those on the waiting list (176). Both analyses agreed that SPK recipients had much higher survival rates than those who remained on the waiting list (175,176).

Our program differs from most in that we have emphasized solitary pancreas transplants from the beginning (7,41), and continued to do so (79). A few other programs have also emphasized solitary pancreas transplants beginning nearly a decade ago (237,256), with results now (239,242,243) equivalent to our own (40,155,156). It is also apparent from the most recent Registry analysis that the number of solitary pancreas transplants is increasing, and that as PAK numbers increase with the emphasis on LD kidney transplants to preempt dialysis in patients with advancing diabetic nephropathy there may be sligltly fewer SPK transplants as DD are other utilized (156).

Otherwise, there are very few aspects of our program that are original, and much of what we have done has been adapted from the pioneering efforts of others. One aspect that is original at Minnesota includes the first use of a LD for a pancreas transplant in 1979 (47), with extension to identical twin donors in 1980 (41,66). The LD option has been exercised only by a few other centers (257,258), but includes the use of identical twin donors (257,259). Our own experience now includes 124 LD pancreas transplants, and we continue to do follow-up studies on the donors (153) and continue to do the procurement of the distal pancreas from LDs laparoscopically (168).

Our splitting of a DD pancreas to give a segment to each of two recipients (108) appears not to have been duplicated in the literature. However, our initiation of LD kidney transplants simultaneous with a DD pancreas (6) has been used in a large number of cases elsewhere (242,260). The introduction of immediate retransplantation for a primary technical (e.g. thrombosis) failure (261) has been adopted by other groups (262,263). Even our use of ED pancreas transplantation to correct exocrine deficiency (94,264) has been duplicated (265). Indeed, in our series of more than 130 total pancreatectomies and islet autotransplants for chronic pancreatitis as of 2005 (266,267), if the islet yield is inadequate to prevent diabetes, some of the patients have gone on to have a pancreas transplant, in which case both endocrine and exocrine deficiency can be corrected (264).

In regard to surgical techniques, segmental pancreas transplantation has largely disappeared except from LDs, as has the use of duct management techniques other than BD or ED, though we continue to occasionally do DI for a segmental graft in which ED or BD would be difficult. In the last decade, many groups have compared outcome with ED versus BD and have concluded that the results with the two techniques are equivalent, at least for SPK transplants (232,268–273). Although portal drainage of pancreas graft venous effulent was done in a few cases at several centers in the 1980s (274–276) including our own (57), Rosenlof et al. (277) reported its routine use for SPK transplants in 1992, stimulating others to adopt the technique as well (232,237,278,279). Portal drainage has to be more physiological than systemic drainage and the metabolic perturbations of systemic drainage include psuedohyperinsulinemia (114), but the relevance is unknown. The latest advance in portal drainage is from the Pisa group using an intraretroperitoneal approach (249).

Surgical complications of pancreas transplantation decreased at our center as we went from era (92) to era (125) to era (125,142) and took special precautions for such problems as recipient obesity (143) and prolonged preservation (146). The reduction in surgical complication incidence is also paralleled by reports from other centers (240,269,280). Chronic complications of BD, however, have persisted (281–283) and our rate of conversion to ED was >10% throughout the 1990s (174) and has not changed in the current era. Both BD and ED have an irreducible incidence of complications (284) and we continue to use both in our program for maximum flexibility in the approach to individual patients.

The most immediate and frequent posttransplant complication is pancreas graft thrombosis (285). Some groups have not found that heparinization reduces the risk (286), while in our experience it seems to have helped (125).

Infections after pancreas transplantation can be local or systemic. Our incidence of local infections has been reduced (125), but can necessitate graft removal (287,288). New immunosuppressive protocols can be associated with reappearance of infectious complications (289). The most common systemic infection is with CMV or Epstein–Barr virus (EBV) infections. We showed that drug prophylaxis is effective in reducing the incidence of CMV infections in pancreas transplant recipients (140,290), as have others (291). The risk of PTLD following EBV infection is a risk in all organ allograft recipients. Our incidence of PTLD after pancreas transplantation has been <2%, including only 0.6% in PTA recipients (164,292). Other groups report a similarly low rate of PTLD following pancreas transplantation (293–297).

In regard to immunosuppression, our center (124) evolved to use Tac and/or MMF in all recipient categories during Era 4, with pretransplant immunosuppression in PTA recipients

(137). Rapamyacin was first used for pancreas transplantation by McAlister (298), and we have also used in patients who did not tolerate MMF (163). We also have use antiT cell therapy routinely for induction, while its use is variable at other centers (231–233,299–306). Indeed in Era 5, we used antiT-cell not only for induction, but for mainetance immunosuppression allowing patients to be both steroid- and CI-free (162); the protocol was most successful in the PAK category, while in the PTA category there was an increased incidence of rejection (163).

Early treatment of REs is important. SPK recipients of grafts from the SD can be monitored by serum creatinine. For solitary pancreas transplant recipients, serum creatinine cannot be used as a surrogate marker for rejection. Thus, we still favor BD and use a decline in UA as a marker for rejection (101). A decline in UA is sometimes preceded or accompanied by a rise in serum pancreatic enzyme levels (307), but we have seen several rejection episodes where only the UA declined and would have been missed by relying on serum enzyme levels alone (8). Thus, UA makes immunological monitoring of solitary BD pancreas transplants relatively easy, and should be considered especially for young PTA recipients, who are particularly prone to rejection episodes both early and late posttransplant (8).

Pancreas allograft biopsies and pathological assessment are less important in SPK recipients than in solitary pancreas transplants for the reasons mentioned above. However, for solitary pancreas transplants, a pancreas graft biopsy has the same utility as for renal allografts. We have employed pancreas allograft biopsies for solitary pancreas transplants by one technique or another since the early 1980s (62,63,101), but it was the introduction of the percutaneous needle technique by Allen et al. (308) and Gaber et al. (309) in the early 1990s that made routine biopsies practical. Pathological features and histological grading of pancreatic allograft biopsies have been well described by many groups (293,310–318), including our own for both acute (101,319), and chronic (141) rejection. Our use of pancreas graft biopsies in the 1980s was critical in identifying recurrence of disease (autoimmune isletitis) (67). Recurrence of disease is also occasionally seen in DD pancreas allografts (320), and its incidence may be underestimated (321).

In SPK recipients, documented discordant rejections (only one organ is involved) are rare, but they do occur (322,323) and in our experience can lead to discordant graft loss as well (97). HLA matching reduced rejection failures in solitary pancreas transplants at a time when the overall results were not as good as now (324). However, our own data reported here, as well as that of the Registry (325), indicates that HLA matching, particularly at the B locus, is still beneficial in the FK/MMF eras, not withstanding the disclaimers of others on a small number of cases (326).

If graft loss does occur for any reason, pancreas retransplantation is feasible. Although some have considered retransplantation a high-risk procedure (327), we have not been deterred (144). We have had a large number of candidates for retransplants because of the low success rate with primary transplants in the early eras. Pancreas GSRs were significantly lower for retransplants than for primary transplants in each era, but the current retransplant success rate is much higher than the primary pancreas transplant success rate in earlier eras. Thus, we have no hesitation in offering retransplantation as a routine to recipients whose primary grafts fail.

Even apart from retransplantation, there are many risk factors that influence outcome. Multivariate analyses have been done by others, looking at both recipient (328) and donor (329) risk factors, but with many fewer patients than in our analyses. Some groups have assessed individual risk factors, such as obesity (330) or recipient race (331); the former has a moderate impact, but the latter does not seem to influence outcome.

The question as to whether early SPK transplants to preempt dialysis gives an advantage in nephropathic diabetics (332) seems answered by our good results in never-dialyzed patients (8). Other questions, such as impact of VD in the recipients on outcome have been well studied by some (255), but most groups have excluded vasculopathic patients from pancreas transplantation consideration in the first place (333). We have not, and as can be seen from our analyses in this chapter recipients with VD can have good outcomes, even if patient and GSRs are not as high as those without VD, but without transplantation almost all of these patients would have an even higher mortality rate, particularly those that are uremic (175,176). In our program, nearly all uremic diabetic patients undergo coronary angiography followed by intervention (bypass or angioplasty) if indicated before a pancreas transplant (112,157). Although patient survival rates are less for those with versus those without preexisting VD, correcting diabetes is beneficial for both groups. A few other centers also do pancreas transplants in diabetics with coronary artery disease (334,335), and believe it safe. Even uremic patients with Type II diabetes have routinely received SPK transplants in some programs (336). We, too, have found no difference in insulin independence rates in the Type 2 diabetics, patients we transplanted (166).

As important as recipient are donor risk factors (329). Although pancreas grafts from both pediatric (337,338) and older donors (339,340) have been successfully transplanted,(110), we (110) and others have also made the case to be selective (341,342). Whatever the age range, one group has shown that the outcomes for paired grafts from the SD are very similar in KTA and SPK recipients (343).

Restoration of normal metabolism is the immediate goal of pancreas transplantation. Although we have described a delayed endocrine function (344), most recipients become insulin independent immediately posttransplant. Nearly all are euglycemic and have normal glycosolated hemoglobin levels as long as the graft functions, as also described in the results section on metabolism. Several other groups have also performed sophisticated metabolic studies on postpancreas transplant (345–353). Even though metabolic perturbations are described, it is interesting to note that recipient lipid profiles usually improve following successful pancreas transplantation (354–356); whether the improvement in lipid profiles translates into a lower risk for VD in pancreas transplant recipients has not been determined. It is clear from our studies described in the section on secondary complications, and from the studies of other groups, which microangiopathy can improve following successful pancreas transplantation (213,214,357) including retinopathy if the intervention is early enough (71,215). Of course, advanced retinopathy is difficult to influence as we (71) and others (358) have found.

Every group that has reported on neuropathic studies has shown improvement (202,216,359,360). Even autonomic defects (361), such as vesicopathy (362) and gastropathy (363), can improve.

As expected, diabetic nephropathy does not recur in renal graft recipients with sustained insulin independence after an SPK transplant (203). Of highest significance in the area of renal disease is our finding that advanced lesions of diabetic nephropathy in native kidneys can resolve over time following a successful PTA (134) and that structural remodeling of the kidney occurs (169).

The benefits of metabolism on secondary complications occur in conjunction with improvement in day-to-day QOL. Many groups have done QOL studies in their pancreas transplant recipients (364–370) and all have the same findings as the independent studies done in our own patients (180–186,371). Recipients are more satisfied before than after the pancreas transplant (364–366).

Pancreas transplantation is a highly effective therapy for diabetes mellitus. There are surgical complications, and immunosuppression is required, but the QOL is improved. Pancreas transplantation, at least in the short run, is more expensive than exogenous insulin treatment (372) but better treatment is worth the higher cost. The economics of pancreas transplantation in the short term has been studied (373–377) but the long-term overall economic impact that prevention or amelioration of secondary complications may provide toward recouping initial start up costs have only been projected (372). Nevertheless, pancreas transplantation is so effective that the American Diabetes Association (ADA) position statement (378,379) says that SPK and PAK should be routine in diabetic kidney transplants recipients and that PTA is appropriate therapy for nonuremic labile diabetic patients.

Our own program is more liberal than the ADA, and we have done pancreas transplants as prophylaxis for secondary complications or for adult patients, who would rather manage immunosuppression and its risks than diabetes and its risks (165). We take it as a matter of informed consent as to which route the patients want to take, the diabetic route or the immunosuppression route. There are risks with each, but the benefits are greater with the transplant route.

Of course if immunosuppression is required for other reasons in a diabetic patient, a pancreas transplant might as well be done, even to children (170). Certainly, the current ADA guidelines are appropriate for children. Whatever hesitation there may be to recommend endocrine transplantation as a treatment for diabetes, it will be less with free grafts of islets because of the elimination of surgical complications (225,380). If tolerance-inducing protocols become successful clinically (223), either pancreas or islet transplantation could be performed without the fear of immunosuppressive complications. If islets are as successful as the pancreas transplant technically, in the absence of immunosuppression (tolerance) virtually every diabetic would want to be treated. Because of the limited supply of human DD donors, to treat all diabetes would require the development of propagated beta cell lines that are suitable for transplantation (381,382) or the application of xenografts of which our results with pig islet to nonhuman primates are quite promising for clinical application (383). Ultimately, neither strategy may be needed if beta cell regeneration can be induced in the native pancreas (384) and the autoimmune threat thwarted (385).

Although the minimally invasive approach of islet transplantation is desirable for beta cell replacement and will undoubtedly expand as further advances are made, pancreas transplantation is highly successful and can be done on a large scale, as we and others have shown. Until other approaches, preventative, regenerative, can be fully applied to obviate or cure diabetes, beta cell replacement will remain the only therapy that can establish insulin-independence in those otherwise, and pancreas transplantation remains the most efficient method as this chapter is written, notwithstanding its surgical complications.

## ACKNOWLEDGMENTS

The authors thank Barbara Bland, M.S., M.L.I.S., B.A.N., R.N. for assistance with the database, and Shannon Pinc for preparation of the tables and manuscript. The authors also greatly appreciate the roles of Barbara Elick, R.N. and the nurse transplant coordinators in facilitating our Pancreas Transplant Program over the years.

## REFERENCES

1. Kelly WD, Lillehei RC, Merkel FK. Allotransplantation of the pancreas and duodenum along with the kidney in diabetic nephropathy. Surgery 1967; 61:827–835.
2. Gruessner AC, Sutherland DE. Pancreas transplant outcomes for United States (US) and non-US cases as reported to the United Network for Organ Sharing (UNOS) and the International Pancreas Transplant Registry (IPTR) as of June 2004. Clin Transplant 2005; 19:433–455.
3. Lillehei RC, Simmons RL, Najarian JS, et al. Pancreatico-duodenal allotransplantation: experimental and clinical experience. Ann Surg 1970; 172:405–436.
4. Sutherland DE, Goetz FC, Najarian JS. One hundred pancreas transplants at a single institution. Ann Surg 1984; 200:414–440.
5. Sutherland DE, Dunn DL, Goetz FC, et al. A 10-year experience with 290 pancreas transplants at a single institution. Ann Surg 1989; 210:274–285.
6. Sutherland DE, Gores PF, Farney AC, et al. Evolution of kidney, pancreas, and islet transplantation for patients with diabetes at the University of Minnesota. Am J Surg 1993; 166:456–491.
7. Lillehei RC, Ruiz JO, Aquino C, Goetz FC. Transplantation of the pancreas. Acta Endocrin 1976; 83(suppl 205):303–320.
8. Sutherland DE, Gruessner RW, Dunn DL, et al. Lessons learned from more than 1,000 pancreas transplants at a single institution. Ann Surg 2001; 233:463–501.
9. Gliedman ML, Gold M, Whittaker J, et al. Clinical segmental pancreatic transplantation with ureter-pancreatic duct anastomosis for exocrine drainage. Surgery 1973; 74:171–180.
10. Dubernard JM, Traeger J, Neyra P, Touraine JL, Traudiant D, Blanc-Brunat N. A new method of preparation of segmental pancreatic grafts for transplantation: trials in dogs and in man. Surgery 1978; 84:633–640.
11. Groth CG, Collste H, Lundgren G. Successful outcome of segmental human pancreatic transplantation with enteric exocrine diversion after modifications in technique. Lancet 1982; 2:522–524.
12. Sollinger HW, Cook K, Kamps D. Clinical and experimental experience with pancreaticocystostomy for exocrine pancreatic drainage in pancreas transplantation. Transplant Proc 1984; 16:749–751.
13. Starzl TE, Iwatsuki S, Shaw BW Jr., et al. Pancreaticoduodenal transplantation in humans. Surg Gynecol Obstet 1984; 159:265–272.
14. Nghiem DD, Corry RJ. Technique of simultaneous pancreaticoduodenal transplantation with urinary drainage of pancreatic secretion. Am J Surg 1987; 153:405–406.
15. Belzer FO. Clinical organ preservation with UW solution. Transplantation 1989; 47:1097–1098.
16. Calne RY, Rolles K, White DJ, et al. Cyclosporin A initially as the only immunosuppressant in 34 recipients of cadaveric organs: 32 kidneys, 2 pancreases, and 2 livers. Lancet 1979; 2:1033–1036.
17. Starzl TE, Todo S, Fung J, Demetris AJ, Venkataramman R, Jain A. FK 506 for liver, kidney, and pancreas transplantation. Lancet 1989; 2:1000–1004.
18. Rayhill SC, Kirk AD, Odorico JS, et al. Simultaneous pancreas-kidney transplantation at the University of Wisconsin. Clinical Transplants 1995; 261–269.

19. Vincent F, Kirkman R, Light S, et al. Interleukin-2-receptor blockade with daclizumab to prevent acute rejection in renal transplantation. Daclizumab Triple Therapy Study Group. N Engl J Med 1998; 338:161–165.
20. Bruce DS, Sollinger HW, Humar A, et al. Multicenter survey of daclizumab induction in simultaneous kidney-pancreas transplant recipients. Transplantation 2001; 72:1637–1643.
21. Kjellstrand CM, Simmons RL, Goetz FC, et al. Renal transplantation in patients with insulin-dependent diabetes. Lancet 1973; 2:4–8.
22. Najarian JS, Kjellstrand CM, Simmons RL, Buselmeier TJ, Von Hartitzch B, Goetz FC. Renal transplantation for diabetic glomerulosclerosis. Ann Surg 1973; 4:477–484.
23. Najarian JS, Sutherland DE, Simmons RL, et al. Ten year experience with renal transplantation in juvenile onset diabetics. Ann Surg 1979; l90:487–500.
24. Sutherland DE, Morrow CE, Fryd DS, Ferguson RM, Simmons RL, Najarian JS. Improved patient and primary renal allograft survival in uremic diabetic recipients. Transplantation 1982; 34:319–325.
25. Sutherland DE, Goetz FC, Carpenter AM, Najarian JS, Lillehei RC. Pancreaticoduodenal grafts: clinical and pathological observations in uremic versus nonuremic recipients. Amsterdam-Oxford: Excerpta Medica, 1979:190–195.
26. Gliedman ML, Tellis VA, Soberman R. Long-term effects of pancreatic transplant function in patients with advanced juvenile onset diabetes. Diabetes Care 1978; 1:1–9.
27. Matas AJ, Sutherland DE, Najarian JS. Current status of islet and pancreas transplantation in diabetes. Diabetes 1976; 25:785–795.
28. Younoszai R, Sorenson RL, Lindall AW. Homotransplantation of isolated pancreatic islets. Diabetes (suppl) 1970; 19:406.
29. Hering BJ, Ricordi C, Sutherland DE, Bluestone JA. Islet transplantation: at the forefront of clinical research on immune tolerance. In: Norman D, Suki WN, eds. Primer on Transplantation. Thorofare, NJ: American Society of Transplant Physicians, 2000.
30. Sutherland DE, Matas AJ, Najarian JS. Pancreatic islet cell transplantation. Surg Clin North Am 1978; 58:365–382.
31. Sutherland DE, Matas AJ, Goetz FC, Najarian JS. Transplantation of dispersed pancreatic islet tissue in humans: autografts and allografts. Diabetes (suppl) 1980; 29:3l–44.
32. Najarian JS, Sutherland DE, Baumgartner D, et al. Total or near total pancreatectomy and islet autotransplantation for treatment of chronic pancreatitis. Ann Surg 1980; 192:526–542.
33. Sutherland DE. Pancreas and islet transplantation. I. Experimental studies. Diabetologia 1981; 20:161–185.
34. Sutherland, DE. Pancreas and islet transplantation. II. Clinical trials. Diabetologia 1981; 20:435–450.
35. Gores PF, Najarian JS, Stephanian E, Lloveras JJ, Kelley SL, Sutherland DE. Insulin independence in type I diabetes after transplantation of unpurified islets from a single donor using 15-deoxyspergualin. Lancet 1993; 341:19–21.
36. Hering BJ, Kandaswamy R, Harmon JV, et al. Transplantation of cultured islets from two-layer preserved pancreases in type 1 diabetes with anti–CD3 antibody. Am J Transplant 2004; 4:390–401.
37. Hering BJ, Kandaswamy R, Ansite JD, Eckman PM, et al. Single-donor, marginal-dose islet transplantation in patients with type 1 diabetes. JAMA 2005; 293:830–835.
38. Kyriakides GK, Sutherland DE, Miller JB, Najarian JS. Segmental pancreatic transplantation in dogs after suppression of exocrine function by intraductal injection of neoprene. Transplant Proc 1979; 11:530–532.
39. Sutherland DE, Goetz FC, Najarian JS. Intraperitoneal transplantation of immediately vascularized segmental pancreatic grafts without duct ligation: a clinical trial. Transplantation 1979; 28:485–49l.
40. Gruessner RW, Sutherland DE, Najarian JS, Dunn DL, Gruessner A. Solitary pancreas transplantation for nonuremic patients with labile insulin-dependent diabetes mellitus. Transplantation 1997; 64:1572–1577.
41. Sutherland DE, Goetz FC, Rynasiewicz JJ, et al. Segmental pancreas transplantation from living related and cadaver donors: a clinical experience. Surgery 1981; 90:159–169.
42. Sutherland DE, Goetz FC, Elick BA, Najarian JS. Experience with 49 segmental pancreas transplants in 45 diabetic patients. Transplantation 1982; 34:330–338.
43. Kyriakides GK, Nuttall FQ, Miller J. Segmental pancreatic transplantation in pigs. Surgery 1979; 85:154–158.
44. Najarian JS, Gruessner AC, Drangsteveit MB, Gruessner RW, Goetz FC, Sutherland DE. Insulin independence for more than 10 years in 32 pancreas transplant recipients from a historical era. Transplant Proc 1998; 30:279.
45. Sutherland DE, Moudry K. Report of the Pancreas Transplant Registry. Clinical Transplant 1986; 7–15.
46. Najarian JS, Simmons RL, Condie RM, et al. Seven years' experience with antilymphoblast globulin for renal transplantation from cadaver donors. Ann Surg 1976; 184:352–367.
47. Sutherland DE, Goetz FC, Najarian JS. Living-related donor segmental pancreatectomy for transplantation. Transplant Proc 1980; 12:19–25.
48. Simmons RL, Kjellstrand CM, Condie RM, et al. Parent-to-child and child-to-parent kidney transplants: experience with 101 transplants at one center. Lancet 1976; 1:321–324.

49.  Simmons RL, Van Hook EJ, Yunis EJ, et al. 100 sibling kidney transplants followed 2 to 7 1/2 years: a multifactorial analysis. Ann Surg 1977; 185:196–204.
50.  Sutherland DE, Goetz FC, Najarian JS. Pancreas transplants from related donors. Transplantation 1984; 38:625–633.
51.  Sutherland DE. Pancreas transplantation in non-uremic diabetic patients. Transplant Proc 1986; 18:1747–1749.
52.  Sutherland DE, Kendall D, Goetz FC, Najarian JS. Pancreas transplantation. Surg Clin North Am 1986; 66:557–582.
53.  Prieto M, Sutherland DE, Goetz FC, Rosenberg ME, Najarian JS. Pancreas transplant results according to the technique of duct management: bladder versus enteric drainage. Surgery 1987; 102:680–691.
54.  Prieto M, Sutherland DE, Fernandez-Cruz L, Heil JE, Najarian JS. Urinary amylase monitoring for early diagnosis of pancreas allograft rejection in dogs. J Surg Res 1986; 40:597–604.
55.  Prieto M, Sutherland DE, Fernandez-Cruz L, Heil JE, Najarian JS. Experimental and clinical experience with urine amylase monitoring for early diagnosis of rejection in pancreas transplantation. Transplantation 1987; 43:71–79.
56.  Sutherland DE, Baumgartner D, Najarian JS. Free intraperitoneal drainage of segmental pancreas grafts: clinical and experimental observations on technical aspects. Transplant Proc 1980; 12:26–32.
57.  Sutherland DE, Goetz FC, Moudry KC, Abouna GM, Najarian JS. Use of recipient mesenteric vessels for revascularization of segmental pancreas grafts: technical and metabolic considerations. Transplant Proc 1987; 19:2300–2304.
58.  Sutherland DE, Ascher NL. Whole pancreas donation from a cadaver. In: Simmons RL, Finch ME, Ascher NL, Najarian JS, eds. Manual of Vascular Access, Organ Donation, Transplantation. New York: Springer-Verlag, 1984:144–152.
59.  Sutherland DE, Moudry KC, Najarian JS. Pancreas transplantation. In: Cerilli J, ed. Organ transplantation and replacement. Philadelphia: JB Lippincott Company, 1987:535–574.
60.  Florack G, Sutherland DE, Heise JW, Najarian JS. Successful preservation of human pancreas grafts for 28 hours. Transplant Proc 1987; 19:3882–3885.
61.  Abouna GM, Sutherland DE, Florack G, Najarian JS. Function of transplanted human pancreatic allografts after preservation in cold storage for 6 to 26 Hours. Transplantation 1987; 43:630–636.
62.  Sutherland DE, Casanova D, Sibley RK. Role of pancreas graft biopsies in the diagnosis and treatment of rejection after pancreas transplantation. Transplant Proc 1987; 19:2329–2331.
63.  Sibley RK, Sutherland DE. Pancreas transplantation: an immunohistologic and histopathologic examination of 100 grafts. Am J Pathol 1987; 128:151–170.
64.  Sutherland DE. Cyclosporine versus azathioprine in pancreas transplantation: a comparison. Transplant Immunol 1985; 2:1–3.
65.  Sutherland DE, Goetz FC, Najarian JS. Improved pancreas graft survival by use of multiple drug combination immunotherapy. Transplant Proc 1986; 18:1770–1773.
66.  Sutherland DE, Sibley RK, Xu XZ, et al. Twin-to-twin pancreas transplantation: reversal and reenactment of the pathogenesis of Type I diabetes. Trans Assoc Am Physicians 1984; 97:80–87.
67.  Sibley RK, Sutherland DE, Goetz FC, Michael AF. Recurrent diabetes mellitus in the pancreas iso- and allograft: a light and electron microscopic and immunohistochemical analysis of four cases. Lab Invest 1985; 53:132–144.
68.  Eisenbarth GS. Type I diabetes mellitus: a chronic autoimmune disease. N Engl J Med 1986; 314:1360–1368.
69.  Sutherland DE, Sibley RK. Recurrence of disease in pancreas transplants. In: van Schilfgaarde R, Hardy MA, eds. Transplantation of the Endocrine Pancreas in Diabetes Mellitus. Amsterdam: Elsevier Science Publishers BV, 1988:60–66.
70.  Sutherland DE, Najarian JS, Greenberg BZ, et al. Hormonal and metabolic effects of a pancreatic endocrine graft: vascularized segmental transplantation in insulin-dependent diabetic patients. Ann Intern Med 1981; 95:537–541.
71.  Ramsay RC, Goetz FC, Sutherland DE, et al. Progression of diabetic retinopathy after pancreas transplantation for insulin-dependent diabetes mellitus. N Engl J Med 1988; 318:208–214.
72.  Van der Vliet JA, Navarro X, Kennedy WR, Goetz FC, Najarian JS, Sutherland DE. The effect of pancreas transplantation on diabetic polyneuropathy. Transplantation 1988; 45:368–370.
73.  Mauer SM, Steffes MW, Ellis EN, Sutherland DE, Brown DM, Goetz FC. Structural-functional relationships in diabetic nephropathy. J Clin Invest 1984; 74:1143–1155.
74.  Sutherland DE. Effect of pancreas transplants on secondary complications of diabetes: review of observations of a single institution. Transplant Proc 1992; 24:859–860.
75.  Dubernard JM, Traeger J. Pancreas and islet transplantation workshop. Transplant Proc 1980; 12:1–2.
76.  Land W. Clinical pancreas transplantation. Transplant Proc 1987; 19:1–2.
77.  Land W, Landgraf R. The world experience in clinical pancreas transplantation. Transplant Proc 1987; 19(suppl 4):1–2.
78.  Sutherland DE, Goetz FC, Najarian JS. Pancreas transplantation at the university of Minnesota: donor and recipient selection, operative and postoperative management, and outcome. Transplant Proc 1987; 19(suppl 4):63–74.

79. Sutherland DE, Kendall DM, Moudry KC, et al. Pancreas transplantation in nonuremic, Type I diabetic recipients. Surgery 1988; 104:453–464.
80. Sutherland DE, Moudry KC, Dunn DL, Goetz FC, Najarian JS. Pancreas transplant outcome in relation to presence or absence of end-stage renal disease, timing of transplant, surgical technique, and donor source. Diabetes 1989; 38(suppl 1):10–12.
81. Frey DJ, Matas AJ, Gillingham KJ, et al. Sequential therapy—a prospective randomized trial of MALG versus OKT3 for prophylactic immunosuppression in cadaver renal allograft recipients. Transplantation 1992; 54:50–56.
82. Wilson LG. The crime of saving lives. The FDA, John Najarian, Minnesota ALG. Arch Surg 1995; 130:1035–1039.
83. Sutherland DE. Immunosuppression for clinical pancreas transplantation. Clin Transplant (Spec issue) 1991; 5:549–553.
84. Morel P, Brayman KL, Goetz FC, et al. Long-term metabolic function of pancreas transplants and influence of rejection episodes. Transplantation 1991; 51:990–1000.
85. Barrou B, Barrou Z, Gruessner A, Moudry-Munns KC, Gruessner RW, Sutherland DE. Probability of retaining endocrine function (insulin independence) after definitive loss of exocrine function in bladder-drained pancreas transplants. Transplant Proc 1994; 26(2):473–474.
86. Gruessner RW, Sutherland DE, Troppmann C, et al. The surgical risk of pancreas transplantation in the cyclosporine era: an overview. J Am Coll Surg 1997; 185:128–144.
87. Morel P, Schlumpf R, Dunn DL, Moudry-Munns K, Najarian JS, Sutherland DE. Pancreas retransplants compared with primary transplants. Transplantation 1991; 51:825–833.
88. Sutherland DE, Dunn DL, Moudry-Munns KC, Gillingham KJ, Najarian JS. Pancreas transplants in non-uremic and post-uremic diabetic patients. Transplant Proc 1992; 24(No. 3):780–781.
89. Sollinger HW. Mycophenolate mofetil for the prevention of acute rejection in primary cadaveric renal allograft recipients. U.S. Renal Transplant Mycophenolate Mofetil Study Group. Transplantation 1995; 60:225–232.
90. Sutherland DE, Gruessner RW, Moudry-Munns KC, Gruessner A, Najarian JS. Pancreas transplants from living related donors. Transplant Proc 1994; 26(2):443–445.
91. Morel P, Gillingham KJ, Schlumpf RB, et al. Effect of simultaneous liver retrieval, retrieval team, and preservation time on cadaver whole-organ, bladder-drained pancreatic allograft survival rates. Transplant Proc 1991; 23:1640–1642.
92. Gruessner RW, Sutherland DE. Simultaneous kidney and segmental pancreas transplants from living related donors - the first two successful cases. Transplantation 1996; 61:1265–1268.
93. Gruessner RW, Dunn DL, Tzardis PJ, et al. An immunological comparison of pancreas transplants alone in nonuremic patients versus simultaneous pancreas/kidney transplants in uremic diabetic patients. Transplant Proc 1990; 22(No. 4):1581.
94. Gruessner RW, Manivel DC, Dunn DL, Sutherland DE. Pancreaticoduodenal transplantation with enteric drainage following native total pancreatectomy for chronic pancreatitis: a case report. Pancreas 1991; 6:479–488.
95. Gruessner RW, Dunn DL, Tzardis PJ, et al. Simultaneous pancreas and kidney transplants versus single kidney transplants and previous kidney transplants in uremic patients and single pancreas transplants in nonuremic diabetic patients: comparison of rejection, morbidity, and long-term outcome Transplant Proc 1990; 22 (No.2):622–623.
96. Gruessner RW, Nakhleh RE, Tzardis P, et al. Rejection patterns after simultaneous pancreaticoduodenal-kidney transplants in pigs. Transplantation 1994; 57:756–760.
97. Sutherland DE, Gruessner RW, Moudry-Munns KC, Gruessner A. Discordant graft loss from rejection of organs from the same donor in simultaneous pancreas-kidney recipients. Transplant Proc 1995; 27(No. 1):907–908.
98. Gruessner RW, Nakhleh RE, Tzardis P, et al. Differences in rejection grading after simultaneous pancreas and kidney transplantation in pigs. Transplantation 1993; 56:1357–1364.
99. Jones JW, Nakhleh RE, Casanova D, Sutherland DE, Gruessner RW. Cystoscopic transduodenal pancreas transplant biopsy: a new needle. Transplant Proc 1994; 26(2):527–528.
100. Nakhleh RE, Sutherland DE, Benedetti E, Goswitz JJ, Gruessner RW. Diagnostic utility and correlation of duodenal and pancreas biopsy tissue in pancreaticoduodenal transplants with emphasis on therapeutic use. Transplant Proc 1995; 27(No. 1):1327–1328.
101. Benedetti E, Najarian JS, Gruessner A, et al. Correlation between cystoscopic biopsy results and hypoamylasuria in bladder-drained pancreas transplants. Surgery 1995; 118:864–872.
102. Burke GW, Gruessner RW, Dunn DL, Sutherland DE. Conversion of whole pancreaticoduodenal transplants from bladder to enteric drainage for metabolic acidosis or dysuria. Transplant Proc 1990; 22(No. 2):651–652.
103. Stephanian E, Gruessner RW, Brayman KL, et al. Conversion of exocrine secretions from bladder to enteric drainage in recipients of whole pancreaticoduodenal transplants. Ann Surg 1992; 216(No. 6):663–672.
104. Gruessner RW, Stephanian E, Dunn DL, Gruessner A, Najarian JS, Sutherland DE. Cystoenteric conversion after whole pancreaticoduodenal transplantation: indications, risk factors, and outcome. Transplant Proc 1993; 25(No. 1):1179–1181.

105. Pescovitz MD, Dunn DL, Sutherland DE. Use of the circular stapler in construction of the duodenoneocystostomy for drainage into the bladder in transplants involving the whole pancreas. Surg Gynecol Obstet 1989; 169:169–171.
106. Marsh CL, Perkins JD, Sutherland DE, Corry RJ, Sterioff S. Combined hepatic and pancreaticoduodenal procurement for transplantation. Surg Gynecol Obstet 1989; 168:254–258.
107. Dunn DL, Schlumpf RB, Gruessner RW, et al. Maximal use of liver and pancreas from cadaveric organ donors. Transplant Proc 1990; 22(No. 2):423–424.
108. Sutherland DE, Morel P, Gruessner RW. Transplantation of two diabetic patients with one divided cadaver donor pancreas. Transplant Proc 1990; 22(No. 2):585.
109. Morel P, Moudry-Munns KC, Najarian JS, Gruessner RW, Dunn DL, Sutherland DE. Influence of preservation time on outcome and metabolic function of bladder-drained pancreas transplants. Transplantation 1990; 49:294–303.
110. Gores PF, Gillingham KJ, Dunn DL, Moudry-Munns KC, Najarian JS, Sutherland DE. Donor hyperglycemia as a minor risk factor and immunologic variables as major risk factors for pancreas allograft loss in multivariate analysis of a single institution's experience. Ann Surg 1992; 215:217–230.
111. Gruessner RW, Dunn DL, Gruessner A, Matas AJ, Najarian JS, Sutherland DE. Recipient risk factors have an impact on technical failure and patient and graft survival rates in bladder-drained pancreas transplants. Transplantation 1994; 57:1598–1606.
112. Manske CL, Wang Y, Rector T. Coronary revascularization in insulin-dependent diabetic patients with chronic renal failure. Lancet 1992; 340:998.
113. Sutherland DER, Goetz FC, Sibley RK. Recurrence of disease in pancreas transplants. Diabetes 1989; 38(suppl 1):85–87.
114. Diem P, Abid M, Redmon JB, Sutherland DE, Robertson RP. Systemic venous drainage of pancreas allografts as independent cause of hyperinsulinemia in Type I diabetic recipients. Diabetes 1990; 39:534–540.
115. Morel P, Goetz FC, Moudry-Munns KC, Freier EF, Sutherland DE. Serial glycosylated hemoglobin levels in diabetic recipients of pancreatic transplants. Transplant Proc 1990; 22(No. 2):649–650.
116. Diem P, Redmon JB, Abid M, et al. Glucagon, catecholamine and pancreatic polypeptide secretion in Type I diabetic recipients of pancreas allografts. J Clin Invest 1990; 86:2008–2013.
117. Morels P, Goetz FC, Moudry-Munns KC, Freier EF, Sutherland DE. Long term glucose control in patients with pancreatic transplants. Ann Intern Med 1991; 115:694–699.
118. Robertson RP, Kendall DM, Sutherland DE. Long-term metabolic control with pancreatic transplantation. Transplant Proc 1994; 26(2):386–387.
119. Kennedy WR, Navarro X, Goetz FC, Sutherland DE, Najarian JS. Effects of pancreatic transplantation on diabetic neuropathy. N Engl J Med 1990; 322:1031–1037.
120. Navarro X, Kennedy WR, Loewensen RB, Sutherland DE. Influence of pancreas transplantation on cardiorespiratory reflexes, nerve conduction, and mortality in diabetes mellitus. Diabetes 1990; 39:802–806.
121. Bilous RW, Mauer SM, Sutherland DE, Najarian JS, Goetz FC, Steffes MW. The effects of pancreas transplantation on the glomerular structure of renal allografts in patients with insulin-dependent diabetes. N Engl J Med 1989; 321:80–85.
122. Gruessner RW, Sutherland DE, Drangstveit MB, Troppmann C, Gruessner A. Use of FK506 in pancreas transplantation. Transplant Intern 1996; 9:251–258.
123. Gruessner RW, Sutherland DE, Drangstveit MB, Wrenshall LE, Humar A, Gruessner A. Mycophenolate mofetil in pancreas transplantation. Transplantation 1998; 66:318–323.
124. Gruessner RW, Sutherland DE, Drangstveit MB, West M, Gruessner A. Mycophenolate mofetil and tacrolimus for induction and maintenance therapy after pancreas transplantation. Transplant Proc 1998; 30:518–520.
125. Humar A, Kandaswamy R, Granger DK, Gruessner RW, Gruessner A, Sutherland DE. Decreased surgical risks of pancres transplantation in the modern era. Ann Surg 2000; 231:269–275.
126. Laftavi MR, Gruessner A, Bland BJ, et al. Diagnosis of pancreas rejection. Transplantation 1998; 65:528–532.
127. Laftavi MR, Gruessner A, Bland BJ, et al. Significance of pancreas graft biopsy in detection of rejection. Transplant Proc 1998; 30:642–644.
128. Robertson RP, Sutherland DE, Kendall DM, Teuscher AU, Gruessner RW, Gruessner A. Characterization of long-term successful pancreas transplants in type I diabetes. J Invest Med 1996; 44:549–555.
129. Robertson RP, Sutherland DE, Lanz KJ. Normoglycemia and preserved insulin secretory reserve in diabetic patients 10–18 years after pancreas transplantation. Diabetes 1999; 48:1737–1740.
130. Kennedy WR, Navarro X, Sutherland DE. Neuropathy profile of diabetic patients in a pancreas transplantation program. Neurology 1995; 45:773–780.
131. Fioretto P, Steffes MW, Mihatsch MJ, Strom EH, Sutherland DE, Mauer SM. Cyclosporine associated lesions in native kidneys of diabetic pancreas transplant recipients. Kidney Int 1995; 48:489–495.
132. Navarro X, Sutherland DE, Kennedy WR. Long-term effects of pancreatic transplantation on diabetic neuropathy. Ann Neurology 1997; 42:727–736.
133. Navarro X, Kennedy WR, Aeppli D, Sutherland DE. Neuropathy and mortality in diabetes: influence of pancreas transplantation. Muscle Nerve 1996; 19:1009–1016.

134. Fioretto P, Steffes MW, Sutherland DE, Goetz FC, Mauer SM. Reversal of lesions of diabetic nephropathy after pancreas transplantation. N Engl J Med 1998; 339:69–75.
135. Schulz T, Martin D, Heimes M, Klempnauer J, Buesing M. Tacrolimus/mycophenolate mofetil/steroid-based immunosuppression after pancreas-kidney transplantation with single shot antithymocyte globulin. Transplant Proc 1998; 30:1533–1535.
136. Sutherland DE, Gruessner RW, Humar A, et al. Pancreas (PX) transplantation (Tx) alone (PTA) for non-uremic diabetic patients: a 20 year experience. Transplantation 2000; 69:S268.
137. Sutherland DE, Gruessner RG, Humar A, et al. Pretransplant immunosuppression for pancreas transplants alone in nonuremic diabetic recipients. Transplant Proc 2001; 33:1656–1658.
138. Humar A, Parr E, Drangstveit MB, Kandaswamy R, Gruessner A, Sutherland DE. Steroid withdrawal in pancreas transplant recipients. Clin Transplant 2000; 14:75–78.
139. Gruessner RW, Sutherland DE, Parr E, Humar A, Gruessner AC. A prospective, randomized, open-label study of steroid withdrawal in pancreas transplantation-a preliminary report with 6-month follow-up. Transplant Proc 2001; 33:1663–1664.
140. Denny R, Asolati M, Dunn D, Sutherland D, Gillingham K, Matas A. Potent immunosuppression, CMV prophylaxis, and CMV risk [abstr]. Am J Transplant 2002; 2(suppl 3):404.
141. Humar A, Khwaja K, Ramcharan T, et al. Chronic rejection: the next major challenge for pancreas transplant recipients. Transplantation 2003; 76:918–923.
142. Humar A, Ramcharan T, Kandaswamy R, Gruessner RW, Gruessner AC, Sutherland DE. Technical failures after pancreas transplants: why grafts fail and the risk factors—a multivariate analysis. Transplantation 2004; 78:1188–1192.
143. Humar A, Ramcharan T, Kandaswamy R, Gruessner RW, Gruessner AG, Sutherland DE. The impact of donor obesity on outcomes after cadaver pancreas transplants. Am J Transplant 2004; 4:605–610.
144. Humar A, Kandaswamy R, Drangstveit MB, Parr E, Gruessner AG, Sutherland DE. Surgical risks and outcome of pancreas retransplants. Surgery 2000; 127:634–640.
145. Florack G, Sutherland DE, Morel P, Condie RM, Najarian JS. Effective preservation of human pancreas grafts. Transplant Proc 1989; 21(No. 1):1369–1371.
146. Humar A, Kandaswamy R, Drangstveit MB, Parr E, Gruessner AG, Sutherland DE. Prolonged preservation increases surgical complications after pancreas transplants. Surgery 2000; 127: 545–551.
147. Tanioka Y, Sutherland DE, Kuroda Y, et al. Excellence of the two-layer method (University of Wisconsinn solution/perfluorochemical in pancreas preservation before islet isolation. Surgery 1997; 122:435–442. Ref Type: Journal (Full).
148. Matsumoto S, Kandaswamy R, Sutherland DE, et al. Clinical application of the two-layer (University of Wisconsin Solution/Perfluorochemical plus O2) method of pancreas preservation before transplantation. Transplantation 2000; 70:771–774.
149. Matas AJ, Humar A, Kandaswamy R, Payne WD, Gruessner RW, Sutherland DE. Kidney and pancreas transplantation without a crossmatch in select circumstances—it can be done. Clin Transplant 2001; 15:236–239.
150. Kandaswamy R, Sutherland DE, Humar A, Payne WD, Gruessner RW, Matas AJ. Transplantation without a final crossmatch-it can be done. Transplant Proc 2001; 33:1234.
151. Khwaja K, Wijkstrom M, Gruessner A, Noreen H, Sutherland D, Gruessner R. Pancreas transplantation in cross-match-positive recipients using cyclosporine- or tacrolimus-based immunosuppression. Transplant Proc 2002; 34:1901.
152. Khwaja K, Wijkstrom M, Gruessner A, et al. Pancreas transplantation in crossmatch-positive recipients. Clin Transplant 2003; 17:242–248.
153. Gruessner RW, Sutherland DE, Drangstveit MB, Bland BJ, Gruessner AC. Pancreas transplants from living donors: short- and long-term outcome. Transplant Proc 2001; 33:819–820.
154. Gruessner RW, Kandaswamy R, Denny R. Laparoscopic simultaneous nephrectomy and distal pancreatectomy from a live donor. J Am Coll Surg 2001; 193:333–337.
155. Humar A, Ramcharan T, Kandaswamy R, et al. Pancreas after kidney transplants. Am J Surg 2001; 182:155–161.
156. Gruessner AC, Sutherland DE, Dunn DL, et al. Pancreas after kidney transplants in posturemic patients with type I diabetes mellitus. J Am Soc Nephrol 2001; 12:2490–2499.
157. Molina JE, Sutherland DE, Wang Y, Gruessner AC, Bland BJ. Coronary bypass before simultaneous pancreas-kidney transplants for type 1 diabetics in renal failure. World J Surg 2004; 28: 1036–1039.
158. Paty BW, Lanz K, Kendall DM, Sutherland DE, Robertson RP. Restored hypoglycemic counterregulation is stable in successful pancreas transplant recipients for up to 19 years after transplantation. Transplantation 2001; 72:1103–1107.
159. Robertson RP, Lanz KJ, Sutherland DE, Seaquist ER. Relationship between diabetes and obesity 9 to 18 years after hemipancreatectomy and transplantation in donors and recipients. Transplantation 2002; 73:736–741.
160. Robertson RP, Sutherland DE, Seaquist ER, Lanz KJ. Glucagon, catecholamine, and symptom responses to hypoglycemia in living donors of pancreas segments. Diabetes 2003; 52:1689–1694.

161. Sutherland DE, Kandaswamy R, Humar A, Gruessner RG. Calcineurin-inhibitor free protocols: use of the anti-T-cell agent campath H-1 for maintenance immunosuppression in pancreas and pancreas kidney recipients [abstr]. Clin Transplant 2004; 18(suppl 13):14–15.

162. Gruessner RW, Kandaswamy R, Humar A, Gruessner AC, Sutherland DE. Calcineurin inhibitor- and steroid-free immunosuppression in pancreas-kidney and solitary pancreas transplantation. Transplantation 2005; 79:1184–1189.

163. Gruessner RW, Kandaswamy R, Dunn T, Humar A, Gruessner AC, Sutherland DE. Calcineurin inhibitor-free and steroid-free immunosuppression in pancreas-kidney and solitary pancreas transplantation [abstr]. Am J Transplant 2005; 5(11):267.

164. Paraskevas S, Coad JE, Gruessner A, et al. Posttransplant lymphoproliferative disorder in pancreas transplantation: a single-center experience. Transplantation 2005; 80:613–622.

165. Sutherland DE. Pancreas and islet transplant population. In: Gruessner RW, Sutherland DE, eds. Transplantation of the Pancreas. New York: Springer-Verlag, 2004:91–102.

166. Nath DS, Gruessner AC, Kandaswamy R, Gruessner RW, Sutherland DE, Humar A. Outcomes of pancreas transplants for patients with type 2 diabetes mellitus. Clin Transplant 2005; 19: 792–797.

167. Nath DS, Gruessner A, Kandaswamy R, Gruessner RW, Sutherland DE, Humar A. Late anastomotic leaks in pancreas transplant recipients - clinical characteristics and predisposing factors. Clin Transplant 2005; 19:220–224.

168. Tan M, Kandaswamy R, Sutherland DE, Gruessner RW. Laparoscopic donor distal pancreatectomy for living donor pancreas and pancreas-kidney transplantation. Am J Transplant 2005; 5:1966–1970.

169. Fioretto P, Sutherland DE, Najafian B, Mauer M. Remodeling of renal interstitial and tubular lesions in pancreas transplant recipients. Kidney Int 2006; 69:907–912.

170. Bendel-Stenzel, MR, Kashtan CE, Sutherland DE, Chavers BM. Simultaneous pancreas-kidney transplant in two children with hemolytic-uremic symptom. Pediatr Nephrol 1997; 11:485–487.

171. LaPorte RE, Matsushima M, Chang YF. Prevalence and incidence of insulin-dependent diabetes. In: Harris MI, ed. Diabetes in America. Washington DC: NIH, 1995:37–46.

172. Kendall DM, Sutherland DE, Najarian JS, Goetz FC, Robertson RP. Effects of hemipancreatectomy on insulin secretion and glucose tolerance in healthy humans. N Engl J Med 1990; 322:898–903.

173. Seaquist ER, Kahn SE, Clark PM, Hales CN, Porte D Jr., Robertson P. Hyperproinsulinemia is associated with increased beta cell demand after hemipancreatectomy in humans [abstr]. J Clin Invest 1996; 97:455–460.

174. West M, Gruessner A, Metrakos P, Sutherland DE, Gruessner RW. Conversion from bladder to enteric drainage after pancreaticoduodenal transplantations. Surgery 1998; 124:883–893.

175. Venstrom JM, McBride MA, Rother KI, Hirshberg B, Orchard TJ, Harlan DM. Survival after pancreas transplantation in patients with diabetes and preserved kidney function. JAMA 2003; 290:2817–2823.

176. Gruessner RW, Sutherland DE, Gruessner AC. Mortality assessment for pancreas transplants. Am J Transplant 2004; 4:2018–2026.

177. Matas AJ, Gillingham KJ, Humar A, Dunn DL, Sutherland DE, Najarian JS. Immunologic and non-immunologic factors: different risks for cadaver and living donor transplantation [see comments]. Transplantation 2000; 69:54–58.

178. Matas AJ, Payne WD, Sutherland DE, et al. 2,500 living donor kidney transplants: a single-center experience. Ann Surg 2001; 234:149–164.

179. Sutherland DE, Gruessner RW, Dunn DC, et al. Lessons Learned from more than 1,000 Pancrea transplants at a single institution. Ann. Surg. 2001, 233(4), April 2001, 463–501.

180. Zehrer CL, Gross CR. Quality of life of pancreas transplant recipients. Diabetologia 1991; 34(suppl 1):S145–S149.

181. Gross CR, Zehrer CL. Health-related quality of life outcomes of pancreas transplant recipients. Clin Transplant 1992; 6(3):165–171.

182. Gross CR, Zehrer CL. Impact of the addition of a pancreas to quality of life in uremic diabetic recipients of kidney transplants. Transplant Proc 1993; 25(No. 1):1293–1295.

183. Zehrer CL, Gross CR. Pevalence of "low blood glucose" symptoms and quality of life in pancreas transplant recipients. Clin Transplant 1993; 7:312–319.

184. Zehrer CL, Gross CR. Patient perceptions of benefits and concerns following pancreas transplantation. Diabetes Educ 1994; 20:216–220.

185. Gross CR, Kangas JR, Lemieux AM, Zehrer CL. One-year change in quality-of-life profiles in patients receiving pancreas and kidney transplants. Transplant Proc 1995; 27:3067–3068.

186. Gross CR, Limwattananon C, Matthees BJ. Quality of life after pancreas transplantation: a review. Clin Transplant 1998; 12:351–361.

187. Morel P, Chau C, Brayman KL, et al. Quality of metabolic control 2 to 12 years after a pancreas transplant. Transplant Proc 1992; 24:835–838.

188. Robertson P. Pancreatic and islet transplantation for diabetes: cures or curiosities? N Engl J Med 1992; 327:1861–1868.

189. Katz H, Homan M, Velosa J, Robertson P, Rizza R. Effects of pancreas transplantation on postprandial glucose metabolism. N Engl J Med 1991; 325:1278–1283.

190. Seaquist ER, Robertson RP. Effects of hemipancreatectomy on pancreatic alpha and beta cell function in healthy human donors. J Clin Invest 1992; 89:1761–1766.
191. Robertson RP. Seminars in medicine of the Beth Israel Hospital, Boston: pancreatic and islet transplantation for diabetes—cures or curiosities? [see comments]. N Engl J Med 1992; 327:1861–1868.
192. Barrou B, Seaquist ER, Robertson P. Pancreas transplantation in diabetic humans normalizes hepatic glucose production during hypoglycemia. Diabetes 1994; 43:661–666.
193. Kendall DM, Rooney DP, Smets YF, Salazar Bolding L, Robertson P. Pancreas transplantation restores epinephrine response and symptom recognition during hypoglycemia in patients with long-standing type I diabetes and autonomic neuropathy. Diabetes 2000; 46:249–257.
194. Teuscher AU, Seaquist ER, Robertson P. Diminished insulin secretory reserve in diabetic pancreas transplant and nondiabetic kidney transplant recipients. Diabetes 1994; 43:593–598.
195. Pyzdrowski KL, Kendall DM, Halter JB, Nakhleh RE, Sutherland DER, Robertson RP. Preserved insulin secretion and insulin independence in recipients of islet autografts. N Engl J Med 1992; 327:220–226.
196. Wahoff DC, Papalois BE, Najarian JS, et al. Autologous islet transplantation to prevent diabetes after pancreatic resection. Ann Surg 1995; 22(4):562–579.
197. Kendall DM, Teuscher AU, Robertson P. Defective glucagon secretion during sustained hypoglycemia following successful islet allo- and autotransplantation in humans. Diabetes 1997; 46:23–27.
198. Gupta V, Wahoff DC, Rooney DP, et al. The defective glucagon response from transplanted intrahepatic pancreatic islets during hypoglycemia is transplantation site-determined. Diabetes 1997; 46: 28–33.
199. Teuscher AU, Kendall DM, Smets YF, Leone JP, Sutherland DE, Robertson RP. Successful islet autotransplantation in humans: functional insulin secretory reserve as an estimate of surviving islet cell mass. Diabetes 1998; 47:324–330.
200. Sutherland DER. Effect of pancreas transplantation on secondary complications of diabetes. In: Dubernard JM, Sutherland DER, eds. International Handbook of Pancreas Transplantation. Boston: Kluwer Academic Publishers, 1989:257–289.
201. DCCT Research Group Diabetes control and complications trial (DCCT): the effect of intensive diabetes treatment in long term complications in IDDM. N Engl J Med 1993; 329:977–986.
202. Solders G, Tydén G, Persson A, Groth CG. Improvement of nerve conduction in diabetic neuropathy: a follow-up study 4 years after combined pancreatic and renal transplantation. Diabetes 1992; 41:946–951.
203. Wilczek H, Jaremko G, Tydén G, Groth CGA. Pancreatic graft protects a simultaneously transplanted kidney from developing diabetic nephropathy: a 1–6 year follow-up study. Transplant Proc 1993; 25:1314–1315.
204. Mauer SM, Steffes MW, Connett J, Najarian JS, Sutherland DER, Barbosa JJ. The development of lesions in the glomerular basement membrane and mesangium after transplantation of normal kidneys to diabetic patients. Diabetes 1983; 32:948–952.
205. Morel P, Sutherland DER, Almond PS, et al. Assessment of renal function in Type I diabetic patients after kidney, pancreas, or combined kidney-pancreas transplantation. Transplantation 1991; 51:1184–1189.
206. Mauer SM, Barbosa J, Vernier RL, et al. Development of diabetic vascular lesions in normal kidneys transplanted into patients with diabetes mellitus. N Engl J Med 1976; 295:916–920.
207. Mauer SM, Goetz FC, McHugh LE, et al. Long-term study of normal kidneys transplanted into patients with type I diabetes. Diabetes 1989; 38:516–523.
208. Najarian JS, Kaufman DB, Fryd DS, et al. Long-term survival following kidney transplantation in 100 Type I diabetic patients. Transplantation 1989; 47:106–113.
209. Fioretto P, Mauer SM, Bilous RW, Goetz FC, Sutherland DER, Steffes MW. Effects of pancreas transplantation on glomerular structure in insulin-dependent diabetic patients with their own kidneys. Lancet 1993; 342:1193–1196.
210. Troppmann C, Gruessner RWG, Matas AJ, et al. Results with renal transplants performed after previous solitary pancreas transplants. Transplant Proc 1994; 26(2):448–449.
211. DCCT Research Group Diabetes control and complications trial (DCCT): update. Diabetes Care 1990; 13:427–433.
212. DCCT Research Group Lifetime benefitsand costs of intensive therapy as practiced in the diabetes control and complications trial. The Diabetes Control and Complications Trial Research Group. JAMA 1997; 277:372.
213. Cheung AT, Perez RV, Chen PC. Improvements in diabetic microangiopathy after successful simultaneous pancreas-kidney transplantation: a computer-assisted intravital microscopy study on the conjunctival microcirculation. Transplantation 1999; 68:927–932.
214. Abendroth D, Landgraf R, Pfeiffer M, Reininger J, Seidel D, Land W. Diabetic microangiopathy and blood viscosity changes after pancreas and kidney transplantation. Transplant Proc 1994; 26:491–492.
215. Chow VC, Pai RP, Chapman JR, et al. Diabetic retinopathy after combined kidney-pancreas transplantation. Clin Transplant 1999; 13:356–362.
216. Allen RD, Al Harbi IS, Morris JG, et al. Diabetic neuropathy after pancreas transplantation: determinants of recovery. Transplantation 1997; 63:830–838.
217. Hering BJ, Ricordi C. Islet transplantation for patients with type I diabetes. Graft 1999; 2:12–27.

218. Matsumoto S, Noguchi H, Yonekawa Y, et al. Pancreatic islet transplantation for treating diabetes. Expert Opin Biol Ther 2006; 6:23–37.
219. Hering BJ. Achieving and maintaining insulin independence in human islet transplant recipients. Transplantation 2005; 79:1296–1297.
220. Shapiro AM, Lakey JR, Paty BW, Senior PA, Bigam DL, Ryan EA. Strategic opportunities in clinical islet transplantation. Transplantation 2005; 79:1304–1307.
221. Ricordi C, Strom TB. Clinical islet transplantation: advances and immunological challenges. Nat Rev Immunol 2004; 4:259–268.
222. Robertson RP. Islet transplantation as a treatment for diabetes - a work in progress. N Engl J Med 2004; 350:694–705.
223. Shapiro AM, Nanji SA, Lakey JR. Clinical islet transplant: current and future directions towards tolerance. Immunol Rev 2003; 196:219–236.
224. Cohen DJ, St ML, Christensen LL, Bloom RD, Sung RS. Kidney and pancreas transplantation in the United States, 1995–2004. Am J Transplant 2006; 6:1153–1169.
225. Stock PG, Bluestone JA. Beta-cell replacement for type I diabetes. Annu Rev Med 2004; 55: 133–156.
226. Shapiro AMJ, Lakey JRT, Ryan E, et al. Insulin independence after solitary islet transplantation in type I diabetic patients using steroid free immunosuppression. N Engl J Med 2000; 343:230–238.
227. Ryan EA, Paty BW, Senior PA, et al. Five-year follow-up after clinical islet transplantation. Diabetes 2005; 54:2060–2069.
228. Froud T, Ricordi C, Baidal DA, et al. Islet transplantation in type 1 diabetes mellitus using cultured islets and steroid-free immunosuppression: Miami experience. Am J Transplant 2005; 5:2037–2046.
229. Toso C, Baertschiger R, Morel P, et al. Sequential kidney/islet transplantation: efficacy and safety assessment of a steroid-free immunosuppression protocol. Am J Transplant 2006; 6:1049–1058.
230. Matsumoto S, Okitsu T, Iwanaga Y, et al. Insulin independence after living-donor distal pancreatectomy and islet allotransplantation. Lancet 2005; 365:1642–1644.
231. Corry RJ, Chakrabarti PK, Shapiro R, et al. Simultaneous administration of adjuvant donor bone marrow in pancreas transplant recipients. Ann Surg 1999; 230:372–379.
232. Stratta RJ, Gaber AO, Shokouh-Amiri MH, et al. Evolution in pancreas transplantation techniques: simultaneous kidney-pancreas translantation using portal-enteric drainage without antilymphocyte induction. Ann Surg 2000; 229:701–708.
233. Kaufman DB, Leventhal JR, Stuart J, Abecassis MM, Fryer JP, Stuart FP. Mycophenolate mofetil and tacrolimus as primary maintenance immunosuppression in simultaneous pancreas-kidney transplantation: initial experience in 50 consecutive cases. Transplantation 1999; 67:586–593.
234. Tyden G, Bolinder J, Solders G, Brattstrom C, Tibell A, Groth CG. Improved survival in patients with insulin-dependent diabetes mellitus and end-stage diabetic nephropathy 10 years after combined pancreas and kidney transplantation. Transplantation 1999; 67:645–648.
235. Sollinger HW, Odorico JS, Knechtle SJ, D'Alessandro AM, Kalayoglu M, Pirsch JD. Experience with 500 simultaneous pancreas-kidney transplants. Ann Surg 1998; 228:284–296.
236. Henry ML, Elkhammas EA, Bumgardner GL, Pelletier RP, Ferguson RM. Outcome of 300 consecutive pancreas-kidney transplants. Transplant Proc 1998; 30:291.
237. Bartlett ST, Schweitzer EJ, Johnson LB, et al. Equivalent success of simultaneous pancreas kidney and solitary pancreas transplantation. A prospective trial of tacrolimus immunosuppression with percutaneous biopsy. Ann Surg 1996; 224:440–449.
238. Di Landro D, Koenigsrainer A, Oefner D, Aichberger C, Romagnoli GF, Margreiter R. Experience with 100 combined pancreatic renal transplantations in a single center. Nephron 1996; 72: 547–551.
239. Stratta RJ, Rohr MS, Adams PL, et al. Kidney and pancreas transplantation at Wake Forest University Baptist Medical Center. Clinical Transplants 2003; 229–245.
240. Di CA, Odorico JS, Leverson GE, et al. Long-term outcomes in simultaneous pancreas-kidney transplantation: lessons relearned. Clinical Transplants 2003; 215–220.
241. Elkhammas EA, Henry ML, Akin B, et al. Simultaneous pancreas-kidney transplantation at a single center. Clinical Transplants 2003; 221–227.
242. Philosophe B, Farney AC, Schweitzer EJ, et al. Simultaneous pancreas-kidney (SPK) and pancreas living-donor kidney (SPLK) transplantation at the University of Maryland. Clinical Transplants 2000; 211–216.
243. Stratta RJ, Shokouh-Amiri MH, Egidi MF, et al. A prospective comparison of simultaneous kidney-pancreas transplantation with systemic-enteric versus portal-enteric drainage. Ann Surg 2001; 233:740–751.
244. Jordan ML, Chakrabarti P, Luke P, et al. Results of pancreas transplantation after steroid withdrawal under tacrolimus immunosuppression. Transplantation 2000; 69:265–271.
245. Kaufman DB, Leventhal JR, Gallon LG, Parker MA. Alemtuzumab induction and prednisone-free maintenance immunotherapy in simultaneous pancreas-kidney transplantation comparison with rabbit antithymocyte globulin induction - long-term results. Am J Transplant 2006; 6:331–339.
246. Freise CE, Kang SM, Feng S, Hirose R, Stock P. Excellent short-term results with steroid-free maintenance immunosuppression in low-risk simultaneous pancreas-kidney transplantation. Arch Surg 2003; 138:1121–1125.

247. Cantarovich D, Karam G, Hourmant M, et al. Steroid avoidance versus steroid withdrawal after simultaneous pancreas-kidney transplantation. Am J Transplant 2005; 5:1332–1338.
248. Fernandez LA, Di CA, Odorico JS, et al. Simultaneous pancreas-kidney transplantation from donation after cardiac death: successful long-term outcomes. Ann Surg 2005; 242:716–723.
249. Boggi U, Vistoli F, Signori, S, et al. A technique for retroperitoneal pancreas transplantation with portal-enteric drainage. Transplantation 2005; 79:1137–1142.
250. Philosophe B, Farney AC, Schweitzer E, et al. The superiority of portal venous drainage over systemic venous drainage in pancreas transplantation. Ann Surg 2001; 234:689–696.
251. Rayhill SC, D'Alessandro AM, Odorico JS, et al. Simultaneous pancreas-kidney transplantation and living related donor renal transplantation in patients with diabetes: is there a difference in survival? Ann Surg 2000; 231:417–423.
252. Becker BN, Pintar TJ, Becker Y. Simultaneous pancreas kidney transplantation reduces excess mortality in Type I diabetes patients with ESRD. Kidney Int 2000; 57:2129–2135.
253. Smets YF, Westendorp RG, van der Pijl JW, et al. Effect of simultaneous pancreas-kidney transplantation on mortality of patients with type-1 diabetes mellitus and end-stage renal failure. Lancet 1999; 353:1915–1919.
254. Tyden G, Tollemar J, Bolinder J. Combined pancreas and kidney transplantation improves survival in patients with end-stage diabetic nephropathy. Clin Transplant 2000; 14:505–508.
255. Biesenbach G, Konigsrainer A, Gross C, Margreiter R. Progression of macrovascular diseases is reduced in type 1 diabetic patients after more than 5 years successful combined pancreas-kidney transplantation in comparison to kidney transplantation alone. Transpl Int 2005; 18:1054–1060.
256. Stratta RJ, Weide LG, Sindhi R, et al. Solitary pancreas transplantation. Experience with 62 consecutive cases. Diabetes Care 1997; 20:362–368.
257. Zielinski A, Nazarewski S, Bogetti D, et al. Simultaneous pancreas-kidney transplant from living related donor: a single-center experience. Transplantation 2003; 76:547–552.
258. Sammartino C, Pham T, Panaro F, et al. Successful simultaneous pancreas kidney transplantation from living-related donor against positive cross-match. Am J Transplant 2004; 4:140–143.
259. Benedetti E, Dunn T, Massad MG, et al. Successful living related simultaneous pancreas-kidney transplant between identical twins. Transplantation 1999; 67:915–918.
260. Farney AC, Cho E, Schweitzer E, et al. Simultaneous cadaver pancreas living donor kidney transplantation (SPLK): a new approach for the type 1 diabetic uremic patient. Ann Surg 2000; 232:696–703.
261. Boudreaux JP, Corry RJ, Dickerman R, Sutherland DER. Combined experience with immediate pancreas retransplantation. Transplant Proc 1991; 23:1628–1629.
262. Fernandez-Cruz L, Gilabert R, Sabater L, Saenz A, Astudillo E. Pancreas graft thrombosis: Prompt diagnosis and immediate thrombectomy or retransplantation. Clin Transplant 1993; 7:230.
263. Sansalone CV, Aseni P, Follini ML, et al. Early pancreas retransplantation for vascular thrombosis in simultaneous pancreas-kidney transplants. Transplant Proc 1998; 30:253–254.
264. Gruessner RW, Sutherland DE, Dunn DL, et al. Transplant options for patients undergoing total pancreatectomy for chronic pancreatitis. J Am Coll Surg 2004; 198:559–567.
265. Stern RC, Mayes JT, Weber FL Jr., Blades EW, Schulak JA. Restoration of exocrine pancreatic function following pancreas-liver-kidney transplantation in a cystic fibrosis patient. Clin Transplant 1994; 8:1–4.
266. Sutherland DER, Gruessner RG, Jie T, et al. Pancreatic islet auto-transplantation for chronic pancreatitis [abstr]. Clinical Transplantation 2004; 18(suppl 13):17–18.
267. Jie T, Hering BJ, Ansite JD, et al. Pancreatectomy and auto-islet transplant in patients with chronic pancreatitis [abstr]. J Am Coll Surg 2005; 201(suppl 3):S14.
268. Kuo PC, Johnson LB, Schweitzer EJ, Bartlett ST. Simultaneous pancreas/kidney transplantation—a comparison of enteric and bladder drainage of exocrine pancreatic secretions. Transplantation 1997; 63:238–243.
269. Pirsch JD, Odorico JS, D'Alessandro AM, Knechtle SJ, Becker BN, Sollinger HW. Posttransplant infection in enteric versus bladder-drained simultaneous pancreas-kidney transplant recipients. Transplantation 1998; 66:1746–1750.
270. Feitosa Tajra LC, Dawhara M, Benchaib M, Lefrancois N, Martin X, Dubernard JM. Effect of the surgical technique on long-term outcome of pancreas transplantation. Transpl Int 1998; 11:295–300.
271. Sugitani A, Gritsch HA, Shapiro R, Bonham CA, Egidi MF, Corry RJ. Surgical complications in 123 consecutive pancreas transplant recipients: comparison of bladder and enteric drainage. Transplant Proc 1998; 30:293–294.
272. Douzdjian V, Rajagopalan PR. Primary enteric drainage of the pancreas allograft revisited. J Am Coll Surg 1997; 185:471–475.
273. Tyden G, Tibell A, Sandberg J, Brattstrom C, Groth CG. Improved results with a simplified technique for pancreaticoduodenal transplantation with enteric exocrine drainage. Clin Transplant 1996; 10:306–309.
274. Calne RY. Paratopic segmental pancreas grafting: a technique with portal venous drainage. Lancet 1984; 1:595–597.
275. Gil-Vernet JM, Fernandez-Cruz L, Caralps A, Andreu J, Figuerola D. Whole organ and pancreaticoureterostomy in clinical pancreas transplantation. Transplant Proc 1985; 17:2019–2022.

276. Tyden G, Brattstrom C, Lundgren G, et al. Pancreatic transplantation with enteric exocrine diversion—the Stockholm experience. Transplant Proc 1987; 19:86–91.
277. Rosenlof LK, Earnhardt RC, Pruett TL, et al. Pancreas transplantation: an initial experience with systemic and portal drainage of pancreatic allografts. Ann Surg 1992; 215:586–595.
278. Stratta RJ, Gaber AO, Shokouh-Amiri MH, et al. Experience with portal-enteric pancreas transplant at the University of Tennessee-Memphis. Clinical Transplants 1998; 239–253.
279. Bruce DS, Newell KA, Woodle ES, et al. Synchronous pancreas-kidney transplantation with portal venous and enteric exocrine drainage: outcome in 70 consecutive cases. Transplant Proc 1998; 30:270–271.
280. Reddy KS, Stratta RJ, Shokouh-Amiri MH, Alloway R, Egidi MF, Gaber AO. Surgical complications after pancreas transplantation with portal-enteric drainage. J Am Coll Surg 1999; 189:305–313.
281. Kaplan B, Wang Z, Abecassis MM, Fryer JP, Stuart FP, Kaufman DB. Frequency of hyperkalemia in recipients of simultaneous pancreas and kidney transplants with bladder drainage. Transplantation 1996; 62:1174–1175.
282. Sindhi R, Stratta RJ, Lowell JA, et al. Experience with enteric conversion after pancreatic transplantation with bladder drainage. J Am Coll Surg 1997; 184:281–289.
283. Ploeg RJ, Eckhoff DE, D'Alessandro AM, et al. Urological complications and enteric conversion after pancreas transplantation with bladder drainage. Transplant Proc 1994; 26:458–459.
284. Nath D, Gruessner A, Kandaswamy R, Gruessner R, Sutherland D, Humar A. Late anastomotic leaks in pancreas transplant recipients—clinical charactersistics and predisposing factors [abstr]. Am J Transplant 2004; 4(8):381.
285. Troppmann C, Gruessner A, Benedetti E, et al. Vascular graft thrombosis after pancreatic transplantation: Univariate and multivariate operative and nonoperative risk factor analysis. J Am Coll Surg 1996; 182:285–316.
286. Sollinger H. Pancreatic transplantation and vascular graft thrombosis (Editorial). J Am Coll Surg 1996; 182:362.
287. Benedetti E, Gruessner AC, Troppmann C, et al. Intra-abdominal fungal infections after pancreatic transplantation: incidence, treatment, and outcome (see comments). J Am Coll Surg 1996; 183:307–316.
288. Benedetti E, Troppmann C, Gruessner AC, Sutherland DE, Dunn DL, Gruessner WG. Pancreas graft loss caused by intra-abdominal infection. A risk factor for a subsequent pancreas retransplantation. Arch Surg 1996; 131:1054–1060.
289. Nath DS, Kandaswamy R, Gruessner R, Sutherland DE, Dunn DL, Humar A. Fungal infections in transplant recipients receiving alemtuzumab. Transplant Proc 2005; 37:934–936.
290. Dunn DL, Gillingham KJ, Kramer MA, et al. A prospective randomized study of acyclovir versus ganciclovir plus human immune globulin prophylaxis of cytomegalovirus infection after solid organ transplantation. Transplantation 1994; 57(6):876–884.
291. Somerville T, Hurst G, Alloway R, Gaber A, Shokouh-Amiri MH, Stratta R. Superior efficacy of oral ganciclovir over oral acyclovir for cytomegalovirus prophylaxis in kidney-pancreas and pancreas alone recipients. Transplant Proc 1998; 30:1546–1548.
292. Hassoun A, Humar A, Kandaswamy R, et al. The low incidence of PTLD after pancreas and simultaneous kidney-pancreas transplant [abstr]. Transplantation 1999; 67:S208.
293. Drachenberg CB, Abruzzo LV, Klassen DK, et al. Epstein-Barr virus-related posttransplantation lymphoproliferative disorder involving pancreas allografts: histological differential diagnosis from acute allograft rejection. Hum Pathol 1998; 29:569–577.
294. Keay S, Oldach D, Wiland A, et al. Posttransplantation lymphoproliferative disorder associated with OKT3 and decreased antiviral prophylaxis in pancreas transplant recipients. Clin Infect Dis 1998; 26:596–600.
295. Darenkov IA, Marcarelli MA, Basadonna GP, et al. Reduced incidence of Epstein-Barr virus-associated posttransplant lymphoproliferative disorder using preemptive antiviral therapy. Transplantation 1997; 64:848–852.
296. Martinenghi S, Dell'Antonio G, Secchi A, Di CV, Pozza G. Cancer arising after pancreas and/or kidney transplantation in a series of 99 diabetic patients. Diabetes Care 1997; 20:272–275.
297. Sasaki TM, Pirsch JD, D'Alessandro AM, et al. Increased beta 2-microglobulin (B2M) is useful in the detection of post- transplant lymphoproliferative disease (PTLD). Clin Transplant 1997; 11:29–33.
298. McAlister VC, Gao Z, Peltekian K, Domingues J, Mahalati K, MacDonald AS. Sirolimus-tacrolimus combination immunosuppression [letter]. Lancet 2000; 355:376–377.
299. Jordan ML, Shapiro R, Gritsch HA, et al. Long-term results of pancreas transplantation under tacrolius immunosuppression. Transplantation 1999; 67:266–272.
300. Odorico JS, Pirsch JD, Knechtle SJ, D'Alessandro AM, Sollinger HW. A study comparing mycophenolate mofetil to azathioprine in simultaneous pancreas-kidney transplantation. Transplantation 1998; 66:1751–1759.
301. Peddi VR, Kamath S, Munda R, Demmy AM, Alexander JW, First MR. Use of tacrolimus eliminates acute rejection as a major complication following simultaneous kidney and pancreas transplantation. Clin Transplant 1998; 12:401–405.
302. Stratta RJ. Sequential pancreas after kidney transplantation: is anti-lymphocyte induction therapy needed? Transplant Proc 1998; 30:1549–1551.

303. Burke GW, Ciancio G, Alejandro R, et al. Use of tacrolimus and mycophenolate mofetil for pancreas-kidney transplantation with or without OKT3 induction. Transplant Proc 1998; 30: 1544–1545.

304. Elkhammas EA, Yilmaz S, Henry ML, et al. Simultaneous pancreas/kidney transplantation: comparison of mycophenolate mofetil versus azathioprine. Transplant Proc 1998; 30:512.

305. Peddi VR, Kamath S, Schroeder TJ, Munda R, First MR. Efficacy of OKT3 as primary therapy for histologically confirmed acute renal allograft rejection in simultaneous kidney and pancreas transplant recipients. Transplant Proc 1998; 30:285–287.

306. Demirbas A, Ciancio G, Burke G, et al. FK 506 in simultaneous pancreas/kidney transplantation: the University of Miami experience. Transplant Proc 1997; 29:2903.

307. Sugitani A, Egidi MF, Gritsch HA, Corry RJ. Serum lipase as a marker for pancreatic allograft rejection. Clin Transplant 1998; 12:224–227.

308. Allen RD, Wilson TG, Grierson JM, et al. Percutaneous biopsy of bladder-drained pancreas transplants. Transplantation 1991; 51:1213–1216.

309. Gaber AO, Gaber L, Shokouh-Amiri MH, Hathaway D. Percutaneous biopsy of pancreas transplants. Transplantation 1992; 54:548–550.

310. Drachenberg CB, Klassen DK, Weir MR, et al. Islet cell damage associated with tacrolimus and cyclosporine: morphological features in pancreas allograft biopsies and clinical correlation. Transplantation 1999; 68:396–402.

311. Papadimitriou JC, Drachenberg CB, Wiland A, et al. Histologic grading of acute allograft rejection in pancreas needle biopsy: correlation to serum enzymes, glycemia, and response to immunosuppressive treatment. Transplantation 1998; 66:1741–1745.

312. Drachenberg CB, Papadimitriou JC, Klassen DK, Weir MR, Bartlett ST. Distribution of alpha and beta cells in pancreas allograft biopsies: correlation with rejection and other pathologic processes. Transplant Proc 1998; 30:665–666.

313. Drachenberg CB, Papadimitriou JC, Klassen DK, et al. Evaluation of pancreas transplant needle biopsy: reproducibility and revision of histologic grading system. Transplantation 1997; 63:1579–1586.

314. Egidi MF, Corry RJ, Sugitani A, et al. Enteric-drained pancreas transplants monitored by fine-needle aspiration biopsy. Transplant Proc 1997; 29:674–675.

315. Gill IS, Stratta RJ, Taylor RJ, et al. Correlation of serologic and urinary tests with allograft biopsy in the diagnosis of pancreas rejection. Transplant Proc 1997; 29:673.

316. Kuo PC, Johnson LB, Schweitzer EJ, et al. Solitary pancreas allografts. The role of percutaneous biopsy and standardized histologic grading of rejection. Arch Surg 1997; 132:52–57.

317. Klassen DK, Hoen-Saric EW, Weir MR, et al. Isolated pancreas rejection in combined kidney pancreas tranplantation. Transplantation 1996; 61:974–977.

318. Drachenberg CB, Papadimitriou JC, Farney A, et al. Pancreas transplantation: the histologic morphology of graft loss and clinical correlations. Transplantation 2001; 71:1784–1791.

319. Nakhleh RE, Benedetti E, Gruessner A, et al. Cystoscopic biopsies in pancreaticoduodenal transplantation. Are duodenal biopsies indicative of pancreas dysfunction? Transplantation 1995; 60:541–546.

320. Tyden G, Reinholt FP, Sundkvist G, Bolinder J. Recurrence of autoimmune diabetes mellitus in recipients of cadaveric pancreatic grafts [see comments] [published erratum appears in N Engl J Med 1996; 335(23):1778]. N Engl J Med 1996; 335:860–863.

321. Burke GW, Ciancio G, Laughlin E, Allende G, Nepom G, Pugliese A. Recurrence of autoimmunity in simultaneous pancreas kidney pancreas transplantation is associated with autoantibodies and autoreactive T cells [abst]. Am J Transplant 2005; 5(11):268.

322. Stratta RJ. Patterns of graft loss following simultaneous kidney-pancreas transplantation. Transplant Proc 1998; 30:288.

323. Hawthorne WJ, Allen RD, Greenberg ML, et al. Simultaneous pancreas and kidney transplant rejection: separate or synchronous events? Transplantation 1997; 63:352–358.

324. So SKS, Moudry-Munns KC, Gillingham KJ, Minford EJ, Sutherland DER. Short-term and long-term effects of HLA matching in cadaveric pancreas transplantation. Transplant Proc 1991; 23:1634–1636.

325. Gruessner A, Sutherland DER. Analyses of pancreas transplant outcomes for United States cases reported to the United Network for Organ Sharing (UNOS) and non-US cases reported to the International Pancreas Transplant Registry. In: Cecka JM, Terasaki PI, eds. Clinical Transplant - 1999. Los Angeles: UCLA Immunogenetics Center, 2000:51–69.

326. Basadonna GP, Auersvald LA, Oliveira SC, Friedman AL, Lorber MI. Pancreas after kidney transplantation: HLA mismatch does not preclude success. Transplant Proc 1997; 29:667.

327. Stratta RJ, Lowell JA, Sudan D, Jerius JT. Retransplantation in the diabetic patient with a pancreas allograft. Am J Surg 1997; 174:759–762.

328. Douzdjian V, Rice JC, Carson RW, Gugliuzza KG, Fish JC. Renal allograft failure after simultaneous pancreas-kidney transplantation: univariate and multivariate analyses of donor and recipient risk factors. Clin Transplant 1996; 10:271–277.

329. Douzdjian V, Gugliuzza KG, Fish JC. Multivariate analysis of donor risk factors for pancreas allograft failure after simultaneous pancreas-kidney transplantation. Surgery 1995; 118:73–81.

330. Bumgardner GL, Henry ML, Elkhammas E, et al. Obesity as a risk factor after combined pancreas/kidney transplantation. Transplantation 1995; 60:1426–1430.

331. Douzdjian V, Thacker LR, Blanton JW. Effect of race on outcome following kidney and kidney-pancreas transplantation in type I diabetics: the South-Eastern Organ Procurement Foundation experience. Clin Transplant 1997; 11:470–475.

332. Stratta RJ, Taylor RJ, Lowell JA, et al. Preemptive combined pancreas-kidney transplantation: is earlier better? Transplant Proc 1994; 26:422–424.

333. Mellinghoff AC, Reininger AJ, Land W, Abendroth D, Hepp KD, Landgraf R. Cardiovascular risk profile after simultaneous pancreas and kidney transplantation. Exp Clin Endocrinol Diabetes 1998; 106:460–464.

334. Schweitzer EJ, Anderson L, Kuo PC, et al. Safe pancreas transplantation in patients with coronary artery disease. Transplantation 1997; 63:1294–1299.

335. Kim SI, Elkhammas EA, Henry ML, Davies EA, Bumgadner GL, Ferguson RM. Outcome of combined kidney/pancreas transplantation in recipients with coronary artery disease. Transplant Proc 1995; 27:3071.

336. Sasaki TM, Gray RS, Ratner RE, et al. Successful long-term kidney-pancreas transplants in diabetic patients with high C-peptide levels. Transplantation 1999; 67:586A.

337. Van der Werf WJ, Odorico J, D'Alessandro AM, et al. Utilization of pediatric donors for pancreas transplantation. Transplant Proc 1999; 31:610–611.

338. Fernandez LA, Turgeon NA, Odorico JS, et al. Superior long-term results of simultaneous pancreas-kidney transplantation from pediatric donors. Am J Transplant 2004; 4:2093–2101.

339. Kapur S, Bonham CA, Dodson SF, Dvorchik I, Corry RJ. Strategies to expand the donor pool for pancreas transplantation. Transplantation 1999; 67:284–290.

340. Stratta RJ, Sundberg AK, Farney AC, Rohr MS, Hartmann EL, Adams PL. Successful simultaneous kidney-pancreas transplantation from extreme donors. Transplant Proc 2005; 37:3535–3537.

341. Odorico JS, Heisey DM, Voss BJ, et al. Donor factors affecting outcome after pancreas transplantation. Transplant Proc 1998; 30:276–277.

342. Stratta RJ. Donor age, organ import, and cold ischemia: effect on early outcomes after simultaneous kidney-pancreas transplantation. Transplant Proc 1997; 29:3291–3292.

343. Cosio FG, Elkhammas EA, Henry ML, et al. Function and survival of renal allografts from the same donor transplanted into kidney-only or kidney-pancreas recipients. Transplantation 1998; 65:93–99.

344. Troppmann C, Gruessner AC, Papalois BE, et al. Delayed endocrine pancreas graft function after simultaneous pancreas-kidney transplantation. Incidence, risk factors, and impact on long-term outcome. Transplantation 1996; 61:1323–1330.

345. Secchi A, Taglietti MV, Socci C, et al. Insulin secretory patterns and blood glucose homeostasis after islet allotransplantation in IDDM patients: comparison with segmental- or whole-pancreas transplanted patients through a long term longitudinal study. J Mol Med 1999; 77:133–139.

346. Nankivell BJ, Chapman JR, Bovington KJ, O'Connell PJ, Allen RD. Glucose homeostasis standards for pancreas transplantation. Clin Transplant 1998; 12:434–438.

347. Tyden G, Bolinder J, Brattstrom C, Tibell A, Grott CG. Long-term metabolic control in recipients of segmental or whole-organ pancreatic grafts with enteric exocrine diversion and function beyond 5 years. Transplant Proc 1998; 30:634.

348. La Rocca E, Gobbi C, Ciurlino D, Di CV, Pozza G, Secchi A. Improvement of glucose/insulin metabolism reduces hypertension in insulin-dependent diabetes mellitus recipients of kidney-pancreas transplantation. Transplantation 1998; 65:390–393.

349. Tibell A, Tyden G, Bolinder J, Larsson M, Groth CG. Metabolic control in recipients of segmental pancreatic grafts functioning beyond 8 years. Transplant Proc 1995; 27:3029–3030.

350. Krebs TL, Daly B, Wong JJ, Chow CC, Bartlett ST. Vascular complications of pancreatic transplantation: MR evaluation. Radiology 1995; 196:793–798.

351. Battezzati A, Luzi L, Perseghin G, et al. Persistence of counter-regulatory abnormalities in insulin-dependent diabetes mellitus after pancreas transplantation. Eur J Clin Invest 1994; 24:751–758.

352. Christiansen E, Tibell A, Volund A, et al. Insulin secretion, insulin action and non-insulin-dependent glucose uptake in pancreas transplant recipients. J Clin Endocrinol Metab 1994; 79:1561–1569.

353. Osei K, Henry M, Ferguson R. Differential effects of systemic insulin delivery and prednisone on tissue glucose and insulin sensitivity in insulin-dependent diabetes mellitus pancreas recipients. Transplant Proc 1994; 26:480–482.

354. Konigsrainer A, Foger B, Steurer W, et al. Influence of hyperinsulinemia on lipoproteins after pancreas transplantation with systemic insulin drainage. Transplant Proc 1998; 30:637–638.

355. Foger B, Konigsrainer A, Palos G, et al. Effects of pancreas transplantation on distribution and composition of plasma lipoproteins. Metabolism 1996; 45:856–861.

356. Foger B, Konigsrainer A, Palos G, et al. Effect of pancreas transplantation on lipoprotein lipase, postprandial lipemia, and HDL cholesterol. Transplantation 1994; 58:899–904.

357. Hawthorne WJ, Wilson TG, Williamson P, et al. Long-term duct-occluded segmental pancreatic autografts: absence of microvascular diabetic complications. Transplantation 1997; 64:953–959.

358. Wang Q, Klein R, Moss SE, et al. The influence of combined kidney-pancreas transplantation on the progression of diabetic retinopathy. A case series. Ophthalmology 1994; 101:1071–1076.

359. Klassen DK, Weir MR, Schweitzer EJ, Bartlett ST. Isolated pancreas rejection in combined kidney-pancreas transplantation: results of percutaneous pancreas biopsy. Transplant Proc 1995; 27:1333–1334.

360. Laftavi MR, Chapuis F, Vial C, et al. Diabetic polyneuropathy outcome after successful pancreas transplantation: 1 to 9 year follow up. Transplant Proc 1995; 27:1406–1409.

361. Gaber AO, el Gebely S, Sugathan P, et al. Changes in cardiac function of type I diabetics following pancreas-kidney and kidney-alone transplantation. Transplant Proc 1995; 27:1322–1323.

362. Martin X. Improvement of diabetic vesicopathy after pancreatic transplantation. Transplant Proc 1995; 27:2441–2443.

363. Gaber AO, Hathaway DK, Abell T, Cardoso S, Hartwig MS, el Gebely S. Improved autonomic and gastric function in pancreas-kidney versus kidney-alone transplantation contributes to quality of life. Transplant Proc 1994; 26:515–516.

364. Secchi A, Martinenghi S, Castoldi R, Giudici D, Di CV, Pozza G. Effects of pancreas transplantation on quality of life in type I diabetic patients undergoing kidney transplantation. Transplant Proc 1998; 30:339–342.

365. Piehlmeier W, Bullinger M, Kirchberger I, Land W, Landgraf R. Evaluation of the quality of life of patients with insulin-dependent diabetes mellitus before and after organ transplantation with the SF 36 health survey. Eur J Surg 1996; 162:933–940.

366. Nakache R, Tyden G, Groth CG. Long-term quality of life in diabetic patients after combined pancreas-kidney transplantation or kidney transplantation. Transplant Proc 1994; 26:510–511.

367. Adang EM, Engel GL, van Hooff JP, Kootstra G. Comparison before and after transplantation of pancreas-kidney and pancreas-kidney with loss of pancreas–a prospective controlled quality of life study. Transplantation 1996; 62:754–758.

368. Kiebert GM, Kaasa S. Quality of life in clinical cancer trials: experience and perspective of the European Organization for Research and Treatment of Cancer. J Natl Cancer Inst Monogr 1996; (20) 91–95.

369. Esmatjes E, Ricart MJ, Fernandez-Cruz L, Gonzalez-Clemente JM, Saenz A, Astudillo E. Quality of life after successful pancreas-kidney transplantation. Clin Transplant 1994; 8:75–78.

370. Nathan DM, Fogel H, Norman D, et al. Long-term metabolic and quality of life results with pancreatic/renal transplantation in insulin-dependent diabetes mellitus. Transplantation 1991; 52:85–91.

371. Zehrer CL, Gross CR. Comparison of quality of life between pancreas/kidney transplant recipients and kidney transplant recipients: one year follow-up. Transplant Proc 1994; 26:508–509.

372. Stratta RJ. The economics of pancreas transplantation. Graft 2000; 3:19.

373. Douzdjian V, Escobar F, Kupin WL, Venkat KK, Abouljoud MS. Cost-utility analysis of living-donor kidney transplantation followed by pancreas transplantation versus simultaneous pancreas-kidney transplantation. Clin Transplant 1999; 13:51–58.

374. Douzdjian V, Ferrara D, Silvestri G. Treatment strategies for insulin-dependent diabetics with ESRD: a cost- effectiveness decision analysis model. Am J Kidney Dis 1998; 31:794–802.

375. Gruessner A, Troppmann C, Sutherland DER, Gruessner RWG. Donor and recipient risk factors significantly affect cost of pancreas transplants. Transplant Proc 1997; 29:656–657.

376. Stratta R, Bennett L. Pancreas underutilization according to united network for organ sharing. Transplant Proc 1998; 30:264.

377. Stratta RJ, Cushing KA, Frisbie K, Miller SA. Analysis of hospital charges after simultaneous pancreas-kidney transplantation in the era of managed care. Transplantation 1997; 64:287–292.

378. American Diabetes Association. Pancreas transplantation for patients with type 1 diabetes. Diabetes Care 2000; 23:S85.

379. Robertson RP, Davis C, Larsen J, Stratta R, Sutherland DE. Pancreas and islet transplantation in type 1 diabetes. Diabetes Care 2006; 29:935.

380. Hering BJ, Wijkstrom M, Eckman PM. Islet transplantation. In: Gruessner RWG, Sutherland DER, eds. Transplantation of the Pancreas. New York: Springer-Verlag, 2004:583–626.

381. Ramiya VK, Maraist M, Arfors KE, Schatz DA, Peck AB, Cornelius JG. Reversal of insulin-dependent diabetes using islets generated in vitro from pancreatic stem cells [see comments]. Nat Med 2000; 6:278–282.

382. Kahan BW, Jacobson LM, Hullett DA, et al. Pancreatic precursors and differentiated islet cell types from murine embryonic stem cells: an in vitro model to study islet differentiation. Diabetes 2003; 52:2016–2024.

383. Hering BJ, Wijkstrom M, Graham ML, et al. Prolonged diabetes reversal after intraportal xenotransplantation of wild-type porcine islets in immunosuppressed nonhuman primates. Nat Med 2006; 12:301–303.

384. Suarez-Pinzon WL, Lakey JR, Brand SJ, Rabinovitch A. Combination therapy with epidermal growth factor and gastrin induces neogenesis of human islet (beta)-cells from pancreatic duct cells and an increase in functional (beta)-cell mass. J Clin Endocrinol Metab 2005; 90:3401–3409.

385. Chase HP, Hayward AR, Eisenbarth GS. Clinical trials for the prevention of type 1 diabetes. Adv Exp Med Biol 2004; 552:291–305.

# 27 | Pancreas Transplantation: The University of Wisconsin Experience

Jon S. Odorico, Stuart J. Knechtle, and Hans W. Sollinger
*Division of Organ Transplantation, Department of Surgery, University of Wisconsin Medical School, Madison, Wisconsin, U.S.A.*

## INTRODUCTION

Pancreas transplantation, more than any other current therapy, effectively achieves normal glucose homeostasis in patients with type I insulin-dependent diabetes mellitus. Immuno-suppressive strategies for pancreas transplantation now rely on newer, more potent immunosuppressive agents, particularly tacrolimus, mycophenolate mofetil, and rapamycin. Substantially lower rates of allograft rejection and improved graft survival have been achieved over the past 10 years. Regimens designed to avoid nephrotoxicity or spare corticosteroid ther-apy are emerging, as the number of drug options grows. Solitary pancreas (SP) transplants have become more successful because of fewer technical graft losses and the development of safe biopsy techniques permitting histologic diagnosis of rejection. Such improvements have allowed solitary pancreas allografts (with historically poor long-term graft survival) to become almost as successful as combined kidney–pancreas transplants. As a result of these advances, the American Diabetes Association endorses pancreas transplantation in diabetics who have received previous successful kidney transplants, and who have life-threatening lability of their glucose homeostasis.

## RATIONALE

The discovery of insulin in 1921 by Banting and Best was immediately hailed as the cure for diabetes. Insulin rapidly led to increased life expectancy among diabetics, and definitively altered the natural history of the disease by preventing death from diabetic keto-acidosis and coma. However, as diabetic patients lived longer, previously unseen complications developed in other vital organs. Diabetes is now the leading cause of renal failure in the United States and associated retinopathy commonly contributes to blindness. Debilitating neuropathies and enteropathy also contribute to morbidity, and accelerated atherosclerosis involving the cerebrovascular and cardiovascular systems contributes to mortality.

Replacement of islets of Langerhans is the most effective means of restoring physiologic glucose metabolism for diabetic patients dependent on exogenous insulin for survival. This is best accomplished with either pancreatic islet or whole pancreaticoduodenal transplantation. The goal of transplantation is to establish insulin independence and, secondarily, to improve quality of life. Since the first successful pancreas transplant performed at the University of Minnesota in 1966, these goals have been met (1). Improvement in end-organ complications has been more challenging to demonstrate perhaps because an extended period of normo-glycemia is necessary to reverse diabetic microangiopathy. Furthermore, many patients who receive transplants already have fixed end-organ disease.

Advances in pancreas transplantation have resulted in a growing population of stable, euglycemic allograft recipients who are being thoroughly studied to determine the benefits of long-term normalization of glucose metabolism. Prospective longitudinal studies have shown that renal, neural, and ocular manifestations of microangiopathy can, in part, be reversed by long-standing euglycemia following pancreas transplantation (2–18). Several recent studies also document that pancreas transplantation reduces mortality in type I dia-betics and prolongs life (Fig. 1) (19–24). Because mortality in diabetes is strongly related to cardiac disease, it is not surprising then that euglycemia also has salutary effects on vascular physiology, atherosclerotic risk factors, and cardiac function (25–30). Furthermore, improved

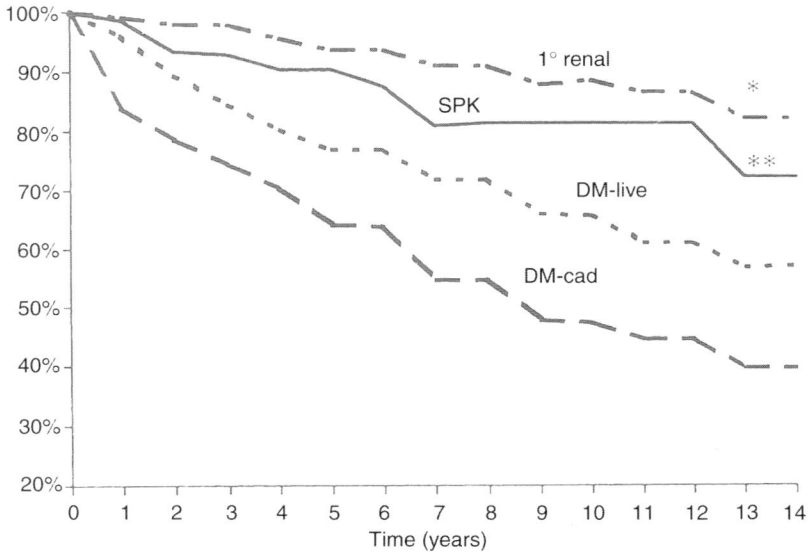

**Figure 1** Comparison of patient survival of simultaneous pancreas–kidney recipients to that of age-range matched cohorts of diabetic renal transplant recipients. $^*p = 0.0029$, 1°, renal versus all others; $^{**}p = 0.004$, SPK versus DM-Cad, DM-Live. *Abbreviations*: SPK, simultaneous pancreas–kidney; DM-Cad, cadaveric kidney transplant in patient with diabetes mellitus (DM) type I; DM-Live, live-donor kidney transplant in patient with type I DM; 1°, renal, nondiabetic renal transplant recipients. *Source*: From Ref. 19.

glycemic control in diabetics may reduce health care costs (31–39). These provocative clinical data complement earlier experimental observations that speak to the profound physiologic benefits of re-establishing precise glucose homeostasis.

The potential surgical complications of pancreas transplantation are well known (40–42). Adding a pancreas transplant to a simultaneously transplanted kidney certainly adds surgical risk, but adds little long-term functional risk for the transplanted kidney (43,44). In other words, simultaneous pancreas–kidney (SPK) transplants have similar, if not better, long-term survival rates compared to cadaver and haplotype-identical living donor kidneys transplanted alone (43,45). Only human leukocyte antigen (HLA)-identical kidneys have better long-term survival than SPK transplants (43). Furthermore, pancreas after kidney (PAK) transplantation represents minimal or no immunologic risk to the previously transplanted kidney, and excellent long-term kidney function is possible (46,47). Until islet or other cell-based transplantation therapy is routinely successful, the risks of the surgical procedure of pancreas transplantation must be weighed against the benefits of restoration of normoglycemia.

## INDICATIONS FOR TRANSPLANTATION

SP or SPK is indicated for selected type I diabetics. The risks of long-term immunosuppression should be weighed against the benefits of reversing uremia, reducing the risk of hypoglycemia, and halting the progression of secondary complications including neuropathy, retinopathy, and nephropathy. In young uremic diabetics, an SPK transplant has little added long-term risk compared to a kidney transplant alone (43,44,48).

The success of pancreas transplantation relies heavily on proper patient selection. At our center, type I insulin-dependent diabetics less than 55 years old are considered potential candidates. Mortality in diabetics is most often secondary to myocardial infarction and stroke; therefore, patients with advanced uncorrected coronary artery disease are excluded. A positive stress test is generally considered a contraindication to pancreas transplantation (Fig. 2). If a patient has had a successful coronary intervention and is expected to have a good long-term functional outcome, then the patient may be expected to live long enough to benefit from restoration of normoglycemia (50,51). Active smoking and severe obesity are generally viewed as relative contraindications to pancreas transplantation (52). Severe visual impairment or

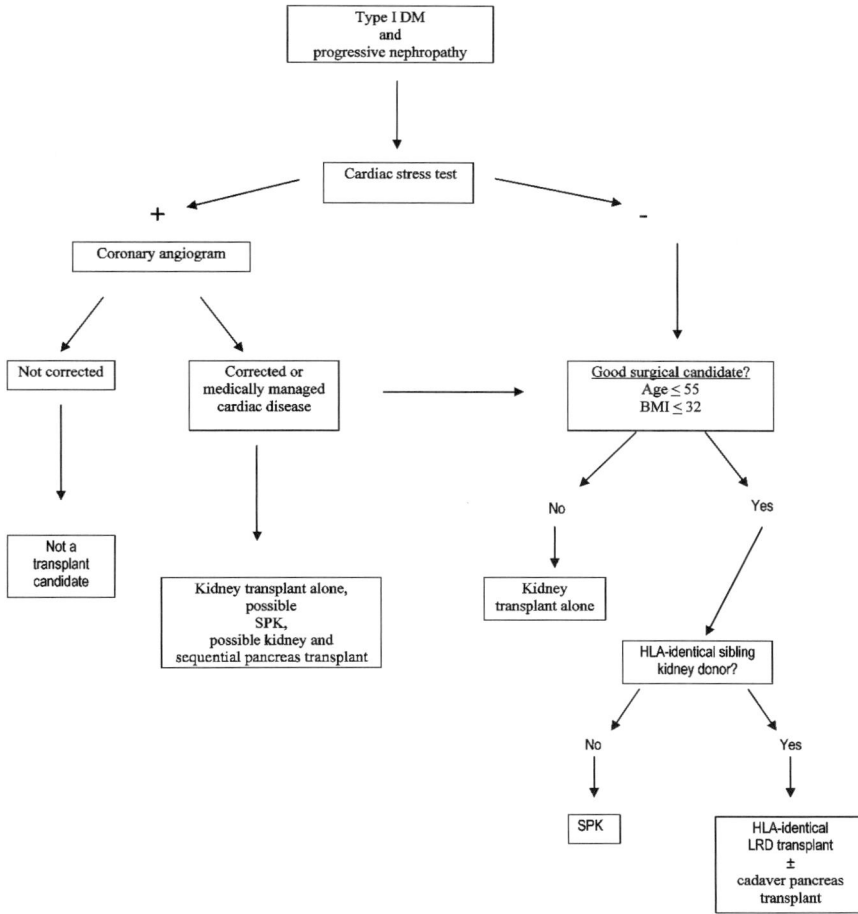

**Figure 2** Algorithm of surgical options in patients with type I diabetes mellitus and renal insufficiency. Options offered are also dependent on expected waiting time for a cadaveric pancreas at a particular center. *Source*: From Ref. 49.

major amputations resulting from severe peripheral vascular disease are not absolute contra-indications, particularly if the patient is uremic. However, not only are these patients unlikely to derive improvement in end-organ function from restoration of glucose homeostasis, but iliac atherosclerotic disease may also complicate technical aspects of the procedure.

Pancreas transplantation is most commonly performed in three different settings: pancreas transplantation alone (PTA) in the nonuremic diabetic without overt diabetic nephro-pathy; pancreas transplantation after successful kidney transplantation (PAK), and pancreas transplantation performed simultaneously with a kidney transplant (SPK) in the uremic patient.

More than 1500 pancreas transplants are performed annually worldwide. Of these, approximately 82% are performed as SPK transplants (53). For the uremic diabetic, options include an SPK or a living donor renal transplant alone. At most centers, SPK transplantation is considered the procedure of choice. However, the young diabetic patient may also receive an HLA-identical living-related renal transplant, if available, since this option offers superior long-term results with less immunosuppression (Fig. 2). The results of haplo-identical or living-unrelated kidney transplantation, on the other hand, are comparable to SPK transplan-tation with respect to kidney graft survival, and the decision of which option to pursue should be based on patient preference and projected waiting time (43,48). After a successful renal transplant, the patient may be offered a PAK graft. This is becoming an increasingly attractive option as waiting times increase, such that PAK transplants now account for 18% of pancreas transplants performed annually (53). If the waiting time for a cadaver SPK is prolonged, another option is a simultaneous cadaver pancreas transplant and living-donor renal transplant (54). In summary, if the patient is an acceptable candidate for a pancreas transplant and has no live donors available, then SPK should be considered the primary treatment option with the dual goals of establishing insulin independence and providing renal replacement therapy.

For diabetics who have undergone prior living-related or cadaveric renal transplantation and who have stable renal function, but have end-organ complications of diabetes, a PAK transplant is a good option. A PTA transplant can be offered to diabetics having normal native renal function and at least two diabetic complications. Other indications for PAK or PTA grafting in nonuremic diabetics would include evidence of glucose hyperlability, including frequent episodes of hypoglycemia without overt symptoms or poor glycemic control despite insulin pump therapy. Patients with marginal function of their transplanted or native kidneys or significant proteinuria should not be considered for solitary pancreas transplantation because high doses of calcineurin inhibitors used postoperatively may precipitate renal failure. Instead, SPK transplantation should be considered in these individuals. Rapamycin may be a useful adjunctive immunotherapeutic agent to mitigate the nephrotoxic effect of calcineurin inhibitors in this setting (55).

## RISK FACTORS

Analysis of donor and recipient risk factors and their effect on outcomes is best evaluated in large series that have statistical power (46,53). A large single-center retrospective study (46) and an update of the International Pancreas Transplant Registry (IPTR) have recently been published (53). Summarizing a large amount of data, these studies came to the following conclusions. Older ($\geq$45 years of age) SPK patients have slightly poorer patient survival than younger patients owing to more advanced cardiovascular disease of older diabetics. Likewise, graft survival is slightly worse for older SPK recipients. This observation was also seen in PAK recipients but not in PTA patients. In fact, older PTA patients may be less likely to reject their graft and outcomes may be improved in general (46,53). In contrast, the technical failure rate is not dependent on age (46,53). As predicted, recipient vascular disease is also a risk factor for poor patient survival, as well as reduced pancreas and kidney graft survival (46,53). Although graft survival rates do not differ between modes of dialysis pre-transplant, prior peritoneal dialysis may be a risk factor for the development of posttransplant intra-abdominal fluid collections (56) and infections (57). For these reasons and in order to avoid dialysis, early referral for transplantation is recommended (58). Re-transplantation and high panel-reactive antibody ($\geq$20%) are factors that correlate with reduced graft survival due to a combination of technical and immunological factors (46,53). A correlation between graft rejection rates and degree of HLA-B and -DR mismatch has been shown in some but not all studies (46,53,59).

## PANCREAS DONOR OPERATION

Cadaver donors aged five to 55 are considered for pancreas donation (60–62). Donors exhibiting grossly diseased pancreata, including fibrosis, excessive fatty infiltration, trauma, or saponification are not considered. Donors who have diabetes of any type, have used insulin, or are morbidly obese are also not considered for pancreas donation. On the other hand, isolated hyperglycemia or hyperamylasemia in the absence of gross organ disease should not be considered contraindications, as these organs have been shown to function satisfactorily (63). Likewise, pancreata procured from controlled non-heart beating donors can be used and have excellent short- and long-term function (64,65). Because the current need for organs is not being met, all available pancreases should be recovered and utilized for whole organ transplantation or islet transplantation whenever possible (66,67). University of Wisconsin solution currently provides an excellent, simple flushout and cold storage preservation method. Other methods of preservation, such as the two-layer method and histidine–tryptophan–ketoglutarate solution are being evaluated for efficacy (68,69).

The pancreatic graft is harvested en bloc with the liver and is then separated and prepared on the back table in University of Wisconsin solution at 4°C. The spleen is first removed by ligating the splenic artery and vein in the splenic hilum. The duodenal segment is shortened to approximately 8–10 cm. The final length of the duodenum is not critical, but care is taken to avoid injury to the head of the pancreas and the ampulla of Vater. If necessary, the common bile duct can be opened and cannulated to confirm patency of the ampulla of Vater. The duodenal staple lines are inverted without tension to avoid duodenal segment leaks. Peripancreatic fat is trimmed, and neural and lymphatic tissues in the region of the celiac axis are ligated. The portal vein is dissected back to the superior mesenteric vein and splenic vein confluence to maximize length. Arterial reconstruction using an end-to-end anastomosis of the donor iliac "Y" graft to the splenic artery and superior mesenteric artery is generally the preferred reconstructive technique; however, other techniques have also been used in specific settings (Fig. 3). A replaced right hepatic artery is not considered a contraindication to using the pancreas, and after the SMA origin and replaced right hepatic artery are dissected and preserved with the liver, the reconstruction proceeds in the usual manner. The head of the pancreas and duodenum have not been found to be ischemic in this setting, since the inferior pancreaticoduodenal arcade vessels can usually be preserved and ample intrapancreatic collaterals between head and tail circulations are commonly present. Careful handling of the pancreas is crucial to avoid posttransplant pancreatitis.

## PANCREAS TRANSPLANT OPERATION

The recipient operation is performed via a midline transabdominal incision. Intra-abdominal placement is associated with a lower incidence of lymphoceles and peripancreatic fluid collection compared to retroperitoneal placement (70,71). The pancreas is preferentially placed into the right iliac fossa, while the kidney, if transplanted simultaneously, is implanted on the left side lateral to the sigmoid colon. In PAK candidates with a prior right-sided kidney transplant, the pancreas can be implanted cephalad to the kidney by establishing arterial inflow through the proximal right common iliac artery without significant risk to the kidney. In our opinion, this is preferable and easier than left-sided placement. The presence of cross circulation in the pelvis, and the use of intravenous mannitol and intra-arterial heparin, allows renal function to be preserved. In the majority of PAK transplants performed at our institution, we have used this technique without any episodes of postoperative renal insufficiency or thrombosis. A tension-free portal vein anastomosis that will accommodate posttransplant graft swelling is critical regardless of whether one chooses systemic or portal venous drainage, or left- or right-sided placement. This is almost always possible without the use of an interposition graft, which may increase the risk of thrombosis (72,73). In order to achieve more physiologic insulin metabolism and avoid hyperinsulinemia associated with systemic drainage, several centers routinely perform portal venous drainage of the pancreas transplant (74–78). The arterial anastomosis is then performed between the reconstructed donor iliac artery "Y" graft and the common iliac artery. We do not routinely give systemic heparin or low

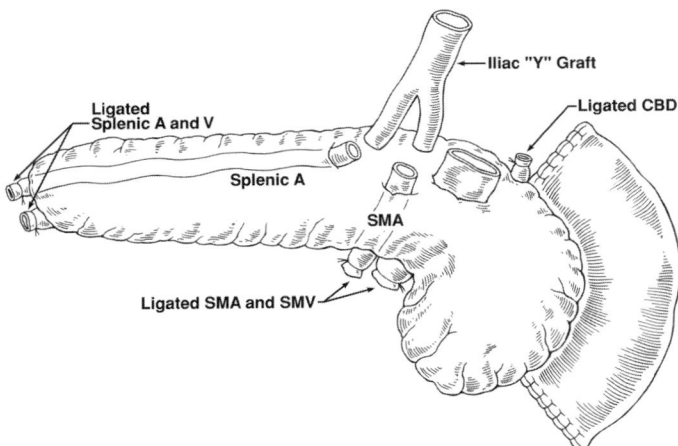

**Figure 3** Vascular reconstruction of the pancreas graft. *Abbreviations*: A, artery; and V, vein; SMA, superior mesenteric artery; SMV, superior mesenteric vein; CBD, common bile duct. *Source*: From Ref. 49.

molecular weight dextran during the anastomoses in either uremic or nonuremic recipients (47,79). These measures may be associated with increased postoperative bleeding (73).

Following reperfusion, the pancreas secretes pancreatic juice into the closed duodenal segment, which should not be allowed to distend. If bladder drainage (BD) is chosen, a pancreaticoduodenocystostomy is performed in a side-to-side fashion to the dome of the bladder (Fig. 4). If enteric drainage (ED) is performed, a side-to-side duodenoenterostomy is performed to the proximal jejunum approximately 1–2 ft from the ligament of Treitz (Fig. 5). Alternatively, a roux-en-y may be used to drain the exocrine secretions of the pancreas, and may be anastomosed end to end to the distal portion of the graft duodenal segment. A roux-en-y does not appear to significantly improve graft survival, nor does it appear to reduce the risk of leak or technical complications (53). Patients generally become euglycemic less than 12 hours postoperatively, without the need for postoperative insulin therapy.

## Bladder Drainage vs. Enteric Drainage

Formerly, the most widely used duct management technique for pancreas transplantation was BD. The duct injection technique, which was widely used in Europe, has been abandoned. In 1996 in the United States, two-thirds of pancreas transplants were performed with BD, while one-third were enterically drained (53). Now, however, nearly 70% of U.S. pancreas transplants are performed with ED, and a roux-en-y is used in combination with ED in approximately a quarter of these cases.

BD permits monitoring of urinary amylase to assess rejection and avoids a bowel anastomosis, which can result in peritoneal contamination (80). The principal advantage of the ED technique is avoidance of postoperative urologic and metabolic complications that occur in many patients, often requiring late surgical conversion to ED (Table 1) (81–85). Other benefits include less chronic dehydration and a reduced need for bicarbonate replacement therapy (86), early removal of the Foley catheter, more physiologic handling of secretions in conjunction with potential treatment of concomitant exocrine insufficiency, and more options for the vascular site of implantation, including portal venous drainage.

A retrospective comparison of bladder drainage with enteric drainage at the University of Maryland noted equivalent one-year graft survival rates without increased morbidity or leaks (87). Likewise, long-term outcomes also appear to be equivalent (53,88). Comparing 1541 BD SPK transplants reported to the IPTR from 1996 to 1999 to 1940 ED allografts, no

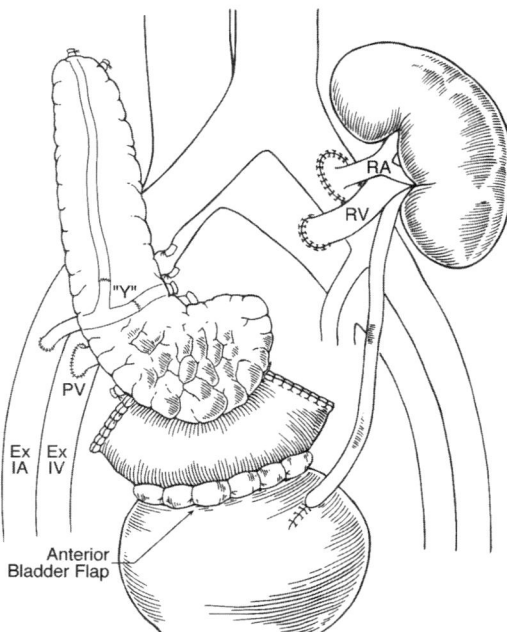

**Figure 4** Combined pancreas–kidney transplant performed with bladder drainage. Duodenocystostomy performed with running absorbable suture and reinforced with an anterior bladder flap. *Abbreviations*: RA and RV, renal artery and vein; ExIA and ExIV, external iliac artery and vein; PV, portal vein. *Source*: From Ref. 49.

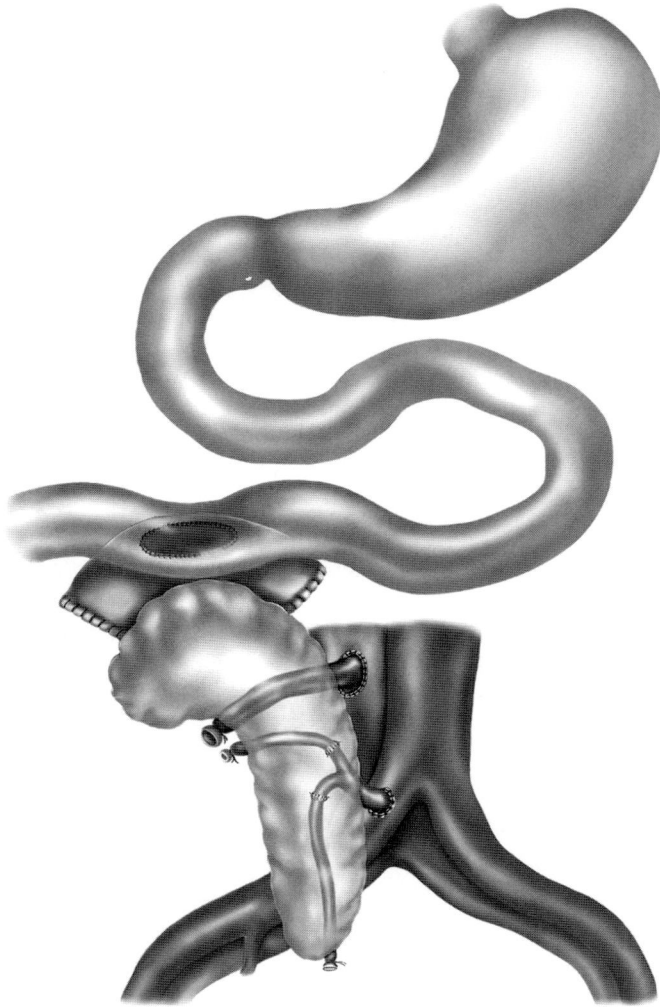

**Figure 5** Combined pancreas–kidney transplant performed with enteric drainage of exocrine secretions using a side-to-side jejunostomy. *Source*: From Ref. 49.

**Table 1** Complications Related to Drainage Technique in Simultaneous Pancreas–Kidney Transplantation at the University of Wisconsin: Comparison Between ED/BD

| Complication | ED | BD | *p* |
|---|---|---|---|
| Urinary tract infection (at least one) | 16% | 67% | < 0.0001 |
| Pancreatic enzyme leak | 5% | 18% | 0.05 |
| Bicarbonate replacement (% pts) | 16% | 65% | 0.001 |
| Mean dose (g/day) | 3.8 | 8.8 | 0.0004 |
| Urologic complications[a] | 0 | 20% | NS |
| Intestinal bleeding[b] | 3.6% | 0 | NS |
| Surgical conversion of drainage route | 0 | Up to 25% | < 0.001 |
| Abdominal infection | 12.1% | 16.4% | NS |
| Pancreatitis | 7.3% | 3.6% | NS |

[a]Urethritis, urethral disruption or digestion and hematuria.
[b]Putative source is enteric anastomosis.
*Abbreviations*: ED, enteric drainage; BD, bladder drainage; NS, not significant.

difference was found in long-term pancreas graft survival (84% vs. 83%, respectively) (53). IPTR data also failed to reveal a difference in kidney graft survival or immunologic pancreas graft loss rates (both 2%) in ED versus BD SPK transplants. According to this large series, adding a roux-en-y anastomosis does not alter graft survival rates compared to non-roux-en-y cases (53).

However, based on IPTR data, PAK and PTA transplants have slightly better graft survival with BD than with ED (53). One-year PAK graft survival is 77% in BD grafts and 67% in ED grafts; for PTA cases, graft survival is 75% in BD grafts and 65% in ED grafts. Since immunological graft loss rates are the same (PAK, 6% BD vs. 7% ED; PTA, 7% BD vs. 9% ED), the difference in graft survival between these techniques is unlikely to be related to the ability to detect rejection by urinary amylase monitoring in BD grafts alone. Instead, the difference in graft survival in SP transplants between BD and ED may be due to significant differences in thrombosis rates. The reported thrombosis rate for PAK cases is 9% in ED transplants versus 5% in BD transplants and for PTA cases is 16% with ED versus 5% with BD (53). The precise reasons for higher rates of thrombosis are not clear, though it is possible that some of these cases represent unrecognized rejection with secondary thrombosis (53). In contrast, the thrombosis rate of SPK transplants was not dependent on exocrine drainage technique (53).

## Venous Drainage: Systemic vs. Portal

Portal venous drainage was first described by both Calne and Tyden et al. in separate reports in 1984 (89,90). The frequency of this technique appears to be increasing such that last year portal venous drainage was used in approximately 20% of ED pancreas transplants performed in the United States and, at some centers, it is routinely applied in all patients (53). With growing experience, several studies have now definitively demonstrated that portal venous drainage is at least equivalent to systemic venous drainage, regarding patient and short-term graft survival rates, as well as technical complication rates (53,75–78,91–93). A retrospective study shows tantalizing reductions in rejection rates in portally drained grafts compared to systemically drained grafts (93). However, whether these observations will be borne out in a prospective randomized trial are unknown. Venous thrombosis of the graft does not appear to be more common than with systemically drained grafts and widespread thrombosis of the recipient visceral circulation has not occurred (94). If systemic venous implantation sites are not accessible due to prior transplants, venous thrombosis, inferior vena caval filter placement, etc., venous drainage into the portal circulation may be the only option. Those experienced in this procedure, however, do report that portal venous drainage is relatively contraindicated in obese patients having a thickened mesentery or a small-diameter superior mesenteric vein (76). Importantly, the arterial anastomosis is reported to be more cumbersome, and absolutely requires an iliac Y graft for length (76). Another important disadvantage of portally drained grafts is their relative inaccessibility to percutaneous biopsy, a factor that is particularly relevant for SP transplants (93). Moreover, the long-term results of this procedure in comparison to systemically drained allografts in a large well-controlled series of patients are not known.

Compared to systemic venous drainage, portal venous drainage may offer some advantages metabolically (95,96). Improved serum lipid profiles (29,97–103) and reduced hyperinsulinemia (104–107) are demonstrated in many such patients. However, it is not clear whether hyperinsulinemia observed following systemically drained pancreas transplantation is due entirely to systemic drainage, as nondiabetic transplant recipients receiving corticosteroids are frequently found to be hyperinsulinemic (95,108–111) and some systemically drained pancreas transplant patients are not hyperinsulinemic (112,113). Nonetheless, hyperinsulinemia following transplantation and immunosuppressive therapy is potentially problematic in view of its known atherogenic effects (114). Whether hyperinsulinemia can be reduced significantly or eliminated in individual pancreas transplant patients by conversion to portal drainage is not known. On the other hand, relative hyperinsulinemia may provide better prolonged glucose control in patients with deteriorating graft function (115). Moreover, hyperinsulinemia is rarely clinically meaningful. Long-term follow-up is needed of a large group of patients with detailed and carefully controlled metabolic studies evaluating lipid parameters, atherosclerosis, hypertension, and obesity. As pancreas transplant recipients live longer, the atherogenic effects of hyperinsulinemia may become a more prominent management issue. Overall, portal venous drainage appears to be an appropriate technique for selected patients and should remain an available option in the pancreas transplant surgeon's armamentarium.

## IMMUNOSUPPRESSION AND POSTOPERATIVE MONITORING

Acute rejection occurs in 70% to 80% of patients following pancreas transplantation, an incidence that is higher than that in patients after isolated renal transplantation (43,116,117). Although the reasons for this have not been clearly defined, this difference requires a strategically different approach that balances aggressive immunosuppression against risks of infection. A quadruple drug regimen, including polyclonal or monoclonal anti-T-cell antibody, mycophenolate mofetil (MMF), tacrolimus (TAC), and a rapid steroid taper, has evolved to be standard immunosuppressive therapy at many centers. Basiliximab, daclizumab or antithymocyte globulin are now used most commonly, and these are first given preoperatively or intraoperatively (53,88,118–123). Analysis of United Network for Organ Sharing registry data comparing SPK recipients induced with antibody therapy versus no anti-T-cell agents failed to demonstrate a benefit in graft survival (53); however, rejection rates were not analyzed. Moreover, there was no difference in graft survival among daclizumab, antithymocyte globulin, or OKT3-treated patients (53). However, several smaller retrospective comparative trials suggest that anti-T-cell antibody induction immunosuppression may lessen the severity and delay the onset of rejection and improve short-term graft survival in SPK (124,125) and SP (126) recipients.

MMF has improved kidney and pancreas graft survival over the last several years by providing more potent immunosuppression than azathioprine (AZA) (127). In addition to inhibiting lymphocyte proliferation and DNA synthesis, MMF also inhibits upregulation of adhesion molecules, and reduces proliferation of human arterial smooth muscle cells, which may, in part, contribute to its ability to control the immune response (127). MMF is associated with somewhat less global bone marrow suppression and less pancreatitis than AZA, and is not thought to be mutagenic for DNA as is AZA. Moreover, MMF may potentiate the anti-herpes virus effects of acyclovir and ganciclovir, thereby also exerting a protective effect (128), but also may be associated with more organ invasive cytomegalovirus (CMV) disease (129,130). However, because enterocytes are also somewhat dependent on inosine monophosphate dehydrogenase and de novo purine synthesis for DNA synthesis, MMF has significant gastrointestinal toxicity. Experience with MMF in pancreas transplantation has been favorable, such that MMF is now considered standard immunosuppression at many pancreas transplant centers in the United States. Numerous studies have reported excellent short-term pancreas and kidney graft survival results and reduced rejection rates with MMF (116,131–138).

A large, single-center retrospective analysis of consecutive SPK transplants compared outcomes of patients who received MMF-Neoral maintenance therapy to those who received AZA–cyclosporin (CSA)/Neoral (116). Actuarial two-year kidney allograft survival was significantly better in MMF-treated patients (95% MMF vs. 86% AZA, $p = 0.02$). Pancreas allograft survival was also significantly better in MMF patients (95% MMF vs. 83% AZA, $p = 0.016$). This study also found that MMF reduced the incidence of biopsy-proven kidney allograft rejection (75% AZA vs. 31% MMF) and steroid refractory acute rejection requiring OKT3, antilymphocyte globulin, or antithymocyte globulin immunotherapy (53% AZA vs. 15% MMF). Improved graft survival did not appear to increase patient morbidity. The incidence of fungal, bacterial, Epstein-Barr virus, and CMV infection was not higher in MMF-treated patients in this study because all patients received CMV prophylaxis. The risk of pancreatic enzyme leaks following SPK was not greater in MMF-treated patients; neither was the risk of posttransplant lymphoproliferative disorder significantly higher (three patients in AZA group vs. none in MMF group).

TAC induction, maintenance, and rescue therapy are effective in pancreas transplantation (78,138–145). Despite the routine use of TAC, excellent results and low acute rejection rates can be achieved with a Neoral–MMF-based regimen (Table 2) (88,116). This suggests that if TAC-related islet toxicity and glucose intolerance develops posttransplantation, it is safe to convert patients to Neoral-based immunosuppression in the setting of MMF without an excessive risk of immunologic rejection. Improved results in solitary pancreas transplantation are

**Table 2**  Rates of Acute Rejection in 588 Primary SPK Transplant Recipients and 47 Solitary Pancreas Transplant Recipients at the University of Wisconsin at One-Year Posttransplant

|  | *n* | Kidney (%) | Pancreas (%) |
|---|---|---|---|
| Primary SPK |  |  |  |
| a. Overall | 588 | 61 | 25 |
| b. TAC–MMF | 69 | 23 | 1.4 |
| c. Neoral–MMF | 160 | 34 | 10 |
| d. CSA/Neoral–AZA | 336 | 78 | 34 |
| e. CSA, AZA, ALG | 72 | 86 | 51 |
| f. CSA, AZA, OKT3 | 273 | 77 | 31 |
| g. Neoral, MMF, ATG | 110 | 34 | 10 |
| h. Neoral, MMF, OKT3 | 30 | 37 | 10 |
| i. Neoral, MMF, SIM | 20 | 35 | 5 |
| j. TAC, AZA, OKT3 | 17 | 59 | 24 |
| k. TAC, MMF, SIM | 27 | 22 | 0 |
| l. TAC, MMF, ZEN | 39 | 21 | 3 |
| Solitary pancreas |  |  |  |
| Overall | 47 | — | 43 |
| TAC–MMF | 24 | — | 29 |
| CSA–AZA | 23 | — | 57 |

*Notes*: Log rank test— (b) versus (c) (kidney), $p = $ NS; (b) versus (c) (pancreas), $p = 0.04$; (c) versus (d) (kidney), $p = 0.0001$; (c) versus (d) (pancreas), $p = 0.0001$; (e) versus (f) versus (g) versus (h) versus (i) versus (j) versus (k) versus (l) (kidney and pancreas), $p = 0.0001$; (n) versus (o) (pancreas), $p = 0.001$; (b) versus (n) (pancreas), $p = 0.001$.
*Abbreviations*: SPK, simultaneous pancreas–kidney; TAC, tacrolimus; MMF, mycophenolate mofetil; CSA, cyclosporine; AZA, azathioprine; ALG, antilymphocyte globulin; ATG, antithymocyte globulin; SIM, Simulect or basiliximab; ZEN, Zenapax or daclizumab.

possible with a TAC–MMF combination (47,139). At the University of Wisconsin, use of this combination regimen results in a very low incidence of rejection for both SPK and isolated pancreas transplantation (Table 2).

Patients should be closely monitored when using a TAC–MMF combination because of the risk of over immunosuppression. Several studies have highlighted the effect of TAC on mycophenolic acid levels, the active metabolite of MMF (146–148). Compared to Neoral, TAC coadministration with MMF significantly increases mycophenolic acid levels and augments the apparent exposure to MMF. Therefore, when used in combination with TAC, the maximum recommended dose of MMF is 2 g/day. However, diarrhea and other symptoms of gastrointestinal toxicity are commonly seen with a TAC–MMF regimen and, in many patients, additional dose adjustments are necessary.

## DIAGNOSIS AND TREATMENT OF REJECTION

In SPK patients, rejection of the pancreas graft alone is unusual, occurring in less than 10% of all rejection episodes (149,150). More commonly, pancreas rejection occurs simultaneously with or lags behind kidney rejection. Thus, after SPK transplantation, the diagnosis of rejection relies almost entirely on serum creatinine, $\beta_2$-microglobulin, and renal biopsy. However, in the setting of PAK or PTA transplantation, or after simultaneous living donor kidney and cadaver pancreas transplantation where isolated pancreas rejection occurs, an ideal serum screening test for rejection of the pancreas allograft, analogous to creatinine for kidney rejection, does not exist. Consequently, numerous putative serum and urinary markers of pancreas allograft rejection have been studied, including serum immunoreactive anodal trypsinogen (151), pancreas-specific protein (152), urinary cytology (153), pancreatic juice cytology (154), neopterin (155), and others (156). However, their clinical usefulness remains to be demonstrated. Decreased endogenous insulin levels and hyperglycemia occur sufficiently late after onset of rejection to preclude their utility as a monitoring tool. Serial histologic studies of pancreas rejection have shown that lymphocytic infiltrates initially involve the exocrine portion of the gland, while islet cell tissue becomes involved later (157). As a result, exocrine dysfunction is frequently the first sign of rejection. An elevated amylase or lipase will frequently, but not always, presage rejection, although these markers are not specific for immunologically mediated allograft dysfunction. In bladder-drained allografts, a decrease in exocrine secretions is often an early indicator of dysfunction and can be detected by a decrease in urinary amylase. A consistent drop in urinary amylase levels of greater than 25% strongly suggests the possibility of rejection of the pancreas (80). A study in which pancreas biopsies were obtained because of hypoamylasuria demonstrated that only 55% of patients exhibiting hypoamylasuria had biopsy evidence of rejection (158). Therefore, although a stable urinary amylase level essentially rules out rejection, a decreasing urinary amylase measurement is not necessarily a reliable indicator of rejection. Since a sensitive and specific marker for pancreatic allograft rejection is not yet available, the early and accurate diagnosis of rejection remains a challenging task that requires a high index of suspicion.

Since the development of safe and reliable percutaneous pancreas biopsy techniques, empiric treatment of pancreas rejection is not advisable in view of the significant risks of unnecessary immunosuppression. The focused use of anti-rejection therapy guided by allograft biopsy has contributed to improved pancreas graft survival (159). Stratta et al. showed that serial protocol biopsies in stable, asymptomatic SP transplant recipients may positively impact graft survival (160). A diagnosis of rejection is dependent on biopsy of either the kidney or pancreas allograft in SPK recipients (whichever organ exhibits dysfunction) or of the pancreas allograft in SP recipients. In the setting of concomitant organ dysfunction in SPK patients, the kidney is usually biopsied. Indications for pancreas allograft biopsy to rule out rejection include elevated amylase or lipase, unexplained fever, and glucose intolerance. In our opinion, histopathologic evidence of immunologic graft injury should be sought in nearly all cases of graft dysfunction. It is equally important to rule out infectious and/or anatomic causes of pancreas graft dysfunction with appropriate radiologic studies (161). By specifically identifying the etiology of graft dysfunction, appropriate treatment is assured and the devastating consequences of empiric immunosuppression is avoided.

A number of safe techniques of pancreas allograft biopsy have been described. Fine-needle aspiration cytology has met with limited success (149,162). Two identified limitations of fine-needle aspiration biopsy are the inability to discern vascular rejection and the difficulty in scoring the severity of rejection. Percutaneous core biopsies of the pancreas allograft with real-time ultrasound or CT guidance have been shown to be safe and reliable, and are now considered standard of care at many pancreas transplant centers (159,162,163). In patients with bladder-drained allografts, cystoscopic transduodenal needle-core biopsy with ultrasound guidance offers the opportunity to biopsy both the pancreas and duodenum (164,165). With both techniques, the use of an automated biopsy needle, and real-time ultrasound guidance has improved the safety and efficacy (166).

The pancreas becomes firmly adherent to surrounding structures. This reduces the risk of biopsy-related complications, particularly bleeding and pancreatic duct leak. Whereas gross hematuria is reported to occur after transcystoscopic biopsy in up to 10% of patients, this complication is rare after the percutaneous approach. Asymptomatic hyperamylasemia following biopsy may be more common following transcystoscopic biopsy than percutaneous biopsy (12–29% vs. 0–5%) (150,162,163,166,167). Other infrequent complications of the percutaneous technique include hematoma or intra-abdominal bleeding, pancreatitis, fistula, and abscess. Complications requiring reoperation or resulting in graft loss are fortunately rare. In our experience with over 90 ultrasound-guided percutaneous pancreas transplant biopsies, the complication rate has been very low. One rectus muscle hematoma occurred and two episodes of post-biopsy hyperamylasemia have been the only complications observed. None of these required treatment.

Nakhleh and Sutherland initially defined histologic criteria for grading rejection of the pancreas allograft (168). This scheme was modified by Papadimitriou et al. and Drachenberg et al. (Table 3) (169,170). Several pathologic features correlate with the earliest phases of acute rejection, including septal and acinar inflammation, the presence of activated lymphocytes and eosinophils, and endothelialitis (169). Conversely, ductal pathology without inflammation correlates with graft pancreatitis rather than rejection and does not necessitate anti-rejection therapy (169). This revised grading system is useful in that it is able to prognosticate outcome and response to therapy (170). There appears to be a strong correlation between duodenal and pancreatic pathology during the rejection process, and duodenal rejection rarely occurs independently of pancreas rejection (165,171,172). As a consequence, biopsy of the acinar gland is usually performed.

Grade I rejection, or inflammation of undetermined significance, generally does not warrant treatment and has an excellent outcome. The treatment of Grade II minimal rejection is usually bolus corticosteroids. However, some episodes of pancreas allograft rejection appear

**Table 3** University of Maryland Histologic Grading System for Pancreas Rejection and Estimated Graft Prognosis

| Histologic grade | Severity | % Graft loss |
|---|---|---|
| 0 | Normal | 0 |
| I | Indeterminate inflammation | 0 |
| II | Minimal | 11.5 |
| III | Mild | 17.3 |
| IV | Moderate | 37.5 |
| V | Severe | 100 |

Major characteristics of each grade:
I—Rare, purely septal mononuclear infiltrate without venous endothelialitis or acinar inflammation.
II—Septal inflammation with endothelialitis, or if absent, then evidence for three or four of the following features: activated lymphocytes, eosinophils, ≤2 acinar foci of inflammation and/or ductal inflammation.
III—Septal and prominent acinar inflammation.
IV—Grade III features plus arterial endothelialitis and/or necrotizing arteritis.
V—Extensive inflammatory acinar infiltrates, and confluent acinar necrosis.
*Source*: From Refs. 169,170.

to be resistant to bolus steroid immunotherapy (167,170). Corticosteroids may worsen already compromised glycemic control, and, as a result, many centers choose to treat Grade II and higher rejection with a course of antilymphocyte antibody therapy in addition to corticosteroids. In addition to steroid-refractory rejection, recurrent and moderate to severe rejections are best treated with antibody therapy, although this has not been formally studied. A significant rejection episode may merit a change in immunosuppression. Most commonly, TAC is employed as rescue therapy, TAC dosage is optimized, or rapamycin is used. Irreversible allograft rejection, a frequent occurrence several years ago, is now an unusual event, occurring in fewer than 5% of patients. If diagnosed before the onset of hyperglycemia, most rejection episodes can be treated successfully with antibody therapy. On the other hand, the success of anti-rejection treatment is far less if initiated after the development of hyperglycemia (168).

## RESULTS

At the University of Wisconsin from 1985 through 1999, 653 pancreas transplants have been performed. Tables 4 and 5 show donor and recipient demography for this series of patients. The number of pancreas transplants performed in each year of this era is shown in Figure 6.

**Table 4** Demographics of Pancreas Donors

| Characteristic | *n* | Value or % |
|---|---|---|
| Age (yr) | 653 | 29± 13 (3–60)[a] |
| Gender (M:F) | 653 | 63:37 |
| Weight (kg) | 597 | 72± 19 (15–159) |
| Serum amylase (SU) | 255 | 93± 190 (2–2002) |
| Plasma glucose (mg/dL) | 618 | 190± 90 (6–824) |
| Pancreas cold ischemia (hr) | | |
|     SPK | 606 | 16± 4 (3–29) |
|     SP | 47 | 13± 7 (2.5–24) |
| Kidney cold ischemia (hr) | | |
|     SPK | 606 | 17± 5 (3.5–30) |
| Cause of death | | |
|     Trauma | 380 | 58.2 |
|     Aneurysm/ICB | 213 | 32.6 |
|     Anoxic brain injury | 52 | 8.0 |
|     Other | 8 | 1.2 |
| Donor status | | |
|     Heart beating | 633 | 96.9 |
|     Non-heart beating | 20 | 3.1 |
| Procured at UW | | |
|     SPK | 584/606 | 96.4 |
|     SP | 32/47 | 68.1 |

[a]Value± standard deviation (range).
*Abbreviations*: SPK, simultaneous pancreas–kidney; SP, solitary pancreas; UW, University of Wisconsin; ICB, intracranial bleeding.

**Table 5**   Recipient Demographics of 653 Pancreas Transplants at the University of Wisconsin Since 1985

| Characteristic | n | Value or % |
|---|---|---|
| Age (yr) | 640 | 36± 6 (18–55)[a] |
| Gender (M:F) | 653 | 62:38 |
| Weight (kg) | 632 | 70± 12 (42–123) |
| Duration of diabetes (yr) | 653 | 24± 6 (8–48) |
| Dialysis pretransplant | | |
| Peritoneal dialysis | 147 | 22.5 |
| Hemodialysis | 189 | 28.9 |
| Both | 35 | 5.4 |
| None | 282 | 43.2 |
| Type of transplant | | |
| SPK | 606 | 92.8 |
| PAK | 35 | 5.4 |
| PASPK | 7 | 1.1 |
| PTA | 5 | 0.8 |
| Transplant no. | | |
| 1 | 593 | 90.8 |
| 2 | 53 | 8.1 |
| 3 | 5 | 0.8 |
| ≥4 | 2 | 0.4 |
| Pancreatic exocrine management | | |
| BD | 410 | 62.8 |
| ED without roux-en-y | 235 | 36.0 |
| ED with roux-en-y | 8 | 1.2 |
| Pretransplant amputations | | |
| Toe | 19 | 2.9 |
| Foot | 2 | 0.3 |
| BKA | 12 | 1.8 |
| Total | 33 | 5.0 |
| Total HLA match | 642 | 1.3± 1.0 (0–6) |

[a]Value± standard deviation (range).
*Abbreviations*: SPK, simultaneous pancreas–kidney; PASPK, pancreas after SPK; PAK, pancreas after kidney; PTA, pancreas transplantation alone; ED, enteric drainage; BD, bladder drainage; HLA, human leukocyte antigen; BKA, below knee amputation.

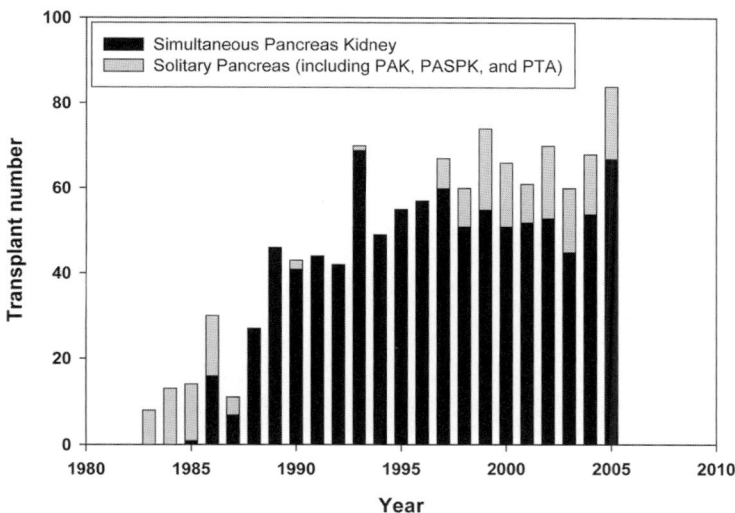

**Figure 6**   Solitary pancreas (SP) and simultaneous pancreas–kidney (SPK) transplants performed annually from 1983 to present at the University of Wisconsin. Due to high morbidity in an early experience, SP transplantation was abandoned in favor of SPK transplantation until advances in immunosuppression and biopsy techniques permitted a return to this procedure. *Abbreviations*: PAK, pancreas after kidney; PASPK, pancreas after SPK; PTA, pancreas transplantation alone.

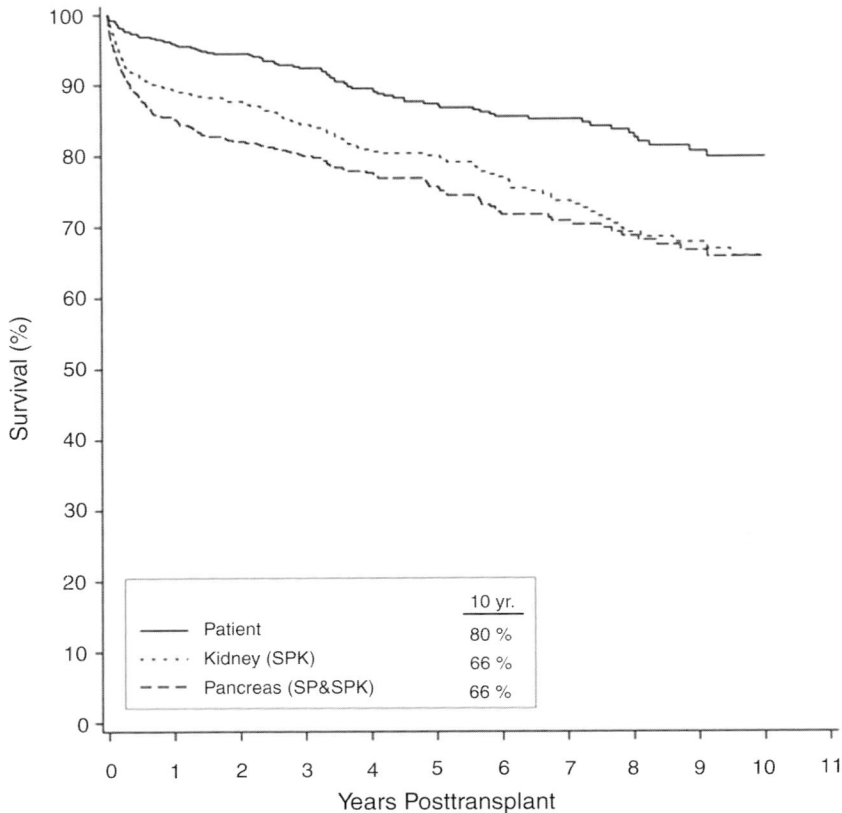

**Figure 7** Overall patient, pancreas graft and kidney graft survival at the University of Wisconsin: 653 pancreas transplants performed from 1985 to 2000. *Abbreviations*: SPK, simultaneous pancreas–kidney; SP, solitary pancreas. *Source*: From Ref. 88.

The five- and 10-year Kaplan–Meier patient survival rates were 87% and 80%, respectively (Fig. 7). Two well-controlled studies with long-term follow-up (19,22) corroborate these data and show that the life span of young patients with type I diabetes and end stage renal disease is significantly increased by combined pancreas and kidney transplantation. By restoring normal glucose homeostasis, pancreas transplantation can have a profound impact on the overall health of type I diabetics. This benefit may be due to long-term euglycemia, which can alter the natural history of end-organ complications. Despite the benefits of pancreas transplantation, the principal causes of death in this series of 653 pancreas transplants were cardiovascular and cerebrovascular disease (40%). The majority of the remaining deaths resulted from sepsis (19%) and malignancy (6%).

Pancreas and kidney graft survival have improved steadily over the past decade. Overall, five- and 10-year pancreas graft survival rates were 76% and 66%, respectively; likewise, five- and 10-year rates for kidney graft survival were 80% and 66%, respectively (Fig. 7). With respect to short-term (one year) graft survival, SPK transplants have consistently done well over this era from 1985 to present time (Fig. 8). On the other hand, three-year graft survival of all SPK transplants at our institution has shown steady improvement over time (Fig. 8). A comparison of pancreas graft survival among SP transplants, primary SPK transplants, and SPK re-transplants is shown in Figure 9. Traditionally, SP transplants and re-transplants represent high-risk groups. Several factors, including advances in immunosuppression, improved preservation with University of Wisconsin solution, and the ability to safely biopsy the grafted pancreas, have resulted in improved function of SP transplants in an era. SP transplants performed since 1997 at our institution enjoy an 86% one-year graft survival, while SP

(A)

(B)

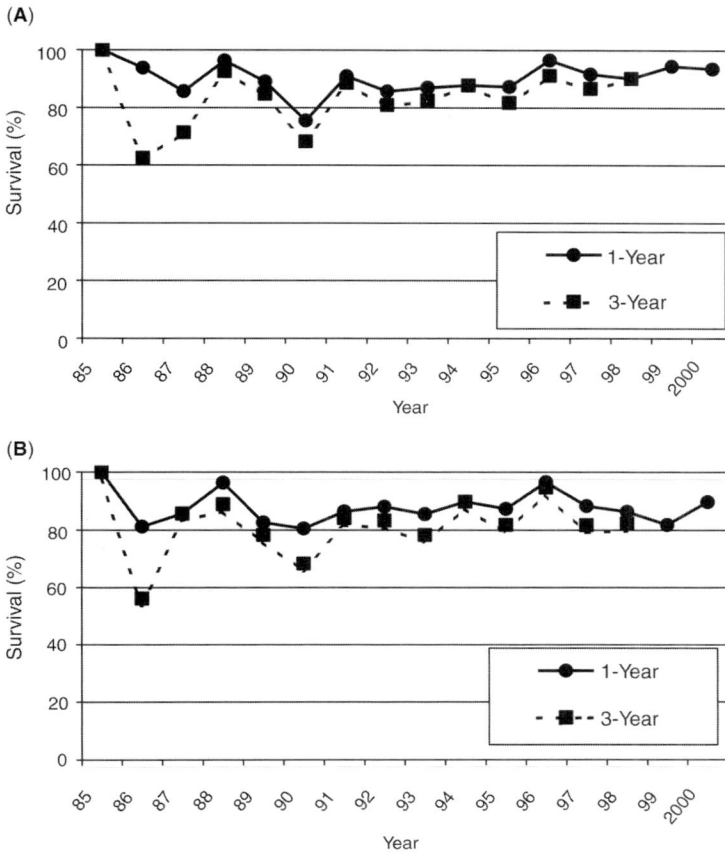

**Figure 8**  One- and three-year Kaplan–Meier graft survival rates by year of transplant for all simultaneous pancreas–kidney transplants performed at the University of Wisconsin from 1985 to 2000. (**A**) Kidney graft survival; (**B**) pancreas graft survival.

transplants performed prior to 1992 had a one-year graft survival of 20% (47). Currently, with TAC–MMF-based immunosuppression, short-term SP transplant graft survival is comparable to that of primary SPK transplants (Fig. 10).

Urologic and metabolic complications occur frequently in BD pancreas transplant recipients, and, at our center, up to 25% of BD pancreas allografts ultimately underwent enteric conversion for these complications (65). In July 1996, ED became the standard primary means of managing pancreatic exocrine secretions at our center. Since that time, nearly all SP and SPK transplants have been performed with ED without a roux-en-y, except in cases of tenuous duodenal segments or anastomoses. The IPTR/United Network for Organ Sharing database demonstrates that an increasing number of centers (nearly 80% currently) and an increasing number of pancreas transplants in the United States are being performed with ED (173). We compared pancreas and kidney graft survival of primary SPK transplants between ED and BD allografts. The results for pancreas graft survival are shown in Figure 11. In agreement with IPTR data, there is no difference in long-term graft survival between drainage procedures. Similarly, kidney graft survival is similar between ED and BD allografts. At the University of Wisconsin, all SP transplants were performed with ED. Although others have advocated the continued use of BD for SP transplants for the advantages of being able to monitor urinary amylase levels as an indicator of rejection, in our experience this is not a critical monitoring tool (174). Not only is this test cumbersome for patients, it is also not reliably predictive of allograft rejection. An equally sensitive noninvasive assessment of graft dysfunction is the serum amylase, and the diagnosis of rejection should ultimately rely on histopathology.

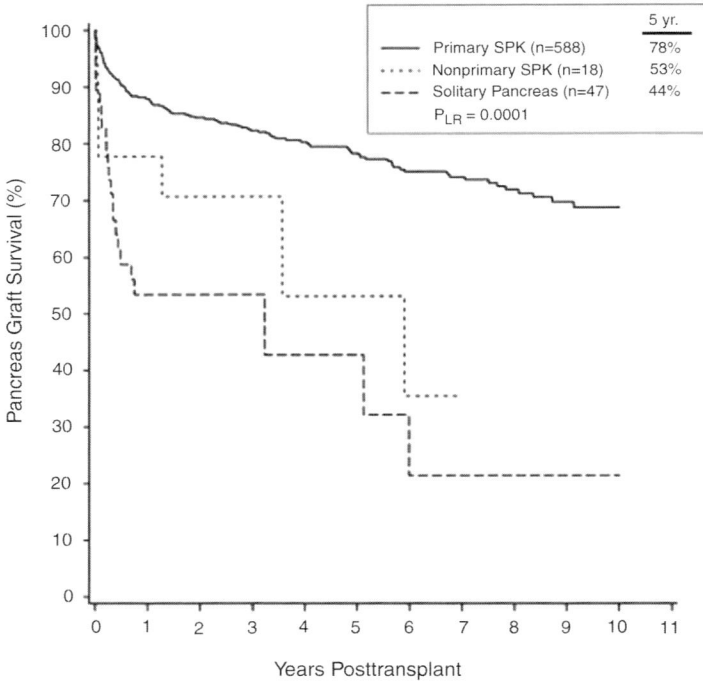

**Figure 9**  Comparison of pancreas graft survival between primary simultaneous pancreas–kidney (SPK) transplants, nonprimary SPK transplants, and solitary pancreas transplants (1985–2000). *Abbreviation*: SPK, simultaneous pancreas–kidney. *Source*: From Ref. 88.

Moreover, ED has several potential advantages in SP transplants. First, ED removes reflux pancreatitis from the differential diagnosis of hyperamylasemia, thereby simplifying the evaluation of graft dysfunction. Second, by eliminating the potential for repeated episodes of pancreatic inflammation, graft function should be optimized by reducing the incidence of acute rejection and chronic fibrosis. Third, ED avoids the metabolic acidosis and dehydration associated with bicarbonate loss through the urinary tract, which can predispose to graft

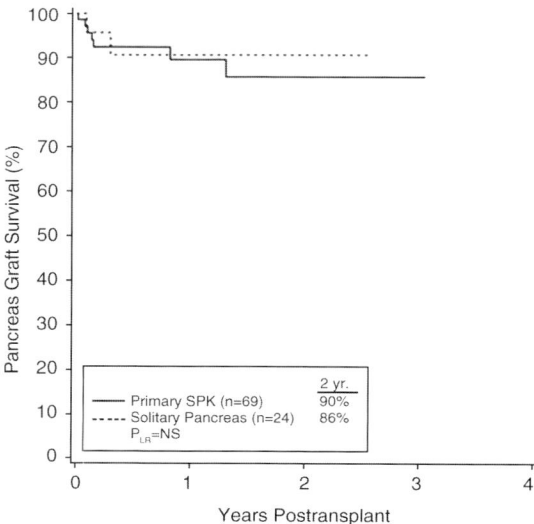

**Figure 10**  Comparison of pancreas graft survival between primary simultaneous pancreas–kidney transplants and solitary pancreas transplants in tacrolimus–mycophenolate mofetil-treated patients. *Abbreviation*: SPK, simultaneous pancreas–kidney. *Source*: From Ref. 88.

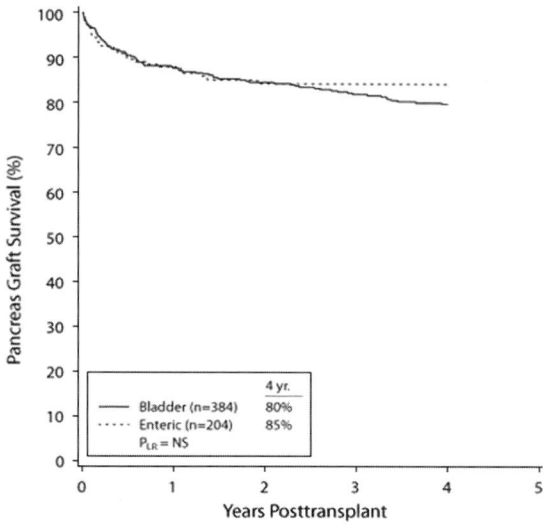

**Figure 11** Comparison of pancreas graft survival in primary simultaneous pancreas–kidney transplants: bladder vs. enteric drainage. *Source*: From Ref. 88.

thrombosis, a problem that continues to plague SP transplants more commonly than SPK transplants. Fourth, ED allows more flexibility for vascular implantation of the allograft, commonly necessary for pancreas re-transplants or PAK transplants.

The technical complication rate has remained low throughout this series (Table 6) and is not different between ED and BD pancreas allografts. The change in the exocrine management technique to ED at our institution has not led to increased technical complication rates, including graft thrombosis, primary nonfunction, or enzyme leaks. A prior analysis of BD versus ED showed that ED was associated with a significant decrease in urinary tract infections within the first year and a reduced length of hospital stay. Enzyme leaks and intra-abdominal infections were not increased compared with BD pancreases (79).

Few SPK re-transplants were performed during this period. The pancreas and kidney graft survival is poorer for SPK re-transplants compared with primary transplants (Fig. 9), a result in keeping with registry data. Whereas the five-year kidney graft survival in primary SPK recipients was 80%, it was 69% in recipients of secondary SPK transplants. Similarly, five-year pancreas graft survival for primary SPK transplants was 78%, whereas for SPK re-transplants it was 53%. Overall, poorer graft survival occurred in this small group of SPK re-transplants despite slightly lower rates of rejection (one-year pancreas rejection: 25% for primary transplants vs. 14% for re-transplants; one-year kidney rejection: 61% for primary transplants vs. 30% for re-transplants). These results highlight the greater technical risks associated with re-transplants.

Optimal immunosuppressive drug regimens for induction and maintenance in SPK and SP transplants are rapidly evolving. In SPK transplants, the lowest rates of acute rejection

**Table 6** Outcomes of 653 Pancreas Transplants Related to Method of Handling Exocrine Secretions

|  | Overall (*n* = 653) (%) | Enteric drained (*n* = 243) (%) | Bladder drained (*n* = 410) (%) |
|---|---|---|---|
| Primary nonfunction[a] |  |  |  |
|    Kidney | 1 (0.2) | 1 (0.4) | 0 |
|    Pancreas | 1 (0.2) | 0 | 1 (0.2) |
| Graft thrombosis[a] |  |  |  |
|    Kidney | 4 (0.7) | 2 (0.8) | 2 (0.5) |
|    Pancreas | 15 (2.3) | 6 (2.5) | 9 (2.2) |
| Acute tubular necrosis[b] | 29 (4.8) | 14 (6.4) | 15 (3.8) |

[a]Resulting in graft loss.
[b]As defined by acute dialysis need during first posttransplant week.

were achieved utilizing a TAC–MMF-based immunosuppressive protocol (Table 2). Although there is limited experience to date, the rates of acute renal and pancreas allograft rejection did not differ between daclizumab- and basiliximab-treated primary SPK patients receiving TAC and MMF. Experience with these agents to date suggests that they are safe and effective in SPK patients. A comparison of immunosuppressive regimens regarding kidney and pancreas allograft survival reveals a survival advantage for TAC–MMF-treated SPK patients receiving an anti-CD25 monoclonal antibody compared to Neoral-, AZA-, or OKT3-based regimens (88). The benefits of TAC–MMF therapy on graft survival parallel the improved rates of rejection seen in this group of patients (Table 2) (88). Thymoglobulin is also an effective induction agent in SPK and SP transplantation. Despite optimal immunosuppression and an aggressive policy of performing either kidney or pancreas allograft biopsies when indicated, the incidence of acute renal allograft rejection remains higher ($\sim$20–25%) than pancreas allograft rejection ($<$5%) in SPK recipients. The reason for this observation is unclear.

A TAC–MMF combination also results in a low rate of acute rejection in SP transplants (one-year acute rejection rates: CSA/AZA—57% vs. TAC–MMF—29%, Table 2). It is interesting that, despite improved immunosuppression and nearly equivalent graft survival, the incidence of acute pancreas allograft rejection remains significantly higher in SP transplants (29%) than in SPK transplants ($<$5%) (Table 2) (88).

In summary, an immunosuppressive regimen including TAC and MMF in both SP and SPK transplants effectively reduced the rate of acute rejection and improved graft survival. In the TAC–MMF era, pancreas graft survival in recipients of SP transplants is essentially equivalent to that in SPK recipients, and excellent short-term graft survival can be achieved in SP transplants using enteric drainage. Finally, anti-interleukin-2 receptor monoclonal antibodies are safe and effective in pancreas transplantation.

The results of pancreas transplantation have markedly improved in the last decade. Proper patient selection, better organ preservation, refinements in surgical technique, and the early diagnosis and treatment of rejection have all contributed to this progress, but none more than the routine use of new immunosuppressive drugs, including MMF and tacrolimus. The transplant procedure of choice for most uremic diabetic patients with stable cardiovascular status is SPK transplantation. Graft and patient survival rates are now comparable to those of other organ transplants, especially when the pancreas is transplanted simultaneously with a kidney. Important advances in SP transplantation have also emerged. As results continue to improve, isolated pancreas transplantation is being offered with increasing frequency to diabetics with normal renal function to prevent or reverse end-organ complications, to prevent life-threatening hypoglycemic episodes, and to improve quality of life.

# REFERENCES

1. Kelly WD, Lillehei RC, Merkel FK, Idezuki Y, Goetz FC. Allotransplantation of the pancreas and duodenum along with the kidney and diabetic nephropathy. Surgery 1967; 61:827–837.
2. Hawthorne WJ, Wilson TG, Williamson P, et al. Long-term duct-occluded segmental pancreatic autografts: absence of microvascular diabetic complications. Transplantation 1997; 64:953–959.
3. Fioretto P, Steffes MW, Sutherland DER, Goetz FC, Mauer M. Reversal of lesions of diabetic nephropathy after pancreas transplantation. N Engl J Med 1998; 339:69–75.
4. Fioretto P, Mauer SM, Bilous RW, Goetz FC, Sutherland DER, Steffes MW. Effects of pancreas transplantation on glomerular structure in insulin-dependent diabetic patients with their own kidneys. Lancet 1993; 342:1193–1196.
5. Wilczek HE, Jaremko G, Tyden G, Groth CG. Evolution of diabetic nephropathy in kidney grafts. Evidence that a simultaneously transplanted pancreas exerts a protective effect. Transplantation 1995; 59:51–57.
6. Muller-Felber W, Landgraf R, Scheuer R, et al. Diabetic neuropathy 3 years after successful pancreas and kidney transplantation. Diabetes 1993; 42:1482–1486.
7. Solders G, Tyden G, Persson A, Groth CG. Improvement of nerve conduction in diabetic nephropathy: a follow-up study 4 yr after combined pancreatic and renal transplantation. Diabetes 1992; 41:946–951.
8. Hathaway DK, Abell T, Cardoso S, Hartwig MS, Gebely SE, Gaber AO. Improvement in autonomic and gastric function following pancreas–kidney versus kidney-alone transplantation and the correlation with quality of life. Transplantation 1994; 57:816–822.

9. The Diabetes Control and Complications Trial Research Group. The effect of intensive treatment of diabetes on the development and progression of long-term complications in insulin-dependent diabetes mellitus. N Engl J Med 1993; 329:977–986.
10. Wang Q, Klein R, Moss SE, et al. The influence of combined kidney–pancreas transplantation on the progression of diabetic retinopathy. A case series. Ophthalmology 1994; 101:1071–1076.
11. Esmatjes E, Adan A, Ricart MJ, et al. Long-term evolution of diabetic retinopathy and renal function after pancreas transplantation. Transplant Proc 1992; 24:12–13.
12. Esmatjes E, Ricart MJ, Fernandez-Cruz L, Gonzalez-Clemente JM, Saenz A, Astudillo E. Quality of life after successful pancreas–kidney transplantation. Clin Transplant 1994; 8:75–78.
13. Kiebert GM, van Oosterhout ECAA, van Bronswijk H, Lemkes HHPJ, Gooszen HG. Quality of life after combined kidney–pancreas or kidney transplantation in diabetic patients with end-stage renal disease. Clin Transplant 1994; 8:239–245.
14. Nakache R, Tyden G, Groth CG. Long-term quality of life in diabetic patients after combined pancreas–kidney transplantation or kidney transplantation. Transplant Proc 1994; 26:510–511.
15. Piehlmeier W, Bullinger M, Kirchberger I, Land W, Landgraf R. Evaluation of the quality of life of patients with insulin-dependent diabetes mellitus before and after organ transplantation with the SF 36 health survey. Eur J Surg 1996; 162:933–940.
16. Navarro X, Sutherland DE, Kennedy WR. Long-term effects of pancreatic transplantation on diabetic neuropathy. Ann Neurol 1997; 42:727–736.
17. Kennedy WR, Navarro X, Goetz FC, Sutherland DE, Najarian JS. Effects of pancreatic transplantation on diabetic neuropathy. N Engl J Med 1990; 322:1031–1037.
18. Cheung ATW, Perez RV, Chen PCY. Improvements in diabetic microangiography after successful simultaneous pancreas–kidney transplantation: a computer-assisted intravital microscopy study on the conjunctival microcirculation. Transplantation 1999; 68:927–932.
19. Becker BN, Brazy PC, Becker YT, et al. Simultaneous pancreas–kidney transplantation reduces excess mortality in type 1 diabetic patients with end-stage renal disease. Kidney Int 2000; 57: 2129–2135.
20. Smets YF, van dPJW, Ringers J, de FJW, Lemkes HH. Mortality of cadaveric kidney transplantation versus combined kidney-pancreas transplantation in diabetic patients. Lancet 1996; 347: 826–827.
21. Smets YF, Westendorp RG, van der Pijl JW, et al. Effect of simultaneous pancreas–kidney transplantation on mortality of patients with type-1 diabetes mellitus and end-stage renal failure. Lancet 1999; 353:1915–1919.
22. Tyden G, Bolinder J, Solders G, Brattstrom C, Tibell A, Groth CG. Improved survival in patients with insulin-dependent diabetes mellitus and end-stage diabetic nephropathy 10 years after combined pancreas and kidney transplantation. Transplantation 1999; 67:645–648.
23. Douzdjian V, Rice JC, Gugliuzza KK, Fish JC, Carson RW. Renal allograft and patient outcome after transplantation: pancreas–kidney versus kidney-alone transplants in type 1 diabetic patients versus kidney-alone transplants in nondiabetic patients. Am J Kidney Dis 1996; 27:106–116.
24. Ojo AO, Meier-Kriesche H-U, Hanson JA, et al. The impact of simultaneous pancreas–kidney transplantation on long-term patient survival. Transplantation 2001; 71:82–90.
25. Fiorina P, La Rocca E, Venturini M, et al. Effects of kidney–pancreas transplantation on atherosclerotic risk factors and endothelial function in patients with uremia and type 1 diabetes. Diabetes 2001; 50:496–501.
26. La Rocca E, Fiorina P, Astorri E, et al. Patient survival and cardiovascular events after kidney-pancreas transplantation: comparison with kidney transplantation alone in uremic IDDM patients. Cell Transplant 2000; 9:929–932.
27. Fiorina P, La Rocca E, Astorri E, et al. Reversal of left ventricular diastolic dysfunction after kidney–pancreas transplantation in type 1 diabetic uremic patients. Diabet Care 2000; 23:1804–1810.
28. Gfesser M, Nusser J, Muller-Felber W, Abendroth D, Land W, Landgraf R. Cross-sectional study of peripheral microcirculation in diabetic patients with microangiopathy: influence of pancreatic and kidney transplantation. Acta Diabetol 1993; 30:79–84.
29. Foger B, Konigsrainer A, Palos G, et al. Effect of pancreas transplantation on lipoprotein lipase, postprandial lipemia, and HDL cholesterol. Transplantation 1994; 58:899–904.
30. Gaber AO, El-Gebely S, Sugathan P, et al. Early improvement in cardiac function occurs for pancreas–kidney but not diabetic kidney-alone transplant recipients. Transplantation 1995; 59: 1105–1112.
31. Wagner EH, Sandhu N, Newton KM, McCulloch DK, Ramsey SD, Grothaus LC. Effect of improved glycemic control on health care costs and utilization. JAMA 2001; 285:182–189.
32. Stratta RJ, Cushing KA, Frisbie K, Miller SA. Analysis of hospital charges after simultaneous pancreas–kidney transplantation in the era of managed care. Transplantation 1997; 64:287–292.
33. Kiberd B, Larson T. Estimating the benefits of solitary pancreas transplantation in nonuremic patients with type 1 diabetes mellitus: a theoretical analysis. Transplantation 2000; 70: 1121–1127.
34. Whiting J, Martin J, Cohen D, et al. Economic outcome of simultaneous pancreas kidney transplantation compared with kidney transplantation alone. Transplant Proc 2001; 33:1923.

35. Douzdjian V, Ferrara D, Silvestri G. Cost-utility analysis of pancreas transplantation compared to other treatment options for type 1 diabetics with end-stage renal disease. Transplant Proc 1998; 30:278.
36. Douzdjian V, Escobar F, Kupin W, Venkat K, Aboujjoud M. Cost-utility analysis of living-donor kidney transplantation followed by pancreas transplantation versus simultaneous pancreas–kidney transplantation. Clin Transplant 1999; 13:51–58.
37. Douzdjian V, Ferrara D, Silvestri G. Treatment strategies for insulin-dependent diabetics with ESRD: a cost-effectiveness decision analysis model. Am J Kidney Dis 1998; 31:794–802.
38. Stratta RJ. The economics of pancreas transplantation. Graft 2000; 3:19–24.
39. Holohan TV. Cost-effectiveness modeling of simultaneous pancreas–kidney transplantation. Int J Technol Assess Health Care 1996; 12:416–424.
40. Stratta RJ, Taylor RJ, Ozaki CF, et al. The analysis of benefit and risk of combined pancreatic and renal transplantation versus renal transplantation alone. Surg Gynecol Obstet 1993; 177: 163–171.
41. Humar A, Kandaswamy R, Granger D, Gruessner RW, Gruessner AC, Sutherland DE. Decreased surgical risks of pancreas transplantation in the modern era. Ann Surg 2000; 231:269–275.
42. Douzdjian V, Abecassis MM, Cooper JL, Smith JL, Corry RJ. Incidence, management and significance of surgical complications after pancreatic transplantation. Surg Gynecol Obstet 1993; 177: 451–456.
43. Rayhill SC, D'Alessandro AM, Odorico JS, et al. Simultaneous pancreas–kidney transplantation and living related donor renal transplantation in patients with diabetes: is there a difference in survival? Ann Surg 2000; 231:417–423.
44. Odorico JS, Rayhill SC, Heisey DM, et al. Immunologic risk of combined kidney–pancreas transplantation. Transplant Proc 1998; 30:249–250.
45. Cosio FG, Elkhammas EA, Henry ML, et al. Function and survival of renal allografts from the same donor transplanted into kidney-only or kidney–pancreas recipients. Transplantation 1998; 65:93–99.
46. Sutherland DE, Gruessner RW, Dunn DL, et al. Lessons learned from more than 1,000 pancreas transplants at a single institution. Ann Surg 2001; 233:463–501.
47. Odorico JS, Becker YT, Groshek M, et al. Improved solitary pancreas transplant graft survival in the modern immunosuppressive era. Cell Transplant 2000; 9:919–927.
48. Gruessner RWG, Dunn DL, Tzardis PJ, et al. Simultaneous pancreas and kidney transplants versus single kidney transplants and previous kidney transplants in uremic patients and single pancreas transplants in non-uremic diabetic patients: comparison of rejection, morbidity, and long-term outcome. Transplant Proc 1990; 22:622–623.
49. Odorico JS, Sollinger HW. Technical and immunosuppressive advances in transplantation for insulin-dependent diabetes mellitus. World J Surg 2002; 26:194–211.
50. Schweitzer EJ, Anderson L, Kuo PC, et al. Safe pancreas transplantation in patients with coronary artery disease. Transplantation 1997; 63:1294–1299.
51. Kim SI, Elkhammas EA, Henry ML, Davies EA, Bumgadner GL, Ferguson RM. Outcome of combined kidney/pancreas transplantation in recipients with coronary artery disease. Transplant Proc 1995; 27:3071.
52. Bumgardner GL, Henry ML, Elkhammas E, et al. Obesity as a risk factor after combined pancreas/kidney transplantation. Transplantation 1995; 60:1426–1430.
53. Gruessner A, Sutherland DER. Pancreas transplant outcomes for United States (US) cases reported to the United Network for Organ Sharing (UNOS) and non-US cases reported to the International Pancreas Transplant Registry (IPTR) as of October, 2000. In: Cecka JM, Terasaki PI, eds. Clinical Transplants 2000. Los Angeles: UCLA Immunogenetics Center, 2001:45–72.
54. Farney AC, Cho E, Schweitzer EJ, et al. Simultaneous cadaver pancreas living-donor kidney transplantation: a new approach for the type 1 diabetic uremic patient. Ann Surg 2000; 232:696–703.
55. Odorico JS, Pirsch JD, Becker YT, Becker BN, Sollinger HW. Experience with rapamycin in pancreas transplantation. Acta Chir Austriaca 2001; 33(suppl 174):23.
56. Douzdjian V, Abecassis M. Deep wound infections in simultaneous pancreas–kidney transplant recipients on peritoneal dialysis. Nephrol Dial Transplant 1995; 10:533–536.
57. Passalacqua JA, Wiland AM, Fink JC, Bartlett ST, Evans DA, Keay S. Increased incidence of postoperative infections associated with peritoneal dialysis in renal transplant recipients. Transplantation 1999; 68:535–540.
58. Stratta RJ, Taylor RJ, Ozaki CF, et al. A comparative analysis of results and morbidity in type I diabetics undergoing preemptive versus postdialysis combined pancreas–kidney transplantation. Transplantation 1993; 55:1097–1103.
59. Basadonna GP, Auersvald LA, Oliveira SC, Friedman AL, Lorber MI. Pancreas after kidney transplantation: HLA mismatch does not preclude success. Transplant Proc 1997; 29:667.
60. Abouna GM, Kumar MS, Miller JL, et al. Combined kidney and pancreas transplantation from pediatric donors into adult diabetic recipients. Transplant Proc 1994; 6:441–442.
61. Van der Werf WJ, Odorico J, D'Alessandro AM, et al. Utilization of pediatric donors for pancreas transplantation. Transplant Proc 1999; 31:610–611.
62. Kapur S, Bonham CA, Dodson SF, Dvorchik I, Corry RJ. Strategies to expand the donor pool for pancreas transplantation. Transplantation 1999; 67:284–290.

63. Odorico JS, Heisey DM, Voss BJ, et al. Donor factors affecting outcome after pancreas transplantation. Transplant Proc 1998; 30:276–277.

64. D'Alessandro AM, Hoffmann RM, Knechtle SJ, et al. Successful extrarenal transplantation from non-heart-beating donors. Transplantation 1995; 59:977–982.

65. D'Alessandro AM, Odorico JS, Knechtle SJ, et al. Simultaneous pancreas–kidney (SPK) transplantation from controlled non-heart-beating donors (NHBDs). Cell Transplant 2000; 9:889–893.

66. Stratta RJ, Bennett L. Pancreas underutilization according to United Network for Organ Sharing data. Transplant Proc 1998; 30:264.

67. Odorico JS. Underutilization of the potential for cadaver pancreas donation. Transplant Proc 1998; 29:3311–3312.

68. Hiraoka K, Trexler A, Eckman E, et al. Successful pancreas preservation before islet isolation by the simplified two-layer cold storage method. Transplant Proc 2000; 33:952–953.

69. Troisi R, Meester D, Regaert B, et al. Physiologic and metabolic results of pancreatic cold storage with histidine–tryptophan–ketoglutarate—HTK solution (Custodiol) in the porcine autotransplantation model. Transplant Int 2000; 13:98–105.

70. Tesi RJ, Henry ML, Elkhammas EA, Sommer BG, Ferguson RM. Decreased wound complications of combined kidney–pancreas transplants using intra-abdominal pancreas graft placement. Clin Transplant 1990; 4:287–291.

71. Schweitzer EJ, Bartlett ST. Wound complications after pancreatic transplantation through a kidney transplant incision. Transplant Proc 1994; 26:461.

72. Troppmann C, Gruessner AC, Benedetti E, et al. Vascular graft thrombosis after pancreatic transplantation: univariate and multivariate operative and nonoperative risk factor analysis. J Am Coll Surg 1996; 182:285–316.

73. Sollinger HW. Pancreatic transplantation and vascular graft thrombosis. J Am Coll Surg 1996; 182:362–363.

74. Gaber AO, Shokouh-Amiri MH, Hathaway DK, et al. Results of pancreas transplantation with portal venous and enteric drainage. Ann Surg 1995; 221:613–624.

75. Cattral MS, Bigam DL, Hemming AW, et al. Portal venous and enteric exocrine drainage versus systemic venous and bladder exocrine drainage of pancreas grafts: clinical outcome of 40 consecutive transplant recipients. Ann Surg 2000; 232:688–695.

76. Stratta RJ, Shokouh-Amiri MH, Egidi MF, et al. A prospective comparison of simultaneous kidney–pancreas transplantation with systemic-enteric versus portal-enteric drainage. Ann Surg 2001; 233: 740–751.

77. Petruzzo P, Da S, Feitosa LC, et al. Simultaneous pancreas–kidney transplantation: portal versus systemic venous drainage of the pancreas allografts. Clin Transplant 2000; 14:287–291.

78. Bruce DS, Newell KA, Woodle ES, et al. Synchronous pancreas–kidney transplantation with portal venous and enteric exocrine drainage: outcome in 70 consecutive cases. Transplant Proc 1998: 30: 270–271.

79. Sollinger HW, Odorico JS, Knechtle SJ, D'Alessandro AM, Kalayoglu M, Pirsch JD. Experience with 500 simultaneous pancreas–kidney transplants. Ann Surg 1998; 228:284–296.

80. Prieto M, Sutherland DER, Fernandez-Cruz L, Heil J, Najarian JS. Experimental and clinical experience with urine amylase monitoring for early diagnosis of rejection in pancreas transplantation. Transplantation 1987; 43:73–79.

81. Van der Werf WJ, Odorico JS, D'Alessandro AM, et al. Enteric conversion of bladder drained pancreas allografts: experience in 95 patients. Transplant Proc 1998; 30:441–442.

82. Sollinger HW, Messing EM, Eckhoff DE, et al. Urological complications in 210 consecutive simultaneous pancreas-kidney transplants with bladder drainage. Ann Surg 1993; 218:561–570.

83. Elkhammas EA, Sethi PS, Henry ML, Williams PA, Bennett WF, Ferguson RM. Urologic complications following pancreas transplantation. Transplant Rev 1997; 11:1–8.

84. Pirsch JD, Odorico JS, D'Alessandro AM, Knechtle SJ, Becker BN, Sollinger HW. Posttransplant infection in enteric versus bladder-drained simultaneous pancreas–kidney transplant recipients. Transplantation 1998; 66:1746–1750.

85. Stephanian E, Gruessner RWG, Brayman KL, et al. Conversion of exocrine secretions from bladder to enteric drainage in recipients of whole pancreaticoduodenal transplants. Ann Surg 1992; 216:663–672.

86. Pearson TC, Santamaria PJ, Routenberg KL, et al. Drainage of the exocrine pancreas in clinical transplantation: comparison of bladder versus enteric drainage in a consecutive series. Clin Transplant 1997; 11:201–205.

87. Kuo PC, Johnson LB, Schweitzer EJ, Bartlett ST. Simultaneous pancreas/kidney transplantation—a comparison of enteric and bladder drainage of exocrine pancreatic secretions. Transplantation 1997; 63:238–243.

88. Odorico JS, Leverson GE, Becker YT, et al. Pancreas transplantation at the University of Wisconsin. In: Cecka JM, Terasaki PI, eds. Clinical Transplants 1999. Los Angeles: UCLA Immunogenetics Center, 2000:199–210.

89. Calne RY. Paratopic segmental pancreas grafting: a technique with portal venous drainage. Lancet 1984; 1:595–597.

90. Tyden G, Wilczek HE, Lundgren G, et al. Experience with 21 intraperitoneal segmental pancreatic transplants with enteric and gastric exocrine diversion in humans. Transplant Proc 1985; 17: 331–335.
91. Newell KA, Woodle ES, Millis JM, et al. Pancreas transplantation with portal venous drainage and enteric exocrine drainage offers early advantages without compromising safety or allograft function. Transplant Proc 1995; 27:3002–3003.
92. Gaber AO, Shokouh-Amiri H, Grewal HP, Britt LG. A technique for portal pancreatic transplantation with enteric drainage. Surg Gynecol Obstet 1993; 177:417–419.
93. Philosophe B, Farney AC, Schweitzer EJ, et al. Superiority of portal venous drainage over systemic venous drainage in pancreas transplantation: a retrospective study. Ann Surg 2001; 234:689–696.
94. Reddy KS, Stratta RJ, Shokouh-Amiri MH, Alloway R, Egidi MF, Gaber AO. Surgical complications after pancreas transplantation with portal-enteric drainage. J Am Coll Surg 1999; 189:305–313.
95. Hawthorne WJ, Griffin AD, Lau H, Ekberg H, Allen RD. The effect of venous drainage on glucose homeostasis after experimental pancreas transplantation. Transplantation 1996; 62:435–441.
96. Shokouh-Amiri MH, Rahimi-Saber S, Andersen HO, Jensen SL. Pancreas autotransplantation in pig with systemic or portal venous drainage. Effect on the endocrine pancreatic function after transplantation. Transplantation 1996; 61:1004–1009.
97. Carpentier A, Patterson BW, Uffelman KD, et al. The effect of systemic versus portal insulin delivery in pancreas transplantation on insulin action and VLDL metabolism. Diabetes 2001; 50:1402–1413.
98. Hughes TA, Gaber AO, Amiri HS, et al. Kidney–pancreas transplantation. The effect of portal versus systemic venous drainage of the pancreas on the lipoprotein composition. Transplantation 1995; 60:1406–1412.
99. Bagdade JD, Teuscher AU, Ritter MC, Eckel RH, Robertson RP. Alterations in cholesteryl ester transfer, lipoprotein lipase, and lipoprotein composition after combined pancreas–kidney transplantation. Diabetes 1998; 47:113–118.
100. Bagdade JD, Ritter MC, Kitabchi AE, et al. Differing effects of pancreas–kidney transplantation with systemic versus portal venous drainage on cholesteryl ester transfer in IDDM subjects. Diabet Care 1996; 19:1108–1112.
101. Konigsrainer A, Foger B, Steurer W, et al. Influence of hyperinsulinemia on lipoproteins after pancreas transplantation with systemic insulin drainage. Transplant Proc 1998; 30:637–638.
102. Konigsrainer A, Foger BH, Miesenbock G, Patsch JR, Margreiter R. Pancreas transplantation with systemic endocrine drainage leads to improvement in lipid metabolism. Transplant Proc 1994; 26:501–502.
103. Foger B, Konigsrainer A, Palos G, et al. Effects of pancreas transplantation on distribution and composition of plasma lipoproteins. Metab Clin Exp 1996; 45:856–861.
104. Gaber AO, Shokouh-Amiri H, Hathaway DK, et al. Pancreas transplantation with portal venous and enteric drainage eliminates hyperinsulinemia and reduces postoperative complications. Transplant Proc 1993; 25:1176–1178.
105. Luck R, Klempnauer J, Ehlerding G, Kuhn K. Significance of portal venous drainage after whole-organ pancreas transplantation for endocrine graft function and prevention of diabetic nephropathy. Transplantation 1990; 50:394–398.
106. Elian N, Carnot F, Bailbe D, Cugnenc P, Altman JJ. Total pancreatico-duodenal transplantation with portal venous drainage: metabolic assessments in diabetic rats. Eur Surg Res 2000; 32:120–124.
107. Diem P, Abid M, Redmon JB, Sutherland DE, Robertson RP. Systemic venous drainage of pancreas allografts as independent cause of hyperinsulinemia in type I diabetic recipients. Diabetes 1990; 39:534–540.
108. Esmatjes E, Fernandez-Cruz L, Ricart MJ, Casamitjana R, Lopez-Boado MA, Astudillo E. Metabolic characteristics in patients with long-term pancreas graft with systemic or portal venous drainage. Diabetologia 1991; 34(suppl 1):S40–S43.
109. Ost L, Tyden G, Fehrman I. Impaired glucose tolerance in cyclosporine–prednisolone-treated renal graft recipients. Transplantation 1988; 46:370–372.
110. Katz H, Homan M, Velosa J, Robertson P, Rizza R. Effects of pancreas transplantation on postprandial glucose metabolism. N Engl J Med 1991; 325:1278–1283.
111. Christiansen E, Vestergaard H, Tibell A, et al. Impaired insulin-stimulated nonoxidative glucose metabolism in pancreas–kidney transplant recipients. Dose-response effects of insulin on glucose turnover. Diabetes 1996; 45:1267–1275.
112. Martin X, Petruzzo P, Dawahra M, et al. Effects of portal versus systemic venous drainage in kidney–pancreas recipients. Transplant Int 2000; 13:64–68.
113. Pfeffer F, Nauck MA, Erb M, Benz S, Hopt UT. Absence of severe hyperinsulinemia after pancreas/ kidney transplantation with peripheral venous drainage. Transplant Proc 1997; 29:645–646.
114. Despres JP, Lamarche B, Mauriege P, et al. Hyperinsulinemia as an independent risk factor for ischemic heart disease. N Engl J Med 1996; 334:952–957.
115. Christiansen E, Roder M, Tibell A, Hales CN, Madsbad S. Effect of pancreas transplantation and immunosuppression on proinsulin secretion. Diabet Med 1998; 15:739–746.
116. Odorico JS, Pirsch JD, Knechtle SJ, D'Alessandro AM, Sollinger HW. A study comparing mycophenolate mofetil to azathioprine in simultaneous pancreas–kidney transplantation. Transplantation 1998; 66:1751–1759.

117. Tesi RJ, Henry ML, Elkhammas EA, Davies EA, Ferguson RM. The frequency of rejection episodes after combined kidney–pancreas transplant—the impact on graft survival. Transplantation 1994; 58:424–430.
118. Bruce DS, Sollinger HW, Humar A, et al. Multicenter survey of daclizumab induction in simultaneous kidney–pancreas transplant recipients. Transplantation 2001; 72:1637–1643.
119. Hesse UJ, Troisi R, Jacobs B, et al. A single center's clinical experience with quadruple immunosuppression including ATG or IL2 antibodies and mycophenolate mofetil in simultaneous pancreas-kidney transplants. Clin Transplant 2000; 14:340–344.
120. Cantarovich D, Giral-Classe M, Hourmant M, et al. Low incidence of kidney rejection after simultaneous kidney–pancreas transplantation after antithymocyte globulin induction and in the absence of corticosteroids: results of a prospective pilot study in 28 consecutive cases. Transplantation 2000; 69:1505–1508.
121. Wiland AM, Fink JC, Philosophe B, et al. Peripheral administration of thymoglobulin for induction therapy in pancreas transplantation. Transplant Proc 2000; 33:1910.
122. Stratta RJ, Alloway RR, Lo A, Hodge E. A multicenter trial of two daclizumab dosing strategies versus no antibody induction in simultaneous kidney–pancreas transplantation: interim analysis. Transplant Proc 2000; 33:1692–1693.
123. Rasaiah SB, Light JA, Sasaki TM, Currier CB. A comparison of daclizumab to ATGAM induction in simultaneous pancreas–kidney transplant recipients on triple maintenance immunosuppression. Clin Transplant 2000; 14:409–412.
124. Wadstrom J, Brekke B, Wramner L, Ekberg H, Tyden G. Triple versus quadruple induction immunosuppression in pancreas transplantation. Transplant Proc 1995; 27:1317–1318.
125. Brayman KL, Egidi MF, Naji A, et al. Is induction therapy necessary for successful simultaneous pancreas and kidney transplantation in the cyclosporine era? Transplant Proc 1994; 26:2525–2527.
126. Stegall MD, Kim DY, Prieto M, et al. Thymoglobulin induction decreases rejection in solitary pancreas transplantation. Transplantation 2001; 72:1671–1675.
127. Allison AC, Eugui EM. Mycophenolate mofetil, a rationally designed immunosuppressive drug. Clin Transplant 1993; 7:96–112.
128. Neyts J, Andrei G, De Clercq E. The novel immunosuppressive agent mycophenolate mofetil markedly potentiates the antiherpesvirus activities of acyclovir, ganciclovir, and penciclovir in vitro and in vivo. Antimicrob Agents Chemother 1998; 42:216–222.
129. ter Meulen CG, Wetzels JF, Hilbrands LB. The influence of mycophenolate mofetil on the incidence and severity of primary cytomegalovirus infections and disease after renal transplantation. Nephrol Dial Transplant 2000; 15:711–714.
130. Sarmiento JM, Dockrell DH, Schwab TR, Munn SR, Paya CV. Mycophenolate mofetil increases cytomegalovirus invasive organ disease in renal transplant patients. Clin Transplant 2000; 14:136–138.
131. Stegall MD, Simon M, Wachs ME, Chan L, Nolan C, Kam I. Mycophenolate mofetil decreases rejection in simultaneous pancreas–kidney transplantation when combined with tacrolimus or cyclosporine. Transplantation 1997; 64:1695–1700.
132. Gruessner RWG, Sutherland DER, Drangstveit MB, Wrenshall L, Humar A, Gruessner AC. Mycophenolate mofetil in pancreas transplantation. Transplant 1998; 66:318–323.
133. Merion RM, Henry ML, Melzer JS, Sollinger HW, Sutherland DE, Taylor RJ. Randomized, prospective trial of mycophenolate mofetil versus azathioprine for prevention of acute renal allograft rejection after simultaneous kidney–pancreas transplantation. Transplantation 2000; 70:105–111.
134. Schulz T, Konzack J, Busing M. Mycophenolate mofetil/prednisolone/single-shot ATG with tacrolimus or cyclosporine in pancreas/kidney transplantation: first results of an ongoing prospective randomized trial. Transplant Proc 1999; 31:591–592.
135. Ciancio G, Lo M, Buscemi G, Miller J, Burke GW. Use of tacrolimus and mycophenolate mofetil as induction and maintenance in simultaneous pancreas–kidney transplantation. Transplant Int 2000; 13(suppl 1):S191–S194.
136. Kaufman DB, Leventhal JR, Koffron A, et al. Simultaneous pancreas–kidney transplantation in the mycophenolate mofetil/tacrolimus era: evolution from induction therapy with bladder drainage to noninduction therapy with enteric drainage. Surgery 2000; 128:726–737.
137. Rigotti P, Cadrobbi R, Baldan N, et al. Mycophenolate mofetil (MMF) versus azathioprine (AZA) in pancreas transplantation: a single-center experience. Clin Nephrol 2000; 53:52–54.
138. Kaufman DB, Leventhal JR, Stuart J, Abecassis MM, Fryer JP, Stuart FP. Mycophenolate mofetil and tacrolimus as primary maintenance immunosuppression in simultaneous pancreas–kidney transplantation: initial experience in 50 consecutive cases. Transplantation 1999; 67:586–593.
139. Bartlett ST, Schweitzer EJ, Johnson LB, et al. Equivalent success of simultaneous pancreas kidney and solitary pancreas transplantation. A prospective trial of tacrolimus immunosuppression with percutaneous biopsy. Ann Surg 1996; 224:440–449.
140. Gruessner RW, Burke GW, Stratta R, et al. A multicenter analysis of the first experience with FK506 for induction and rescue therapy after pancreas transplantation. Transplantation 1996; 61:261–273.
141. Gruessner RW, Sutherland DE, Drangstveit MB, Troppmann C, Gruessner AC. Use of FK 506 in pancreas transplantation. Transplant Int 1996; 9(suppl 1):S251–S257.
142. Corry RJ, Egidi MF, Shapiro R, et al. Pancreas transplantation with enteric drainage under tacrolimus induction therapy. Transplant Proc 1997; 29:642.

143. Stratta RJ, Taylor RJ, Castaldo P, et al. FK506 induction and rescue therapy in pancreas transplant recipients. Transplant Proc 1996; 28:1001–1002.
144. Stratta RJ, Egidi F, Corry RJ et al. Simultaneous use of FK506 and mycophenolate mofetil in combined pancreas–kidney transplant recipients: a multi-center report. Transplant Proc 1997; 29: 654–655.
145. Jordan ML, Shapiro R, Gritsch HA, et al. Long-term results of pancreas transplantation under tacrolimus immunosuppression. Transplantation 1999; 67:266–272.
146. Zucker K, Rosen A, Tsaroucha A, et al. Augmentation of mycophenolate mofetil pharmacokinetics in renal transplant patients receiving Prograf and CellCept in combination therapy. Transplant Proc 1997; 29:334–336.
147. Pirsch JD, Bekersky I, Vincenti F, et al. Coadministration of tacrolimus and mycophenolate mofetil in stable kidney transplant patients: pharmacokinetics and tolerability. J Clin Pharmacol 2000; 40: 527–532.
148. Zucker K, Rosen A, Tsaroucha A, et al. Unexpected augmentation of mycophenolic acid pharmacokinetics in renal transplant patients receiving tacrolimus and mycophenolate mofetil in combination therapy, and analogous in vitro findings. Transplant Immunol 1997; 5:225–232.
149. Hawthorne WJ, Allen RD, Greenberg ML, et al. Simultaneous pancreas and kidney transplant rejection: separate or synchronous events? Transplantation 1997; 63:352–358.
150. Klassen DK, Hoehn-Saric EW, Weir MR et al. Isolated pancreas rejection in combined kidney pancreas transplantation. Transplantation 1996; 61:974–977.
151. Perkal M, Marks C, Lorber MI, Marks WH. A three-year experience with serum anodal trypsinogen as a biochemical marker for rejection in pancreatic allografts: false positives, tissue biopsy, comparison with other markers, and diagnostic strategies. Transplantation 1992; 53:415–419.
152. Fernstad R, Tyden G, Brattstrom C, et al. Pancreas specific protein. New serum marker for graft rejection in pancreas-transplant recipients. Diabetes 1989; 38:55–56.
153. Radio SJ, Stratta RJ, Taylor RJ, Linder J. The utility of urine cytology in the diagnosis of allograft rejection after combined pancreas–kidney transplantation. Transplantation 1993; 55:509–516.
154. Kubota K, Reinholt FP, Tyden G, Groth CG. Recent experience with pancreatic juice cytology in monitoring pancreatic graft rejection. Transplant Proc 1989; 21:3643–3645.
155. Konigsrainer A, Tilg H, Reibnegger G, et al. Pancreatic juice neopterin excretion—a reliable marker of pancreas allograft rejection. Transplant Proc 1992; 24:907–908.
156. Linder R, Sziegoleit A , Brattstrom C, Tyden G, Groth CG. Pancreatic elastase 1 after pancreatic transplantation. Pancreas 1991; 6:31–36.
157. Tyden G. Pancreatic graft rejection. In: Groth CG, ed. Pancreatic Transplantation. Philadelphia: W.B. Saunders, Co., 1988.
158. Benedetti E, Najarian JS, Gruessner AC, et al. Correlation between cytoscopic biopsy results and hypoamylasuria in bladder-drained pancreas transplants. Surgery 1995; 118:864–872.
159. Kuo PC, Johnson LB, Schweitzer EJ, et al. Solitary pancreas allografts. The role of percutaneous biopsy and standardized histologic grading of rejection. Arch Surg 1997; 132:52–57.
160. Stratta RJ, Taylor RJ, Grune MT, et al. Experience with protocol biopsies after solitary pancreas transplantation. Transplantation 1995; 60:1431–1437.
161. Pozniak MA, Propeck PA, Kelcz F, Sollinger HW. Imaging of pancreas transplants. Radiol Clin North Am 1995; 33:581–594.
162. Allen RDM, Wilson TG, Grierson JM, et al. Percutaneous biopsy of bladder-drained pancreas transplants. Transplantation 1991; 51:1213–1216.
163. Gaber AO, Gaber LW, Shokouh-Amiri MH, Hathaway D. Percutaneous biopsy of pancreas transplants. Transplantation 1992; 54:548–550.
164. Lowell JA, Bynon JS, Nelson N, et al. Improved technique for transduodenal pancreas transplant biopsy. Transplantation 1994; 57:752–753.
165. Nakhleh RE, Benedetti E, Gruessner A, et al. Cytoscopic biopsies in pancreaticoduodenal transplantation. Are duodenal biopsies indicative of pancreas dysfunction? Transplantation 1995; 60:541–546.
166. Kuhr CS, Davis CL, Barr D, et al. Use of ultrasound and cystoscopically guided pancreatic allograft biopsies and transabdominal renal allograft biopsies: safety and efficacy in kidney–pancreas transplant recipients. J Urol 1995; 513:316–321.
167. Klassen DK, Weir MR, Schweitzer EJ, Bartlett ST. Isolated pancreas rejection in combined kidney–pancreas transplantation: results of percutaneous pancreas biopsy. Transplant Proc 1995; 27:1333–1334.
168. Nakhleh RE, Sutherland DER. Pancreas rejection: significance of histopathologic findings with implication for classification of rejection. Am J Surg Pathol 1992; 16:1098–1107.
169. Drachenberg CB, Papadimitriou JC, Klassen DK, et al. Evaluation of pancreas transplant needle biopsy: reproducibility and revision of histologic grading system. Transplantation 1997; 63:1579–1586.
170. Papadimitriou JC, Drachenberg CB, Wiland A, et al. Histologic grading of acute allograft rejection in pancreas needle biopsy: correlation to serum enzymes, glycemia, and response to immunosuppressive treatment. Transplantation 1998; 66:1741–1745.

171. Nakhleh RE, Gruessner RWG, Tzardis PJ, Dunn DL, Sutherland DER. Pathology of transplanted human duodenal tissue: a histologic study with comparison to pancreatic pathology in resected pancreaticoduodenal transplants. Clin Transplant 1991; 5:241–247.
172. Nakhleh RE, Sutherland DE, Tzardis P, Schechner R, Gruessner RW. Correlation of rejection of the duodenum with rejection of the pancreas in a pig model of pancreaticoduodenal transplantation. Transplantation 1993; 56:1353–1356.
173. Sutherland DER, Gruessner A, Bland B, et al. Int Pancreas Transplant Registry (IPTR) Newslett 1999; 11:1–19.
174. Odorico JS, Pirsch JD, Becker YT, et al. Results of solitary pancreas transplantation with enteric drainage: is there a benefit from monitoring urinary amylase levels? Transplant Proc 2000; 33:1700.

# 28 | Experience with Portal-Enteric Pancreas Transplantation at the University of Tennessee Memphis

**Robert J. Stratta**

*Department of General Surgery, Wake Forest University School of Medicine, Winston-Salem, North Carolina, U.S.A.*

**M. Hosein Shokouh-Amiri**

*Department of Surgery, College of Medicine, The University of Tennessee Health Science Center, Memphis, Tennessee, U.S.A.*

**M. Francesca Egidi**

*The University of Tennessee Health Science Center, Methodist University, Transplant Institute, Memphis, Tennessee, U.S.A.*

**Hani P. Grewal**

*Mayo Clinic, Jacksonville, Florida, U.S.A.*

**A. Tarik Kizilisik**

*Vanderbilt University Medical Center, Kidney/Pancreas Transplant Program, Nashville, Tennessee, U.S.A.*

**Donna K. Hathaway**

*Department of Surgery, College of Medicine, The University of Tennessee Health Science Center, Memphis, Tennessee, U.S.A.*

**Lillian W. Gaber**

*Department of Pathology, College of Medicine, The University of Tennessee Health Science Center, Memphis, Tennessee, U.S.A.*

**A. Osama Gaber**

*Department of Surgery, Cornell University, and The Methodist Hospital, Houston, Texas, U.S.A.*

## INTRODUCTION

Vascularized pancreas transplantation (PTX) was first developed as a means to reestablish endogenous insulin secretion responsive to normal feedback controls. PTX is currently the only available form of autoregulating total endocrine replacement therapy that reliably establishes an insulin-independent euglycemic state and normal glucose homeostasis resulting in the successful treatment of diabetes mellitus. With improvements in organ retrieval and preservation technology, refinements in diagnostic technology and surgical techniques, advances in clinical immunosuppression and antimicrobial prophylaxis, and experience in donor and recipient selection, success rates for PTX have steadily increased. From 1966 through July 2000, over 14,000 PTXs were performed worldwide and reported to the International Pancreas Transplant Registry (IPTR) (1). In the United States, over 1200 PTXs are performed annually, with 83% being simultaneous kidney-PTXs (SKPTs). The current one-year actuarial patient, kidney, and pancreas (with complete insulin independence) graft survival rates after SKPT are 95%, 92% and 84%, respectively (1). Solitary PTXs comprise the remaining activity, including either sequential pancreas after kidney transplants (PAKT, 12%) or PTX alone (PA, 5%). The current one-year actuarial pancreas graft survival rates are 73% for PAKT and 70% for PA (1). With the advent of Medicare coverage, SKPT and PAKT have become accepted as preferred treatment options in selected patients with insulin-dependent diabetes mellitus (IDDM) and advanced nephropathy.

According to IPTR data, most PTXs are performed with systemic venous delivery of insulin and either bladder [systemic-bladder (S-B)] or enteric [systemic-enteric (S-E)] drainage of the exocrine secretions (2). From 1988 through 1995, more than 90% of PTX procedures were performed by the standard technique of S-B drainage using a duodenal segment conduit.

Although well tolerated in most PTX recipients, S-B drainage was associated with a finite and troublesome rate of unique metabolic and urologic complications resulting from altered physiology. When these complications became persistent or refractory, conversion from bladder to enteric drainage (enteric conversion) was often necessary and successful (3). Because of a favorable experience with enteric conversion, coupled with advances in preservation, donor selection, and immunosuppression that placed the duodenal segment at a lower risk for ischemic or immunologic injury, a resurgence of interest occurred in primary enteric drainage in an effort to avoid the complications of bladder drainage.

Since 1995, the number of PTX procedures performed with primary enteric drainage has steadily increased, accounting for 60% of cases in 1999 (1). In the last few years, the results of SKPT with enteric drainage have improved and are now comparable to SKPT with bladder drainage (2). Despite an evolution in surgical techniques, the majority of PTXs with enteric drainage are performed with systemic venous delivery of insulin, resulting in peripheral hyperinsulinemia. In the nontransplant setting, chronic hyperinsulinemia has been associated with insulin resistance, dyslipidemia, accelerated atherosclerosis, and macroangiopathy. To improve the physiology of PTX, a new surgical technique was developed at our center combining portal venous delivery of insulin with enteric drainage of the exocrine secretions [portal-enteric (P-E)] (4–6). In a recent survey of surgical techniques among PTX centers, seven reported experience with the P-E technique, of which five used a diverting Roux limb (7). Table 1 provides a list of centers that have reported experience in PTX with P-E drainage. Many of these centers have adopted the P-E technique as their preferred method of PTX. However, the proportion of cases with P-E drainage has remained low and represents only 15% to 20% of enteric-drained PTXs (1,2). In the most recent IPTR analysis including PTXs performed between 1996 and 1999, the one-year pancreas graft survival rates were similar for P-E versus S-E drainage, 83% and 84%, respectively (2).

## HISTORICAL BACKGROUND

The history of clinical PTX largely revolves around the development and application of various surgical techniques. Experience in PTX with portal venous delivery of insulin dates back to the mid-1980s. Initial attempts employed segmental PTX with either gastric (23), pyelic (24), or jejunal (25,26) drainage. Whole organ PTX using the P-E technique was first described clinically by our group in 1992 (4) and was based on experimental work by Shokouh-Amiri et al. in a porcine model (27–29). This new technique employed a tributary of the superior mesenteric vein to reestablish portal venous drainage and differed substantially from other initial reports of whole organ PTX with portal venous drainage. In 1990, Muhlbacher et al. described a technique involving an end-to-side anastomosis between the distal splenic vein of the donor and

**Table 1** Recent Experience in Pancreas Transplantation with Portal-Enteric Drainage

| Center | No. of cases | References |
|---|---|---|
| University of Tennessee Memphis | >100 | (8–12) |
| University of Chicago | >100 | (13–16) |
| University of Maryland | >100 | (17,18) |
| Lyon, France | >20 | (19) |
| Toronto | >20 | (20) |
| Louisiana State University | >15 | (21) |
| University of Virginia | >10 | (22)[a] |
| Duke University | >10 | [a] |
| University of Massachusetts | >10 | [a] |
| Northwestern University | >5 | [a] |

[a]Personal communication.

the recipient's portal vein in combination with bladder drainage (30). In 1992, Rosenlof et al. applied Calne's original technique to whole organ PTX using an end-to-side anastomosis between the donor portal vein and the recipient's splenic vein coupled with enteric drainage (22). In each of these other series, however, the procedure was not widely applied because of technical problems associated with the vascular reconstruction (31).

We have previously reported our initial experience with P-E drainage, including both retrospective and prospective comparisons to control groups of patients who underwent SKPT with either S-B or S-E drainage (6,8,9,32–34). We have also reported our initial experience in solitary PTX with P-E drainage, including a retrospective comparison to a control group of solitary PTX recipients with S-B drainage (35). In 1995, Ncwell et al. from the University of Chicago reported their initial experience with a similar P-E technique in 12 SKPT recipients compared to a retrospective control group of 12 SKPT patients with S-B drainage (13). Six-month patient and graft survival rates were comparable, and the P-E group had less acidosis, dehydration, hematuria, rejection, and need for enteric conversion. There were no differences in technical complications, and renal and pancreas allograft functions were similar. In 1996, Newell et al. presented 12-month follow-up on the same two groups with similar findings (14). In addition, the initial length of stay and total hospital days in the first year after SKPT were slightly lower in the P-E group. There were no significant differences in costs, no delay in the diagnosis of rejection, and the authors concluded that their initial results confirmed the safety and efficacy of this new technique.

In 1998, Bruce et al. from the University of Chicago reported their experience with 70 consecutive SKPTs with P-E drainage performed between January 1992 and August 1997 (15). They compared this group to a "historical" control group of 70 SKPTs with S-B drainage performed between January 1987 and December 1994. One-year patient, kidney, and pancreas graft survival rates were comparable between groups. There were no significant differences in technical or immunologic graft failure rates, as no enteric or anastomotic leaks were reported in the series. Renal and pancreas allograft functions at one year were similar. However, the total number of hospital days and operative complications in the first year were significantly higher in the S-B group, with the difference in these results almost entirely accounted for by a 21% rate of enteric conversion in patients with S-B drainage. In addition, the authors noted a possible "learning curve" effect, with improved results in the latter 35 versus the former 35 SKPTs with P-E drainage. In 1998, Busing et al. reported on 70 consecutive SKPTs without anastomotic complications, including two with P-E drainage (36). Busing et al. later updated his experience to 10 SKPTs with P-E drainage, including none using a Roux limb (37). Kidney and pancreas survival rates were both 90%, with one graft lost due to thrombosis. Buell et al. likewise updated the University of Chicago experience, including 16 SKPTs with P-E drainage without a Roux limb (16). This group also reported good initial results with the P-E technique in the absence of a diverting Roux limb.

In 1999, Philosophe et al. from the University of Maryland reported their initial experience with 66 PTXs with P-E drainage compared to 183 PTXs with S-E drainage (17). Graft survival rates for SKPT, PAKT, and PA recipients were similar according to technique. However, when stratified for human leukocyte antigen (HLA) matching, the incidence of rejection was lower in patients with P-E drainage. In a follow-up report in 2000, Philosophe et al. compared 117 solitary PTXs with P-E drainage versus 70 with S-E drainage (18). The authors noted not only an improvement in the pancreas graft survival rate, but also a decrease in the incidence and severity of rejection in patients with P-E drainage. The authors concluded that P-E drainage may be associated with an immunologic advantage.

In 2000, the Lyon group reported a prospective study of 34 SKPT recipients randomized to either S-E or P-E drainage with a Roux limb (19). Patient and graft survival rates and morbidity were similar between groups. Also in 2000, Cattral et al. prospectively studied 20 SKPTs with S-B drainage followed by a sequential cohort of 20 consecutive SKPTs with P-E drainage (20). One-year patient and graft survival rates were similar between groups. However, medical morbidity, cytomegalovirus (CMV) infections, and acute rejection were more common in the S-B group. Zibari et al. reported their initial experience with 17 SKPTs with P-E drainage and a Roux-en-y venting jejunostomy to monitor for rejection and prevent anastomotic leak (21). Patient, kidney, and pancreas graft survival rates were 100%, 100% and 94%, respectively, after a mean follow-up of 16 months. In each of these studies, the authors concluded that SKPT with P-E drainage can be performed with excellent short-term outcomes and minimal morbidity.

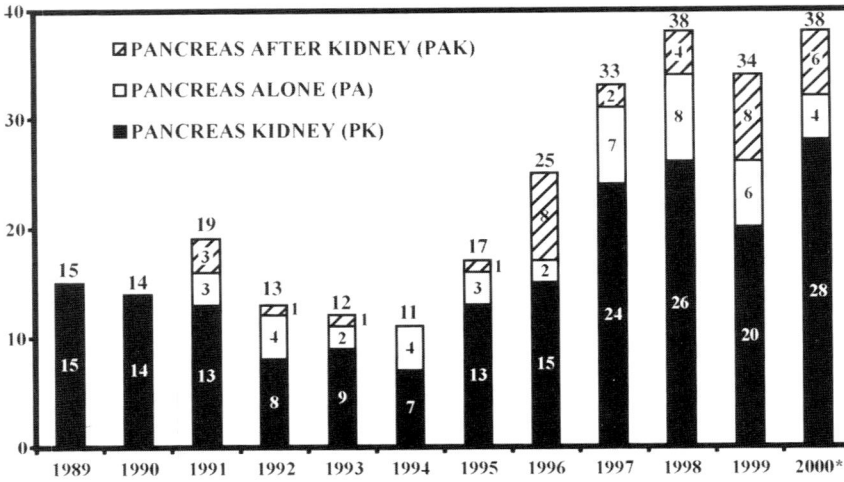

**Figure 1** University of Tennessee Memphis pancreas transplant experience by year according to type of transplant (∗, through Sept. 15, 2000.).

Herein we report the chronology of our nine-year single center experience with 126 PTXs with P-E drainage spanning different immunosuppressive eras.

## PROGRAM OVERVIEW

The University of Tennessee (UT), Memphis, PTX program began in 1989 (Fig. 1) (9). Between April 1989 and September 1990, 24 consecutive SKPTs were performed with S-B drainage (Fig. 2). The first SKPT with P-E drainage was performed in October 1990, and this patient continues to enjoy excellent dual allograft function over 10 years later. Also in 1990, the first solitary PTXs were performed at our program including both sequential PAKT and PA (Fig. 1).

From October 1990 through December 1994, we performed 42 SKPTs, including 26 with P-E and 16 with S-B drainage (Fig. 2). During the same interval, a total of 18 solitary PTXs were performed with S-B drainage, including 13 PA and 5 PAKT (Fig. 1). In 1995 and 1996, 42 consecutive PTXs (29 SKPT, 9 PAKT, and 4 PA) were performed exclusively with P-E drainage (Fig. 2). From February 1997 through March 1998, we compared 32 consecutive PTXs performed with either S-B or P-E drainage (32). From April 1998 through May 2000, 54 consecutive SKPT recipients were entered into a prospective study of S-E versus P-E drainage at our center (Fig. 2) (33). From 1989 through 1999, we performed a total of 231 PTXs, including 126 with P-E, 76 with S-B, and 29 with S-E drainage (Fig. 3). This overall experience accumulated over a decade includes 163 SKPTs, 39 PA, and 29 PAKTs (Fig. 4). The UT Memphis PTX program is

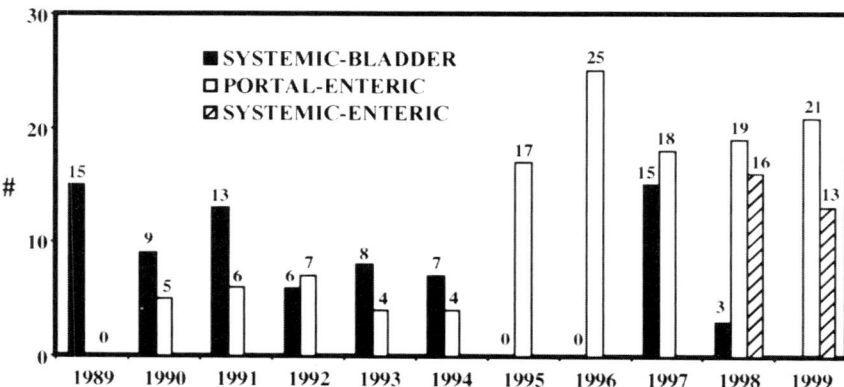

**Figure 2** University of Tennessee Memphis pancreas transplant experience by year according to technique of transplant.

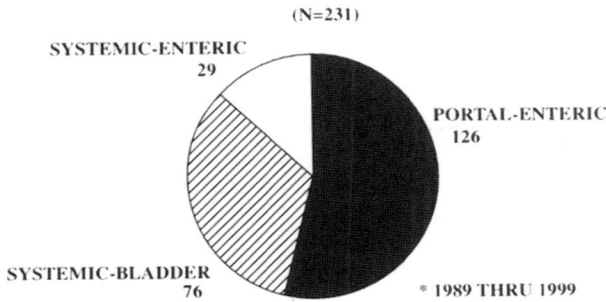

(N=231)

SYSTEMIC-ENTERIC
29

PORTAL-ENTERIC
126

SYSTEMIC-BLADDER
76

* 1989 THRU 1999

**Figure 3** Total number of pancreas transplants at the University of Tennessee Memphis according to type of transplant.

currently one of the seven largest centers in the United States and recently became the 13th center worldwide to perform 250 PTXs. To date, we have one of the largest single center experiences with the P-E technique, including 126 PTXs (90 SKPT, 18 PAKT, and 18 PA) with P-E drainage (Fig. 5). This report represents a case series and our collective experience with the P-E technique.

## Organ Procurement, Preservation, and Preparation

Donor selection and organ procurement were recognized to be of paramount importance to the success of the new procedure. Most heart-beating donors who have been declared brain dead and are appropriate for kidney, heart, lung, and liver donation are also suitable for pancreas donation (Table 2). Although there is some evidence to suggest that donor hyperglycemia may have an adverse affect on initial and long-term allograft function, the presence of hyperglycemia or hyperamylasemia as such are not contraindications for pancreas donation. In general, ideal pancreas donors range in age from 10 to 40 years and range in weight from 30 to 80 kg (38). Management of the multiple organ donor includes aggressive resuscitation to maintain hemodynamic stability, organ perfusion, and oxygenation. Resuscitative efforts usually result in significant hyperglycemia, and intensive control with insulin may have a favorable effect on initial allograft function and survival. Intravenous colloid fluids and mannitol are given to minimize pancreatic edema. Judicious administration of vasopressors, such as dopamine, is indicated to maintain a systolic blood pressure above 90 mmHg and promote diuresis.

The pancreas and/or kidney were procured from heart-beating cadaveric donors in conjunction with multiple organ retrieval using standardized techniques (39). We believe that combined liver, kidney, and whole organ pancreaticoduodenal retrieval can be safely performed in virtually all donors regardless of vascular anatomy. Whole organ pancreaticoduodenosplenectomy was performed by an en bloc technique (39). In cases in which a replaced or accessory hepatic artery originated from the superior mesenteric artery, we were either able to dissect the superior mesenteric artery in situ to include the accessory hepatic

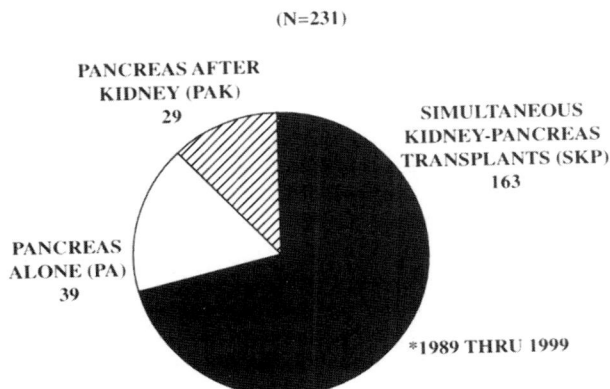

(N=231)

PANCREAS AFTER
KIDNEY (PAK)
29

SIMULTANEOUS
KIDNEY-PANCREAS
TRANSPLANTS (SKP)
163

PANCREAS
ALONE (PA)
39

*1989 THRU 1999

**Figure 4** Total number of pancreas transplants at the University of Tennessee Memphis according to type of transplant.

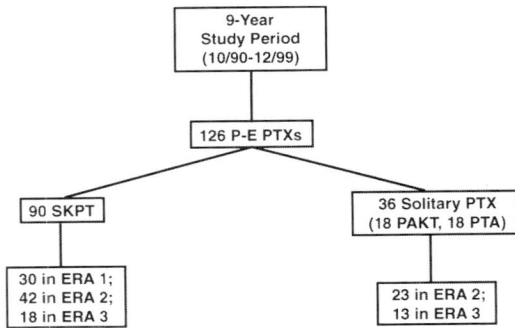

**Figure 5** Overall experience in pancreas transplantation with portal-enteric drainage spanning different immunosuppressive eras. *Abbreviations*: P-E, portal-enteric; PTXs, pancreas transplants; SKPT, simultaneous kidney-pancreas transplantation; PAKT, pancreas after kidney transplant.

**Table 2**  Cadaveric Pancreas Organ Donation

Indications
    Declaration of brain death
    Informed consent
    Age 6–55 yr (ideal 10–40)
    Weight 30–100 kg (ideal 30–80)
    Hemodynamic stability with adequate perfusion and oxygenation
    Normal glycosylated hemoglobin level (only needed in cases of severe
      hyperglycemia, extreme obesity, or positive family history of diabetes)
    Absence of infectious or transmissible diseases (i.e., tuberculosis, syphilis,
      hepatitis, AIDS)
    Negative aerology (HIV; hepatitis B and C)
    Absence of malignancy (unless skin or low grade brain cancer)
    Absence of pancreatic disease
Contraindications
    History of diabetes mellitus (type 1, 2, or gestational)
    Previous pancreatic surgery
    Moderate to severe pancreatic trauma
    Pancreatitis (active acute or chronic)
    Significant intra-abdominal contamination
    Major (active) infection
    Chronic alcohol abuse
    Recent history of intravenous drug abuse
    Recent history of homosexuality
    Prolonged hypotension or hypoxemia with evidence for significant end organ
      (kidney, liver) damage
    Severe atherosclerosis
    Inexperienced retrieval team
    Severe fatty infiltration
    Severe pancreatic edema
    Severe obesity ( >150% ideal body weight)
Risk factors
    Massive transfusions
    Prior splenectomy
    Mild to moderate obesity ( <150% ideal body weight)
    Aberrant hepatic artery anatomy
    Positive VDRL/RPR serology
    Prolonged length of hospital stay
    Donor age above 45 yr
    Cardiovascular or cerebrovascular cause of brain death
    Mild to moderate fatty infiltration
    Mild to moderate pancreatic edema
    Donor instability
    Mild pancreatic trauma
    Mild to moderate atherosclerosis

*Abbreviations*: VDRL, venereal disease research laboratory; RPR, rapid plasma reagin.

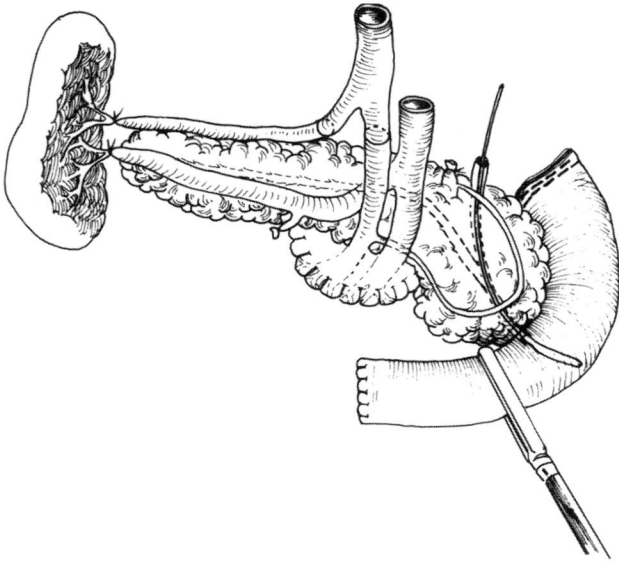

**Figure 6** Bench reconstruction of pancreas allograft. See text for details.

artery with the liver or alternatively (and preferentially) performed combined en bloc hepaticopancreatico-duodenosplenectomy followed by back table ex vivo separation of the liver and pancreas (40). University of Wisconsin (UW) solution was used for both in situ flush and preservation of all organs under cold storage conditions. Cold ischemia was kept to a minimum, and pancreas preservation times were below 24 hours in all cases and below 12 hours in about 1/3 of cases. The mean pancreas cold ischemia time was 13 hours. In a retrospective analysis of our data, we found that steroid administration to the donor resulted in a significant reduction in postreperfusion pancreatitis (41). In the same analysis, we demonstrated that postreperfusion pancreatitis increased significantly when cold ischemia exceeded 12 hours. Moreover, by using calcium channel blockers in the early postoperative period, we were able to significantly decrease the incidence of posttransplant pancreatitis (41). Because of these observations, whenever possible, we attempt to limit preservation times and administer steroids to the donor and calcium channel blockers to the recipient.

Prior to transplantation, the pancreas was reconstructed on the back table with a donor iliac artery bifurcation Y-graft to the splenic and superior mesenteric arteries (Fig. 6) (40). The P-E procedure requires that the arterial bifurcation graft be constructed intentionally long for subsequent arterialization. The donor portal vein was mobilized and dissected back to the splenic and superior mesenteric venous confluence without the need for a venous extension graft. The proximal duodenal staple line (just distal to the pylorus) was inverted with suture, and the distal duodenal closure incorporated the third and a variable length of the fourth portion of the duodenum, as previously described (9). The closure of the mesenteric root was reinforced with a running suture. The spleen was left attached to the tail of the pancreas to be used as a handle, but in some cases, the splenic hilar structures were ligated in continuity before revascularization. The kidney was likewise prepared using standard techniques. The pancreaticoduodenal graft was repackaged separately and in sterile fashion in cold UW solution prior to implantation.

## RECIPIENT SELECTION AND PRETRANSPLANT EVALUATION

Indications for PTX at UT Memphis include the presence of IDDM (Type 1 or Type 2) and the predicted abilities to tolerate the operative procedure, the requisite immunosuppression after transplantation, and possible associated complications (Table 3) (9,38,42). Patient selection is aided by a comprehensive medical evaluation before transplantation (Table 4) performed by a multidisciplinary team that confirms the diagnosis of IDDM, determines the patient's ability to withstand the operative procedure, establishes the absences of any exclusion criteria (Table 5), and documents end-organ complications for future tracking after transplantation

**Table 3**  Indications for Pancreas Transplantation: Eligibility Guidelines

Medical necessity
   Presence of insulin-treated diabetes mellitus:
      Documentation of insulin dose
      Type 1 or 2 diabetes
   Ability to withstand surgery and immunosuppression (as assessed by pretransplant medical evaluation):
      Adequate cardiopulmonary function
         Cardiac stress testing± coronary angiography to rule out significant
            coronary artery disease or other cardiac contraindications
         Patients with significant coronary artery disease should have it corrected
            pretransplant
      Absence of other organ system failure (other than kidney)
   Emotional and sociopsychological suitability
   Presence of well-defined diabetic complications (any two):
      Proliferative retinopathy
      Nephropathy (hypertension, proteinuria, or decline in GFR)
      Symptomatic peripheral or autonomic neuropathy
      Microangiopathy
      Accelerated atherosclerosis (macroangiopathy)
      Glucose hyperlability, insulin resistance, or hypoglycemia unawareness with a
         significant impairment in quality of life
   Absence of any contraindications
   Financial resources
Type of pancreas transplant
   Specific entry criteria based on degree of nephropathy:
      Simultaneous kidney–pancreas transplant: creatinine clearance below
         30 mL/min
      Sequential pancreas after kidney transplant: creatinine clearance
         ≥40 mL/min (on calcineurin inhibitor)
      Pancreas transplant alone: creatinine clearance above 60 mL/min
   Primary determinants for recipient selection are the presence of diabetic
      complications, degree of nephropathy, and cardiovascular risk

*Abbreviation*: GFR, glomerular filtration rate.

(9,38). The primary determinants for recipient selection are the presence of diabetic complications, degree of nephropathy, and cardiovascular risk (Table 3) (42).

     We believe that SKPT should be at least considered in all IDDM patients with advanced nephropathy, defined as those who are dialysis dependent or dialysis imminent with a creatinine clearance less than 30 mL/min or failure of a previous kidney transplant. We encourage kidney-transplantation alone (KTA) in all patients who have a living donor, particularly if the potential donor is a 6-antigen HLA-match. We also offer diabetic patients with uremia, the opportunity to be listed either for KTA or SKPT in order to take advantage of zero antigen HLA mismatch sharing. Patients with IDDM and impending or end stage renal disease (ESRD) who have minimal or limited secondary complications of diabetes (usually between the ages of 20 and 40 years) are considered optimal candidates for SKPT (38,42). However, not all diabetic patients with ESRD are acceptable candidates. In our experience, about two-thirds of diabetic patients screened are actually accepted for SKPT. In contrast to some centers, we do not regard blindness, history of major amputation, or history of cardiac disease as absolute contraindications for SKPT. Although these diabetes-related problems are certainly irreversible, a number of patients are well adjusted to these complications and can lead productive lives after dual organ transplantation with facilitated rehabilitation. With increasing experience in PTX, previous absolute contraindications have become relative contraindications, and relative contraindications have become risk factors for a successful outcome (38). Inclusion and exclusion criteria for PTX are listed in Tables 3 and 5.

     Selection criteria for solitary PTX are based on the presence of early diabetic complications associated with either hypoglycemia unawareness or exogenous insulin failure with hyperlabile diabetes and a significant impairment in quality of life (38,42). Diabetic patients with a creatinine clearance above 60 mL/min and evidence of overt diabetic complications or unawareness of hypoglycemic symptoms are potential candidates for PA (Table 3). Diabetic patients that have previously received a renal allograft, whether from a living or a cadaveric

**Table 4** Evaluation of the Pancreas Transplant Candidate

Interviews and consults
    History and physical examination by nephrologist, endocrinologist, and
       transplant surgeon
    Ophthalmology evaluation including visual acuity, fluorescein angiography,
       retinal fundus photography with retinopathy score, and slit-lamp examination
    Transplant coordinator and medical social worker interview including
       completion of quality of life questionnaire
    Gynecology consultation for all females (pelvic examination with Pap smear)
    Dental evaluation
    When indicated, additional evaluations may be required by orthopedic surgery,
       podiatry, psychology, psychiatry, neurology, or gastroenterology
Cardiovascular, respiratory, and peripheral vascular evaluations
    Standard testing includes orthostatic vital signs, 12 lead electrocardiogram, chest
       radiograph, echocardiography, and exercise treadmill, stress thallium, or
       dobutaminc stress echocardiography
    Additional studies may include arterial blood gases, 24 hr Holter monitoring,
       autonomic and peripheral vasomotor reflexes, Doppler arterial studies,
       ankle/brachial index, transcutaneous oxygen monitoring, plethysmography,
       carotid Doppler examination, aortography with run-off, or pulmonary function
       tests as indicated
    Cardiology consultation with or without coronary angiography as indicated
Metabolic and endocrine evaluation
    Standard testing includes fasting blood glucose, glycohemoglobin, and fasting
       lipid panel (cholesterol, triglycerides, and HDL-cholesterol)
    Fasting and stimulated C-peptide levels are used to assess type of diabetes
       if needed
    Additional studies may include oral or intravenous glucose challenge, anti-insulin
       and islet cell antibodies, proinsulin level, and lipoprotein profile
Genitourinary/renal evaluation
    Standard testing includes electrolytes, blood urea nitrogen, serum creatinine,
       urinalysis with culture, and 24 hr urine for protein and creatinine clearance
    Voiding cystourethrogram and urodynamics when indicated
    Radiometric glomerular filtration rate if needed
    In addition, kidney biopsy, or evaluation of erectile dysfunction may be indicated
    Calcineurin inhibitor challenge test when indicated
    Hormonal profiles as indicated
Serology and immunology evaluation
    ABO blood type and HLA tissue type
    Cytotoxic antibodies
    Viral liters (Epstein–Barr virus, herpes simplex virus, varicella-zoster virus,
       human immunodeficiency virus, hepatitis B virus, hepatitis C virus, and
       cytomegalovirus); PCR quantitation when indicated
    VDRL/FTA test for syphilis
Other laboratory tests
    Complete blood count with differential and platelets, prothrombin time, partial
       thromboplastin time, chemistry profile, amylase, lipase
    Abdominal ultrasound of kidneys and gallbladder
    Mammography in females over 35 yr
Hemoccull ×3; contrast studies or endoscopy when indicated
When indicated, nerve conduction studies, gastric emptying scan,
    electromyography
Hypercoagulable work-up (when indicated)

*Abbreviations*: HDL, high density lipoprotein; PCR, polymerase chain reaction; VDRL, venereal disease research laboratory; FTA, fluorescent treponemal antibody, HLA, human leukocyte antigen.

donor, are considered potential candidates for PAKT if the creatinine clearance is above 40 mL/min on either cyclosporine (CYA) or tacrolimus (TAC) immunosuppression (Table 3).

The cardiac status of each candidate must be assessed carefully because significant (and silent) coronary artery disease is not uncommon in this population (43). The cardiac evaluation consists of a noninvasive functional assessment such as an exercise or pharmacologic stress test in addition to echocardiography (38,42). Coronary angiography is reserved for specific indications such as age over 45 years, diabetes for more than 25 years, a positive smoking history, longstanding hypertension, previous major amputation due to peripheral vascular

**Table 5**  Absolute and Relative Contraindications and Risk Factors for Pancreas Transplantation

Absolute contraindications
    Insufficient cardiovascular reserve; one or more of the following:
        Coronary angiographic evidence of significant noncorrectable or unbeatable
         coronary artery disease
        Recent myocardial infarction
        Ejection fraction below 30%
    Active infection
    History of malignancy diagnosed within past three years (excluding
      nonmelanoma skin cancer)
    Positive HIV serology
    Positive hepatitis B surface antigen serology
    Active, untreated peptic ulcer disease
    Ongoing substance abuse (drug or alcohol)
    Major ongoing psychiatric illness
    Recent history of noncompliance
    Inability to provide informed consent
    Any systemic illness that would severely limit life expectancy or
      compromise recovery
    Significant, irreversible hepatic or pulmonary dysfunction
    Positive crossmatch
Relative contraindications
    Age less than 18 or greater than 65 yr
    Recent retinal hemorrhage
    Symptomatic cerebrovascular or peripheral vascular disease
    Absence of appropriate social support network
    Extreme obesity (greater than 150% ideal body weight)
    Active smoking
    Severe aorto-iliac vascular disease
Risk factors
    History of myocardial infarction, congestive heart failure, previous open heart
      surgery, or cardiac intervention
    History of major amputation or peripheral bypass graft
    History of cerebrovascular event or carotid endarterectomy
    History of hypercoagulable syndrome

disease, history of cerebrovascular disease, or cases in which the history, physical examination, or noninvasive cardiac studies reveal an abnormality. A history of previous myocardial infarction, angioplasty, stenting, or coronary artery bypass grafting is not necessarily contraindications for PTX. We have found that pharmacologic stress cardiac imaging is an excellent screening tool, with only about one-third of our evaluants undergoing coronary angiography. However, sudden cardiac death, in the absence of significant structural heart disease, continues to be a major cause of mortality after PTX (44). For this reason, cardiac autonomic function is currently measured by two methods; laboratory evoked cardiovascular tests and 24-hour heart rate variability measurements (43,44). These methods are able to detect alterations in autonomic function prior to the onset of disabling symptoms.

In general, we consider age over 60 years, active smoking, a left ventricular fraction below 30%, and severe obesity (greater than 150% ideal body weight) as contraindications for PTX (Table 5). We accept most patients younger than 45 years for PTX, provided that no significant coronary artery disease is present. A history of compliance with medication regimens and scheduled follow-up is an important factor in our patient selection. Other exclusion criteria that are applicable to all solid organ transplant recipients include the presence of active infection or recent malignancy, active substance abuse or dependence, recent history of noncompliance or psychiatric illness, and positive human immunodeficiency virus or hepatitis B virus serology (Table 5).

Because of the impact that PTX has on quality of life, we are conducting comprehensive, prospective studies examining quality of life changes in this patient population (45,46). The dramatic increase in posttransplant patient and graft survival rates over the last decade has resulted in great interest in quality of life. This is of particular importance for those patients with ESRD and IDDM who not only have symptoms associated with uremia, but complications related to longstanding diabetes. Quality of life is a multidimensional construct reflecting an individual's perception of health, well being, and happiness. Since 1990, UT Memphis has included three measurements of quality of life in order to capture as many dimensions as possible. Functional disability is measured by the Sickness Impact Profile, whereas a more positive view of health is measured by the Quality of Life index. Psychoemotional dimensions are measured with the Adult Self-image Scale (45,46). Each instrument has been used in the transplant population and has documented reliability and validity. All patients are asked to participate by completing a battery of quality of life instruments that provide a multi-dimensional assessment of this construct. Combined, the instruments yield over 20 scores reflecting specific dimensions of quality of life such as mobility, work, family, anxiety, and independence; composite scores that group specific dimensions into five categories (health-related, physical, psychological, disability, and self-esteem); and one global measure of quality of life that does not separate specific dimensions. These instruments are repeated at 6 and 12 months after PTX and yearly thereafter. This provides us with prospective, longitudinal data regarding the influence of PTX on quality of life.

## OPERATIVE PROCEDURE

Patients were selected for transplantation based on ABO blood type compatibility, period of time on the waiting list, and a negative T-lymphocytotoxic crossmatch, in accordance with United Network for Organ Sharing guidelines. HLA-matching was not part of the allocation algorithm. After preparation of the organs, the recipient operation was performed through a midline intraperitoneal approach. The surgical technique of P-E drainage has been previously described in detail by our group (Fig. 7) (4–6,8,9,32). The portal vein of the pancreas graft was anastomosed end-to-side to a major tributary of the superior mesenteric vein. The donor iliac bifurcation graft was brought through a window made in the distal ileal mesentery and anastomosed end-to-side to the right common iliac artery. The transplant duodenum was ana-stomosed to a diverting Roux-en-y limb of recipient jejunum. Splenectomy was performed after revascularization, and an attempt was made to anchor the tail of the pancreas to the anterior abdominal wall with interrupted sutures. These anchoring sutures permitted subsequent per-cutaneous, ultrasound-guided pancreas allograft biopsies to be performed as needed (47).

When applicable, the kidney transplant was performed in the left iliac fossa, with end-to-side vascular anastomoses between the renal vessels and left external iliac vessels. Fol-lowing an extra-vesical ureteroneocystostomy by standard techniques, the renal allograft was then "retroperitonealized" by anchoring the sigmoid colon mesentery to the lateral peritoneal reflection with interrupted sutures. A nasogastric tube, central venous line, and urethral cath-eter were placed at the beginning of the surgical procedure, and two closed suction drains

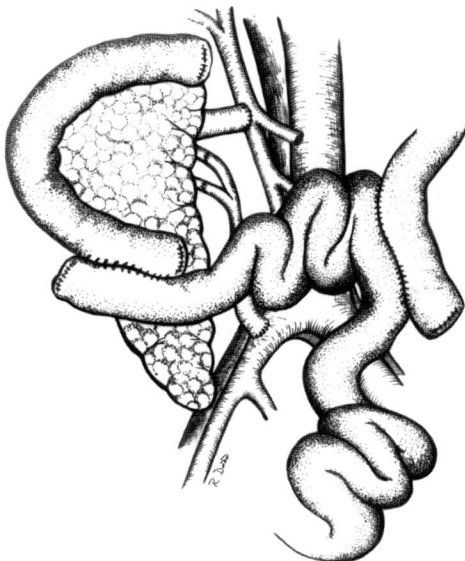

**Figure 7** Technique of pancreas transplantation with portal-enteric drainage. See text for details.

were placed medial and lateral to the pancreas allograft near the end of the procedure prior to wound closure.

## PERIOPERATIVE MANAGEMENT

Perioperative antibiotic prophylaxis consisted of a preoperative dose, an intra operative dose, and three postoperative doses of Cefazolin (1 g intravenous). All patients received single-strength Sulfamethoxazole/Trimethoptim one tablet/day for 12 months as prophylaxis for *Pneumocystis* pneumonia. Patients allergic to sulfa medications received inhaled Pentamidine therapy. Antifungal prophylaxis consisted of either oral nystatin (Era 1) swish and swallow 5 cc four times daily or oral fluconazole (Eras 2 and 3) 200 mg/day for three months (48). Antiviral prophylaxis consisted of either oral acyclovir for three months (Era 1), intravenous ganciclovir followed by oral acyclovir for three months (Era 2), or intravenous ganciclovir (2.5–5 mg/kg twice daily) during the initial hospitalization followed by oral ganciclovir (Era 3) 1 g three times daily for three months (for six months if the donor was seropositive for CMV and the recipient was seronegative) (48–50).

Patients were monitored in the intensive care unit for 24 to 36 hours before being transferred to the transplant unit. Nasogastric tube decompression was maintained for two to three days, closed-suction drainage for three to five days, and urethral catheter drainage for five to seven days. Antiplatelet therapy consisting of oral aspirin (81 mg/day) was administered to all patients. In addition, 2000 to 3000 units of intravenous Heparin was administered as a single dose during surgery before implantation of the pancreas. In selected cases (Era 2), Heparin prophylaxis was continued after surgery (5000 units subcutaneously twice daily) for three to five days. In most cases (Era 3), Heparin prophylaxis was continued after surgery (continuous infusion of 300 U/hr for 24 hours, then 400 U/hr for 24 hours, then 500 U/hr until postoperative day 5). Oral Coumadin (Era 3) in a single dose of 1 mg/day was administered to patients requiring prolonged vascular access or those with subsequent placement of a permanent central venous catheter. A number of management protocols evolved over time including: (i) donor selection restricted to ideal situations, particularly in solitary PTX; (ii) protective CMV matching (seronegative donor organs transplanted into a seronegative recipient); (iii) minimizing cold ischemia, particularly for nonideal donors (41); (iv) routine anticoagulation and HLA-matching, especially in re-transplants and solitary PTX; (v) routine ganciclovir and fluconazole prophylaxis (48–50); and (vi) surveillance pancreas biopsy monitoring (particularly for solitary PTX recipients) (51).

## IMMUNOSUPPRESSION

According to IPTR data, rejection accounts for 32% of graft failures in the first year after PTX (2). Most PTX centers use quadruple drug immunosuppression with antilymphocyte induction (ALI) because of a high incidence of rejection and the general impression that the pancreas is a highly immunogenic organ. The evolution of surgical techniques has been, in large part, facilitated by the rapid changes in immunosuppressive therapy. With the recent commercial availability of potent immunosuppressive agents such as TAC and mycophenolate mofetil (MMF), the need for routine ALI therapy after PTX has been questioned (10,52).

From October 1990 through June 1995 (Era 1), 30 SKPTs with P-E drainage were performed at our center with quadruple therapy consisting of OKT3 induction in combination with CYA-Sandimmune, Prednisone, and Azathioprine (Fig. 8) (8). CYA dosing was titrated to achieve a target 12-hour trough level of greater than 300 ng/mL for the first three months after transplant and greater than 200 ng/mL thereafter. Azathioprine dosing was 1 to 2 mg/kg/day, Prednisone was tapered to achieve a dose of 10 mg/day by one year and 5 mg/day by two years after transplant.

From July 1995 through May 1998 (Era 2), 42 SKPTs and 23 solitary PTXs (11 PAKT and 12 PA) with P-E drainage received TAC, Prednisone, and MMF triple therapy without antibody induction (10,35,52). TAC dosing was titrated to a 12-hour trough level of 15 to 25 ng/mL by IMX assay for the first three months after transplant. After three months, TAC blood levels were maintained at 10 to 15 ng/mL in the absence of rejection. Oral MMF was begun immediately after transplant at 2 to 3 g/day in two to four divided doses. The MMF dose was reduced in patients with gastrointestinal intolerance (nausea, vomiting, and diarrhea)

ERA 1 (10/90-6/95):
- **30 SKPTs with P-E drainage received OKT3 induction, CSA-Sandimmune, prednisone (Pred), and azathioprine**

ERA 2 (7/95-5/98):
- **42 SKPTs and 23 solitary PTXs (11 PAKT, 12 PTA) received tacrolimus (TAC), Pred, and mycophenolate mofetil (MMF) w/o antibody induction**

ERA 3 (6/98-12/99):
- **18 SKPTs and 13 solitary PTXs (7 PAKT, 6 PTA) received TAC, MMF, and Pred ± either Basiliximab or Daclizumab induction**

**Figure 8** Chronology of experience at the University of Tennessee Memphis in pancreas transplantation with portal-enteric drainage according to immunosuppressive era. *Abbreviations*: SKPTs, simultaneous kidney-pancreas transplants; P-E, portal-enteric; PTXs, pancreas transplants; PAKT, pancreas after kidney transplant.

or when the total white blood cell count was less than 3000/mm (3). MMF was discontinued temporarily in patients with active CMV infection or septicemia, or when the total white blood cell count was less than 2,000/mm (3); it was restarted later at a reduced dose. Prednisone was gradually tapered to achieve a dose of 5 mg/day at one year.

From June 1998 through December 1999 (Era 3), 18 SKPTs and 13 solitary PTXs (seven PAKT and six PA) with P-E drainage received TAC, MMF, and Prednisone immunosuppression with or without either Simulect (Basiliximab) or Zenapax (Daclizumab) antibody induction (Fig. 9) (53). Half of the SKPT and all of the solitary PTX recipients received either Basiliximab (20 mg intravenous on day 0 and 4) or Daclizumab (1 mg/kg on day 0 and then at two week intervals for a total of five doses) as induction therapy.

## POSTOPERATIVE MONITORING

After transplantation, duplex ultrasonography of the pancreas and/or kidney were performed on the first postoperative day and whenever clinically indicated. Recipients were serially monitored for daily fasting serum glucose, amylase, and lipase levels (54); renal profiles; CYA or TAC levels; and complete blood cell counts. Metabolic control and hormonal profiles were

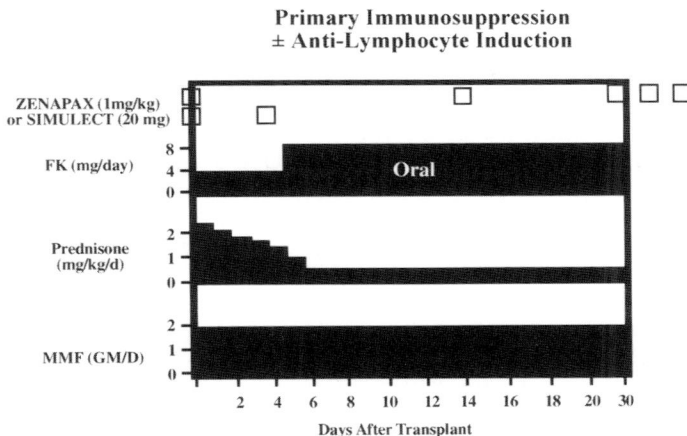

**Primary Immunosuppression ± Anti-Lymphocyte Induction**

**Figure 9** Regimen of immunosuppression in Era 3 with selective use of monoclonal antibodies directed against the interleukin-2 receptor (EL2R) as induction therapy. Maintenance immunosuppression was triple therapy with tacrolimus (FK), mycophenolate mofetil and steroids. *Abbreviation*: MMF, mycophenolate mofetil.

assessed by intravenous glucose tolerance testing, fasting and stimulated C-peptide levels, lipid profiles, and glycosylated hemoglobin levels (55).

The diagnosis of rejection was based on clinical criteria (56), renal allograft dysfunction, serum amylase and lipase levels (54), serum glucose levels, a change in the slope of glucose disappearance (55), and renal or pancreas allograft histopathology (47,51). Renal allograft rejection was suggested by an unexplained rise in serum creatinine of 0.3 mg/dL or greater and confirmed by ultrasound-guided percutaneous biopsy. Because of our concern regarding the ability to diagnose rejection after enteric drainage, we developed a safe outpatient technique of percutaneous pancreas allograft biopsy (47). Pancreas allograft rejection was suggested by an unexplained elevation in serum amylase, lipase, or glucose and confirmed by ultrasound-guided percutaneous biopsy (47,51,54). The severity of rejection was defined according to the BANFF criteria (57) for kidney biopsies and by a modification of the Maryland classification (58) of allograft rejection for pancreas biopsies. Mild renal allograft rejection was treated with intravenous methylprednisolone 500 to 1000 mg/day for three doses. Antilymphocyte therapy with OKT3, ATGAM, or Thymoglobulin for 5 to 10 days was used as the initial treatment for moderate or severe renal allograft rejection or for any pancreas allograft rejection. Steroid-resistant mild renal allograft rejection was also treated with anti-lymphocyte therapy.

CMV infection was defined as a positive blood culture, antigenemia, or IGM titer (50). Invasive CMV infection (CMV disease) was defined as symptomatic CMV infection or histologic evidence of tissue invasion. Treatment of CMV infection consisted of intravenous ganciclovir for two to four weeks and a reduction in immunosuppression (50). Oral Acyclovir or Ganciclovir was given for a variable period after treatment of a documented CMV infection. Other infections were recorded, with major infection defined as the need for hospitalization for diagnosis or treatment.

## LONG-TERM FOLLOW-UP AND STATISTICAL ANALYSIS

Long-term post-transplant follow-up is designed to document changes in metabolic and target organ function that could be attributed to the pancreas allograft. To achieve this goal, all pretransplant evaluations were replicated at regular posttransplant intervals. All tests are performed not only for the pancreas recipients but also on a comparable group of diabetic patients who only receive a kidney allograft. This enables us to consider the influence that correction of uremia alone might have on the secondary complications of diabetes.

Data arc reported as mean and range. Renal allograft loss was defined as death with function, transplant nephrectomy, return to dialysis or to the pre-transplant serum creatinine level. Pancreas graft loss was defined as death with function, transplant pancreatectomy, or the need for daily scheduled insulin therapy.

## RESULTS
### Systemic-Bladder vs. Portal-Enteric Drainage

In our early P-E experience (four patients), the pancreas was placed retroperitoneally with an end-to-side duodeno-enterostomy (4). This procedure was revised to an intraperitoneal placement of the allograft with exocrinc drainage into a Roux-en-y limb (Fig. 7) (5). In 1993, our group studied nine SKPT recipients having undergone the revised P-E procedure in comparison with a matched group of 12 SKPT recipients with S-B drainage (6). The results of this initial study indicated that P-E PTX with Roux limb diversion not only achieves acceptable metabolic control and eliminates hyperinsulinemia, but is associated with reduced postoperative complications. Although glucose homeostasis improved in both groups, insulin kinetics was more normal with P-E drainage. Moreover, SB drainage was associated with a higher incidence of urinary tract infections, hematuria, metabolic acidosis, and dehydration.

In 1995, we compared 19 patients undergoing SKPT with the P-E technique versus a retrospective and concurrent control group of 28 patients receiving SKPT with the conventional S-B technique (8). Actual patient and graft survival rates at one and three years were no different in the two groups. Metabolic and urologic complications and urinary tract infections were more common in the S-B group. Metabolic control was comparable between groups and peripheral hyperinsulinemia did not occur in patients with P-E drainage.

In 1997, Nymann et al. from our group reported improving outcomes with increased experience with the P-E technique (34). Two groups were compared: 23 SKPTs with P-E drainage performed during 1991–1994 versus 23 P-E PTXs (17 SKPT, 3 PA, and 3 PAKT) performed during 1995–1996. The latter group received TAC-based immunosuppression, while the former group was managed with CYA. Cold ischemia time and perioperative blood transfusions were significantly lower in the latter group. In addition, the incidence of technical graft loss was reduced from 26% to 9%. Consequently, one-year patient and pancreas graft survival rates were improved in the most recent era. In a subsequent study, Nymann et al. analyzed 47 SKPTs with graft function at one month, including 30 with S-B and 17 with P-E drainage (56). All patients were managed with quadruple immunosuppression with CYA-based therapy. The two groups were comparable for HLA mismatches, cold ischemia times, and level of immunosuppression at the time of rejection. We noted comparable patient and graft survival and surgical complication rates, but demonstrated that the incidence of rejection, graft loss due to rejection, and the density of rejection were all lower in patients with P-E drainage. In the S-B group, the incidence of kidney and pancreas rejection per patient was 1.04 and 0.90, respectively, whereas the P-E group experienced 0.53 kidney and 0.47 pancreas rejection episodes per patient, respectively. The S-B group also had a significantly higher density of both kidney and pancreas rejection. In addition, even though 6 of 30 (20%) pancreas and 4 of 30 (13%) kidney grafts were lost due to irreversible rejection in the S-B group, only one pancreas and one kidney graft (6% each) were lost due to rejection in the P-E group. These data demonstrated that P-E placement of the pancreas allograft affects the rates of acute rejection and immunologic graft loss, implying that there may exist some important immunologic advantages when the pancreas graft is drained into the portal circulation. The reduction in the rate of rejection noted in patients with P-E drainage formed the basis for our subsequent attempts to eliminate ALI therapy from the immunosuppressive regimen.

In 1998, we reported our initial experience with 30 SKPTs receiving TAC, MMF, and steroids without ALL (52). Eighteen patients underwent PTX with P-E and 12 with S-B drainage. All patients experienced immediate function of both kidney and pancreas grafts. One-year actuarial patient, kidney, and pancreas graft survival rates were 93%, 93%, and 90%, respectively. Nine patients (30%) had a total of 13 rejection episodes (12 biopsy proven), including four within two weeks, six between two weeks and three months, and three more than three months after SKPT. Three rejection episodes were treated with steroids alone, whereas 10 were treated with anti-lymphocyte therapy (five OKT3 and five ATGAM). A total of seven patients (23%) received antilymphocyte therapy. Three patients (10%) had more than one rejection episode. Two pancreas grafts (7%) and one kidney graft (3%) were lost from rejection. Four patients (13%) developed CMV infection, but none had tissue-invasive CMV disease. At present, 22 patients with excellent dual graft function (81%) remain on triple immunosuppression with TAC, MMF and Prednisone. In this study, the death-censored kidney and pancreas graft survival rates were 96% and 93%, respectively. The preliminary results of this study suggested that TAC, MMF and steroid immunosuppression without ALT is safe and effective after SKPT.

With preliminary data demonstrating the equivalence of both procedures, we designed a prospective evaluation of PTX with S-B versus P-E drainage (32). During an 11-month period extending from February 1997 to January 1998, 32 consecutive PTXs were performed at our center and patients were alternately assigned to either S-B or P-E drainage. The total of 16 patients were allocated to each technique. The S-B group included 11 SKPT, 1 PAKT, and 4 PA recipients, whereas the P-E group included 12 SKPT, 2 PAKT, and 2 PA recipients. The two groups were well matched for donor and recipient demographic, immunologic, and transplant characteristics (Table 6). All SKPT and PAKT recipients received primary immunosuppression with TAC, MMF, and steroids without ALL PA recipients in both groups received OKT3 induction in addition to the above triple maintenance therapy. Patient, kidney and pancreas graft survival rates were 88% S-B versus 94% P-E, 92% S-B versus 93% P-E, and 81% SB versus 88% P-E, respectively, with a mean follow-up of eight months (minimum of three months) (Table 7). All kidney grafts had immediate function and the incidence of early technical problems related to the pancreas allograft (pancreatitis, thrombosis) was similar in the two groups. There were no graft losses either to immunologic or infectious complications in either group, but the incidence of acute rejection was slightly higher in the S-B group (44% S-B vs. 31% P-E, $P = $ NS). Length of stay and hospital charges for the initial hospitalization

**Table 6**   Group Characteristics

| N | S-B (N = 16) | P-E (N = 16) |
|---|---|---|
| Age (yr) | 38± 6 | 37± 7 |
| Gender | | |
|   Female | 7 (44%) | 7 (44%) |
|   Male | 9 (56%) | 9 (56%) |
| Years of diabetes | 25.5± 6 | 26± 4 |
| Race: Caucasian | 16 (100%) | 16 (100%) |
| Pre-transplant dialysis | 11/11 (100%) | 6/12 (50%)[a] |
| Prior transplant | 1 (6%) | 3 (19%) |
| Current PRA ≥10% | 1 (6%) | 1 (6%) |
| Pancreas ischemia (hr) | 15.1± 3.4 | 13.4± 3.0 |
| HLA match: ABDR | 1.8± 1.3 | 1.8± 1.3 |
| HLA mismatch | 4.2± 1.3 | 4.1± 1.3 |
| Waiting time (mo) | 4.6± 4.3 | 4.4± 3.1 |
| Type of transplant | | |
|   SKPT | 11 (69%) | 12 (75%) |
|   PAKT | 1 (6%) | 2 (12.5%) |
|   PA | 4 (25%) | 2 (12.5%) |

Mean ± SD.
[a]$p = 0.0l$.
*Abbreviations*: PRA, panel reactive antibody; SKPT, simultaneous kidney-pancreas transplantation; PAKT, pancreas after kidney transplants; PA, pancreas alone; S-B, systemic-bladder; P-E, portal-enteric; HLA, human leukocyte antigen.

were similar between groups (Table 7). For all patients, the mean length of initial hospital stay was 13 days and initial hospital charges approximated $100,000.

The incidence of urologic complications was doubled in the S-B group (25% S-B vs. 12% P-E, $P = $ NS). The S-B group was also characterized by a higher incidence of urinary tract infections (50% S-B vs. 19% P-E, $P = 0.12$). Metabolic acidosis with oral bicarbonate supplementation was universal in the S-B group, but rarely occurred with P-E drainage. Dehydration with the need for intravenous fluid supplementation and placement of long-term indwelling central venous catheters occurred in all patients with S-B drainage but in only 44% with P-E drainage ($P < 0.01$). The incidence of operative complications was similar, but the relaparotomy rate was higher in the P-E group (two patients in this group required a second reoperation, while no patients in the S-B group received multiple laparotomies). In the P-E

**Table 7**   Results

| | S-B (N = 16)[a] | P-E (N = 16)[a] |
|---|---|---|
| Patient survival | 14 (88%) | 15 (94%) |
| Graft survival | | |
|   Kidney | 11/12 (92%) | 13/14 (93%) |
|   Pancreas | 13 (81%) | 14 (88%) |
| Follow-up (mo) | 7.5± 3.4 | 8.9± 3.8 |
| ATN (dialysis) | 0 | 0 |
| Early technical problems/pancreatitis | 3 (19%) | 3 (19%) |
| Initial LOS (day) | 13.7± 9 | 12.8± 7 |
| Readmissions | 2.6± 1.8 | 1.75± 1.2 |
| Acute rejection | 7 (44%) | 5 (31%) |
| Major infection | 8 (50%) | 10 (62.5%) |
| Re-operations | 4 (25%) | 4 (25%) |
| Initial hospital charges ($) | 100,215± 54,012 | 94,083± 25,873 |
| Urologic complication | 4 (25%) | 2 (12.5%) |
| UTI | 8 (50%) | 3 (19%) |
| Dehydration/acidosis | 16 (100%) | 7 (44%)[b] |
| CMV infection | 2 (12.5%) | 3 (19%) |
| Multiple re-operations | 0 | 2 (12.5%) |

[a]Mean ± SD.
[b]$p < 0.01$.
*Abbreviations*: ATN, acute tubular necrosis; LOS, length of stay; S-B, systemic-bladder; P-E, portal-enteric; UTI, urinary tract infection; CMV, cytomegalovirus.

group, one patient (6%) had an enteric leak with intra-abdominal infection. Two patients underwent enteric conversion in the S-B group. The incidences of major infections and CMV infection were similar between groups.

We believe that this study represented the first prospective analysis comparing PTX performed by a standardized technique of P-E drainage versus the conventional technique of S-B drainage with similar immunosuppression (32). It is important to emphasize that 23 patients (72%) underwent SKPT, whereas the remaining nine (28%) received solitary PTX. The categories of PTX were equally distributed among the two groups. Although our overall numbers are small and follow-up is limited, most of the study outcomes relevant to comparing these two techniques occur in the first three to six months after PTX. Conceding the above limitations in study design, patient, kidney, and pancreas graft survival rates were comparable between groups and no immunologic graft loss occurred. The three deaths that occurred in this series were cardiac in origin and probably related to pre-existing disease. These deaths accounted for five (three pancreas and two renal) of the seven graft losses that occurred in the study. These preliminary results suggested that whole organ PTX with P-E drainage could be performed with results comparable to the conventional technique of S-B drainage.

In 1998, Eubanks et al., from our group compared 12 solitary PTXs with S-B drainage performed during 1991–1995 with 16 solitary PTXs with P-E drainage performed between July 1995 and March 1997 (35). The former group was managed with CYA, whereas the latter group received TAC-based therapy. One patient in each group experienced graft loss due to thrombosis. In the remaining patients, the incidence and density of rejection was lower in the more recent era leading to an improvement in the one-year pancreas survival rate to 80%. These results compared favorably to the results of solitary PTX with the other reported techniques.

In 2000, Lo et al. studied long-term outcomes in 45 SKPT recipients at our center, including 26 with P-E and 19 with S-B drainage (59). All patients were alive with functioning kidney and pancreas grafts at one year after SKPT and had a minimum follow-up of 3.5 years (mean 5.9 years). Demographic, immunologic, and transplant characteristics were similar between the P-E and S-B groups. All patients received OKT3 for induction, and Azathioprine and Prednisone as maintenance immunosuppression. In the P-E group, 48% of the patients received TAC and 52% received CYA-Sandimmune based therapy. In the S-B group, all of the patients received CYA, but 10% of the patients were switched to TAC at a mean of two years posttransplant. At five years, there were no differences in the actual patient, kidney, and pancreas graft survival rates between the P-E and S-B groups; 92% versus 84%, 81% versus 79%, and 88% versus 74%, respectively ($P = $ NS). The 10-year actuarial patient, kidney, and pancreas graft survival rates in the P-E group were 74%, 50%, and 53%, respectively, compared to 37%, 31%, and 32%, in the S-B group, respectively.

During the first year post-transplant, patients in the S-B group had more readmissions, including more readmissions for urinary tract infections and dehydration. Renal and pancreas functions remained stable and comparable between the two groups. Patients in the S-B group received fewer antihypertensive agents than patients in the P-E group. At five years, patients in the P-E group experienced a slight decline in body weight. In contrast, patients in the S-B group had a significant increase in weight over time. At three years, 53% of the patients in the S-B group reported no activity limitation compared to 76% in the P-E group ($P = 0.11$). Irrespective of surgical technique, more patients reported no activity limitations post-transplant than pre-transplant. Improved quality of life was reported in all but one of the scales, with many dimensions showing a significant improvement. At the end of follow-up stabilization in microvascular complications including retinopathy, peripheral neuropathy, and autonomic function were reported in both groups of patients. The results of this study suggested trends toward better patient and graft survival, fewer metabolic complications, less morbidity, and improved quality of life in the P-E group when compared to the S-B group long-term.

### Portal-Enteric Drainage

Paralleling our efforts with P-E PTX were the development of two new immunosuppressive agents, TAC and MMF. With increasing confidence and experience with the P-E technique, we attempted to examine whether it could be performed without ALL From September 1996 to November 1998, we performed 28 primary SKPTs with P-E drainage and no ALL (10). All patients received triple immunosuppression with TAC, MMF, and steroids. The study group included 15 males and 13 females with a mean age of 38 years and a mean pre-SKPT

**Table 8**   Group Characteristics (*N* = 28)

| | |
|---|---|
| Age (yr) | 38.4 (26–54)[a] |
| Gender | |
|    Female | 13 (46%) |
|    Male | 15 (54%) |
| Race | |
|    Caucasian | 26 (93%) |
|    African American | 2 (7%) |
| Years of diabetes | 25.1 (9–35) |
| Total insulin dose (units/day) | 42.5 (15–72) |
| Prior kidney transplant | 4 (14%) |
| Pretransplant dialysis | |
|    None | 11 (39%) |
|    Hemodialysis | 8 (29%) |
|    Peritoneal dialysis | 9 (32%) |
| Duration of dialysis (mo) | 15.2 (6–27) |
| Waiting time (mo) | 4.0 (0.25–10) |
| Current PRA $\geq$ 10% | 4 (14%) |
| HLA | |
|    ABDR match | 1.55 (0–5) |
|    ABDR mismatch | 4.1 (1–6) |
| Cold ischemia (hr) | |
|    Pancreas | 12.9 (6–18) |
|    Kidney | 13.3 (7–21) |
| D/R CMV serologic status | |
|    D+/R− | 3 (11%) |
|    D+/R+ | 11 (39%) |
|    D−/R+ | 3 (11%) |
|    D−/R− | 7 (25%) |
|    Unknown | 4 (14%) |

[a]Mean (range).
*Abbreviations*: PRA, panel reactive antibody; HLA, human leukocyte antigen; CMV, cytomegalovirus; D, donor; R, recipient.

duration of diabetes of 25 years (Table 8). Four patients (1.4%) had prior kidney transplants. Eleven patients (39%) were transplanted preemptively and the remaining 17 (eight hemodialysis, nine peritoneal dialysis) had a mean pre-SKPT duration of dialysis of 15 months. The mean waiting time for SKPT was four months and the mean HLA match was 1.5.

All patients experienced immediate renal allograft function. Actual patient, kidney, and pancreas graft survival rates were 86%, 82%, and 82%, respectively, after a mean follow-up of 12 months. Four patients died including three due to cardiac events unrelated to SKPT. Two of the four deaths occurred in patients with previous pancreas graft loss. All of the deaths were believed to be related to pre-existing autonomic neuropathy, affecting either cardiac or circulatory reflexes. If the three cardiac deaths are censored, patient, kidney, and pancreas graft survival rates were 96%, 92%, and 88%, respectively. Five kidney and five pancreas grafts were lost, including five deaths with function and three due to chronic rejection. The mean length of stay and total charges for the initial hospitalization were 12.5 days and $99,517, respectively (Table 9). Nine patients (32%) were dismissed within eight days of SKPT. The mean number of readmissions was 2.9 and 10 patients (36%) had no readmissions. Six patients (21%) developed acute rejection, with five (18%) receiving anti-lymphocyte therapy. Six patients (21%) underwent relaparotomy, including two (7%) for intra-abdominal infection. Nine patients (32%) had major infections, including three (11%) with CMV infection. There was no graft loss due to acute rejection, and no death or pancreas graft loss from infection. Of the 24 surviving patients, 22 (92%) are both dialysis and insulin free.

This study represented the first prospective analysis of SKPT with P-E drainage in patients not receiving ALI therapy (10). The study demonstrated that only one-fifth of the patients experienced rejection episodes, and that 67% of those were single rejection episodes that responded to initial therapy. Overall, the elimination of induction therapy resulted in reduced hospital costs and earlier hospital dismissal as evidenced by the fact that nearly one-third of the patients were discharged within eight days of SKPT. Considering that the incidence of acute rejection was 21%, 82% of patients were spared exposure to anti-lymphocyte

**Table 9** Results (*N* = 28)

| | |
|---|---|
| Patient survival | 24 (86%)[a] |
| Graft survival | |
|    Kidney | 23 (82%) |
|    Pancreas | 23 (82%) |
| Follow-up (mo) | 12.1 (1–26) |
| Dialysis posttransplant | 0 |
| Initial hospitalization | |
|    Length of stay (day) | 12.5 (6–30) |
|    Total charges ($) | 99,517 (7,146–141,634) |
| Number of re-admissions | 2.9 (0–8) |
| No re-admissions | 10 (36%) |
| Acute rejection | 9 in 6 (21%) |
| Chronic rejection | 3 in 2 (7%) |
| Major infection | 13 in 9 (32%) |
|    CMV infection | 3 |
|    Line sepsis | 3 |
|    Urosepsis | 2 |
|    Intra-abdominal infection | 2 |
|    Other infection | 3 |
| Urinary tract infection | 4 (14%) |
| Relaparotomy | 7 (25%) |
| Multiple re-operations | 3 (11%) |
| Prolonged vascular access | 9 (32%) |

[a]Mean (range).

therapy. There was no renal or pancreas graft loss due to acute rejection; however, there was one renal and two pancreas graft losses due to chronic rejection, each 13 months after SKPT. Moreover, in spite of the administration of TAC immediately after SKPT in order to achieve early therapeutic levels, there were no cases of delayed renal allograft function and no patient required dialysis after transplant. Whether portal delivery of antigen conferred an immunologic advantage above and beyond that achieved with the new immunosuppressants remained to be determined.

In summary, these preliminary results suggested that SKPT with P-E drainage and TAC/MMF/steroid immunosuppression without ALI could be performed with results comparable to other PTX techniques with ALI. We noted a low incidence of metabolic and urologic complications without incurring excessive risk for surgical or infectious complications. In addition, we noted a low immunologic risk without impairment in allograft function. Studies with more patients and longer follow-up are needed to document the beneficial effects of portal venous delivery of insulin on carbohydrate and lipid metabolism. However, due to its physiologic, economic, and immunologic advantages, SKPT with P-E drainage and no ALI may soon become the standard of care in PTX.

There is limited data available on the incidence and outcome of surgical complications following PTX with P-E drainage. We retrospectively studied surgical complications after 83 PTXs in 79 patients (65 SKPT, 10 PAKT, and 8 PA) with P-E drainage (11). Twelve (15%) were retransplants. A surgical complication was defined as the need for relaparotomy within the first three months after PTX, A total of 53 surgical complications requiring relaparotomy (Table 10) occurred in 31 patients (37%). The incidences of surgical complications in SKPT and solitary PTX were 38% and 33%, respectively ($P$ = NS). The most common indications for relaparotomy were: vascular thrombosis 13% (SKPT 14% and solitary PTX 11%), intra-abdominal infection 10% (SKPT 12% and solitary PTX 0), intra-abdominal bleeding 8% (SKPT 8% and solitary PTX 11%), and duodenal allograft leak 4% (SKPT 3%, solitary PTX 6%, all $P$ = NS). The patient survival rates at one and three years with versus without surgical complications were 84% and 80%, versus 94% and 86%, respectively ($P$ = NS), Pancreas graft survival rates at one and three years with versus without surgical complications were 48% and 44%, versus 89% and 76%, respectively ($P < 0.001$).

The incidence of surgical complications was 45% in the first 42 P-E transplants performed between 1990 and 1995, compared to 29% in the next 41 P-E transplants performed during 1996 and 1997 (Fig. 10) (11). The mean number of relaparotomies per patient decreased

**Table 10** Indications for Repeat Laparotomy

| Indication | SKPT (n = 65) | Solitary PTX (n = 18) | Total (N = 83) | |
|---|---|---|---|---|
| | | | n | % |
| Intra-abdominal infection | 13 in 8 | 0 | 8 | 10 |
| Thrombosis (pancreas) | 9 | 2 | 11 | 13 |
| Intra-abdominal bleeding | 7 in 5 | 2 | 7 | 8 |
| Duodenal leak | 5 in 2 | 2 in l | 3 | 4 |
| Other | 12 | 1 | 13 | 16 |
|   Wound dehiscence | 4 | 0 | 4 | 5 |
|   Negative laparotomy | 4 | 0 | 4 | 5 |
|   Thrombosis (kidney) | 1 | 0 | 1 | 1 |
|   Small-bowel obstruction (adhesive) | 1 | 0 | 1 | 1 |
|   Gastrointestinal bleeding | 1 | 0 | 1 | 1 |
|   Leak at small-bowel anastomosis | 1 | 0 | 1 | 1 |
|   Dislodgment of jejunostomy tube | 0 | 1 | 1 | 2 |
| Total | 46 in 25 (38%) | 7 in 6 (33%) | 53 in 31 | 37 |

*Abbreviations*: SKPT, simultaneous kidney-pancreas transplantation; PTX, pancreas transplantation.

from 1.2 in the former group to 0.5 in the latter group ($P$ = NS). The incidence of vascular thrombosis, intra-abdominal infection, and duodenal leak in the former and latter groups were 17% versus 10%, 12% versus 7%, and 2% versus 5%, respectively (all $P$ = NS). These results suggested that surgical complications after PTX were common and their incidence and outcome with P-E drainage were similar to those reported for S-B drainage. The complication rate did not vary according to type of transplant (SKPT or solitary PTX) in this series. Early relaparotomy had no effect on patient survival but was associated with a significant decrease in the pancreas graft survival rate. Increasing experience with the P-E technique resulted in a decreased incidence of surgical complications.

With longer follow-up of P-E transplant recipients, we began to examine long-term outcomes and complications of the procedure. In 1997, Nymann et al. reported an 8% incidence of late duodenal complications occurring after PTX with P-E drainage (60). All four patients were managed operatively and patient and graft survival rates were 100%. Reddy et al. reported our initial experience with P-E retransplantation (61). Five patients initially underwent SKPT with P-E drainage and experienced early pancreas graft loss (four thrombosis and one infection) resulting in allograft pancreatectomy. Pancreas retransplantation with the P-E technique was subsequently performed as a PAKT in each of the cases. Patient and pancreas graft survival rates were 100% after retransplantation with a mean follow-up of two years. In this experience, we did not have any technical or vascular problems with exposure and identification of an adequate length of superior mesenteric vein at the time of retransplantation even

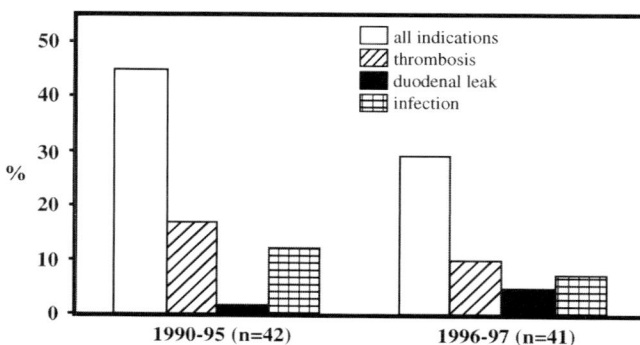

**Figure 10** Incidence of surgical complications according to era.

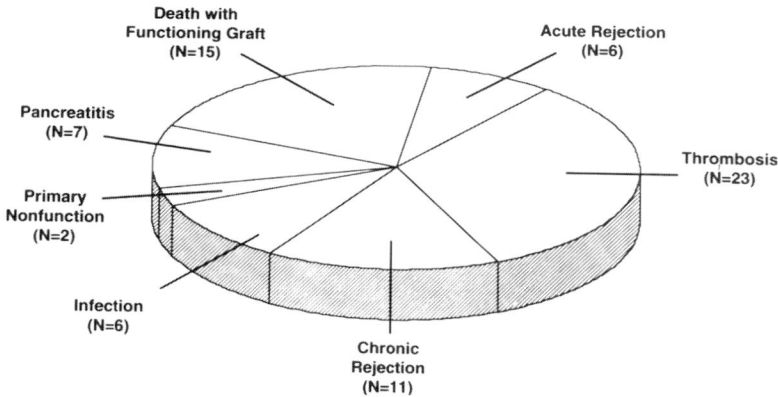

**Figure 11** Causes of pancreas graft failure from 1989 to 1997 ($N = 70$).

though previous dissection had occurred in this area. In most cases, the new site of venous anastomosis was cephalad to the previous anastomotic site. Moreover, we were able to use the previous Roux limb for the enteric reconstruction, thereby avoiding a second bowel anastomosis. This preliminary experience suggested that excellent results in retransplantation with a solitary pancreas graft could be achieved with the P-E technique.

The indications and outcomes of allograft pancreatectomy following PTX were also described by our group (62). From 1989 through 1997, we performed 159 vascularized PTXs, including 117 SKPT, 25 PA, and 17 sequential PAKT. A total of 73 PTXs were performed with S-B and 86 with P-E drainage. A total of 70 (44%) pancreas grafts were lost (Fig. 11), with 37 (23%) resulting in allograft pancreatectomy. Pancreatectomy was performed at a mean of 4.7 months after PTX. Twenty-seven procedures were performed within one month, 30 (81%) within three months, and the remaining seven more than six months after PTX (Fig. 12). The incidence of pancreatectomy did not differ between SKPT, PAKT, or PA. Indications for pancreatectomy were thrombosis (23), rejection (9), infection (3), and pancreatitis (2). Pancreatectomy was directly related to the timing of graft loss; 77% of grafts lost within three months of PTX required pancreatectomy while only 25% of grafts lost after three months (Fig. 12) resulted in pancreatectomy ($P < 0.01$). The incidence of pancreatectomy was similar according to technique of transplant, 26% S-B versus 21% P-E ($P = $NS). In addition, the indications for and timing of pancreatectomy were similar in S-B and P-E PTX recipients. However, the incidence of graft failure resulting in pancreatectomy did differ according to technique of transplant (43% S-B vs. 69% P-E, $P < 0.05$). Moreover, the incidence of pancreatectomy was directly related to the cause of graft loss (thrombosis 100%, infection 80%, rejection 47%, and pancreatitis 29%). Ten patients died at a mean of 19.5 months after pancreatectomy, including five within two months of the procedure. Overall patient survival was 73% after a mean follow-up of 48 months after pancreatectomy. In our experience, pancreatectomy was performed in over half of cases of pancreas allograft loss and was directly related to the timing and cause of graft loss. However, the incidence of pancreatectomy was neither

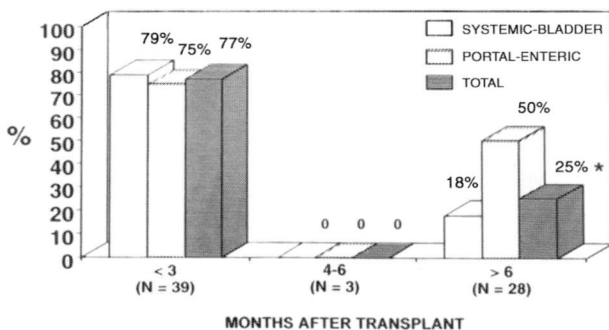

**Figure 12** Incidence of allograft pancreatectomy according to timing of graft loss and technique of transplant.

related to the type nor technique of PTX, indicating that whole organ PTX with P-E drainage does not place the patient at an increased risk for pancreatectomy.

### Systemic-Enteric vs. Portal-Enteric Drainage

As the number of PTXs with enteric drainage has steadily increased, we decided to compare SKPT with S-E versus P-E drainage in a prospective fashion with standardized immuno-suppression (33). During a 26-month period from April 1998 through May 2000, 54 consecutive SKPT recipients were entered into a prospective study of S-E ($N = 27$) versus P-E ($N = 27$) drainage. The technique to be performed was chosen before the transplant with selection determined by an alternating methodology. The two groups were well matched for most donor and recipient demographic, immunologic, and transplant characteristics (Table 11). The racial distribution differed slightly, with African-American patients representing 15% of the S-E and 33% of the P-E group. With regard to immunosuppression, 63% of S-E and 44% of P-E patients were managed with no antibody induction. The remaining S-E patients received either Daclizumab or Basiliximab induction, while the P-E patients received Daclizumab, Basiliximab, or Thymoglobulin in two patients with acute tubular necrosis (ATN). Maintenance immuno-suppression in both groups consisted of TAC, MMF, and steroids.

Results are depicted in Table 12, Patient survival rates were 93% S-E versus 96% P-E, whereas kidney graft survival rates were 93% in both groups. PTX survival (complete insulin independence) was 74% after S-E versus 85% after P-E drainage, with a mean follow-up of 17 months. All but 3 of the 54 transplanted renal allografts had immediate function. ATN, defined as the need for dialysis in the first week after transplant, occurred in one patient after S-E and two patients after P-E drainage. All three of these kidneys eventually functioned. All 54

**Table 11**  Demographic and Transplant Characteristics

|  | S-E: ($N = 27$)[a] | P-E: ($N = 27$)[a] |
|---|---|---|
| Age (yr) | 40.6 (27–57) | 39.2 (26–58) |
| Gender |  |  |
|   Male | 19 (70%) | 16 (59%) |
|   Female | 8 (30%) | 11 (41%) |
|   Weight (kg) | 73.9 (45–103) | 73.3 (49–95) |
| Race |  |  |
|   Caucasian | 22 (81%) | 18 (67%) |
|   African-American | 4 (15%) | 9 (33%) |
|   Asian | 1 (4%) | 0 |
| Pretransplant dialysis: # | 21 (78%) | 18 (67%) |
|   Duration (mo) | 16 (5–36) | 13 (1–46) |
|   Peritoneal dialysis | 7 (26%) | 10 (37%) |
|   Hemodialysis | 14 (52%) | 8 (30%) |
|   None | 6 (22%) | 9 (33%) |
| Hepatitis C positive | 2 (7%) | 1 (4%) |
| Years of diabetes | 24 (4–50) | 23.2 (9–46) |
| Type 2 diabetes | 4 (15%) | 2 (7%) |
| Daily insulin dose (U/day) | 38 (15–80) | 44 (15–80) |
| Prior kidney transplant | 2 (7%) | 3 (11%) |
| PRA > 10% | 2 (7%) | 2 (7%) |
| HLA Match: ABDR | 1.4 (0–4) | 1.4 (0–4) |
| HLA mismatch | 4,6 (2–6) | 4.6 (2–6) |
| CMV D+/R− | 7 (26%) | 5 (19%) |
| Cold ischemia (hr) |  |  |
|   Kidney | 14.3 (8–23) | 15.1 (9.5–2.6) |
|   Pancreas | 14.2 (7.5–22.5) | 15.3 (10.5–23) |
| Waiting time (mo) | 2.8 (0.1–7) | 3 (0.25–8.5) |
| Immunosuppression; FK, MMF, steroids + |  |  |
|   No antibody induction | 17 (63%) | 12 (44%) |
|   Daclizumab | 6 (22%) | 8 (30%) |
|   Basiliximab | 4 (15%) | 5 (19%) |
|   Thymoglobulin | 0 | 2 (7%) |

[a]Mean (range).
*Abbreviations*: FK, tacrolimus; MMF, mycophenolate mofetil; PRA, panel reactive antibody; HLA, human leukocyte antigen; S-E, systemic-enteric; P-E, portal-enteric; $P$ = NS: D, donor; R, recipient; CMV, cytomegalovirus.

**Table 12** Results

| | S-E: (N = 27) | P-E: (N = 27)[a] |
|---|---|---|
| Patient survival | 25 (93%) | 26 (96%) |
| Graft survival | | |
|   Kidney | 25 (93%) | 25 (93%) |
|   Pancreas | 20 (74%) | 23 (85%) |
| Follow-up (mo) | 17.4 (5–30) | 17 (5–29) |
| ATN (post-op dialysis) | 1 (4%) | 2 (7%) |
| Early technical problems | 3 (11%) | 2 (7%) |
| Initial hospital stay (day) | 12.4 (7–30) | 12.8 (7–38) |
| Initial hospital charges ($) | 102,255 | 105,789 |
| No. of re-admissions | 2.8 (0–10) | 2.2 (0–10) |
| No re-admissions | 8 (30%) | 5 (19%) |
| Acute rejection | 9 (33%) | 9 (33%) |
| Anti-T cell therapy | 4 (15%) | 6 (22%) |
| Immunologic pancreas graft loss | 3 (11%) | 1 (4%) |
| Early relaparotomy (<3 mo) | 8 (30%) | 7 (26%) |
| Pancreas thrombosis | 2 (7%) | 1 (4%) |
| Major infection | 14 (52%) | 14 (52%) |
| CMV infection | 1 (4%) | 1 (4%) |
| Intra-abdominal infection | 7 (26%) | 3 (11%) |
| Total hospital days | 33 (9–160) | 24 (8–92) |
| Event-free survival (no rejection, graft loss, or death) | 15 (56%) | 16 (59%) |

[a]Mean (range).
$p$ = NS.
*Abbreviations*: CMV, cytomegalovirus; ATN, acute tubular necrosis; S-E, systemic-enteric; P-E, portal-enteric.

transplanted pancreas allografts had initial function, although three were subsequently lost to thrombosis in the first week after transplant. The incidence of allograft pancreatitis, early leaks, or other technical problems related to the pancreas allograft were similar between groups.

The mean length of initial hospital stay was 12.4 days in the S-E and 12.8 days in the P-E groups, respectively. Mean initial hospital charges were comparable between groups. The S-E group was characterized by a slight increase in the number of readmissions (mean 2.8 S-E vs. 2.2 P-E, $P$ = NS) and total hospital days (mean 33 days S-E vs. 24 days P-E, $P$ = NS). The incidence of acute rejection was similar (33%) in both groups, with immunologic pancreas graft loss occurring in three S-E patients versus one P-E patient. The incidence of major infection was 52% in both groups, with one CMV infection (4%) in each group. The incidence of intra-abdominal infection was slightly higher in the S-E group (26% S-E vs. 11% P-E, $P$ = NS). However, the early relaparotomy rate was similar between groups (30% S-E vs. 26% P-E). The composite endpoint of no rejection, graft loss, or death was attained by 56% of S-E and 59% of P-E patients (Table 12). These results suggested that SKPT with S-E or P-E drainage could be performed with comparable short-term outcomes.

### Overall Results

From October 1990 through December 1999, we performed 126 PTXs with P-E drainage (Fig. 5), including 90 SKPTs and 36 solitary PTXs (18 PAKT and 18 PA) (12). The P-E group included 69 male and 57 female patients with a mean age of 39 years (Table 13). The mean duration of pre-transplant diabetes was 24 years (range 8–50). The majority of recipients were Caucasian, although 15 (12%) were African-American recipients. A total of 13 patients (10%) underwent pancreas re-transplantation with the P-E technique. The majority of patients had poor HLA matching (mean 1.4, range 0–5), and the mean pancreas cold ischemia was 13 hours (range 6–23). Minimum follow-up was 11 months (mean 4.6 years).

Thirty patients underwent SKPT with P-E drainage in Era 1 and were compared to 42 SKPTs performed in Era 2 and 18 in Era 3 (Fig. 8). The patients in Era 1 were managed with CYA while those in Eras 2 and 3 received TAC/MMF. We also compared 23 solitary PTXs (11 PAKT and 12 PA) performed in Era 2 with 13 (seven PAKT and six PA) performed in Era 3 (Fig. 5). One-year patient survival rates after SKPT (Fig. 13) were 77% in Era 1, 93% in Era 2, and 100% in Era 3 ($P$ = 0.03). The one-year kidney graft survival rates were 77% in Era 1.93% in

**Table 13**  Demographic and Transplant Characteristics

| N | 126 |
|---|---|
| Age (yr) | 39 (19–56)[a] |
| Gender | |
|    Female | 57 (45%) |
|    Male | 69 (55%) |
| Race | |
|    Caucasian | 111 (88%) |
|    African American | 15 (12%) |
| Years of diabetes | 24 (8–50)[a] |
| Transplant type | |
|    SKPT | 90 (72%) |
|    PAKT | 18 (14%) |
|    PA | 18 (14%) |
| Prior PTX | 13 (10%) |
| HLA Match: ABDR | 1.4 (0–5)[a] |
| Pancreas cold ischemia (hr) | 13 (6–23)[a] |

[a]Mean (range).
*Abbreviations*: HLA, human leukocyte antigen; SKPT, simultaneous kidney-pancreas transplantation; PAKT, pancreas after kidney transplant; PA, pancreas alone; PTX, pancreas transplantation.

Era 2, and 94% in Era 3 ($P = 0.08$). The one-year pancreas graft survival rates after SKPT (Fig. 13) were 60% in Era 1, and 83% both in Eras 2 and 3 ($P = 0.06$). The most common causes of kidney graft loss were death with function and chronic rejection (Table 14). The overall incidence of kidney graft loss decreased from 56% in Era 1 to 23% in Era 2 to 11% in Era 3 ($P < 0.001$). The most common causes of pancreas graft loss were thrombosis, death with function, chronic rejection, and infection (Table 12). The overall incidence of pancreas graft loss decreased from 60% in Era 1 to 31% in Era 2 to 22% in Era 3 ($P < 0.001$).

The incidences of rejection (63% vs. 33% vs. 39%, $P < 0.001$) and major infection (60% vs. 43% vs. 44%, $P = $ NS) after SKPT were decreased in each successive era (Fig. 14). The rates of thrombosis (20% vs. 7% vs. 6%, $P < 0.001$) and early relaparotomy (47% vs. 31% vs. 33%, $P = $ NS) after SKPT were also decreased in each consecutive era (Fig. 15).

The one-year patient survival rates after solitary PTX were both 100% in Eras 2 and 3, whereas the corresponding pancreas graft survival rates were 61% and 69%, respectively (Table 15). The most common causes of graft loss after solitary PTX were thrombosis and chronic rejection. The overall incidence of pancreas graft loss after solitary PTX decreased from 70% in Era 2 to 31% in Era 3 ($P = 0.02$). The rates of acute rejection (57% vs. 38%), major infection (35% vs. 31%), thrombosis (22% vs. 15%), and relaparotomy (43% vs. 38%) after solitary PTX were all slightly improved in Era 3 compared to Era 2 ($P = $ NS). This overall experience demonstrates that SKPT and solitary PTX with P-E drainage can be performed with improving outcomes.

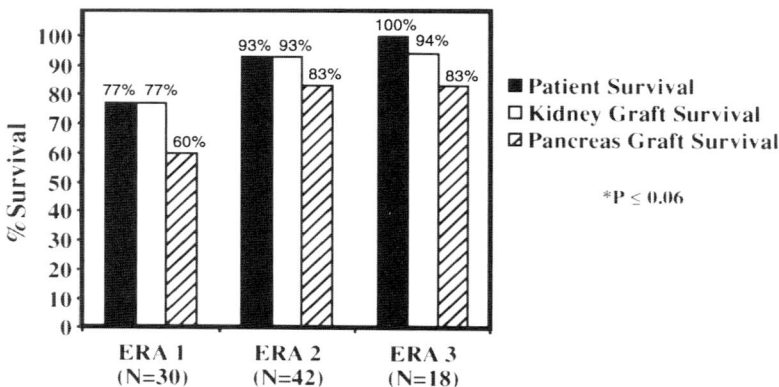

**Figure 13**  One-year patient and graft survival rates after simultaneous kidney-PTX according to immunosuppressive era. Survival rates were similar in Eras 2 and 3 and significantly improved compared to Era 1 for simultaneous kidney-pancreas transplantation.

**Table 14**   Results (Simultaneous Kidney-Pancreas Transplantation)

| | Era 1 (N = 30) | Era 2 (N = 42) | Era 3 (N = 18) | P value |
|---|---|---|---|---|
| *One-year survival* | | | | |
| Patient | 23 (77%) | 39 (93%) | 18 (100%) | 0.03 |
| Kidney | 23 (77%) | 39 (93%) | 17 (94%) | 0.08 |
| Pancreas | 18 (60%) | 35 (83%) | 15 (83%) | 0.06 |
| Acute rejection | 19 (63%) | 14 (33%) | 7 (39%) | <0.001 |
| Major infection | 18 (60%) | 18 (43%) | 8 (44%) | NS |
| Thrombosis | 6 (20%) | 3 (7%) | 1 (6%) | <0.001 |
| Relaparotomy | 14 (47%) | 13 (31%) | 6 (33%) | NS |
| *Overall graft loss* | | | | |
| Kidney | 17 (56%) | 10 (23%) | 2 (11%) | <0.001 |
| Pancreas | 18 (60%) | 13 (31%) | 4 (22%) | <0.001 |
| *Causes of kidney graft loss* | | | | |
| DWFG | 7 (23%) | 5 (12%) | 1 (5.5%) | <0.001 |
| Chronic rejection | 4 (13%) | 3 (7%) | 1 (5.5%) | NS |
| Infection | 2 (7%) | 1 (2%) | 0 | NS |
| Acute rejection | 1 (3%) | 0 | 0 | NS |
| PTLD | 2 (7%) | 1 (2%) | 0 | NS |
| Thrombosis | 1 (3%) | 0 | 0 | NS |
| *Causes of pancreas graft loss* | | | | |
| Thrombosis | 6 (20%) | 3 (7%) | 1 (5.5%) | <0.001 |
| DWFG | 5 (17%) | 2 (5%) | 1 (5.5%) | <0.001 |
| Chronic rejection | 1 (3%) | 5 (12%) | 1 (5.5%) | NS |
| Infection | 3 (10%) | 1 (2%) | 1 (5.5%) | NS |
| PTLD | 2 (7%) | 1 (2%) | 0 | NS |
| Acute rejection | 1 (3%) | 1 (2%) | 0 | NS |

*Abbreviations*: DWFG, death with functioning graft; PTLD, posttransplant lymphoproliferative disease.

Increasing experience with the P-E technique coupled with advances in immunosuppression are associated with: (i) increasing patient, kidney, and pancreas graft survival rates; (ii) less medical morbidity with a decreasing incidence of acute rejection and major infection; and (iii) reduced surgical complications including decreasing rates of thrombosis and relaparotomy. The P-E technique does not appear to incur any additional or unique risks, and can be performed with results comparable to the other standard techniques of PTX. We believe that this technique should be included in the repertoire of PTX, because it offers potential physiologic, metabolic, and immunologic advantages over the other techniques currently available.

## METABOLIC, PHYSIOLOGIC, QUALITY OF LIFE, AND LONG-TERM OUTCOMES

With the improving short-term success of PTX, long-term prognosis after the first year is excellent and at least provides the potential for stabilization of diabetic complications.

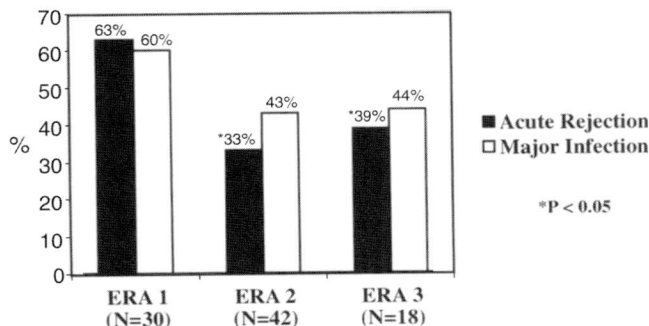

**Figure 14**   The incidence of acute rejection was similar in Eras 2 and 3 and significantly decreased compared to Era 1 for simultaneous kidney-pancreas transplantation.

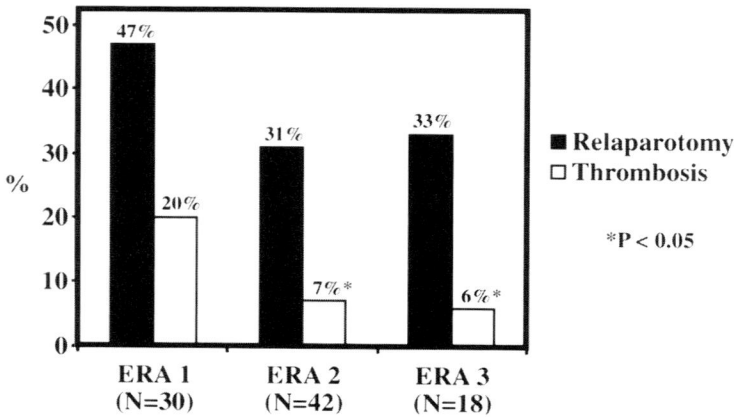

**Figure 15** The incidence of pancreas allograft thrombosis was similar in Eras 2 and 3 and significantly decreased compared to Era 1 for simultaneous kidney-pancreas transplantation.

We retrospectively reviewed remote SKPT recipients with P-E drainage; 26 patients (65%) were alive with functioning grafts one year after SKPT and were followed for a minimum of three years (mean five years) (63). Hospital admissions decreased significantly from a mean of 2.4 admissions per patient in the first year to 0.6 by year four. Mean systolic blood pressure and diastolic blood pressure fell to 132 mmHg ($P = 0.02$) and 80 mmHg ($P = 0.02$) at one-year post-SKPT, respectively, and remained stable thereafter. The daily mean Prednisone dose decreased by 23% at three years, but CYA and TAC doses remained stable. Patients showed a gain in weight from a mean of 68.2 kg at SKPT to 77.3 kg at year 4 ($P = 0.02$). Fasting serum glucose fell to 85 mg/dL at year 1 ($P < 0.01$) and remained stable thereafter. Glycosylated hemoglobin levels decreased to 6.0% at one-year post-SKPT ($P < 0.05$) and 5.8% at year 4. Serum creatinine was 1.6 mg/dL at year 1 and 1.8 mg/dL at year 4 ($P = $ NS). Total cholesterol remained stable over four years (mean 206 mg/dL, HDL greater than 50) but mean triglycerides decreased over time from 224 to 182 mg/dL at year 4. At one-year posttransplant, improvements in most diabetic complications were noted. No activity limitations were reported in 80% of patients at one year after SKPT compared to 23% pre-transplant. Four quality of life surveys that provided 29 scores were completed 6 to 24 months (mean 18 months) after SKPT. Improved quality of life was reported in all but one of the scales. Actual patient,

**Table 15** Results (Solitary Pancreas Transplantation)

|  | Era 2: (*N* = 23) | Era 3: (*N* = 13) | *P* value |
|---|---|---|---|
| PAKT | 11 (48%) | 7 (54%) | NS |
| PA | 12 (52%) | 6 (46%) | NS |
| One-year survival |  |  |  |
| Patient | 23 (100%) | 13 (100%) | NS |
| Pancreas | 14 (61%) | 9 (69%) | NS |
| Acute rejection | 13 (57%) | 5 (38%) | NS |
| Major infection | 8 (35%) | 4 (31%) | NS |
| Thrombosis | 5 (22%) | 2 (15%) | NS |
| Rclaparotomy | 10 (43%) | 5 (38%) | NS |
| Overall pancreas graft loss | 16 (70%) | 4 (31%) | 0.02 |
| Causes of graft loss |  |  |  |
| Thrombosis | 5 (22%) | 2 (15%) | NS |
| Chronic rejection | 4 (17%) | 2 (15%) | NS |
| Infection/PTLD | 3 (13%) | 0 | NS |
| Acute rejection | 2 (9%) | 0 | NS |
| Primary nonfunction | 1 (4%) | 0 | NS |
| DWFG | 1 (4%) | 0 | NS |

*Abbreviations*: DWFG, death with functioning graft; PTLD, posttransplant lymphoproliferative disease; PAKT, pancreas after kidney transplants; PA, pancreas alone.

kidney, and pancreas graft survival rates were 92%, 81%, and 89%, respectively. These results demonstrated that SKPT with P-E drainage is a safe and effective method to treat advanced diabetic nephropathy and is associated with decreasing morbidity, improving rehabilitation and quality of life, and stable metabolic function over time.

In addition to correcting dysmetabolism and freeing the patient from exogenous insulin therapy, data are emerging on the course of secondary diabetic complications after PTX. Besides our work on procedure development and describing the diagnosis of rejection and management strategies, significant work has been published by members of our group regarding various physiologic, metabolic, and quality of life outcomes (43–46).

We demonstrated a decline in the incidence of rejection and graft loss to rejection with P-E drainage in the CYA era (56). This has led to significant interest in research related to portal antigen delivery and its effect on tolerance. In addition to describing utilization of intravenous glucose tolerance as a noninvasive marker for rejection (55), we examined determinants of altered glucose tolerance with TAC immunosuppression in P-E recipients (64). In 1995, Hughes et al. analyzed lipoprotein profiles in 31 SKPT recipients at our center, including 20 with S-B and 11 with P-E drainage (65). By 6 and 12 months after PTX, patients with P-E drainage experienced a significant improvement in lipoprotein profiles and particle composition that was not seen in patients with S-B drainage. This data was further supported by our collaborative work with Bagdade et al.(66). Also in 1995, El-Gebely et al. analyzed renal function two years after transplant in SKPT and diabetic KTA recipients at our center (67). The KTA recipients experienced a mild but significant deterioration in the serum creatinine coincident with the development of microalbuminuria after two years, findings that were not observed in SKPT patients despite significantly higher CYA levels in the latter.

In a study of 28 SKPT versus 20 KTA recipients with IDDM, Nymann et al. from our group reported improvements in motor nerve conduction and sensory nerve amplitude that were exclusive to the SKPT group (68). Although we noted a transitory, beneficial effect of reversal of uremia by KTA on motor nerve conduction in the first 12 months after transplant, only SKPT recipients continued to experience improvement in nerve conduction over time.

Chronic hyperglycemia has been associated with depressed myocardial contractility independent of the effects of hypertension, coronary disease, or renal function. Gaber et al. compared echocardiographic parameters in 20 SKPT, 2 PAKT, and 11 diabetic KTA recipients at 6 and 12 months follow-up (69). In the KTA group, systolic function improved at six months and remained stable thereafter. In comparison, a significant improvement in all echocardiographic measures (systolic function, diastolic function, and left ventricular geometry) occurred at 6 and 12 months after SKPT. Moreover, the improvements that occurred in all echocardiographic measures represented a restoration of normal cardiac function in most SKPT recipients. A follow-up study from our group by Wicks et al. documented sustained improvements in cardiac function at 24 months after SKPT (70).

Autonomic neuropathy is one consequence of IDDM that has been associated with severe morbidity and mortality (43). Both uremia and diabetes cause autonomic dysfunction leading to symptoms that can greatly compromise quality of life (44,71). Autonomic function is currently measured by two methods at our center; laboratory evoked cardiovascular tests and 24-hour rate variability measurement (71). The evoked cardiovascular tests, which include change in heart rate with deep respiration and Valsalva ratio, are performed in a temperature controlled laboratory equipped with computer, data acquisition, and analysis systems to obtain heart rate and blood pressure responsiveness to postural and respiratory maneuvers. Heart rate variability is measured by 24-hour Holter monitoring, with oscillations in R-R intervals examined in both time and frequency domains. Two of the three time domains reflect circadian rhythmicity, with one of these domains being closely associated with cardiac death. The remaining time domain reflects vagal function and is virtually independent of circadian rhythm. The frequency domains estimate parasympathetic and sympathetic control of the variations in the R-R intervals. We have had the unique opportunity to examine the association between quality of life and biologic outcomes longitudinally as well as constructing study designs to determine the degree to which these constructs are correlated and the relative contribution of biologic outcomes to overall quality of life (72,73).

Gaber and co-workers compared autonomic function in SKPT versus diabetic KTA recipients at 6 and 12 months follow-up (72,74). Several parameters were tested to generate an autonomic index or composite autonomic score. These parameters included tests of vasomotor function (total capillary pulse amplitude, reflex vasoconstriction, postural adjustment ratio), cardiorespiratory reflexes, and gastric function. We noted an improvement in nearly all of these autonomic parameters after SKPT versus KTA, although the differences were not always significant. In the one parameter that did not change (R-R respiratory interval variation), stabilization occurred after SKPT whereas continued progression occurred after KTA.

Hathaway et al. from our group demonstrated improvement in the Valsalva ratio but not in the electrocardiographically derived R-R interval respiratory variation after PTX (72). In spite of the improvement in cardiac autonomic function following SKPT, sudden cardiac death continues to be a concern in this population. We evaluated five otherwise healthy diabetic transplant recipients (three SKPT and two KTA) who experienced sudden cardiac death and compared their laboratory evoked cardiac autonomic responses to a group of surviving diabetic transplant recipients ($N = 26$) (44). Autonomic function was also compared to the patients with diabetes who had sudden cardiac death prior to receiving a transplant ($N = 5$). Of those patients that died while waiting, four of the five had extremely compromised Valsalva ratios. Sixteen surviving diabetic patients showed improvement in the Valsalva ratio from before to after transplant. Patients with transplants who experienced sudden cardiac death demonstrated no improvement in the Valsalva ratio. While the study could not categorically state that impaired Valsalva ratio was indicative of a poor transplant outcome, it did suggest that an abnormal Valsalva ratio might become a marker for patients who could be at potential risk for sudden cardiac death, particularly in the absence of improvement after successful transplantation.

We also analyzed laboratory evoked cardiovascular responses as well as 24-hour heart rate variability in nondiabetic and diabetic KTA and SKPT recipients (71,73). The nondiabetic KTA recipients displayed the least improvement in heart rate variability, however, their values were not as severely compromised pretransplant and therefore we were unable to show much improvement. By 12 months after transplant, most measures of heart rate variability for the nondiabetic KTA recipients had, in fact, reached values that approached those seen in healthy adults. Although the number of diabetic KTA recipients was small, it is interesting to note that the heart rate variability actually continued to decline somewhat in this group. This is in contrast to SKPT recipients who, following a slight decline in some measures at six months, showed improvement in heart rate variability at 12 months. Exercise has been associated with improved heart rate variability in a normal male population. We were able to demonstrate that those patients with diabetes who exercised regularly had significantly better heart rate variability than nonexercising diabetic individuals. This finding led us to initiate a prospective study of exercise on heart rate variability in both diabetic and nondiabetic KTA and SKPT recipients.

Improvement in quality of life is one of the major goals of PTX. Current data documents the presence of poor overall quality of life in patients with diabetes as compared to their nondiabetic counterparts. It is interesting to note that the baseline quality of life reported for our more recent diabetic patients has generally improved from previous reports (45,46,72,73). We could only surmise that advances in medical care (erythropoietin) and/or earlier transplant referral may have influenced this outcome. When comparing SKPT to nondiabetic KTA recipients, patients with diabetes pretransplant had a poorer quality of life in two of five measures, primarily reflecting greater physical dysfunction and a less positive view of their overall health. Following transplantation, quality of life improved in four of the five categories for both groups. However, at 24 months, a lingering disparity was still noted between diabetic KTA and SKPT recipients with respect to physical function and overall health perspective.

Numerous studies have demonstrated that a successful SKPT results in improvements in physical function, activities and daily living, energy level, mobility, vocational rehabilitation, social well-being, communication, role function, health perception, health image, pyschologic function, future expectations, sense of well-being, overall satisfaction, diet flexibility, diabetes-related concerns, time to manage health, health impact on family, and autonomy (45,46). The major benefits of PTX are an enhanced quality of life characterized by the following: (i) rehabilitation to "normal" living with physical, social, and psychological well-being with near normal activities and daily living and a self perception of normality; (ii) global improvement in quality of life with the perception of being healthy and having control over one's destiny; and (iii) fewer restrictions and enhanced capacities leading to an improved sense of well-being and independence. Freedom from daily insulin injections and blood glucose monitoring are important advantages in patients with a successful PTX. Although the long-term commitment to immunosuppression is the major trade-off, most patients with diabetes find the transition of transplantation easier than continued insulin therapy because of an improved sense of well-being with fewer dietary and activity restrictions. With the increasing short- and long-term success of PTX, the emphasis has shifted from survival outcomes to health-related quality of life.

Because transplant recipients are living longer, interest in long-term quality of life outcomes is emerging. Given the projection that many recipients will live well into the second decade following transplantation, it is important to know that some forms of neuropathy continue to demonstrate improvements in these later years, that neuropathy is associated with mortality as well as quality of life in the transplant population (72,73), and that some interventions may be available to improve neuropathy long-term. Therefore, it seems apparent that well-designed, longitudinal studies are needed not only to assess quantity but quality of life as well as physiologic function.

## SUMMARY

The UT Memphis group has made a number of important contributions to the field of PTX, including (i) pioneering studies on the effects of PTX on autonomic neuropathy, (ii) comprehensive reports dealing with quality of life after PTX, (iii) seminal studies on the metabolic effects of PTX with portal venous delivery of insulin, (iv) refining and perfecting a novel technique of PTX with portal venous drainage of insulin and primary enteric drainage of the exocrine secretions, (v) describing a safe outpatient percutaneous technique of pancreas allograft biopsy, (vi) developing the use of glucose tolerance for rejection surveillance, and (vii) managing PTX patients with biopsy-directed immunosuppression and no ALI.

The P-E technique has the potential to become the standard of care in the near future because it is more physiologic, normalizes carbohydrate and lipid metabolism, and minimizes complications attributed to the transplant procedure. In addition, we have been actively involved in studying new immunosuppressive regimens in order to improve and simplify the care of the PTX recipient. We believe that PTX will remain an important treatment option for IDDM until other strategies are developed that can provide equal glycemic control with less or no immunosuppression and less overall morbidity.

## ACKNOWLEDGMENTS

We gratefully acknowledge the expertise of Joyce Lariviere and Cassie Heidelberg in preparation of the manuscript.

## REFERENCES

1. Sutherland DER, Gruessner AC. International Pancreas Transplant Registry Update. IPTR Newslett 2000; 12:1–23.
2. Gruessner AC, Sutherland DER. Analyses of pancreas transplant outcomes for United States cases reported to the United Network for Organ Sharing (UNOS) and non-US cases reported to the International Pancreas Transplant Registry (IPTR). In: Cecka JM, Terasaki PI, eds. Clinical Transplants 1999. Los Angeles, CA: UCLA Immunogenetics Center, 2000:51–69.
3. Sindhi R, Stratta RJ, Lowell JA, et al. Experience with enteric conversion after pancreas transplantation with bladder drainage. J Am Coll Surg 1997; 184:281–289.
4. Shokouh-Amiri MH, Gaber AO, Gaber LW, et al. Pancreas transplantation with portal venous drainage and enteric exocrine diversion: a new technique. Transplant Proc 1992; 24:776–777.
5. Gaber AO, Shokouh-Amiri H, Grewal HP, Britt LG. A technique for portal pancreatic transplantation with enteric drainage. Surg Gynecol Obstet 1993; 177:417–419.
6. Gaber AO, Shokouh-Amiri H, Hathaway DK, et al. Pancreas transplantation with portal venous and enteric drainage eliminates hyperinsulinemia and reduces post-operative complications. Transplant Proc 1993; 25:1176–1178.
7. Di Carlo V, Castoldi R, Cristallo M, et al. Techniques of pancreas transplantation through the world: an IPITA center survey. Transplant Proc 1998; 30:231–241.
8. Gaber AO, Shokouh-Amiri MH, Hathaway DK, et al. Results of pancreas transplantation with portal venous and enteric drainage. Ann Surg 1995; 221:613–624.

9. Stratta RJ, Gaber AO, Shokouh-Amiri MH, et al. Experience with portal-enteric pancreas transplant at the University of Tennessee-Memphis. In: Cecka JM, Terasaki PI, eds. Clinical Transplant 1998. Los Angeles, CA: UCLA Tissue Typing Laboratory, 1999:239–253.

10. Stratta RJ, Gaber AO, Shokouh-Amiri MH, et al. Evolution in pancreas transplantation techniques: Simultaneous kidney-pancreas transplantation using portal-enteric drainage without anti-lymphocyte induction. Ann Surg 1999; 229:701–712.

11. Reddy KS, Stratta RJ, Shokouh-Amiri MH, Alloway R, Egidi MF, Gaber AO. Surgical complications after pancreas transplantation with portal-enteric drainage. J Am Coll Surg 1999; 189:305–313.

12. Stratta RJ, Gaber AO, Shokouh-Amiri MH, et al. A 9-year experience with 125 pancreas transplants with portal-enteric drainage. Transplant Proc. In press.

13. Ncwell KA, Woodle ES, Millis JM, et al. Pancreas transplantation with portal venous drainage and enteric exocrine drainage offers early advantages without compromising safety or allograft function. Transplant Proc 1995; 27:3002–3003.

14. Newell KA, Bruce DS, Cronin DC, et al. Comparison of pancreas transplantation with portal venous and enteric exocrine drainage to the standard technique utilizing bladder drainage of exocrine secretions. Transplantation 1996; 62:1353–1356.

15. Bruce DS, Newell KA, Woodle ES, et al. Synchronous pancreas-kidney transplantation with portal venous and enteric exocrine drainage: outcome in 70 consecutive cases. Transplant Proc 1998; 30:270–271.

16. Buell JF, Woodle ES, Siegel C, et al. Portal-enteric drained simultaneous pancreas-kidney transplantation: to Roux or not to Roux? 7th World Congress of the International Pancreas and Islet Transplant Association 1999; 57(A18) [Abstr].

17. Philosophe B, Taylor JP, Schweitzer FJ, et al. Portal venous drainage in pancreas transplantation: is there an immunologic advantage? 7th World Congress of the International Pancreas and Islet Transplant Association 1999; 56(A15) [Abstr].

18. Philosophe B, Farney AC, Schweitzer EJ, et al. The superiority of portal venous drainage over systemic venous drainage in solitary pancreas transplantation. 17th International Congress of the Transplantation Society 2000; 115(AO330) [Abstr].

19. Petruzzo P, Da Silva M, Feitosa LC, et al. Simultaneous pancreas-kidney transplantation: portal versus systemic venous drainage of the pancreas allografts. Clin Transplant 2000; 14:287–291.

20. Cattral MS, Bigam DL, Hemming AW, et al. Portal venous and enteric exocrine drainage versus systemic venous and bladder exocrine drainage of pancreas grafts: clinical outcome of 40 consecutive transplant recipients. Ann Surg 2000; 232:688–695.

21. Zibari GB, Aultman DF, Abreo KD, et al. Roux-en-Y venting jejunostomy in pancreatic transplantation: a novel approach to monitor rejection and prevent anastomotic leak. Clin Transplant 2000; 14:380–385.

22. Rosenlof LK, Earnhardt RC, Pruett TL, et al. Pancreas transplantation: an initial experience with systemic and portal drainage of pancreatic allografts. Ann Sure 1992; 215:586–597.

23. Calne RY. Paratopic segmental pancreas grafting: a technique with portal venous drainage. Lancet 1984; 1:595–597.

24. Gil-Vernet J, Fernandez-Cruz L, Andreu J, Figuerola D, Caraleps A. Clinical experience with pancreaticopyelostomy for exocrine pancreatic drainage and portal venous drainage in pancreas transplantation. Transplant Proc 1985; 17:342–345.

25. Tyden G, Wilczek H, Lundgren G, et al. Experience with 21 intraperitoneal segmental pancreatic transplants with enteric or gastric exocrine diversion in humans. Transplant Proc 1985; 17:331–335.

26. Sutherland DER, Goetz FC, Moudry KC, Abouna GM, Najarian JS. Use of recipient mesenteric vessels for revascularization of segmental pancreas grafts: technical and metabolic considerations. Transplant Proc 1987; 19:2300–2304.

27. Shokouh-Amiri MH, Rahimi-Saber S, Andersen AJ. Segmental pancreatic autotransplantation in the pig. Transplantation 1989; 47:42–44.

28. Shokouh-Amiri MH, Falholt K, Hoist JJ, et al. Pancreas endocrine function in pigs after segmental pancreas autotransplantation with either systemic or portal venous drainage. Transplant Proc 1992; 24:799–800.

29. Shokouh-Amiri MH, Rahimi-Saber S, Anderson HO, Jensen SL. Pancreas autotransplantation in pig with systemic or portal venous drainage: effect on the endocrine pancreatic function after transplantation. Transplantation 1996; 61:1004–1009.

30. Muhlbacher F, Gnant MFX, Auinger M, et al. Pancreatic venous drainage to the portal vein: a new method in human pancreas transplantation. Transplant Proc 1990; 22:636–637.

31. Rees M, Brons IGM. Pancreas transplantation: a historical perspective from a single institution. In: Hakim NS, Stratta RJ, Dubernard JM, eds. Second British Symposium on Pancreatic Transplantation. London, UK: Royal Society of Medicine Press, 1998:85–89.

32. Stratta RJ, Gaber AO, Shokouh-Amiri MH, et al. A prospective comparison of systemic-bladder versus portal-enteric drainage in vascularized pancreas transplantation. Surgery 2000; 127:217–226.

33. Stratta RJ, Shokouh-Amiri MH, Egidi MF, et al. Simultaneous kidney-pancreas transplant with systemic-enteric versus portal-enteric drainage. Transplant Proc. In press.

34. Nymann T, Elmer DS, Shokouh-Amiri MH, Gaber AO. Improved outcome of patients with portal-enteric pancreas transplantation. Transplant Proc 1997; 29:637–638.

35. Eubanks JW, Shokouh-Amiri MH, Elmer D, Hathaway D, Gaber AO. Solitary pancreas transplantation using the portal-enteric technique. Transplant Proc 1998; 30:446–447.
36. Busing M, Martin D, Schultz T, et al. Pancreas-kidney transplantation with urinary bladder and enteric exocrine diversion: 70 cases without anastomotic complications. Transplant Proc l998; 30:434–437.
37. Busing M, Schultz T, Konzack J, Gumprich M, Bloch T. Simultaneous pancreas/kidney transplantation with portal venous and enteric exocrine drainage; First experience in Europe. 7th World Congress of the International Pancreas and Islet Transplant Association 1999; 70(P48) [Abstr].
38. Stratta RJ. Pancreas Transplantation. Prob Gen Surg 1998; 15:43–65.
39. Stratta RJ, Taylor RJ, Spees EC, et al. Refinements in cadaveric pancreas-kidney procurement and preservation. Transplant Proc l99l; 23:2320–2322.
40. Gill IS, Sindhi R, Jerius JT, Sudan D, Stratta RJ. Bench reconstruction of pancreas for transplantation: experience with 192 cases. Clin Transplant 1997; 11:104–109.
41. Grewal HP, Garland L, Novak K, et al. Risk factors for post-implantation pancreatitis and pancreatic thrombosis in pancreas transplant recipients. Transplantation 1993; 56:609–612.
42. Stratta RJ, Taylor RJ, Gill IS. Pancreas transplantation: a managed cure approach to diabetes. Curr Prob Surg 1996; 33:709–816.
43. Hathaway DK, Cashion AK, Mil stead EJ, et al. Autonomic dysregulation in patients awaiting kidney transplantation. Am J Kidney Pis l998; 32:22l–229.
44. Hathaway DK, El-Gebely S, Cardoso S, et al. Autonomic cardiac dysfunction in diabetic transplant recipients succumbing to sudden cardiac death. Transplantation 1995; 59:634–637.
45. Hathaway DK, Hartwig MS, Milstead J, et al. A prospective study of changes in quality of life reported by diabetic recipients of kidney-only and pancreas-kidney allografts. J Transplant Coord 1994; 4:12–17.
46. Hathaway DK, Hartwig MS, Crom DB, Gaber AO. Identification of quality of life outcomes distinguishing diabetic kidney-alone and pancreas-kidney recipients. Transplant Proc l995; 27(6): 3065–3066.
47. Gaber AO, Gaber LW, Shokouh-Amiri MH, Hathaway D. Percutaneous biopsy of pancreas transplants. Transplantation 1992; 54:548–550.
48. Stratta RJ. Ganciclovir/acyclovir and fluconazole prophylaxis after simultaneous kidney-pancreas transplantation. Transplant Proc 1998; 30:2–62.
49. Somerville T, Hurst G, Alloway RR, Shokouh-Amiri MH, Gaber AO, Stratta RJ. Superior efficacy of oral ganciclovir over oral acyclovir for cytomegalovirus prophylaxis in kidney-pancreas and pancreas alone recipients. Transplant Proc 1998; 30:1546–1548.
50. Lo A, Stratta RJ, Egidi MF, et al. Patterns of cytomegalovirus infection in simultaneous kidney-pancreas transplant recipients receiving tacrolimus, mycophenolate mofetil, and prednisone with ganciclovir prophylaxis. Transplant Infect Dis. In press.
51. Gaber LW, Stratta RJ, Lo A, et al. Importance of surveillance biopsy monitoring in solitary pancreas transplant patients receiving tacrolimus and mycophenolate mofetil. Transplant Proc. In press.
52. Reddy KS, Stratta RJ, Shokouh-Amiri H, et al. Simultaneous kidney-pancreas transplantation without anti-lymphocyte induction. Transplantation 2000; 69:49–54.
53. Lo A, Stratia RJ, Alloway RR, et al. Limited benefits of induction with monoclonal antibody to interleukin-2 receptor in combination with tacrolimus, mycophenolate mofetil, and steroids in simultaneous kidney-pancreas transplantation. Transplant Proc. In press.
54. Sugitani A, Egidi MF, Grisch HA, Corry RJ. Serum lipase as a marker for pancreatic allograft rejection. Transplant Proc 1998; 30:645.
55. Elmer DS, Hathaway DK, Abdulkarim AB, et al. Use of glucose disappearance rates (Kg) to monitor endocrine function of pancreas allografts. Clin Transplant 1998; 12:56–64.
56. Nymann T, Hathaway DK, Shokouh-Amiri MH, et al. Patterns of acute rejection in portal-enteric versus systemic-bladder pancreas-kidney transplantation. Clin Transplant 1998; 12:175–183.
57. Solez K, Axelsen RA, Benediksson H, et al. International standardization of criteria for the histologic diagnosis of renal allograft rejection: The BANFF working classification of kidney transplant pathology. Kidney Int 1993; 44:411–424.
58. Kuo PC, Johnson LB, Schweitzer EJ, et al. Solitary pancreas allografts: the role of percutaneous biopsy and standardized histologic grading of rejection. Arch Surg 1997; 132:52–57.
59. Lo A, Stratta RJ, Hathaway DK, et al. Long-term outcomes in simultaneous kidney-pancreas transplant recipients with portal-enteric versus systemic-bladder drainage. Transplant Proc. In press.
60. Nymann T, Shokouh-Amiri MH, Elmer DS, et al. Diagnoses, management, and outcome of late duodenal complications in portal-enteric pancreas transplantation: case reports. J Am Coll Surg 1997; 185:560–566.
61. Reddy KS, Stratta RJ, Shokouh-Amiri H, Gaber AO. Successful reuse of portal-enteric technique in pancreas retransplantation. Transplantation 2000; 69:2443–2445.
62. Stratta RJ, Gaber AO, Shokouh-Amiri MH, et al. Allograft pancreatectomy after pancreas transplantation with systemic-bladder versus portal-enteric drainage. Clin Transplant 1999; 13:465–472.
63. Stratta RJ, Lo A, Hathaway DK, et al. Long-term outcome in simultaneous kidney- pancreas transplant recipients with portal-enteric drainage. 7th World Congress of the International Pancreas and Islet Transplant Association 1999; 71(P52) [Abstr].

64. Elmer DS, Abdulkarim AB, Fraga D, et al. Metabolic effects of FK506 (tacrolimus) versus cyclosporine in portally drained pancreas allografts. Transplant Proc 1998; 30:523–524.
65. Hughes TA, Gaber AO, Shokouh-Amiri H, et al. Kidney-pancreas transplantation: the effect of portal versus systemic venous drainage of the pancreas on the lipoprotein composition. Transplantation 1995; 60:1406–1412.
66. Bagdade JD, Ritter MC, Kitabchi AE, et al. Differing effects of pancreas-kidney transplantation with systemic versus portal venous drainage on cholesterol ester transfer in IDDM subjects. Diabetes Care 1996; 19:1108–1112.
67. El-Gebely S, Hathaway DK, Elmer DS, et al. An analysis of renal function in pancreas-kidney and diabetic kidney-alone recipients at two years following transplantation. Transplantation 1995; 59:1410–1415.
68. Nymann T, Hathaway DK, Bertorini TE, et al. Studies of the impact of pancreas-kidney and kidney transplantation on peripheral nerve conduction in diabetic patients. Transplant Proc 1998; 30:323–324.
69. Gaber AO, El-Gebely S, Sugathan P, et al. Early improvement in cardiac function occurs for pancreas-kidney but not diabetic kidney-alone transplant recipients. Transplantation 1995; 59:1105–1112.
70. Wicks MN, Hathaway DK, Shokouh-Amiri MH, et al. Sustained improvement in cardiac function 24 months following pancreas-kidney transplant. Transplant Proc 1998; 30:333–334.
71. Cashion AK, Hathaway DK, Milstead EJ, Reed L, Gaber AO. Changes in patterns of 24-hour heart rate variability after kidney and kidney-pancreas transplant. Transplantation 1999; 68:1846–1850.
72. Hathaway DK, Abell T, Cardoso S, et al. Improvement in autonomic and gastric function following pancreas-kidney versus kidney-alone transplantation and the correlation with quality of life. Transplantation 1994; 57:816–822.
73. Hathaway DK, Wicks MN, Cashion AK, et al. Heart rate variability and quality of life following kidney and kidney-pancreas transplantation. Transplant Proc 1999; 31:643–644.
74. Gaber AO, Hathaway DK, Abell T, et al. Improved autonomic and gastric function in pancreas-kidney versus kidney-alone transplantation contributes to quality of life. Transplant Proc 1994; 26:515–516.

# 29 | Simultaneous Pancreas–Kidney Transplantation at the Ohio State University

**Elmahdi A. Elkhammas, Alp Demirag, Ginny L. Bumgardner, Ronald P. Pelletier, Ronald M. Ferguson, and Mitchell L. Henry**
*Division of Transplantation, Department of Surgery, College of Medicine, The Ohio State University, Columbus, Ohio, U.S.A.*

## INTRODUCTION

Type I diabetes affects between one and two million people in the United States, with about 30,000 new cases diagnosed every year (1). Although intensified insulin therapy regimens enable normalization of blood glucose levels and related metabolic parameters, these regimens are associated with an increased incidence of hypoglycemic episodes (2). Transplantation of the insulin-producing islet cells would be an ideal approach, but until recently, only a small percentage of patients have achieved long-term insulin independence (3). The major problems in islet cell transplantation are failure of engraftment, rejection of the graft, and recurrence of autoimmune isletitis of the beta cells. Even if these immunologic barriers could be overcome, an important limiting factor for islet allotransplantation is an inadequate islet tissue supply. On the other hand, simultaneous pancreas–kidney transplantation (SPKT) has gained momentum in the last 12 years, and has become one of the standard treatment options for type I diabetic patients with end-stage renal disease. Advances in immunosuppression and better understanding of postoperative complications, as well as improvements in technical aspects, have allowed it to become a successful intervention. Currently, SPKT is the procedure of choice at our center for selected type I diabetic patients with end-stage renal disease. Ninety-four percent (94%) of the pancreatic transplantation at our center has been performed in the setting of SPKT. transplantation. In this chapter, we discuss our experience with 450 patients receiving an SPKT.

## RECIPIENT SELECTION CRITERIA

Careful patient selection is crucial to lowering morbidity and mortality after SPKT. Currently, patients are selected for SPKT based on ABO blood type compatibility, period of time on the waiting list, and a negative T-lymphocytotoxic or flow cross-match, in accordance with United Network for Organ Sharing guidelines. SPKT is not an immediate life-saving procedure; therefore, patient selection is based on achieving an improved quality of life with minimal risk for perioperative mortality. Our center, and many others, offers SPK transplantation to recipients with coronary artery disease once it has been treated either with bypass surgery or with angioplasty/stenting. Approximately 50% of the late mortality after SPKT is related to cardiovascular disease (4). With this in mind, it is not surprising that severe cardiovascular disease is the main limiting criterion for patient selection at our center, similar to other programs (5). We have adopted a relatively aggressive approach of accepting patients with mild-to-moderate coronary artery disease or with surgically treatable disease as candidates for the procedure, as long as they have adequate left ventricular function. Screening by selective angiography and revascularization when appropriate may allow selected patients with treatable coronary artery disease to undergo SPKT. Nevertheless, because of the high incidence of coronary artery disease and autonomic cardiomyopathy in diabetic patients, we have set an upper limit of 60 years for the recipient age. At our center, we make no attempt at human leukocyte antigen matching (6).

## DONOR SELECTION AND RECIPIENT OPERATION

Donors of pancreas grafts are usually younger than 55 years, nonobese, nondiabetic, with no history of severe alcohol abuse (5). We have more recently extended the donor age to 60 years in cases where direct examination by the procuring surgeon has indicated that the pancreas is appropriate for transplantation (7). Hyperamylasemia is a common finding in donors with severe head trauma, and we have not used it as a contraindication by itself for ruling out donors, as has been reported by others (8). Mild hyperglycemia is often associated with stress following head trauma, ischemic brain damage, or glucocorticoid administration. In the absence of a history of diabetes mellitus, we have not considered mild hyperglycemia to be a contraindication to using the pancreatic graft (9). The pancreas is procured from heart-beating cadaveric donors and flushed with University of Wisconsin preservation solution. We try to use only hemodynamically stable donors, with strict organ retrieval techniques, to minimize ischemia-induced complications (10).

In the recipient, we continue to use a systemic (venous)/bladder (exocrine) drainage technique. The portal vein (without a graft) is anastomosed to the recipient's external iliac vein, and the Y-arterial graft to the recipient's external iliac artery. The short duodenal segment is anastomosed to the bladder. Donor splenectomy is performed after revascularization. The kidney is then placed in a peritoneal pocket to keep it extraperitoneal, both to avoid rotation and to allow for easier percutaneous biopsy in the future. We have not seen a need to convert a large number of patients to enteric drainage because of persistent complications. In the first year, the presence of amylase in the urine is an additional tool to help us monitor the occurrence of acute rejection in the pancreatic graft, while safely allowing the elimination of the exocrine secretions.

## IMMUNOSUPPRESSION

Sequential induction therapy with an antilymphocytic preparation [antilymphocyte globulin, antithymocyte globulin (ATG) or OKT3] for 10 days is used in many centers (6). According to International Pancreas Transplant Registry data, antibody induction therapy has been used in 88% of pancreas transplants performed in the United States since 1987 (11). Daclizumab and basiliximab, two recently introduced chimeric monoclonal interleukin-2 receptor antagonists, are currently used as induction agents to reduce rejection rates after kidney transplantation and may also be beneficial in SPKT (12). We have selected basiliximab as the drug of choice for our sequential treatment. It is easy to use, with no cytokine release syndrome. In addition, the incidence of acute rejection has been very acceptable. The regimen has allowed us to delay cyclosporine use in the first few days posttransplantation, while the renal graft is recovering from ischemia-reperfusion injury. Azathioprine (AZA) or more recently mycophenolate mofetil (MMF) is started in the immediate preoperative period and continued for maintenance immunosuppression. MMF has been very effective in reducing acute rejection after SPKT, in combination with either cyclosporine (CsA) or tacrolimus (12). High-dose oral steroids are also started immediately prior to transplantation and are tapered postoperatively. Cyclosporine is added at 8 to 10 mg/kg/day when the serum creatinine falls from 2.5 to 3 mg/dL. Cyclosporine doses are adjusted according to renal function and cyclosporine levels.

## PATIENT AND GRAFT SURVIVAL

Data from the International Pancreas Transplant Registry show that in 1994–1996, 1516 SPKT transplants were performed worldwide, with a one-year patient survival rate of 92% (13). In the United States, overall patient survival rates were 92% at one year and 81% at five years, respectively (12). At our center, the one-, three-, and five-year patient survival rates are 90%, 88%, and 86%, respectively (Fig. 1). In our review, patient survival was not influenced by the presence of retinopathy, gastropathy, neuropathy, or by the loss of the kidney or the pancreas. In our series (14), age greater than 45 years was, however, associated with a lower patient survival rate. According to International Pancreas Transplant Registry data, one-year pancreas graft survival rate was 81% (13). One-year pancreas graft survival for SPKT in United Network for Organ Sharing registry is significantly better in the OKT3 induction group (81%) than in the ATG (78%) induction group and in the group receiving no induction therapy (75%) (11). Similarly, Knechtle et al. (15) found that one-year pancreas graft and

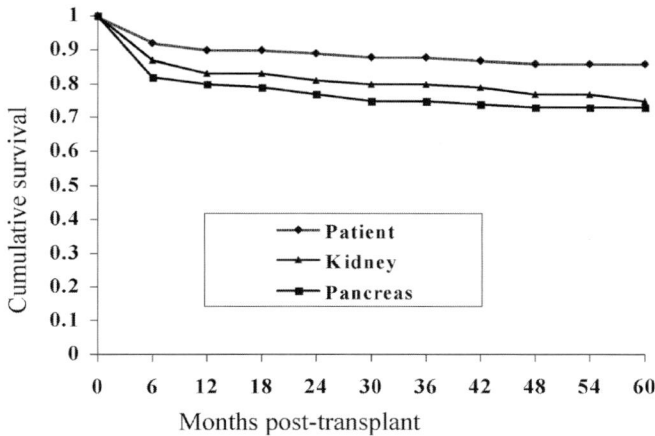

**Figure 1** Overall patient, kidney, and pancreas actuarial survival for 209 recipients of simultaneous pancreas–kidney transplants.

patient actuarial survival were higher in patients treated with OKT3 (89% and 95%, respectively) than in the antilymphocyte globulin group (83% and 91%, respectively). Recently, we reviewed our experience with basiliximab and found that the one-year patient survival rate with basiliximab induction therapy ($n = 36$) was better than in patients who received OKT3 induction ($n = 173$) (100% vs. 88%, $p$-value $= 0.03$) (Fig. 2). In this study, the main cause of death was predominantly cardiac, as shown in Table 1. The overall pancreas survival rate in our series at one, three, and five years was 80%, 75%, and 73%, respectively (Fig. 1). One-year pancreas survival was significantly better in the basiliximab group than for other recipients of antibody induction (92% vs. 76% $p$-value $= 0.045$) (Fig. 3). The loss of the kidney remained a significant factor in predicting shorter survival of the pancreas (14). This reflects our inability to monitor the pancreatic graft adequately, and also may indicate an upregulation of the immune system in such patients. Hopefully, the increase in safety and experience with percutaneous pancreatic allograft biopsy will help in monitoring such high-risk patients. Among the patients who lost their pancreatic graft, causes of graft loss were rejection (44%), death with a functioning graft (38%), thrombosis (31%), and sepsis (8%) (Table 2) (16,17).

Kidney graft survival has been slightly higher at each time point than pancreas survival. Overall, kidney survival rates in our series at one, three, and five years were 84%, 81%, and 75%, respectively (Fig. 1). The presence of retinopathy, gastropathy, and neuropathy had no impact on kidney or pancreas graft survival. One-year kidney graft survival was significantly better in the basiliximab induction group compared to any other antilymphocytic antibody induction (97% vs. 81%, $p$-value $= 0.02$) (Fig. 4). The loss of the pancreas graft had a significant negative impact on the survival of the kidney ($p$-value $= 0.0001$). This may be an indicator of the higher susceptibility of such recipients to immunologic graft loss. The causes of kidney graft loss were similar to those associated with pancreas graft loss.

Induction therapy with monoclonal or polyclonal agents in pancreas transplant recipients may delay the onset and lessen the severity of rejection episodes when compared to no

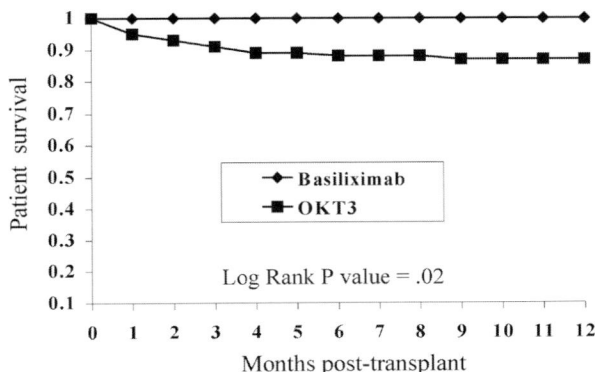

**Figure 2** Actuarial survival of recipients receiving induction with OKT3 or basiliximab.

**Table 1**  Overall Cause of Death in Recipients of Simultaneous Pancreas–Kidney Transplants

| Cause of death | % of deaths |
| --- | --- |
| Cardiac | 36 |
| Infections | 36 |
| Pulmonary embolism | 16 |
| MVA | 4 |
| CVA | 4 |
| PTLD | 4 |

*Abbreviations*: CVA, cerebrovascular accident; PTLD, posttransplant lymphoproliferative disease.

induction (12). Antibody induction therapy has not been found to adversely affect patient survival. Graft survival following SPKT was improved by the use of antibody induction, especially at three to five years after transplantation, in the Sandimmune era (12).

## ACUTE REJECTION

We have previously reported that acute rejection is a significant cause of graft loss in SPKT patients (18). In our center, acute rejection is established by renal biopsy prior to committing the patient to antirejection treatment. Serum creatinine, urine amylase, and serum amylase have been the markers that indicate the need for further workup, which includes an ultrasound and biopsy of the kidney. The overall rate of acute rejection has been 37% (Fig. 5). In the literature, the incidence of acute rejection episodes in patients receiving OKT3 and ATG induction was reported to be 62% to 75% (16,19). Rates of both acute and chronic rejection were lower, however, in patients receiving OKT3 compared with those receiving ATG (12,15,16). Until recently, maintenance immunosuppressive therapy consisted of steroids, cyclosporine, and AZA. With the use of these drugs, our experience was similar to that of other transplant centers, with acute rejection rates ranging from 60% to 80% (12). Over time, our immunosuppression protocol evolved from the use of OKT3 and AZA to OKT3 and MMF, and more recently to basiliximab and MMF. The largest single-center experience with MMF has been described by the University of Wisconsin, where 109 SPKT recipients received MMF and were compared to a historical control group of 249 SPKT patients managed with AZA (16). In this study, all patients received CsA-based immunosuppression in a sequential quadruple induction protocol with either ATG or OKT3. Kidney and pancreas two-year allograft survival rates (95% and 86%, and 95% and 83%, respectively) both were significantly higher in the MMF-treated patients during the follow-up period (16). In addition, the use of MMF was associated with significant reductions in biopsy-proven acute rejection for both kidney allografts (75% vs. 31%) and pancreas allografts (24% vs. 7%) (16). In our AZA group, the incidence of acute rejection was 72%. With the change to MMF, the incidence dropped to 24%. The use of basiliximab has improved the side effect profile, and has been associated with a 22% incidence of acute rejection of 22% under maintenance therapy with CsA, MMF, and

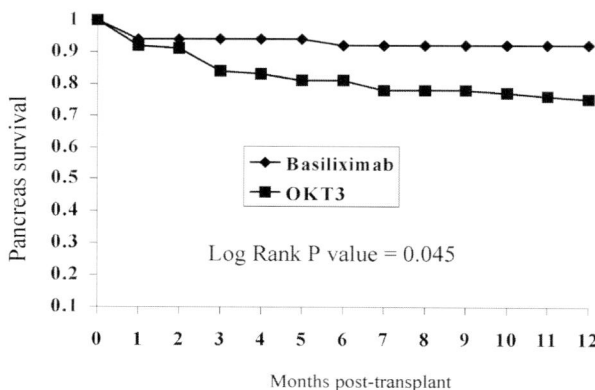

**Figure 3**  The actuarial survival of pancreatic allografts receiving induction with OKT3 or basiliximab.

**Table 2** Causes of Graft Loss in Recipients of Simultaneous Pancreas–Kidney Transplants

| Cause of graft loss | Pancreas (%) | Kidney (%) |
|---|---|---|
| Death | 38 | 53 |
| Thrombosis | 31 | 23 |
| Rejection | 23 | 14 |
| Sepsis | 8 | 2 |
| Unknown | 0 | 8 |

prednisone. This is consistent with our previous publication comparing OKT3 and AZA with OKT3 and MMF (20). Nearly 80% of the acute rejection episodes occurred during the first 90 days following transplantation. The renal allograft is involved in 90% of the rejection episodes. The availability of percutaneous pancreatic biopsy has given us the ability to make an earlier diagnosis and thus intervene in a timely manner.

## ENTERIC CONVERSION

In the literature, the enteric conversion rate has been reported to be between 10% and 49% of the bladder-drained (BD) SPKT recipients (16,17,21). At our center, enteric conversion has been needed in 11% of SPKT recipients. Enteric conversion has been reported to treat complications related to the BD procedure, including hematuria (19–45%), duodenal leak (35–44%), pancreatitis (0–5%), recurrent urinary tract infection (UTI) (4–11%), and severe metabolic acidosis (13,17,22). Our results are consistent with other centers' reports (Fig. 6). Early hematuria has generally responded to medical treatment, but chronic or recurrent hematuria requires enteric conversion (23). In late leaks, it is advisable to perform immediate enteric conversion. Enteric conversion is generally required within the first few years after transplantation (16), and appears to be a safe procedure, but is not without morbidity and mortality.

## UROLOGICAL COMPLICATIONS

Urological complications after kidney–pancreas transplantation are not uncommon. The major noninfectious complication is hematuria (17.7–26%). The etiology of early hematuria is usually bleeding from the suture line, whereas ulcers in the duodenal segment or granulation tissue in the area of the anastomosis can cause chronic hematuria (16,24). At our center, hematuria (15%) has generally been treated conservatively, using Foley catheter drainage and continuous bladder irrigation. For persistent early hematuria, we have also used cystoscopy and cauterization. For late or recurrent hematuria, enteric conversion has been the treatment of choice.

   Leak at the duodenocystostomy has become an uncommon event. Small leaks are managed by Foley catheter drainage. Late leaks have been treated by enteric conversion. In our program, leaks occurred in less than 10% of the recipients. Regarding the kidney, the overall ureteral complication rate is between 5.3% and 6% (16,24). At our center, ureteral strictures are

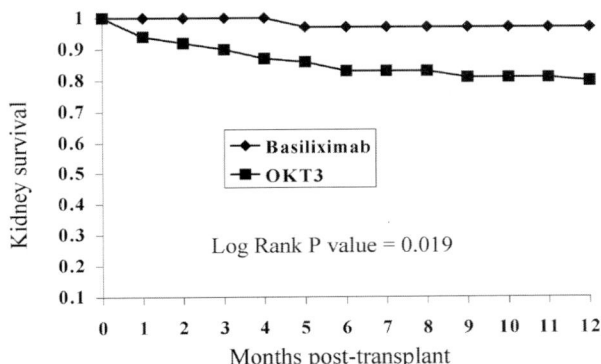

**Figure 4** The actuarial survival of renal allografts receiving induction with OKT3 or basiliximab.

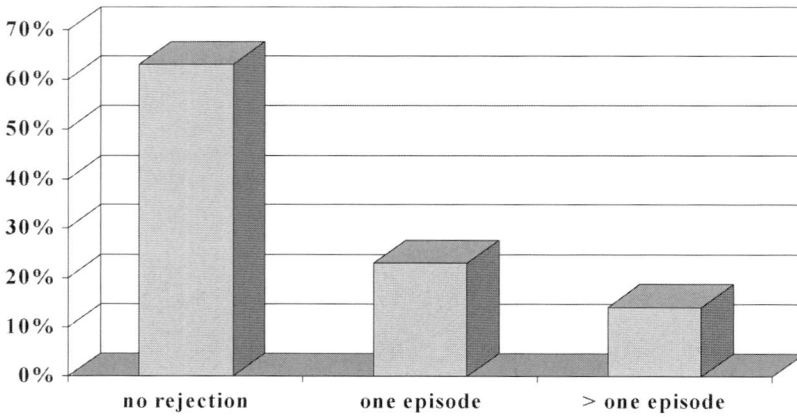

**Figure 5** Incidence of acute rejection episodes in recipients of simultaneous pancreas–kidney transplants.

very uncommon; they are treated with dilatation and stenting, and, in some cases, ureteral resection and reimplantation (16,24).

Other noninfectious complications are urethral disruption and urethral strictures. We have seen such complications in 7% of our recipients. They usually present with dysuria and frequency, and have sterile urine cultures. A retrograde urethrogram is diagnostic. We usually place a Foley catheter for two weeks to divert the urine and give the urothelium a chance to heal. This approach has been very successful, with the exception of a few cases that required enteric conversion.

Reflux pancreatitis has occurred in 10% of the patients after pancreas–kidney transplantation and has responded to the Foley catheter drainage or intermittent catheterization in all patients.

The main infectious complications are recurrent lower UTI, testicular abscess, and epididymitis (15,23,24). UTI is by far the most common complication of BD; it can result in frequent readmission to the hospital, requiring antibiotic therapy (Fig. 7). Some recipients with recurrent UTIs may require native nephrectomy if the native kidney is found to be the source of infection.

## TECHNICAL FAILURE

Technical complications have become very uncommon. There is a learning curve for the program as well as for the individual surgeon. Almost one-third of the pancreatic graft losses and

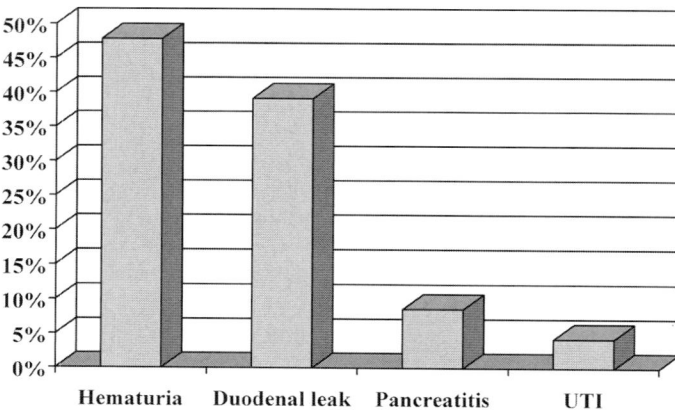

**Figure 6** Indications for enteric conversion in recipients of simultaneous pancreas–kidney transplants. *Abbreviation:* UTI, urinary tract infection.

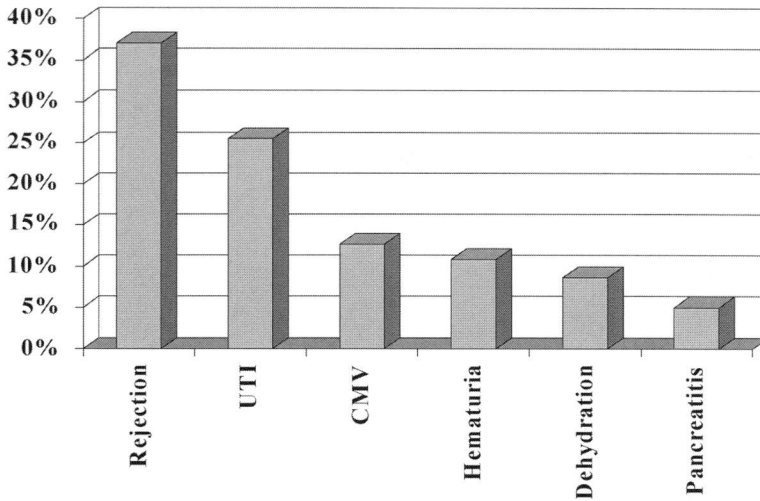

**Figure 7** The most common causes of readmissions in the first year posttransplant in recipients of simultaneous pancreas–kidney transplantation. *Abbreviations:* UTI, urinary tract infection; CMV, cytomegalovirus.

one-quarter of the kidney graft losses were due to graft thrombosis. Some of these occurred early, and were most likely related to donor, preservation, or technical issues, but some occurred late and probably were related to chronic rejection or native inflow abnormalities. Our incidence of pancreatic graft thrombosis has been 3%. Most of the technical problems have been related to the arterial supply, either due to error in the graft arterial reconstruction or underestimation of the arterial disease of the recipient iliac system. Sollinger et al. reported that overall thrombosis rate for the pancreas was 0.8% in their series of 500 SPKTs (16).

The technical failure rate from 1994 to 1998 for cadaveric BD pancreas transplants in the United States was 8% for recipients of SPKT. Heparin is only advised for pre-emptive pancreas transplants (i.e., in patients not on dialysis) to prevent thrombosis. We have been using baby aspirin as part of long-term antiplatelet therapy, which requires no specific monitoring.

## INFECTIONS

Although the technical success rate of SPKT has improved, morbidity remains high due to infection and acute rejection. Peddi et al. (17) reported that lower extremity infections (47.5%), cytomegalovirus (CMV) infections (25.4%), and fungal infections (8.5%) were seen after SPKT. Smets et al. (25) reviewed all infections following 66 consecutive bladder-drained SPK transplants. The overall mean infection rate was 2.9 infections/patient/year with a mean follow-up of 2.3 years, and lower UTIs accounted for 48% of all infections. In our series, UTI is the most common type of infection, occurring in 25% of our recipients during the first year following transplantation (Fig. 7). Of those who developed a UTI, only one episode occurred in two-thirds of the patients. *Enterococcus* was the most common organism cultured from the urine (26). Bacterial infections in general were more common with OKT3 than with basiliximab. In our series, 16% of the patients developed CMV infection, with only four patients having a recurrent CMV infection. DHPG has been a very effective treatment, and we have yet to document viral resistance in SPKT recipients. The occurrence of CMV infection was not different between OKT3 and basiliximab. Other viral infections occurred in 8% of patients, and very few were documented to be related to Epstein-Barr virus or herpes simplex virus.

## SUMMARY

SPKT is the procedure of choice to treat type I diabetic patients with end stage renal disease. The diabetic patient is a high-risk individual, but with improvements in technical skills and immunosuppressive medications the procedure has become relatively safe. Careful evaluation and selection are required to achieve excellent results with these scarce organs. As we have seen in our series, death is the number one cause of graft loss, and thorough preoperative evaluation will continue to be important to lower the mortality rate of SPKT. At our center, long-term patient and graft survival rates have been acceptable, and we will continue to use SPKT as the procedure of choice in appropriate candidates.

## REFERENCES

1. Libman I, Songer T, LaPorte R. How many people in the U.S. have IDDM? Diabet Care 1993; 16(5):841.
2. Orchard TJ. From diagnosis and classification to complications and therapy. DCCT. Part II? Diabetes Control and Complications trial. Diabetes Care 1994; 17:326. (AD—Department of Epidemiology, Graduate School of Public Health, University of Pittsburgh, Pennsylvania, U.S.A.).
3. Inverardi L, Ricordi C. Transplantation of pancreas and islets of Langerhans: a review of progress. Immunol Today 1996; 17:7.
4. Kim SI, Elkhammas EA, Henry ML, Davies EA, Bumgardner GL, Ferguson RM. Outcome of combined kidney/pancreas transplantation in recipients with coronary artery disease. Transplant Proc 1995; 27:3071. (AD—Department of Surgery, Ohio State University, Columbus, U.S.A.).
5. Odorico JS, Becker YT, Van der Werf W, et al. Advances in pancreas transplantation: the University of Wisconsin experience. In: Terasaki CA, ed. Clinical Transplants. Los Angeles, CA: UCLA Tissue Typing Laboratory, 1997:157.
6. Elkhammas EA, Henry ML, Yilmaz S, Pelletier RP, Bumgardner GL, Ferguson RM. Simultaneous pancreas–kidney transplantation at the Ohio State University Medical Center. In: Terasaki CA, ed. Clinical Transplants. Los Angeles, CA: UCLA Tissue Typing Laboratory, 1997:167.
7. Elkhammas EA, Henry ML, Tesi RJ, Ferguson RM. Combined kidney/pancreas transplantation at the Ohio State University Hospitals. In: Terasaki PI, Cecka JM, eds. Clinical Transplants 1992. Los Angeles: UCLA Tissue Typing Laboratory, 1993:191.
8. Sutherland DER, Bartlett ST, Gaber AO, Stock P. Symposium: pancreas transplantation. Contemp Surg 1997; 51(4):253.
9. Shaffer D, Madras PN, Sahyoun AI, Simpson MA, Monaco AP. Cadaver donor hyperglycemia does not impair long-term pancreas allograft survival or function. Transplant Proc 1994; 26(2):439.
10. Stratta RJ, Taylor RJ, Lowell JA, et al. Pancreas transplantation: the Nebraska experience. In: Cecka TA, ed. Clinical Transplants. Los Angeles, CA: UCLA Tissue Typing Laboratory, 1994:265.
11. Gruessner A, Sutherland DER. Pancreas transplantation in the United States (US) and non-US as reported to the United Network for Organ Sharing (UNOS) and the International Pancreas Transplant Registry. In: Terasaki CA, ed. Clinical Transplants. Los Angeles, CA: UCLA Tissue Typing Laboratory, 1996:47.
12. Stratta RJ. Review of immunosuppressive usage in pancreas transplantation. Clin Transplant 1999; 13(1 Pt 1):1.
13. Shapira Z, Yussim A, Mor E. Pancreas transplantation. J Pediatr Endocrinol Metab 1999; 12:3.
14. Tso PL, Elkhammas EA, Henry ML, et al. Risk factors of long-term survivals in combined kidney/pancreas transplantation: a multivariate analysis of 259 recipients. Transplant Proc 1995; 27:3104.
15. Knechtle SJ, Pirsch JD, Groshek M, et al. OKT3 vs ALG induction therapy in combined pancreas–kidney transplantation. Transplant Proc 1991; 23(1):1581.
16. Sollinger HW, Odorico JS, Knechtle SJ, D'Alessandro AM, Kalayoglu M, Pirsch JD. Experience with 500 simultaneous pancreas–kidney transplants. Ann Surg 1998; 228(3):284.
17. Peddi VR, Munda R, Demmy AM, First MR. Long-term outcome in simultaneous kidney and pancreas transplant recipients with functioning allografts at 1-year posttransplantation. Transplant Proc 1999; 31:608.
18. Tesi RJ, Elkhammas EA, Henry ML, Davies EA, Ferguson RM. Pattern of graft loss after combined kidney pancreas transplant. Transplant Proc 1994; 26(2):425.
19. Hasegawa T, Tzakis AG, Todo S, et al. Orthotopic liver transplantation for ornithine transcarbamylase deficiency with hyperammonemic encephalopathy. 30:863.
20. Elkhammas EA, Yilmaz S, Henry ML, et al. Simultaneous pancreas/kidney transplantation: comparison of mycophenolate mofetil versus azathioprine. 1998; 30:512.
21. Sindhi R, Stratta RJ, Taylor RJ, Lowell JA, Sudan D, Castaldo P. Experience with enteric conversion after pancreas transplantation with bladder drainage. Transplant Proc 1995; 27(6):3014.
22. Stratta RJ, Taylor RJ, Lowell JA, et al. OKT3 induction in 100 consecutive pancreas transplants. Transplant Proc 1994; 26(2):546.
23. Baktavatsalam R, Little DM, Connolly EM, Farrell JG, Hickey DP. Complications relating to the urinary tract associated with bladder-drained pancreatic transplantation. Br J Urol 1998; 81:219.
24. Gettman MT, Levy JB, Engen DE, Nehra A. Urological complications after kidney–pancreas transplantation. J Urol 1998; 159:38.
25. Smets YF, van der Pijl JW, van Dissel JT, Ringers J, de Fijter JW, Lemkes HH. Infectious disease complications of simultaneous pancreas kidney transplantation. Nephrol Dial Transplant 1997; 12(4):764.
26. Elkhammas EA, Sethi PS, Henry ML, Williams PA, Bennett FB, Ferguson RM. Urologic complications following pancreas transplantation. Transplant Rev 1997; 11:1.

# 30 | Pancreatic Transplantation at the University of Maryland

**Benjamin Philosophe**
*Division of Transplantation, Department of Surgery, University of Maryland, Baltimore, Maryland, U.S.A.*

**Venkatesh Krishnamurthi and Stephen T. Bartlett**
*Department of Surgery, University of Maryland, Baltimore, Maryland, U.S.A.*

In 1966, Kelly et al. performed the first human pancreatic transplantation at the University of Minnesota, which unfortunately resulted in the death of the recipient (1) (see Chapter 3). Early modifications of the original procedure met with poor success and resulted in a high incidence of intra-abdominal infections, graft loss, and patient death. In these early years, pancreas transplantation was associated with a 60% mortality rate and a 3% one-year success rate (2). In 1984, Sollinger et al. introduced the technique of bladder drainage (BD), a technique that was rapidly accepted because of the marked reduction of the risk of post-transplant sepsis (Fig. 1) (3). This technique, which was modified by Nghiem and Corry (4), was associated with improved outcomes, largely as a result of better monitoring of pancreas rejection. Although still used in many centers today, bladder drainage is largely being replaced by the more physiologic and less morbid technique of enteric drainage (ED). The success rate of pancreatic transplantation has increased so significantly that the procedure has been endorsed by the American Diabetes Association as an accepted treatment for patients with Type 1 diabetes and end-stage renal disease (ESRD) (5). In 1998, more than 1200 pancreas transplants were performed in the United States, a 15% increase from the previous year (6).

In 1991, the pancreas transplant program was initiated at the University of Maryland. Initially, the program was dedicated to establishing the standard simultaneous pancreas and kidney (SPK) transplant technique with the lowest possible morbidity. As the program evolved, solitary pancreas transplantation improved to the point where graft survival was comparable to that seen with SPK transplants. Through January 2000, 434 pancreas transplants have been performed (Fig. 2). This includes 204 SPK transplants for patients with ESRD and Type 1 diabetes mellitus, 124 pancreas after kidney (PAK) transplants for patients with Type 1 diabetes mellitus and a prior successful kidney transplant, 68 pancreas transplants alone (PTA), and 38 simultaneous cadaveric pancreas and living donor kidney (SPLK) transplants.

## THE EVOLUTION OF LAPAROSCOPIC LIVING DONOR NEPHRECTOMY AND ITS INFLUENCE ON PANCREAS TRANSPLANTATION

By the end of 1998, 42,652 patients were on the waiting list for a kidney transplant, with a median waiting time of 936 days. During that year, 13,132 (31%) underwent kidney transplantation, of which 4151 (31.6%) were with living donors (7). Live donor renal transplantation is a potentially underutilized resource that can substantially reduce waiting times and provide improved patient and graft survival. Resistance to living kidney donation can be attributed to concerns by the donors regarding the operation, the necessary hospital stay, prolonged recuperative period, and the financial liability (lost wages, etc.).

Laparoscopic nephrectomy for neoplasms has been proven to reduce postoperative pain, hospital length of stay, and convalescent time compared to the open approach (8). This provided the rationale for the development of minimally invasive living donor nephrectomy. Laparoscopic live donor nephrectomy has been performed at the University of Maryland since March 1996. The morbidity and mortality compare to open donor nephrectomy, but with substantial improvements in donor recovery (9). The sum of these improvements has resulted in a

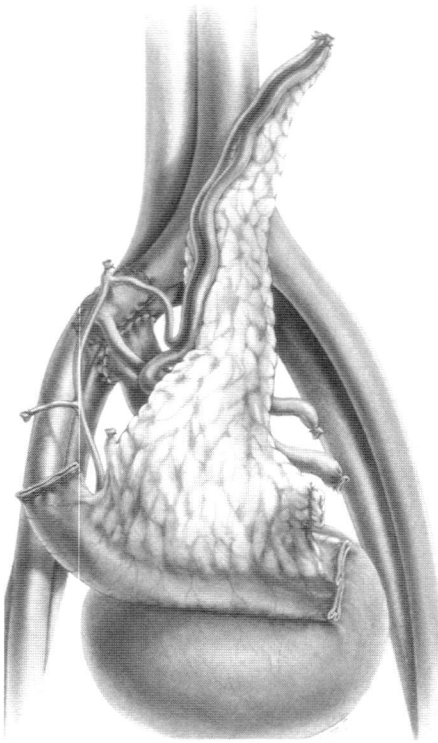

**Figure 1** Simultaneous pancreas–kidney transplantation with systemic venous and bladder exocrine drainage.

significant increase in acceptance of the donor operation, resulting in an expanded pool of potential kidney donors. In 1999, 44% of our renal transplants were from living donors, a significantly higher percentage than the national average. As of June 2000, we performed more than 500 laparoscopic donor nephrectomies.

In contrast, the slower development of pancreas transplantation in the United States has provided a relatively large number of pancreases available for transplantation through national sharing. The heavy reliance on living donor renal transplants to alleviate the cadaveric donor shortage has also resulted in the development of strategies to reduce significantly the waiting time required for Type 1 diabetics with renal failure to receive both a kidney and a

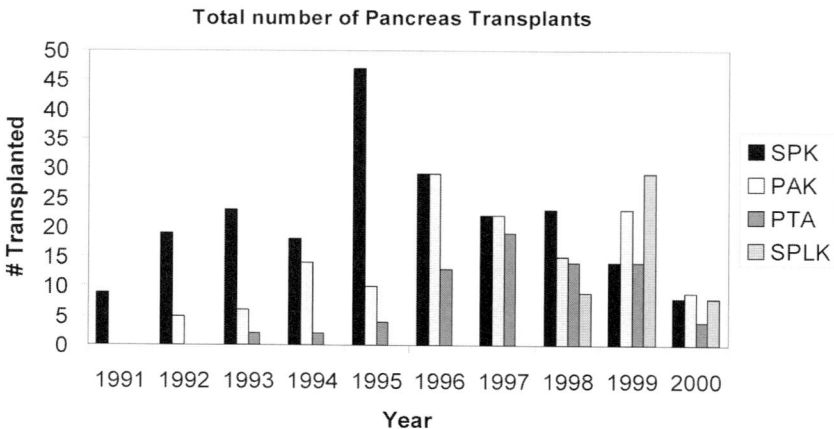

**Figure 2** Number of pancreas transplants performed at the University of Maryland. *Abbreviations*: SPK, simultaneous pancreas–kidney; PAK, pancreas after kidney transplantation; PTA, pancreas transplantation alone; SPLK, simultaneous cadaveric pancreas and living donor kidney.

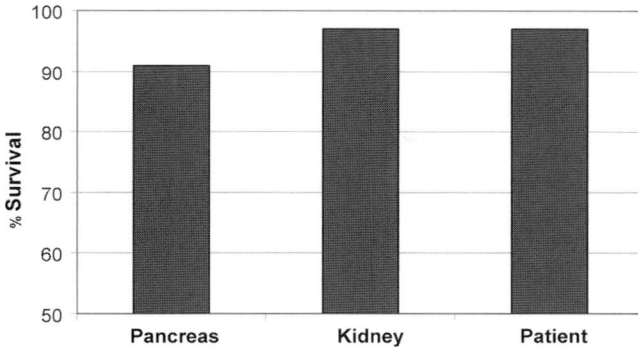

**Figure 3** Pancreas graft, kidney graft, and patient survival for simultaneous cadaveric pancreas and living donor kidney transplants ($n = 46$).

pancreas transplant. To date, 681 living donor renal transplants were performed in our institution, and 108 of those recipients received pancreas transplants either three to six months following the renal transplant or simultaneously as an SPLK.

## SIMULTANEOUS CADAVER PANCREAS–LIVING DONOR KIDNEY TRANSPLANTATION

Because there are currently a theoretically sufficient number of cadaver pancreases available for transplantation, we have questioned the need for living pancreas donors, for the time being. This has been supported by our observation that potential solitary pancreas transplant recipients are transplanted very quickly. In the past, Type 1 diabetics with ESRD who had a living donor had to choose among one of three options. Option 1 was to reject living kidney donation and wait for a cadaver SPK. The recipient's insurance carrier sometimes mandated this choice. Option 2 was to receive a living donor kidney transplant alone and accept life as a diabetic. Option 3 was to have a living donor kidney transplant and then have a PAK procedure, usually three to six months later. We hypothesized that a living donor kidney and cadaver pancreas could be performed together safely, thereby avoiding a second operation and its associated morbidity (10). Our results after 46 cases demonstrated one-year pancreas and kidney graft survival rates of 91% and 97%, respectively, and a patient survival of 97% (Fig. 3). Moreover, the waiting time for SPLK is substantially less than for cadaver SPK. Finally, the cost of SPLK has been less than the combined cost of living donor kidney and PAK transplantation as separate procedures.

## PATIENT SELECTION

Pancreatic transplantation has been reserved for patients with Type 1 diabetes mellitus. In the majority of cases, there has been unequivocal information to confirm the diagnosis of Type 1 diabetes, including a history of juvenile onset (the mean age has been 14 years), past ketoacidosis, lean body habitus, and a requirement for 20 to 80 U of insulin daily. Adult onset, obesity, absence of a history of ketoacidosis, periods of insulin independence or extraordinary insulin requirements may suggest a diagnosis of Type 2 diabetes mellitus. Diagnostic uncertainty is resolved by the administration of a 100 g oral glucose challenge, followed by simultaneous measurement of blood C-peptide and glucose one hour later. A Type 1 diabetic will have undetectable C-peptide levels despite maximal stimulation of the pancreas with a simultaneously elevated blood glucose. Conversely, a Type 2 diabetic will have blood insulin levels that are normal or elevated as a result of insulin resistance. Although some Type 2 diabetics have achieved insulin independence after pancreatic transplantation, there is little published information on the long-term efficacy of pancreatic transplantation in this setting. With only 5000 cadaver donors in the United States annually, it has been our view that extension of pancreatic transplantation to Type 2 diabetics should not be widely applied before the benefits of transplantation in this setting have been established.

The majority of patients evaluated for pancreas transplantation have or have had ESRD. Thus, the patients are on dialysis, approaching dialysis, or have had a successful kidney transplant. In addition to ESRD, most patients have other secondary complications of diabetes, including retinopathy, neuropathy, autonomic neuropathy, gastroparesis, and evidence of accelerated atherosclerosis. The evidence is clear that pancreatic transplantation prevents recurrent diabetic nephropathy in transplanted kidneys (11). This fact alone, combined with the marked improvement in quality of life achieved with a successful pancreas transplant, strongly supports pancreatic transplantation either simultaneously with a kidney transplant or after a kidney transplant, in the Type 1 diabetic with renal failure. It is rare to have ESRD as an isolated secondary complication of diabetes. Thus, the vast majority of candidates have varying degrees of other secondary complications that may be arrested or reversed after pancreatic transplantation.

## PATIENT EVALUATION

At the University of Maryland, all candidates undergo noninvasive cardiac stress testing, such as dobutamine stress echocardiography or adenosine thallium stress scintigraphy. Potential candidates with reversible myocardial defects undergo coronary angiography. Our indications for myocardial revascularization are different in the diabetic population and are addressed accordingly. With modern anesthetic techniques and perioperative monitoring, we believe that pancreas transplantation presents few risks in diabetics with significant, asymptomatic coronary artery disease (12). Therefore, adopting an aggressive policy of coronary angioplasty, stenting, or bypass may not always be warranted.

The presence of aortoiliac occlusive disease that can compromise arterial inflow to the transplanted organs may require pretransplant intervention. Correction of aortoiliac disease with angioplasty, placement of an iliac artery endoluminal stent, or formal aortofemoral bypass usually precedes transplantation. We have successfully transplanted patients after each of these interventions. Similarly, all candidates are screened for hemodynamically significant carotid occlusive disease that may warrant pretransplant carotid endarterectomy.

Contraindications for pancreatic transplantation include the presence of an active infection, recent malignancy, chronic active hepatitis, cirrhosis, psychiatric disease, and active alcohol and drug dependency, which could impair the patient's ability to cooperate with post-transplant management.

The indications for a PTA performed before the development of clinically significant renal insufficiency are obviously different from those patients who have current or prior ESRD. The most common reason to perform a PTA is severely labile diabetes. This is defined clinically as a syndrome of repeated episodes of hypoglycemic coma or seizure, or hypoglycemia requiring third party assistance. Many of these patients have experienced frequent seizure episodes or coma requiring emergency room treatment or hospital admission. Others have had industrial or motor vehicle accidents or accidentally injured children under their care. Occasionally, a PTA is performed because there has been an inexorable decline in the patient's functional status because of a combination of progressive neuropathy, retinopathy, gastroparesis, and proteinuria secondary to early diabetic nephropathy. Except for a lack of proven effect on advanced retinopathy, successful pancreas transplantation can lead to a reversal of many of these secondary complications over time (see Chapter 2).

## TECHNICAL ASPECTS

The various surgical techniques of pancreas transplantation can broadly be classified according to the type of exocrine drainage performed and to the type of venous drainage employed. Exocrine drainage BD continues to be the most common method of duct management, because of the ability to monitor urinary amylase as a marker for rejection. With improvements in immunosuppression and a reduction in the frequency of surgical complications, combined with the unique metabolic and urologic complications posed by BD, increasing numbers of transplant programs are adopting ED as a primary method of duct management. In 1998, ED was used in over 50% of SPK transplants, compared to only 6% in 1994 (6). Pancreas graft survival rates at one year in this patient group were similar between these two duct management techniques (83% for BD and 82% for ED). A significant difference in pancreas graft survival according to the type of duct management continues to be observed in recipients of solitary pancreas transplants, although these differences appear to be a result of a higher technical failure rate.

In a recent survey of 121 active pancreas transplant centers recognized by the International Pancreas and Islet Transplant Association, 78 (64%) reported their preferred surgical technique of pancreas transplantation (13). Thirty different surgical techniques of pancreas transplantation were described; however, these differences were largely variations on the same theme. In addition to the major differences of BD versus ED, subtle modifications, depending on the location of the anastomosis, the use of arterial and venous extension grafts, and "hand-sewn" versus stapled anastomosis of the duodenal segment, account for the large variation in techniques.

## Venous Reconstruction

The preferred method of venous drainage remains controversial. Systemic venous (SV) drainage, the method used in over 90% of reporting centers, is an established surgical technique that is associated with excellent long-term results (13). A theoretical disadvantage of SV drainage, however, relates to the high levels of insulin in the peripheral circulation. Hyperinsulinemia has been shown in experimental systems to be associated with insulin resistance and altered lipid metabolism (14–16). Portal venous (PV) drainage, a more physiologic method that eliminates peripheral hyperinsulinemia, is gaining interest among a few pancreas transplant centers. Following the initial description by Calne in 1984, PV drainage of pancreas allografts has undergone several technical modifications (17,18). The current technique of PV drainage used in most centers is based on the technique described by Shokouh-Amiri et al. (19). Although follow-up is limited, several centers, including ours, have shown excellent graft survival rates and a reduced number of surgical complications with PV drainage (13,20,21).

The technique of SV drainage involves anastomosis of the donor portal vein to the recipient iliac vein or vena cava (Fig. 2). During the back-table preparation, the donor portal vein should be mobilized to the confluence of the splenic and superior mesenteric branches. This often involves division of several pancreaticoduodenal branches. In addition, the recipient common and external iliac veins should be fully mobilized by dividing all internal iliac and lumbar branches, effectively placing this vein anterolateral to the iliac artery on the right side and medial to the external iliac artery, when performed on the left side. This maneuver decreases tension on the venous anastomosis, allows it to be performed under improved exposure, and reduces the risk of venous thrombosis (22–24). In cases of SV drainage, we perform an end-to-side anastomosis directly between the portal vein and the iliac vein using fine (#6-0 or #7-0) polypropylene suture. Several authors have described the use of venous extension grafts to facilitate the venous anastomosis, although others have associated this with a higher incidence of venous thrombosis (23,24).

Portal venous drainage remains our preferred technique for reasons discussed below (Fig. 4). In this technique, the transverse colon is reflected cephalad, exposing the small bowel mesentery. The peritoneum at the root of the mesentery is then incised, the mesenteric lymphatics are divided between ligatures, and the superior mesenteric vein (SMV) is exposed. A sufficient length (3–4 cm) of the SMV is then circumferentially mobilized. This may require division of small draining branches. We typically administer intravenous heparin (50 U/kg) prior to clamping the vein. An end-to-side anastomosis between the portal vein and the SMV is then performed using #7-0 polypropylene suture. Once the venous anastomosis is complete, we occlude the donor portal vein with a bulldog clamp and restore the venous drainage of the bowel. At this point, a tunnel is made in the small bowel mesentery adjacent to the venous anastomosis, through which the arterial graft is passed to the retroperitoneum.

In addition to its potential physiological advantages, PV drainage may be technically easier to perform than SV drainage. Complete mobilization of the iliac vein can be time consuming and technically challenging, particularly in a deep pelvis. With PV drainage, a large tributary of the SMV can be isolated quickly and the anastomosis is generally performed in a well-exposed area of the operative field.

## Arterial Reconstruction

Arterial reconstruction of the pancreas allograft begins with the back-table preparation of the organ. A donor Y-iliac artery extension graft is used to join the superior mesenteric and splenic arteries supplying the pancreas (Fig. 4). In the setting of significant atherosclerosis involving the donor iliac arteries, alternate reconstruction using a donor brachiocephalic and carotid

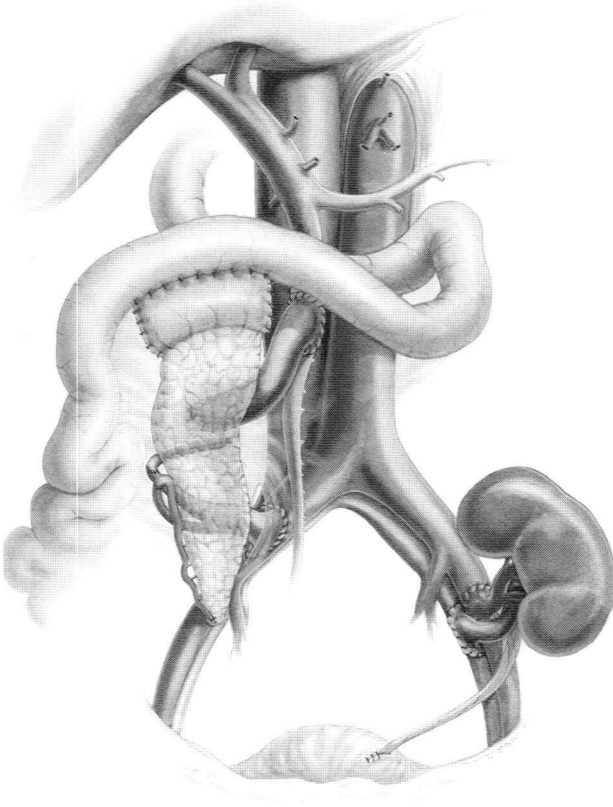

**Figure 4** Simultaneous pancreas–kidney transplantation with portal venous and enteric exocrine drainage.

arterial graft can be performed. Arterial reconstruction with the donor Y-graft is the preferred technique in whole organ pancreatic transplantation, as all other arterial reconstructive techniques are associated with an increased incidence of thrombosis (24).

Arterial revascularization of the pancreas allograft is preferentially performed to the right common iliac or external iliac artery. With SV drainage, use of the right iliac vessels is technically easier because of the more superficial course of the external iliac vein and its relative ease of mobilization as compared to the left iliac vein. When portal venous drainage is used, it is important to have a long Y-graft in order to reach the proximal right common iliac artery without tension. An extension graft may be placed during the back-table preparation of the allograft, if necessary.

## Duct Management

Bladder drainage remains the most common method of managing the exocrine secretions among pancreas transplant centers worldwide. BD is almost exclusively limited to systemically drained pancreas transplants. When performing BD, the donor duodenum should be kept to the minimum possible length, as this avoids metabolic complications related to fluid and bicarbonate loss. The pancreas is oriented with the head positioned caudally and the vascular anastomoses are completed. The bladder is mobilized by dividing the lateral attachments. A location on the dome of the bladder that provides for a tension-free anastomosis is selected. The duodenum is opened along its antimesenteric border and the duodenocystostomy is performed with a two-layer "hand-sewn" approach or, alternatively, with a stapling instrument as described by others (25).

Enteric drainage is increasingly being utilized as a method of managing the exocrine secretions. ED is associated with a significant reduction in urologic and metabolic complications, with no increase in septic complications (21,26). When performing ED, reconstructive options include direct side-to-side anastomosis to the recipient small bowel or anastomosis to a diverting Roux-en-Y limb. The anastomosis to the Roux limb may be performed in either a side-to-side fashion or an end-to-end fashion. Any type of enteric anastomosis can be performed by a "hand-sewn" or stapled technique. The majority of reporting centers perform the enteric anastomosis directly to the recipient bowel (58%) in a hand-sewn fashion (87%) (13). Although a diverting Roux limb has the theoretical advantage of isolating anastomotic complications from the remainder of the bowel, our experience suggests that major complications related to enteric anastomosis are uncommon and that creation of a Roux loop may be unnecessary (26).

## RESULTS: THE IMPACT OF PORTAL VENOUS DRAINAGE ON GRAFT SURVIVAL AND REJECTION

It has long been hypothesized that portal venous drainage of pancreas allografts should offer physiologic benefits. The prevention of hyperinsulinemia and improvement in lipoprotein profiles in patients receiving portal-drained pancreas allografts has been well documented (16,27). In addition, in our program, the improvements in physiologic profiles have been supplemented with lower rejection rates in portal-drained pancreas transplants, resulting in significantly higher graft survival rates following the routine implementation of this technique. We showed that pancreas allografts drained into the portal vein, regardless of whether a kidney was cotransplanted, had a significantly lower incidence of acute rejection compared to allografts that were drained systemically into the iliac vein (Philosophe B, Farney AC, Schweitzer EJ, et al. The superiority of portal venous drainage over systemic venous drainage in pancreas transplantation. Submitted).

With the introduction of mycophenolate mofetil and tacrolimus, allograft survival and rejection rates for both renal and pancreas transplants have significantly improved. In our institution, a multivariate analysis of variables affecting graft survival and rejection following pancreas transplantation since 1991 revealed that tacrolimus and mycophenolate mofetil were the only variables with a significant positive impact (Table 1). Human leukocyte antigen matching has had no effect on either survival or rejection (manuscript in preparation). With these factors in mind, it was important to assess the immunological impact of portal drainage during a period when the immunosuppressive protocol had not varied. Figure 5 depicts the Kaplan–Meier graft survival for portal and systemically drained pancreas transplants during this period. The higher graft survival was also seen for each type of pancreas transplant. Figure 6 depicts the one-year graft survival for SPK, SPLK, PAK, and PTA. In addition to improved patient and graft survival, a lower overall rejection rate with portal venous drainage compared to systemic venous drainage was noted (Fig. 7). This significant difference is evident in each type of pancreas transplant. The one-year cumulative rate of at least one rejection episode for each type of transplant is depicted in Figure 8.

It is clear that immunosuppression by itself could not account for the improved outcome following portal drainage of pancreas transplants. Our center has adopted the routine use of ultrasound-guided percutaneous pancreas biopsy under local anesthesia that has historically yielded tissue in greater than 88% of the cases following systemic drainage (28). However, in that review, the pancreas transplants were placed in the pelvis, where access to percutaneous biopsy was more successful than with portal-drained pancreas transplants. Suspected

**Table 1** Multivariate Analysis of Variables Affecting Graft Survival and Rejection in All Pancreas Transplants

| Variable | Graft survival | | Rejection free | |
|---|---|---|---|---|
| | *p*-Value | RR | *p*-Value | RR |
| Type | 0.62 | | 0.64 | |
| HLA mm | 0.16 | | 0.19 | |
| AB mm | 0.21 | | 0.68 | |
| DR mm | 0.68 | | 0.69 | |
| FK-506 | 0.009 | 0.25 | 0.02 | 0.51 |
| MMF | 0.06 | | 0.03 | 0.53 |

*Abbreviations*: RR, relative risk; HLA, human leukocyte antigen; MMF, mycophenolate mofetil.

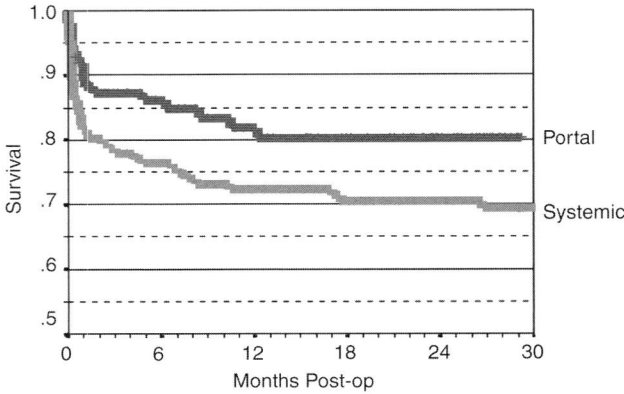

**Figure 5** Overall graft survival following pancreas transplantation. The overall graft survival for all categories of pancreas transplants is significantly higher in the portal venous group, $p = 0.05$. The 30-month graft survival is 70% for systemic venous and 80% for portal venous.

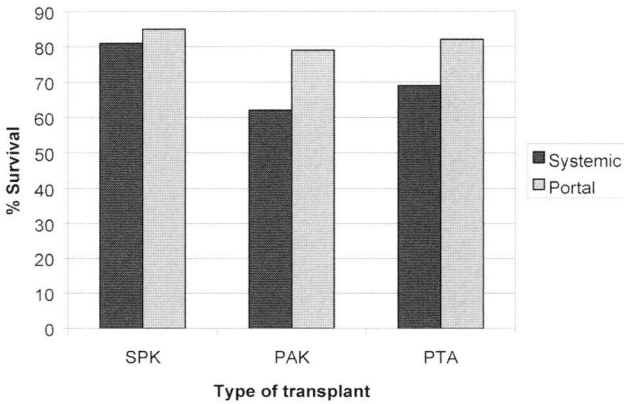

**Figure 6** One-year pancreas graft survival for SPK, PAK and PTA. *Abbreviations*: SPK, simultaneous pancreas–kidney; PAK, pancreas after kidney transplantation; PTA, pancreas transplantation alone.

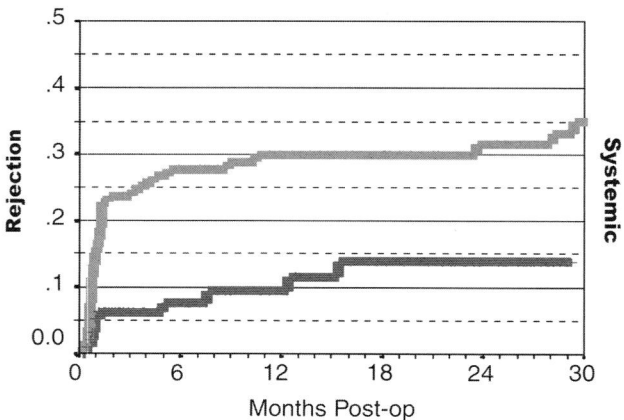

**Figure 7** Cumulative rate of at least one rejection episode following pancreas transplantation. The overall rejection rate for all categories of pancreas transplants is significantly lower in the portal venous group, $p = 0.001$. The 30-month rejection rate is 35% for systemic venous and 15% for portal venous.

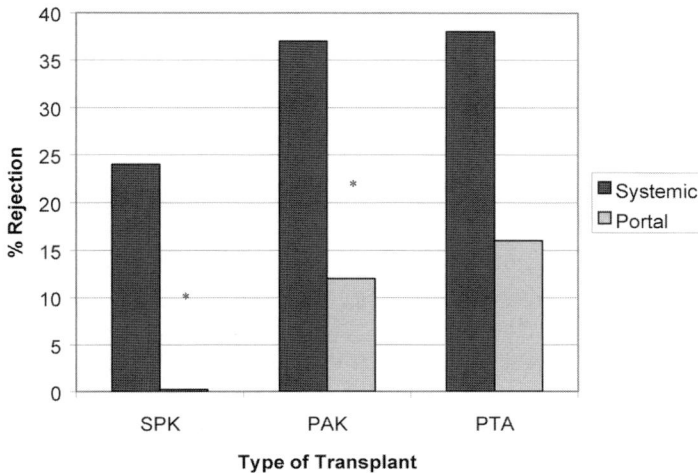

**Figure 8**   The one-year cumulative rate of at least one rejection episode for each type of pancreas transplants. $^{*}p < 0.05$. *Abbreviations*: SPK, simultaneous pancreas–kidney; PAK, pancreas after kidney transplantation; PTA, pancreas transplantation alone.

rejection events based on biochemical analysis that have not been successfully biopsied have been treated and counted as rejection episodes. Elevated serum amylase and lipase correlate with histologic rejection in greater than 85% of the cases, based on previous reports from our institution (20). Therefore, it can be estimated that 15% of the suspected rejections treated and therefore counted are not truly rejections, artificially increasing the rejection rate in the portal-drained group. This difference, however, is small and probably insignificant.

It has been shown experimentally that introduction of donor antigen into the portal vein can enhance allograft survival. In certain rodent strain models, cardiac (29,30) and renal (31) allografts have been prolonged by pre-immunization with donor antigen specifically injected in the portal vein. Drainage of allografts directly into the portal vein has also resulted in prolongation of heart (29,30,32), kidney (31,33), and small bowel allograft survival (34). The liver is rich in migratory passenger leukocytes, including dendritic cells, widely regarded as the primary antigenic component of transplanted organs. The important interaction of the apoptotic cells (experimentally induced by UVB irradiation) presented in the portal vein with the resident hepatic dendritic cells could therefore prove extremely important. The protective effect of the liver in combined kidney and liver transplantation has also been well established clinically (35,36). Although this can be related to the mechanisms proposed above or to the presence of passenger leukocytes, the causal relationship has not been established. In the analysis of our SPK transplants, kidney graft survival was improved and the incidence of rejection was reduced following portal drainage of the pancreas transplant. The introduction of peripancreatic nodal tissue in the portal vein could theoretically induce an immunomodulatory response in the host liver, which could have a protective effect on both organs from the same donor. This is an interesting, albeit unproven concept that is the basis of future investigation.

Although it is tempting to state that portal venous drainage offers lasting immunologic advantages, long-term follow-up is necessary to establish this conclusion. Chronic rejection is a poorly understood entity, which probably involves multiple complex immunologic mechanisms. The correlation between the number or severity of acute rejections and late graft loss has been well documented in other organ transplants. Acute rejection has predicted graft loss secondary to chronic rejection in kidney transplants (37). Based on these observations and results from the rodent models mentioned, we hypothesize that immunomodulation offered by portal venous drainage of the pancreas would also protect the allografts from chronic rejection.

## Postoperative Care of the Pancreas Transplant Patient

Postoperative care, including the immunosuppressive drug strategy, has evolved over the past few years. At the University of Maryland, all patients receive prophylactic intravenous antibiotics. Currently, piperacillin/tazobactam is administered preoperatively and for at least two days following the pancreas transplant. Modifications are made if the patients are penicillin allergic. All recipients, regardless of their (or the donors') cytomegalovirus serologic status, receive intravenous gancyclovir for cytomegalovirus prophylaxis until the patient is able to tolerate oral feeding, at which point oral gancyclovir is administered for 14 weeks following transplantation.

In the immediate postoperative setting, it is important to monitor the pancreas transplant patients closely in a surgical intensive care or step-down unit; this allows continual assessment of graft function, as well as cardiac and hemodynamic parameters. Unless otherwise indicated, the patients are usually transferred to a monitored nursing unit 24 to 48 hours later. Routine laboratory studies include complete blood count, and serum electrolytes, serum amylase, and lipase. Serum glucose levels are checked at hourly intervals during the first 24 hours, every two hours during the next 24 hours, and every six hours thereafter. Blood glucose levels under 200 mg/dL are considered acceptable. The need for insulin or serum glucose values over 200 mg/dL warrants immediate radiographic evaluation. Duplex ultrasonography allows for real-time assessment of the allograft, with particular emphasis on the vascular supply.

As described in detail above, we have been utilizing enteric drainage for all pancreas transplants and as such, nasogastric decompression is maintained until bowel function returns. Following SPK transplants, the urethral catheter is maintained for a minimum of five days.

Since 1998, we have implemented a protocol of low-dose anticoagulation in recipients of solitary pancreas transplants (PAK and PTA) and in pre-uremic SPK or SPLK recipients. Intravenous heparin is administered at a dose of 300 U/hr immediately following surgery and, over the next 24 hours, is increased to 500 U/hr. Heparin is maintained at this dose and the serum hematocrit, platelet count, prothrombin time, and partial thromboplastin time (PTT) are monitored serially. We do not attempt to attain a specific PTT and accordingly decrease the rate of heparin administration when dictated by an abnormal elevation in the PTT, a declining hematocrit, or clinical evidence of bleeding. Although such a practice has resulted in an increased number of re-explorations for postoperative bleeding, the thrombosis rate has been markedly reduced and is now less than 5%.

In addition to the routine post-transplant laboratory studies, close attention is also given to the levels of serum amylase, lipase, and glucose. As the exocrine pancreas is more susceptible to injury from infection or rejection, elevations in blood sugar are usually late findings. An abnormally elevated amylase, lipase, white blood cell count, or unexplained fever comprises indications for radiographic evaluation with computed tomography and possibly percutaneous pancreas biopsy. When present in patients with the above-mentioned indications, peripancreatic fluid collections should be drained, most often by open surgical intervention. If graft dysfunction cannot be explained by peripancreatic collections, percutaneous biopsy of the allograft should be performed.

## Diagnosis of Rejection

The diagnosis of rejection following pancreas transplantation is suggested by any of the following indicators: (i) hyperamylasemia, (ii) hyperlipasemia, (iii) unexplained hyperglycemia, or (iv) unexplained fever or allograft tenderness. If bladder drainage is utilized, hypoamylasuria, described as a 50% drop in the timed urinary amylase output, indicates possible rejection. In SPK or SPLK recipients, a 20% rise in serum creatinine or a failure of the serum creatinine to fall to an appropriate level has been potential signs of rejection that have prompted percutaneous biopsy. After the technique of ultrasound-guided percutaneous pancreas biopsy was established (20), it was used routinely in all cases of suspected pancreas rejection. The percutaneous pancreas biopsy is performed with an 18-gauge automated biopsy needle, utilizing color-flow duplex ultrasound to identify the tail of the pancreas in an area free of overlying bowel and clear of the splenic artery and vein. Occasionally, poor visualization due to overlying loops of bowel may necessitate further attempts with computed tomography or laparoscopy. In patients with chronic rejection, fibrotic changes resulting in a small, shrunken pancreas may require laparotomy to obtain an adequate tissue sample. Interpretation of pancreatic biopsies is based on the scheme listed in Table 2, which was developed by our pathologists (38) (see Chapter 15).

**Table 2** Histologic Classification System for Acute Pancreas Allograft Rejection

| Grade | Class | Histology |
|-------|-------|-----------|
| 0 | Normal | Normal pancreas histology |
| 1 | Borderline | Changes consisting of rare lymphocytic septal infiltrates while the acinar parenchyma is free of inflammation |
| 2 | Mild | Mixed inflammatory septal infiltrates with focal involvement of acinar parenchyma. Ductal inflammation and/or venulitis are often seen. |
| 3 | Moderate | Septal inflammation with multifocal involvement of acinar parenchyma associated with single cell injury, such as vacuolization, necrosis, or apoptosis. |
| 4 | Moderate with vascular rejection | Moderate rejection with areterial endothelitis or vasculitis |
| 5 | Severe | Extensive inflammatory infiltrates with confluent acinar necrosis. |

## Outpatient Follow-Up of the Pancreas Transplant Recipient

Outpatient management of the pancreas transplant recipient varies little from that of the kidney transplant patient. Routine clinical follow-up, serial laboratory studies, and immunosuppressive drug monitoring are the focal points of outpatient management.

## Immunosuppression

The pancreas is among the most immunogenic of the solid organ transplants perhaps because of a large associated lymphoid component. International Pancreas Transplant Registry data suggest that 75% of pancreas transplant centers utilize antilymphocyte induction therapy. Choices include monoclonal OKT3® (Ortho Pharmaceuticals) or a polyclonal antibody such as Thymoglobulin® (Sangstat Pharmaceuticals) or ATGAM® (Pharmacia & Upjohn). The value of the newer humanized or chimeric monoclonal antibodies to the interleukin-2 receptor in pancreas transplantation is not fully established, but many centers have elected to utilize them because of their low toxicity. At the University of Maryland, postoperative antilymphocyte antibody induction is utilized for nearly all pancreas transplants. ATGAM doses were adjusted daily to achieve less than 50 CD3+ lymphocytes per cubic millimeter, and OKT3 was adjusted to keep CD3+ cells less than 5% of the total lymphocyte count. Currently, Thymoglobulin is used preferentially, given its efficacy and apparently fewer cytokine release symptoms. Like ATGAM, it is adjusted daily to achieve less than 50 CD3+ lymphocytes per cubic millimeter.

Mycophenolate mofetil (Cellcept®, Hoffman-La Roche Pharmaceuticals) is a reversible inhibitor of inosine monophosphate dehydrogenase, an enzyme critical for purine synthesis during lymphocyte activation. This drug has proven to be superior to azathioprine, and has replaced it in virtually all of solid organ transplantation. Mycophenolate mofetil is combined with one of the calcineurin inhibitors, either tacrolimus or cyclosporine. While there is no clear advantage of one calcineurin inhibitor over another for SPK transplants, the results for solitary pancreas transplants with cyclosporine have been poor. After April 1994, with the general availability of tacrolimus, our group began a prospective trial of solitary pancreas transplants using tacrolimus-based immunosuppression (20). Based on these encouraging results, tacrolimus-based therapy became our standard in 1995, except in those few circumstances in which Neoral® was used because of tacrolimus intolerance (less than 5%) after transplantation.

The role of the newer cell cycle inhibitor sirolimus has not been established in pancreas transplantation, but its success in islet and kidney transplantation suggests that it will have a significant role in pancreas transplant recipients, at least as a replacement for those patients experiencing unacceptable toxicity with the standard agents.

Our induction therapy for low-risk SPK and SPLK now consists of the chimeric anti-interleukin-2 receptor antibody basiliximab (Simulect®, Novartis Pharmaceuticals), tacrolimus, mycophenolate mofetil, and steroids. Our current maintenance immunosuppression is equivalent for all types of pancreas transplants, and generally includes tacrolimus, mycophenolate mofetil, and a tapering regimen of steroids.

## SUMMARY

Pancreatic transplantation has become an extremely successful procedure. The evolution of portal venous and enteric exocrine drainage, better immunosuppression, and better patient care have all contributed to the dramatically improved results. Moreover, improved monitoring of rejection has allowed a similar success of pancreatic transplantation alone in non-uremic patients with brittle diabetes. The treatment of diabetes mellitus has room for improvement; however, and there is no question that islet and xenotransplantation, and the pursuit of immunologic tolerance, will play extremely important roles in that endeavor.

## REFERENCES

1. Kelly WD, Lillehei RC, Merkel FK, Idezuki Y, Goetz FC. Allotransplantation of the pancreas and duodenum along with the kidney in diabetic nephropathy. Surgery 1967; 61:827.
2. Sutherland DER, Kendall D, Goetz FC, Najarian JS. Pancreas transplantation in humans. In: Flye MW, ed. Principles of Organ Transplantation, 1989. Philadelphia: W.B. Saunders Co, 1989:364.
3. Sollinger HW, Cook K, Kamps D, Glass NR, Belzer FO. Clinical and experimental experience with pancreaticocystostomy for exocrine pancreatic drainage in pancreas transplantation. Transplant Proc 1984; 16:749–751.
4. Ngheim DD, Corry RJ. Transplantation with urinary drainage of pancreatic secretions. Am J Surg 1987; 153:405.
5. American Diabetes Association Position statement. Pancreas transplantation for patients with diabetes mellitus. Diabet Care 1993; 16:21.
6. 1998 Annual Report of the U.S. Scientific Registry of Transplant Recipients and the Organ Procurement and Transplantation Network-Transplant Data: 1988–1998. UNOS, Richmond, VA, and the Division of Transplantation, Bureau of Health Resources and Services Administration, U.S. Department of Health and Human Services, Rockville, MD, 1996.
7. 1999 Annual Report of the U.S. Scientific Registry of Transplant Recipients and the Organ Procurement and Transplantation Network-Transplant Data: 1989–1998. UNOS, Richmond, VA, and the Division of Transplantation, bureau of Health Resources and Services Administration, U.S. Department of Health and Human Services, Rockville, MD.
8. Kavoussi LR, Kerbl K, Capelouto CC, McDougal EM, Clayman RV. Laparoscopic nephrectomy for renal neoplasms. Urology 1993; 42:603.
9. Flower JL, Jacobs S, Cho E, et al. Comparison of open and laparoscopic live donor nephrectomy. Ann Surg 1997; 226:483.
10. Farney AC, Cho E, Schweitzer EJ, et al. Simultaneous cadaver pancreas living donor kidney transplantation (SPLK): a new approach for the type 1 diabetic uremic patient. Ann Surg. In press.
11. Fioretto P, Steffes MW, Sutherland DE, Goetz FC, Mauer M. Reversal of lesions of diabetic nephropathy after pancreas transplantation. N Engl J Med 1998; 339:69–75.
12. Schweitzer E, Anderson L, Kuo P, Johnson LB, et al. Safe pancreas transplantation in patients with coronary artery disease. Transplantation 1997; 63(9):1294–1299.
13. Di Carlo V, Castoldi R, Cristallo M, et al. Techniques of pancreas transplantation through the world: an IPITA Center survey. Transplant Proc 1998; 30:231–241.
14. Luck R, Klempnauer J, Ehlerding G, Kuhn K. Significance of portal venous drainage after whole-organ pancreas transplantation for endocrine graft function and prevention of diabetic nephropathy. Transplantation 1990; 50:394–398.
15. Bagdade JD, Ritter MC, Kitabchi AE, et al. Differing effects of pancreas–kidney transplantation with systemic versus portal venous drainage on cholesteryl ester transfer in IDDM subjects. Diabet Care 1996; 19:1108–1112.
16. Hughes TA, Gaber AO, Amiri HS, et al. Kidney–pancreas transplantation. The effect of portal versus systemic venous drainage of the pancreas on the lipoprotein composition. Transplantation 1995; 60:1406–1412.
17. Calne RY. Paratopic segmental pancreas grafting: a technique with portal venous drainage. Lancet 1984; 1:595–597.
18. Rosenlof LK, Earnhardt RC, Pruett TL, et al. Pancreas transplantation. An initial experience with systemic and portal drainage of pancreatic allografts. Ann Surg 1992; 215:586–595.
19. Shokouh-Amiri MH, Gaber AO, Gaber LW, et al. Pancreas transplantation with portal venous drainage and enteric exocrine diversion: a new technique. Transplant Proc 1992; 24:776–777.
20. Bartlett ST, Schweitzer EJ, Johnson L, et al. Equivalent success of simultaneous pancreas kidney and solitary pancreas transplantation: a prospective trial of tacrolimus immunosuppression with percutaneous biopsy. Ann Surg 1996; 224:440–452.
21. Stratta RJ, Gaber AO, Shokouh-Amiri MH, et al. A prospective comparison of systemic-bladder versus portal-enteric drainage in vascularized pancreas transplantation. Surgery 2000; 127:217–226.
22. Gill IS, Sindhi R, Jerius JT, Sudan D, Stratta RJ. Bench reconstruction of pancreas for transplantation: experience with 192 cases. Clin Transplant 1997; 11:104–109.

23. Sollinger HW. Pancreatic transplantation and vascular graft thrombosis [editorial; comment]. J Am Coll Surg 1996; 182:362–363.
24. Troppmann C, Gruessner AC, Benedetti E, et al. Vascular graft thrombosis after pancreatic transplantation: univariate and multivariate operative and nonoperative risk factor analysis. J Am Coll Surg 1996; 182:285–316.
25. Pescovitz MD, Dunn DL, Sutherland DE. Use of the circular stapler in construction of the duodeno-neocystostomy for drainage into the bladder in transplants involving the whole pancreas. Surg Gynecol Obstet 1989; 169:169–171.
26. Kuo PC, Johnson LB, Schweitzer EJ, Bartlett ST. Simultaneous pancreas/kidney transplantation—a comparison of enteric and bladder drainage of exocrine pancreatic secretions. Transplantation 1997; 63:238–243.
27. Gaber AO, Shokouh-Amiri H, Hathaway DK, et al. Results of pancreas transplantation with portal venous and enteric drainage. Ann Surg 1995; 221(6):613.
28. Klassen DK, Hoehn-Saric EW, Weir MR, et al. Isolated pancreas rejection in combined kidney pancreas transplantation. Transplantation 1996; 61:974–977.
29. Rao VK, Burris DE, Gruel SM, Sollinger HW, Burlingham WJ. Evidence that donor spleen cells administered through the portal vein prolong the survival of cardiac allografts in rats. Transplantation 1988; 45:1145.
30. Lowry RP, Kenick S, Lisbona R. Speculation on the pathogenesis of prolonged cardiac allograft survival following portal venous inoculation of allogeneic cells. Transplant Proc 1987; 19:3451.
31. Yoshimura N, Matsui S, Hamashima T, Lee CJ, Ohsaka Y, Oka T. The effects of perioperative portal venous inoculation with donor lymphocytes on renal allograft survival in the rat. I. Specific prolongation of donor grafts and suppressor factor in the serum. Transplantation 1990; 49:167.
32. Holman JM, Todd R. Enhanced survival of heterotopic rat heart allografts with portal venous drainage. Transplantation 1990; 48:229.
33. Sakai A. Role of the liver in kidney allograft rejection in the rat. Transplantation 1970; 9:333.
34. Gorezynski RM, Chan Z, Chung S, et al. Prolongation of rat small bowel or renal allograft survival by pretransplant transfusion and/or by varying the route of allograft venous drainage. Transplantation 1994; 58:816.
35. Gonwa TA, Nery JR, Husberg BS, Klintmalm GB. Simultaneous liver and renal transplantation in man. Transplantation 1988; 46:690–693.
36. Flye MW, Duffy BF, Phelan DL, Ratner LE, Mohanakumar T. Protective effects of liver transplantation on a simultaneously transplanted kidney in a highly sensitised patient. Transplantation 1990; 50:1051–1054.
37. Matas A. Chronic rejection in renal transplant recipients–risk factors and correlates. Clinical Transplantation 1994; 8:332–335.
38. Drachenberg CB, Papadimetriou JC, Klassen DK, Bartlett ST. Histologic grading of pancreas acute allograft rejection in percutaneous needle biopsies. Transplant Proc 1996; 28:512–513.
39. Nakhleh R, Sutherland DER. Pancreas rejection: significance of histopathologic findings with implications for classification of rejection. Am J Surg Pathol 1992; 16:1098–1107.

# 31 | The Northwestern University Experience in Pancreas Transplantation

**Dixon B. Kaufman**

*Division of Transplantation, Department of Surgery, Feinberg School of Medicine, Northwestern University, Chicago, Illinois, U.S.A.*

The Pancreas Transplantation Program at Northwestern University began in 1993; through June 2006, 429 pancreas transplants have been performed. This included 355 (83%) simultaneous pancreas kidney (SPK) transplants, 31 (7%) pancreas after kidney transplants, and 43 (10%) pancreas transplants alone. We have tried to document our experiences along the way to share insights into what we have learned from the standpoint of surgical techniques, immunosuppression, and infectious disease (1–8).

To do that we have taken a somewhat systematic approach in our SPK transplant program to evaluate key elements of the transplant process by performing a series of nonrandomized, retrospective, sequential studies. When we started, there was controversy about the best site for pancreatic exocrine drainage, the best method of venous drainage, and how to optimally combine the new immunosuppressive agents that were coming on-line.

Prior to 1996, we were consistent in our use of pancreatic exocrine bladder drainage and systemic venous drainage, and the maintenance immunosuppression included various combinations of cyclosporine, azathioprine, prednisone, tacrolimus, and mycophenolate mofetil (MMF). The steps that have led to our current approach to SPK transplantation are as follows:

1. In January 1996, we changed to a consistent protocol of tacrolimus/MMF/prednisone (1).
2. In January 1998, we stopped using the bladder drainage technique and were consistent in our use of primary enteric drainage (without a Roux-en-Y) of the exocrine pancreas, and the patients continued with the tacrolimus/MMF/prednisone maintenance immunosuppression (2).
3. In January 2000, we tested a rapid corticosteroid withdrawal protocol with tacrolimus-based maintenance in combination with antilymphocyte globulin induction (3,4).
4. In November 2001, with enteric drainage and prednisone-free maintenance as our standard of care, we tested alemtuzumab induction in place of antilymphocyte globulin (5).
5. In July 2003, with enteric drainage, alemtuzumab induction, and prednisone-free maintenance as our standard of care, we tested a de novo calcineurin inhibitor-free maintenance protocol consisting of tacrolimus and MMF. Preliminary results have been presented (6) but will not be discussed in this overview.

Along the way we described the benefits of SPK transplantation on hypertension (7), and defined the risks of cytomegalovirus (CMV) infection with the new immunosuppressive combinations (8), including the benefits of avoiding chronic corticosteroids in that context (9). Elaboration of the Northwestern experience in pancreas transplantation follows.

## ADVANCES IN IMMUNOSUPPRESSION

A liberal approach has been taken at our institution in accepting patients for SPK transplantation. This has included a broad recipient (R) age range, 15 to 59 years, with 10% over 45 years of age, and a willingness to transplant patients with coronary revascualization (nearly 25% of the SPK recipients).

A number of additions to the immunopharmacologic armamentarium took place since the initiation of the pancreas transplant program in 1993. We were among the first groups to report on the improvement in SPK transplantation outcome with the combination of tacrolimus and MMF (1). Figure 1 shows the results of our early series of SPK transplants

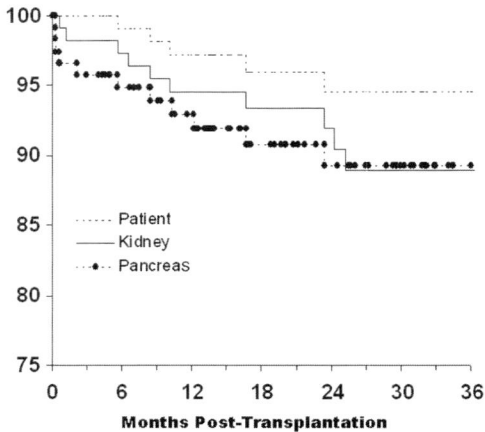

**Figure 1** Actuarial three-year patient and graft survival rates in simultaneous pancreas–kidney transplant recipients given tacrolimus/mycophenolate mofetil maintenance immunosuppression. The one-year patient, kidney, and pancreas survival rates are 97%, 95%, and 93%, respectively.

receiving MMF/tacrolimus/prednisone immunosuppression ($n = 118$) performed through 12/30/1999. The mean follow-up was 28 months; actuarial survival estimates were calculated by Kaplan–Meier life table analysis. Kidney graft failure was defined as removal, return to dialysis, or death with function. Pancreas graft failure was defined as removal, return to exogenous insulin therapy, or death with function. The actuarial one-year patient, kidney, and pancreas survival rates were 97%, 95%, and 93%, respectively. By comparison, the benchmark actuarial one-year patient, kidney, and pancreas survival rates reported by the International Pancreas Transplant Registry for all U.S. cases of SPK transplantation from 1/1998 to 5/2000 were 95%, 92%, and 83%, respectively (10).

In addition to the benefits seen with the use of tacrolimus and MMF as maintenance agents, we were impressed by the efficacy of antibody induction. The overall six-month actuarial rate of rejection using tacrolimus/MMF/prednisone was reduced from 24% to as low as 7%, depending on whether antibody induction was employed. This was a dramatic reduction in rejection and this transformed SPK transplantation into a routinely safe and effective procedure akin to kidney transplantation alone. Figure 2 shows the specific rates of acute rejection in SPK transplant recipients receiving no induction, induction with rabbit antithymocyte globulin (Thymoglobulin[R]), or induction with an interleukin (IL)-2 receptor antagonist (daclizumab, Zenapax[R]). In later reports, the use of alemtuzumab was shown to be as effective in reducing the rejection rate as rabbit antithymocyte globulin.

In 2000, ours was the first U.S. pancreas transplant program to use a rapid corticosteroid withdrawal protocol in SPK transplant recipients. This approach was an extension of our experience with rapid steroid withdrawal, which was successful in our kidney-alone transplant population (11). The main difference was the decision to use rabbit antithymocyte globulin instead of an IL-2 receptor antagonist because of our observation of the relatively high risk of early acute rejection with the latter induction agent.

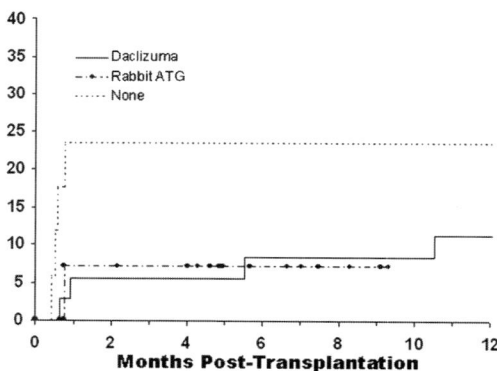

**Figure 2** Rates of acute rejection following simultaneous pancreas–kidney transplantation according to induction therapy.

Forty consecutive SPK transplant recipients were enrolled in a prospective study in which antithymocyte globulin induction and six days of corticosteroids were administered along with tacrolimus and MMF ($n = 20$) or tacrolimus and sirolimus ($n = 20$). Mean $\pm$ S.D. follow-up for recipients receiving tacrolimus/MMF and tacrolimus/sirolimus were $10.7 \pm 3.9$ and $11.4 \pm 2.9$ months, respectively. Patient and graft survival, and rejection rates were compared to an historical control group ($n = 86$; mean follow-up $39.5 \pm 15.4$ months) of SPK recipients that received induction and tacrolimus, MMF, and corticosteroids (3).

In the prednisone-free group, maintenance immunosuppression consisted of tacrolimus (target 12 hour trough concentrations 12–14 ng/mL), and either MMF (target dose of 3 g/day) or sirolimus (4 mg/day, with target 24 hour trough concentrations 5–10 ng/mL). Corticosteroids as six doses of parenteral methylprednisolone (500, 250, 125, 60, 40, and 20 mg) were given on consecutive days beginning at the time of transplantation and then eliminated.

We compared the early outcomes of SPK transplantation in the rapid steroid withdrawal group to a control group ($n = 86$) of SPK transplant recipients who received tacrolimus/MMF/prednisone maintenance immunosuppression and antibody induction with either an equine antithymocyte globulin ($n = 50$) or an IL-2 receptor antagonist ($n = 37$).

The results of the rapid corticosteroid withdrawal protocol were successful, based on the patient and graft survival rates and the low rates of rejection. At the time of the initial publication, the actuarial six-month patient, kidney, and pancreas graft survivals in the rapid steroid withdrawal group was 100%. Rejection occurred in only one patient for an actuarial six-month rejection rate of 3%. All patients in the rapid corticosteroid withdrawal group remain off prednisone. These early results of rapid corticosteroid withdrawal in SPK transplant recipients using induction therapy and either tacrolimus/MMF or tacrolimus/sirolimus were very encouraging. These outcomes compared favorably to a recent report of corticosteroid avoidance in 28 SPK transplants from Institut de Transplantation, Nantes University Hospital, France (12).

Longer-term follow-up with a greater number of patients has recently been reported, which has more clearly defined the role of rapid corticosteroid withdrawal and the optimal induction and maintenance agents (5). We compared the effects of using two T-cell depleting antibodies, alemtuzumab and rabbit antithymocyte globulin, as induction immunosuppression for SPK transplant recipients given a prednisone-free maintenance regimen. We used a single-center, nonrandomized, retrospective, sequential study design to evaluate the efficacy and safety of alemtuzumab ($n = 50$) or antithymocyte globulin ($n = 38$) induction in combination with a prednisone-free, tacrolimus/sirolimus-based immunosuppression protocol. The alemtuzumab treatment group received transplants during the period from November 2001 through June 2003. The minimum follow-up was 26 months posttransplant, with a mean of $29.5 \pm 7.6$ S.D. months (range 22–41 months). The antithymocyte globulin–treated cases included patients who received their transplants during the period from February 2000 through October 2001. The mean $\pm$ S.D. follow-up for recipients receiving antithymocyte globulin was $56.2 \pm 6.2$ months (range 47–67 months).

Kaplan–Meier analyses of long-term patient and graft survivals and rejection rates were determined according to induction agent. Secondary endpoints included the incidence of infectious and malignant complications, and cost considerations.

Overall long-term patient and graft survival rates did not significantly differ between patients treated with alemtuzumab and antithymocyte globulin. The three-year actuarial patient survival rates for recipients who received alemtuzumab and antithymocyte globulin were 91.2% and 92.1%, respectively [$p = $ ns (not significant)]. The three-year actuarial death-censored kidney graft survival rates for recipients who received alemtuzumab and antithymocyte globulin were 90.9% and 86.2%, respectively. The three-year actuarial death-censored pancreas graft survival rates for recipients who received alemtuzumab and antithymocyte globulin were 92% and 97.2%, respectively.

Rejection rates were also nearly equivalent at one and two years. The 12-month actual rejection rates for recipients who received alemtuzumab and antithymocyte globulin were 6.1% and 2.6%, respectively ($p = $ ns). The 24-month actual rejection rates for recipients who received alemtuzumab and antithymocyte globulin were 8.2% and 5.3%, respectively ($p = $ ns).

The etiologies of various infectious diseases were very similar in both induction treatment groups, but the incidence of viral diseases was statistically significantly lower in the alemtuzumab group. For example, the three-year incidence of CMV in high-risk recipients—those who were not previously exposed to CMV but received organs from donors (Ds) with positive CMV serology—in the alemtuzumab and antithymocyte globulin groups were 6.5% and 28.0%, respectively. One recipient in the antithymocyte globulin treatment group acquired posttransplant lymphoproliferative disorder at 13.5 months post transplant and was successfully treated with maintenance of graft function with a reduction in immunosuppression and chemotherapy. No recipients in the alemtuzumab group acquired posttransplant lymphoproliferative disorder. The cost of alemtuzumab induction was lower than antithymocyte globulin.

We concluded that alemtuzumab induction followed by steroid-free maintenance therapy with a tacrolimus/sirolimus-based immunosuppression regimen provided an effective, safe, and cost-conscious approach to SPK transplantation. The alemtuzumab induction protocol combined with prednisone-free immunosuppression continues as our standard immunosuppression regimen. We have used this in nearly 150 SPK transplant recipients, and have extended it to over 30 pancreas transplants alone recipients. Our current interest is to determine whether the alemtuzumab induction protocol combined with prednisone-free immunosuppression will be successful in supporting a de novo calcineurin inhibitor–free protocol.

## Surgical Technique of Pancreas Exocrine Drainage

Avoiding technical complications of pancreas transplantation is related primarily to effective control of pancreatic exocrine drainage. In the past, enteric drainage was associated with high rates of infectious and technical complications. We analyzed the role of bladder ($n = 50$) versus enteric ($n = 50$) exocrine drainage in a nonrandomized, retrospective, sequential study of SPK transplant recipients receiving tacrolimus/MMF/prednisone maintenance immunotherapy (2). Actuarial patient and graft survival and rejection rates at one year were evaluated. We also examined end points pertaining to infectious complications and re-hospitalizations.

Table 1 shows the actuarial one-year patient, kidney, and pancreas survival rates in the bladder and enteric drainage groups. The one-year actuarial patient, kidney, and pancreas survival rates in the bladder drainage group were 98%, 94%, and 94%, respectively. The one-year actuarial patient, kidney, and pancreas survival rates in the enteric drainage group were 97%, 97%, and 89%, respectively. Renal allograft function, as assessed by serum creatinine values, was found to be equivalent in the two groups.

There were more bacterial infections in patients who underwent bladder drainage. Urinary tract infections were seen in 48% of the bladder-drained recipients during the first six months after transplantation. In the enteric drainage group, the incidence of urinary tract infections was 37%. There were no localized or systemic fungal infections.

The length of inpatient hospitalization for transplantation was nearly identical in recipients with bladder ($8.0 \pm 3.0$ days) or enteric ($8.4 \pm 3.3$ days) drainage. However, there were significantly fewer readmissions in enterically drained recipients. The average number of readmissions per SPK transplant recipient with bladder drainage was 1.8, versus 0.9 in recipients with enteric drainage. The proportion of patients requiring re-hospitalization within the first six months after transplantation also favored the enteric drainage group. Seventy-two percent of SPK transplant recipients with bladder drainage required $\geq 2$ re-hospitalizations, compared with 21% of recipients with enteric drainage. The increased readmissions for recipients with bladder drainage were related to more frequent episodes of hematuria and dehydration. Within the enteric drainage group, those not receiving induction therapy had a higher rate of early readmission because of more frequent episodes of early rejection.

What we learned was that use of the newer immunosuppressive agents had decreased the risk of rejection, and that enteric drainage was no longer associated with a high

**Table 1** One-Year Actuarial Patient and Graft Survival Rates in Simultaneous Pancreas–Kidney Transplantation Stratified by to Pancreas Exocrine Drainage and Antibody Induction

| Group (*n*) | Patient (%) | Kidney (%) | Pancreas (%) |
|---|---|---|---|
| All (100) | 98 | 96 | 92 |
| Bladder (50) | 98 | 94 | 94 |
| Enteric (50) | 97 | 97 | 89 |
|   Induction (33) | 93 | 93 | 84 |
|   Non-induction (17) | 100 | 100 | 94 |

complication rate. We have consistently used enteric drainage in SPK transplantation since 1998 and have extended it to include all solitary pancreas transplant recipients a few years later.

## CMV DISEASE IN SIMULTANEOUS PANCREAS–KIDNEY TRANSPLANTATION

CMV is the single most important viral pathogen in solid organ transplantation. The direct and indirect effects of CMV disease have had major deleterious effects on transplant outcomes despite the introduction of more effective prophylactic antiviral agents. Little is known about the rates of CMV in SPK recipients. Several important differences set the population of diabetic, uremic SPK recipients' transplants apart from kidney-alone transplant recipients, even though both groups receive renal allografts. Recipients of SPK transplants are more likely to receive induction therapy and tend to require more intensive maintenance immunosuppression to offset a relatively higher risk of acute rejection. In addition, a recipient of a pancreas allograft is apt to be younger and may have a higher likelihood of being CMV seronegative compared to a recipient of kidney-alone transplant.

We have published two studies pertaining to the risk factors for the development of CMV disease in a group of SPK transplant recipients. In the first study, we described the risks of CMV in 100 consecutive SPK transplant recipients who received a consistent protocol of maintenance immunosuppression with tacrolimus/MMF/prednisone (8). In the second study, we compared the CMV risk in SPK transplant recipients who were on the prednisone-free maintenance protocol with either antilymphocyte globulin induction or alemtuzumab induction (9).

In the first study, we observed that at two years posttransplant, the overall rate of CMV disease was 18.1% (13.1% noninvasive, 5.0% tissue invasive, respectively). Eighteen recipients developed CMV $7.5 \pm 2.4$ months posttransplant (range 3.4–12.2 months). Tissue-invasive CMV occurred in five patients and noninvasive CMV in 13 patients. The rates of CMV were stratified according to donor and recipient CMV serologic status and are illustrated in Figure 3A. The overall two-year incidence of CMV disease in the four groups were as follows: no cases of CMV occurred in the D−/R+ combination; one case (4.8 months posttransplant) occurred in the D−/R− combination (3%); four cases ($6.5 \pm 2.2$ months posttransplant) in the D+/R+ combination (27%); and 14 cases ($8.1 \pm 2.4$ months posttransplant) in the D+/R− combination (44%).

The two-year actuarial rate of CMV in the high-risk recipients (CMV D+/R−) was 40.6% (31.1% noninvasive and 9.5% tissue invasive). In the CMV D+/R+ group, two-year actuarial rate of CMV was 25.6% (13.3% noninvasive and 12.3% tissue-invasive CMV). These rates of CMV disease are no different in frequency or severity from those reported in kidney transplant recipients receiving similar immunosuppression.

Several variables were analyzed to determine their relative predictive value of CMV (tissue invasive and noninvasive) disease: recipient age, gender, diabetes duration, dialysis duration, induction therapy, induction with ATGAM, acute rejection, coronary artery revascularization, donor CMV serologic status, and recipient CMV serologic status. Table 2 shows that there was one significant predictive variable for the development of CMV disease, donor CMV seropositivity. Multivariate analysis confirmed the same variable as a significant risk factor for the development of CMV disease.

In the second study, we examined the impact of a prednisone-free immunosuppressive regimen in SPK recipients on the development of CMV disease and infection. In this retrospective study, 200 consecutive SPK transplant recipients received tacrolimus-based immunosuppression with ($n = 100$) or without ($n = 100$) chronic prednisone therapy. Patients were induced with lymphocyte depleting antibodies or IL-2 receptor blockers and received prophylactic antiviral therapy. CMV antiviral prophylaxis was administered to all recipients posttransplant and after treatment of a rejection episode. Between 7/1995 and 7/2002, recipients received therapeutic doses of intravenous ganciclovir during the inpatient stay. Ganciclovir or valganciclovir was prescribed to all recipients for at least three months posttransplant. In the group of patients treated with prednisone, recipients in the high-risk subgroup (D+/R−) also received CMV hyperimmune globulin over 16 weeks. From 7/2002 to 4/2003 patients were treated exclusively with three months of oral valganciclovir (450 mg/day).

Patient and graft survivals and rejection rates were not statistically significantly different between treatment groups. Figure 3 shows the incidences of CMV according to donor and recipient CMV serologic status stratified by use of prednisone therapy. Avoidance of

**(A)**

**(B)**

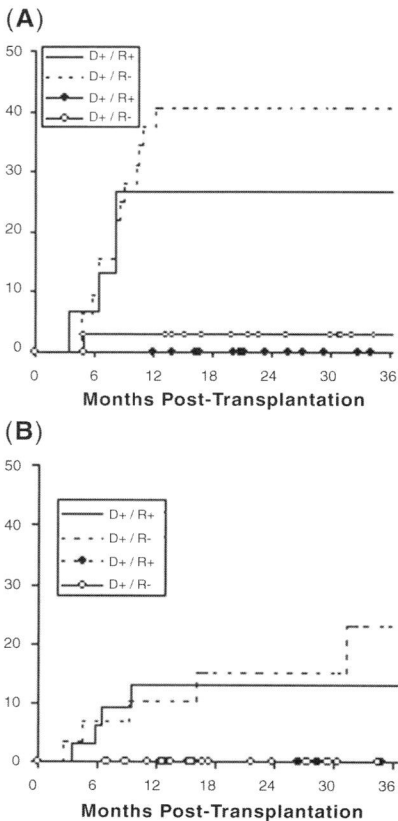

**Figure 3** Incidence of cytomegalovirus disease in simultaneous pancreas–kidney transplant recipients that received prednisone (Pred+) ($n = 100$) (**A**), or in the absence of prednisone (Pred−) ($n = 100$) (**B**), according to donor (D) and recipient (R) cytomegalovirus serologic status.

prednisone treatment was associated with a trend toward a reduction in the overall rate of CMV (8.6% vs. 17%, $p = 0.15$). The rate of noninvasive CMV disease was statistically significantly ($p = 0.05$) reduced in the prednisone-free group (3.1%) versus the prednisone group (12%). Figure 4A illustrates that among the highest-risk patients, those with CMV-positive donors (D+/R− and D+/R+), the overall (noninvasive and tissue invasive) rate of CMV was statistically significantly ($p = 0.05$) reduced in the prednisone-free group (18%, $n = 61$) versus the prednisone-treated group (36%, $n = 48$). The rate of noninvasive CMV disease was statistically significantly ($p = 0.02$) reduced in the prednisone-free group (8.8%) versus the prednisone-treated group (25.6%) (Fig. 4B).

In the multivariate Cox proportional hazard analysis of all 200 SPK recipients, only three factors were found to be associated with an increase in the development of CMV: positive CMV serologic status of the donor [relative risk (RR) 27.927, $p = 0.001$], diabetes duration [RR 1.045 (per year), $p = 0.04$], and prednisone therapy (RR 2.318, $p = 0.04$). Interestingly, in recipients who received the prednisone-free protocol, the incidence of CMV appeared to be less frequent in recipients who received induction with alemtuzuamb versus rabbit antilymphocyte globulin (2.4% vs. 12.6%, $p = 0.14$) (5,9).

We learned that eliminating prednisone immunotherapy did not adversely affect outcomes and was associated with a statistically significantly reduced rate of CMV in SPK recipients of organs from seropositive donors.

## SUMMARY

We believe that the Northwestern pancreas transplant program has made some useful contributions to the field in the following areas: the development of safe and effective immunosuppression, including a new protocol of rapid withdrawal of corticosteroids; analysis of the effects of surgical technique of pancreas exocrine drainage on outcome; and a multi-

**Table 2** Univariate and Multivariate Analyses of Predictors of Cytomegalovirus Disease in Simultaneous Pancreas–Kidney Transplant Recipients

| | | Relative risk | | | |
|---|---|---|---|---|---|
| Predictor | Coefficient | Mean | (95% CI) | t Stat | p-Value |
| Univariate analysis | | | | | |
| Donor positive | 3.131 | 22.89 | (3.05–172.03) | 3.04 | 0.0023 |
| Diabetes duration | 0.051 | 1.05 | (1.00–1.11) | 1.86 | 0.0629 |
| Age | 0.032 | 1.03 | (0.97–1.10) | 1.09 | 0.2752 |
| Recipient positive | −0.513 | 0.60 | (0.20–1.82) | 0.91 | 0.3646 |
| Revascularization | 0.509 | 1.66 | (0.59–4.67) | 0.97 | 0.3337 |
| Male | 0.558 | 1.75 | (0.62–4.90) | 1.06 | 0.2894 |
| Rejection | −0.870 | 0.42 | (0.10–1.82) | 1.16 | 0.2459 |
| Induction ATGAM | −0.173 | 0.84 | (0.33–2.13) | 0.37 | 0.7148 |
| Induction | 0.526 | 1.69 | (0.39–1.35) | 0.70 | 0.4827 |
| Dialysis duration | −0.007 | 0.99 | (0.96–1.03) | 0.32 | 0.7526 |
| Multivariate analysis | | | | | |
| Donor positive | 3.106 | 22.34 | (2.97–168.11) | 3.02 | 0.0026 |

variate analysis of the predictors of CMV disease in SPK transplant recipients. We have found that antibody induction (antilymphocyte globulin or alemtuzumab), with tacrolimus-based immunosuppression (combined with either MMF or sirolimus), allows for rapid elimination of corticosteroids, resulting in excellent patient and graft survival rates with low rates of rejection. In the setting of modern immunosuppression, we have demonstrated that both bladder and enteric drainage are associated with good patient and graft survival rates, with low rates of rejection and comparable rates of infection. The largest difference was a lower rate of complications leading to hospital readmissions in recipients with enteric drainage. Thus, enteric drainage has become our standard. We also observed that CMV disease occurred at rates no different in frequency and severity from those reported in kidney transplant recipients receiving similar protocols of the contemporary immunosuppressive agents. A multivariate analysis showed that the only significant predictive variable for the development of CMV disease occurred in transplantation of organs from a CMV seropositive donor. Even in the high-risk group (D+/R−), no relationship was established that CMV disease could trigger rejection or that the treatment of rejection was associated with CMV disease. Importantly, we learned that the use of prednisone-free protocols in conjunction with appropriate antiviral therapy would reduce the burden of CMV in this transplant population.

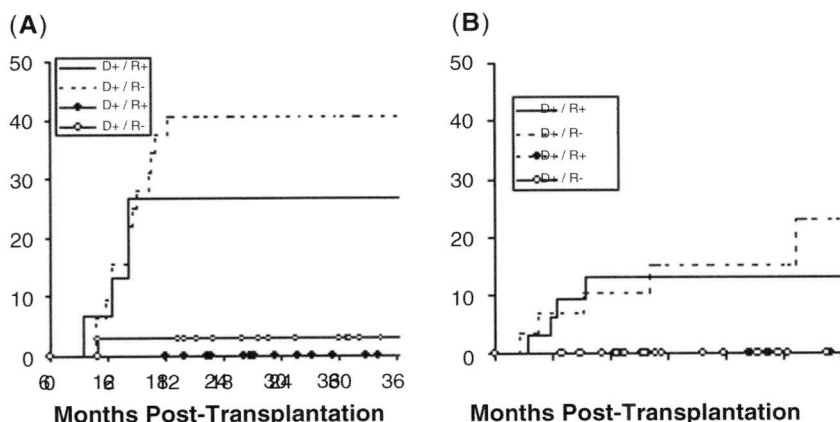

**Figure 4** Incidence of any cytomegalovirus (**A**), and noninvasive cytomegalovirus disease (**B**), in simultaneous pancreas–kidney transplant recipients at high risk (D+/R+, D+/R−), receiving prednisone (Pred+) (n = 100) or in the absence of prednisone (Pred−) (n = 100) therapy. *Abbreviations*: D, donor; R, recipient.

## ACKNOWLEDGMENTS

It is a pleasure to acknowledge the surgical and medical faculty that helped with the transplant surgical procedures and the posttransplant medical care. The nursing and ancillary staffs have contributed greatly to the care of the patients. The clinical research nurses have been instrumental in helping maintain and update the database on a regular basis.

## REFERENCES

1.  Kaufman DB, Leventhal JR, Stuart J, Abecassis MM, Fryer JP, Stuart FP. Mycophenolate mofetil and tacrolimus as primary maintenance immunosuppression in simultaneous pancreas–kidney transplantation: initial experience in 50 consecutive cases. Transplantation 1999; 67:586.
2.  Kaufman DB, Leventhal JR, Koffron AJ, Abecassis MM, Fryer JP, Stuart FP. Simultaneous pancreas–kidney transplantation in the mycophenolate mofetil/tacrolimus era: evolution from induction therapy with bladder drainage to non-induction therapy with enteric drainage. Surgery 2000; 128:726.
3.  Kaufman DB, Leventhal JR, Koffron AJ, et al. A prospective study of rapid corticosteroid elimination in simultaneous pancreas–kidney transplantation: comparison of two maintenance immunosuppression protocols: tacrolimus/mycophenolate mofetil versus tacrolimus/sirolimus. Transplantation 2002; 73:169–177.
4.  Kaufman DB, Leventhal JR, Gallon LG, et al. Technical and immunological progress in simultaneous pancreas-kidney transplantation. Surgery 2002; 132:545–555.
5.  Kaufman DB, Leventhal JR, Gallon LG, Parker MA. Alemtuzumab induction and prednisone-free maintnenace immunotherapy in simultaneous pancreas–kidney transplantation. Comparison with rabbit antilymphocyte globulin induction: long-term results. Am J Transplant 2006; 6:331–339.
6.  Kaufman DB, Leventhal JR, Gallon LG, Baker TB, Parker MA. Calcineurin inhibitor free/steroid-free maintenance immunosuppression in simultaneous pancreas–kidney transplantation. Am J Transplant 2005; 5(suppl 11):266.
7.  Elliott MD, Kapoor A, Parker MA, Kaufman DB, Bonow RO, Gheorghiade M. Improvement in hypertension in patients with diabetes mellitus after kidney/pancreas transplantation. Circulation 2001; 104:563–569.
8.  Kaufman DB, Leventhal JR, Gallon LG, et al. Risk factors and impact of cytomegalovirus disease in simultaneous pancreas–kidney transplantation. Transplantation 2001; 72:1940–1945.
9.  Axelrod D, Leventhal JR, Gallon LG, Parker MA, Kaufman DB. Reduction of CMV disease with steroid-free immunosuppresssion in simultaneous pancreas kidney transplant recipients. Am J Transplant 2005; 5:1423–1429.
10. Gruessner AC, Sutherland DER. Analyses of pancreas transplant outcomes for United States cases reported to the United Network for Organ Sharing (UNOS) and Non-US Cases Reported to the International Pancreas Transplant Registry. In: Cecka JM, Terasaki PI, eds. Clinical Transplants. UCLA Immunogenetics Center, Los Angeles 1999:51–69.
11. Kaufman DB, Leventhal JR, Axelrod D, Gallon LG, Parker MA, Stuart FP. Alemtuzumab induction and prednisone-free maintenance immunotherapy in kidney transplantation. Comparison with basiliximab induction: long-term results. Am J Transplant 2005; 5:2539–2548.
12. Cantarovich D, Giral-Classe M, Hourmant M, et al. Low incidence of kidney rejection after simultaneous kidney–pancreas transplantation after antithymocyte globulin induction and in the absence of corticosteroids: results of a prospective pilot study in 28 consecutive cases. Transplantation 2000; 69:1505.

# 32 | Pancreas Transplantation at Indiana University: A Brief Overview of Recent Progress

Jonathan A. Fridell, Avinash Agarwal, and John A. Powelson
*Department of Surgery, Indiana University School of Medicine, Indianapolis, Indiana, U.S.A.*

## INTRODUCTION

The pancreas transplantation program at Indiana University was started in 1988. Prior to 2001, approximately 8 to 10 pancreas transplants were performed annually, most of which were simultaneous pancreas and kidney transplants (SPK). After 2001, the number of pancreas transplants more than doubled (Fig. 1) so that by 2004 over 50 pancreas transplants were being performed annually, with a growing percentage being pancreas after kidney transplants (PAK) or solitary pancreas transplants [pancreas transplant alone (PTA)]. With the increase in the number of transplants performed, innovations in preservation, techniques, immunosuppressive protocols, and postoperative management were introduced. In addition, new indications for pancreas transplantation were developed. This chapter will summarize the recent outcomes after pancreas transplantation at Indiana University.

## PRESERVATION

As was common in most centers, all pancreas transplants performed at Indiana University were routinely flushed with and preserved in the University of Wisconsin solution. In May 2003, the standard cold preservation solution for all abdominal organ transplants at Indiana University was changed to histidine–tryptophan ketoglutarate (HTK). We published the initial results with the first 10 pancreas transplants preserved with HTK (1) and subsequently have published a follow-up study of 78 pancreas transplants using HTK (2). There was essentially no difference in terms of patient, kidney, or pancreas allograft survival, when compared with previous transplants preserved with University of Wisconsin solution. We have also reported the first series of kidney allografts flushed with HTK at the time of recovery and subsequently preserved on a pulsatile perfusion apparatus with Belzer MPS perfusate (3). This study included 50 renal allografts flushed with HTK, of which 10 were used for simultaneous kidney and pancreas transplantation. The results suggested that the preservation solution used for the initial flush did not affect renal graft function or survival.

## TECHNICAL ASPECTS

The typical pancreas transplant at Indiana University is performed through a midline incision with systemic venous drainage and enteric exocrine drainage. The two modifications introduced at our institution in recent years have included the use of the end-to-end anastomotic stapler for the creation of the duodenoenterostomy for exocrine drainage of the pancreas allograft (Fig. 2) (4) and the ipsilateral placement of both allografts on the right iliac system at the time of simultaneous kidney and pancreas transplantation (Fig. 3) (5). The latter technique has the advantage of a simplified vascular dissection and preservation of the left iliac system for future transplantation, if necessary.

## POSTTRANSPLANT MANAGEMENT AND IMMUNOSUPPRESSION

In terms of postoperative management, we routinely administer dextrose-free intravenous fluids and medications. Any increase in serum glucose levels requires investigation in this

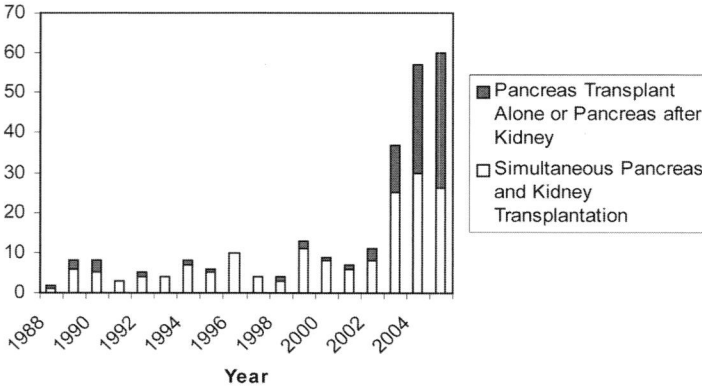

**Figure 1** Volume of pancreas transplants performed at Indiana University by year. There has been a significant increase in the volume of pancreas transplants that began in 2003. The proportion of pancreas transplants that were either pancreas after kidney transplants or isolated pancreas transplants has also grown as the volume has increased.

setting. To date, probably because of relatively short cold ischemia times (6–8 hours) there have not been any episodes of delayed pancreas allograft function.

The immunosuppressive protocol utilized in all cases consists of rabbit antithymocyte globulin (Thymoglobulin) induction for five doses, rapid weaning of corticosteroids over five days, and maintenance immunosuppression with tacrolimus and sirolimus. Interestingly, using this early steroid withdrawal protocol, we have been able to discontinue steroids routinely in kidney transplant patients on long-term prednisone maintenance who undergo PAK (6). Despite concerns based on the renal transplant literature that weaning chronic steroids in kidney transplant recipients leads to an increased rate of acute cellular rejection, there has not been any increased incidence of rejection in this patient population. It appears that the augmentation of immunosuppression at the time of PAK transplantation allows an opportunity in this scenario for safe late weaning of steroids.

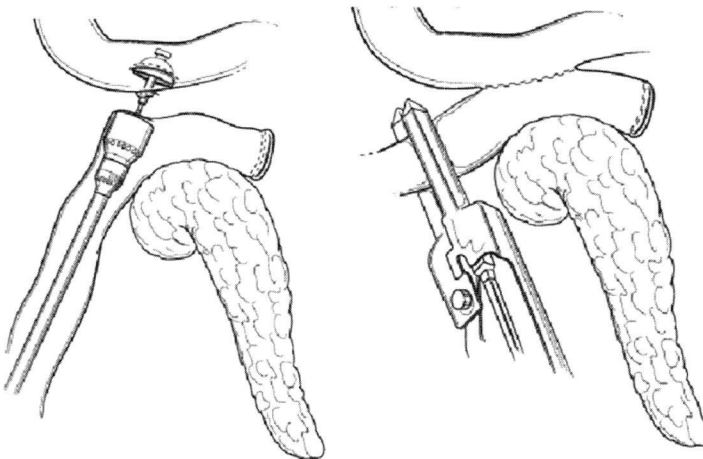

**Figure 2** Creation of the duodenoenterostomy for exocrine drainage using the end-to-end anastomatic (EEA) stapler: the anvil of the EEA stapler is inserted into the jejunum through an enterotomy and secured with a purse-string suture. The EEA stapler device is advanced into the second portion of the donor duodenum through the open jejunal end, mated with the anvil, closed and then fired, creating the anastomosis. The distal donor duodenum and jejunum are then removed with a single fire of a gastrointestinal anstomatic stapler (GIA).

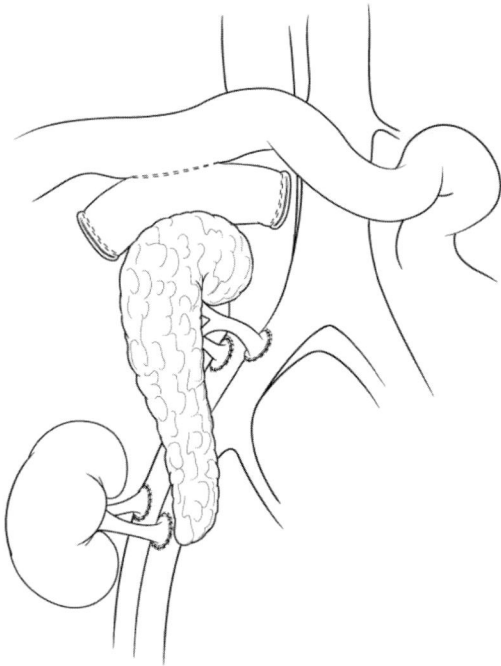

**Figure 3** Ipsilateral placement of simultaneously transplanted pancreas and kidney allografts. The iliac artery extension Y-graft and portal vein from the donor pancreas are anastomosed to the recipient common iliac artery and vein, respectively. The renal artery and vein from the donor kidney are anastomosed to the external iliac artery and vein, respectively.

## RESULTS

Given the relatively short follow-up for the majority of the cases, only one-year outcomes are available. One-year patient survival has been 95% for both SPK and PAK transplants, and 100% for PTA (Table 1). One-year graft survival rates for both the kidney and the pancreas in both SPK and PAK transplants have been between 92% and 95%. The one-year graft survival for the PTA group has been worse, 70%, but two of the three graft losses has been related to recipient noncompliance.

## NEW INDICATIONS

In addition to the typical indications for pancreas transplantation, it has become evident that there are other patient groups who could benefit from pancreas transplantation. Because of improvements in pulmonary therapy, more patients with cystic fibrosis are living long enough to develop extrapulmonary complications. Of these, cirrhosis and pancreatic insufficiency are

**Table 1** Patient and Graft Survival

| Group | N | 1 Yr survival (%) |
|---|---|---|
| Patient survival | | |
|   SPK | 92 | 95 |
|   PTA | 14 | 100 |
|   PAK | 43 | 95 |
| Graft survival | | |
|   SPK | | |
|     Pancreas | | 92 |
|     Kidney | | 94 |
|   PAK | | |
|     Pancreas | | 93 |
|     Kidney | | 95 |
|   PTA | | |
|     Pancreas | | 70 |

*Abbreviations*: SPK, simultaneous pancreas and kidney transplants; PTA, pancreas transplant alone; PAK, pancreas after kidney transplants.

**(A)** **(B)**

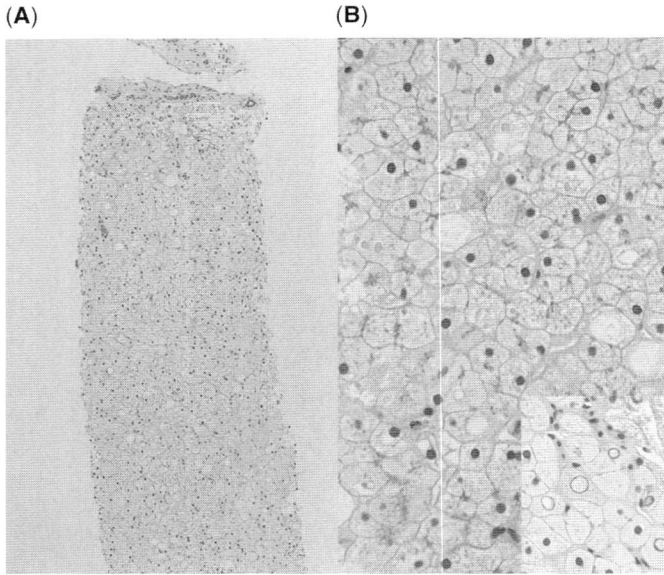

**Figure 4** An hematoxyein and eosin (H&E)-stained pre-pancreas transplant liver biopsy from a patient with glycogen hepatopathy demonstrated a diffuse paleness and unremarkable portal tracts (**A**). The hepatocytes were markedly swollen with occasional vesicles and prominent giant mitochondria (*arrows*) (**B**). Prominent glycogenated nuclei were also noted (*inset*).

common and can impact on the pulmonary reserve of these patients. At present, liver transplantation is the procedure of choice for progressive, irreversible hepatic insufficiency in this setting (7). For a patient with cystic fibrosis and cirrhosis also complicated by diabetes mellitus and pancreatic exocrine insufficiency, the addition of pancreas transplantation with enteric drainage at the time of liver transplantation has the potential advantage of providing normal glucose control and improved nutrition, two major factors felt to influence pulmonary performance in these patients. To date, we have performed two simultaneous liver–pancreas

**(A)** **(B)**

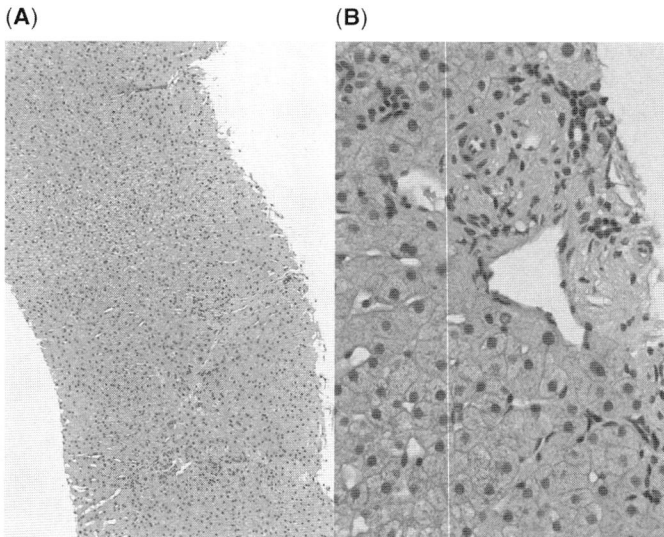

**Figure 5** Post-pancreas transplant and H&E-stained liver biopsy revealed resolution of the pale appearance (**A**). The hepatocyte cytoplasm showed no swelling and the giant mitochondria and glycogenated nuclei had disappeared (**B**).

transplants in patients with cystic fibrosis (8). Both have done extremely well, with excellent graft function, improved body mass index, and improved pulmonary function.

In addition, we have recently performed pancreas transplantation in two diabetics who presented with tender hepatomegaly, right upper quadrant pain, and elevated liver chemistries. These patients had glycogen hepatopathy (GH), a pathological overloading of hepatocytes with glycogen that is associated with poorly controlled diabetes mellitus. Following pancreas transplantation, the hepatomegaly resolved completely, and the liver chemistries normalized (9). Repeat liver biopsies obtained at six months post-transplantation demonstrated dramatic improvement in GH (Figs. 4 and 5). Although not currently recognized as an indication for pancreas transplantation, GH is commonly associated with poorly controlled type 1 diabetes mellitus and has been shown in these two cases to resolve completely after pancreas transplantation.

In conclusion, the pancreas transplant program at Indiana University has benefited from a marked increase in volume over the last three years, and this has allowed the introduction of innovations in preservation techniques and immunosuppressive management, and the development of new indications, with excellent short-term outcomes.

## REFERENCES

1. Fridell JA, Agarwal A, Milgrom ML, Goggins WC, Murdock P, Pescovitz MD. Comparison of histidine–tryptophan–ketoglutarate solution and University of Wisconsin solution for organ preservation in clinical pancreas transplantation. Transplantation 2004; 77(8):1304–1306.
2. Agarwal A, Murdock P, Pescovitz MD, Goggins WC, Milgrom ML, Fridell JA. Follow-up experience using histidine–tryptophan ketoglutarate solution in clinical pancreas transplantation. Transplant Proc 2005; 37(8):3523–3526.
3. Agarwal A, Goggins WC, Pescovitz MD, Milgrom ML, Murdock P, Fridell JA. Comparison of histidine–tryptophan ketoglutarate and University of Wisconsin solutions as primary preservation in renal allografts undergoing pulsatile perfusion. Transplant Proc 2005; 37(5):2016–2019.
4. Fridell JA, Milgrom ML, Henson S, Pescovitz MD. Use of the end-to-end anastomotic circular stapler for creation of the duodenoenterostomy for enteric drainage of the pancreas allograft [corrected]. J Am Coll Surg 2004; 198(3):495–497.
5. Fridell JA, Shah A, Milgrom M, Goggins WC, Leapman SB, Pescovitz MD. Ipsilateral placement of simultaneous pancreas and kidney allografts. Transplantation 2004; 78(7):1074–1076.
6. Fridell JA, Agarwal A, Powelson JA, Goggins WC, Milfrom M, Pescovitz MD, Tector AJ. Steroid withdrawal for pancreas offer kidney transplantation in recipients on maintenance prednisone immunosuppression. Transplanation (in press).
7. Fridell JA, Bond GJ, Mazariegos GV, et al. Liver transplantation in children with cystic fibrosis: a long-term longitudinal review of a single center's experience. J Pediatr Surg 2003; 38(8):1152–1156.
8. Fridell JA, Vianna R, Kwo PY, et al. Simultaneous liver and pancreas transplantation in patients with cystic fibrosis. Transplant Proc 2005; 37(8):3567–3569.
9. Fridell JA, Chalasani NP, Saxena R, Goggins WC, Cummings OW. Complete reversal of glycogen hepatopathy with Pancreas transplantation: Two cases. Transplantation (in press).

# 33 | Pancreas Transplantation: The Stockholm Experience

## Gunnar E. Tydén

*Departments of Transplantation Surgery, Neurophysiology and Medicine, Karolinska University Hospital, Stockholm, Sweden*

In this chapter, the Stockholm experience with 169 pancreatic transplantations in diabetic patients is described. When the program was started in 1974, we elected to drain the exocrine secretion into the patient's bowel by creating a pancreaticoenteric anastomosis. Initially, the enteric drainage technique was associated with a high incidence of technical complications. However, with refinements in the surgical technique, improved techniques for harvesting and procurement, and advances in immunosuppressive therapy, the results have become satisfactory. For many years, segmental pancreatic grafts were used. The reason for this decision was that the use of segmental grafts avoided the duodenum, an organ that was then believed to be dangerous to transplant. Later on, the main reason for using segmental grafts was that they made it possible to harvest the liver as well as the pancreas from a cadaveric donor without creating a conflict over the arterial trunks that led to both organs. This problem was eventually solved, and because pancreaticoduodenal grafts have many potential advantages over segmental grafts, we changed technique in 1988. The cumbersome pancreaticoenteric anastomosis needed for enteric drainage was replaced by a simple bowel-to-bowel anastomosis. Also, the increased blood flow in the whole organ graft reduced the risk of graft thrombosis, making systemic anticoagulation unnecessary. The technique for whole organ pancreaticoduodenal transplantation with enteric exocrine diversion has now evolved into a safe, routine procedure and has been adopted worldwide as the standard procedure for pancreatic transplantation.

## DONORS

From April 1974 through 1999, 169 pancreatic transplantations were performed at Huddinge Hospital. Because brain death was not accepted in Sweden until 1988, the first 103 transplantations were from the so-called controlled non-heart-beating donors. In the non-heart-beating era, it was observed that graft pancreatitis often developed when cold ischemia times were above six hours. For many years, therefore, the aim was to keep the cold ischemia time around four hours. However, as brain death was accepted, and at the same time the University of Wisconsin solution was introduced, cold ischemia times of 12 hours were accepted.

## TECHNIQUE FOR PANCREATIC TRANSPLANTATION WITH PANCREATICOENTEROSTOMY

Except for the first pioneering cases performed before 1980, in which a variety of enteric drainage techniques were explored, all segmental pancreatic grafts have been anastomosed end-to-end to a jejunal roux-en-Y loop (1). A pancreatic duct catheter was used to temporarily exteriorize the pancreatic juice, thus allowing the anastomoses to heal without being exposed to the digestive forces of pancreatic exocrine secretion. The use of a pancreatic duct catheter also facilitated the monitoring of exocrine pancreatic function by analyzing the volume and enzyme content of the pancreatic juice (2). The splenic or celiac artery of the segmental graft was anastomosed end-to-side to the recipient's right common iliac artery and the portal vein end-to-side to the caval vein. All grafts were placed intra- instead of extraperitoneally with the assumption that the conditions for anastomotic healing would thereby be improved.

Since 1988, all transplantations have been performed with pancreaticoduodenal grafts. In most cases, the liver was also harvested from the same donor, and the celiac axis was then taken with the liver. The duodenum and the pancreatic head thus derive their arterial supply from the inferior pancreaticoduodenal artery arising from the superior mesenteric artery, and the pancreatic body and tail derive their arterial supply from the splenic artery. A Y-extension graft from the donor iliac artery bifurcation has been used to join the splenic artery and the superior mesenteric artery. If necessary, the portal vein of the graft was also extended by a graft from the donor iliac vein. Again, all the grafts have been placed intraperitoneally.

The abdomen was entered through a midline incision, and the peritoneum was incised over the common iliac artery from the aortic bifurcation to the internal/external iliac bifurcation. The common iliac artery was then isolated on a vessel loop. All the lymphatics were carefully ligated. The distal caval vein was dissected free at a distance of approximately 5 cm lateral to the aortic bifurcation. The portal vein or iliac vein extension graft was then anastomosed end-to-side to the caval vein, and the iliac artery extension graft was anastomosed end-to-side to the common iliac artery. The pancreaticoduodenal graft consists of the entire pancreas and a 5 to 10 cm segment of the duodenum. The duodenal segment of the pancreaticoduodenal graft was closed by staples before the division distal to the pylorus and proximal to the ligament of Treitz during harvesting. The staple lines on either side of the duodenal segment were later inverted using nonabsorbable or slowly absorbing suture material. An incision approximately 5 cm long was then made along the antemesenteric border of the duodenal segment. In the first seven cases of pancreaticoduodenal transplantation, a roux-en-Y loop was used (3). However, the technique was soon simplified by omitting the roux-en-Y loop and simply anastomosing the duodenal segment side-to-side to the first part of the jejunum approximately 50 cm distal to the ligament of Treitz. Initially, a pancreatic duct catheter was used to protect the bowel anastomosis. However, because the technique for pancreaticoduodenal transplantations with enteric exocrine diversion soon proved to be a very safe and simple technique, the enteric anastomosis did not need protection (4). Furthermore, because the vast majority of the transplantations were performed in conjunction with a renal transplantation, there was no need for monitoring of the exocrine pancreatic function, and the pancreatic duct catheter was therefore omitted. However, in cases with pancreatic transplantation alone or pancreas transplantation after kidney transplantation, the use of a pancreatic duct catheter for exocrine diversion of pancreatic juice could still be a valuable option.

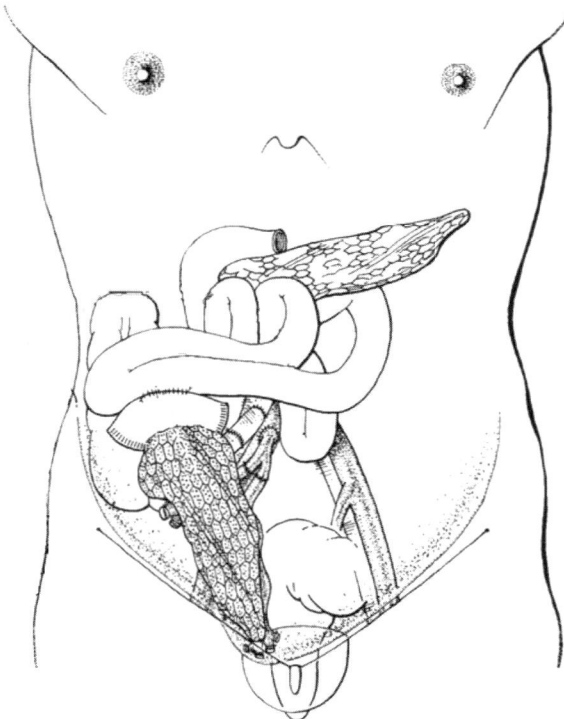

**Figure 1**  Pancreaticoduodenal transplant with exocrine drainage to the proximal jejunum. A Y-extension graft from the donor iliac artery bifurcation is used to join the splenic artery and the superior mesenteric artery and then anastomosed to the recipient common iliac artery. The portal vein is anastomosed to the recipient vena cava.

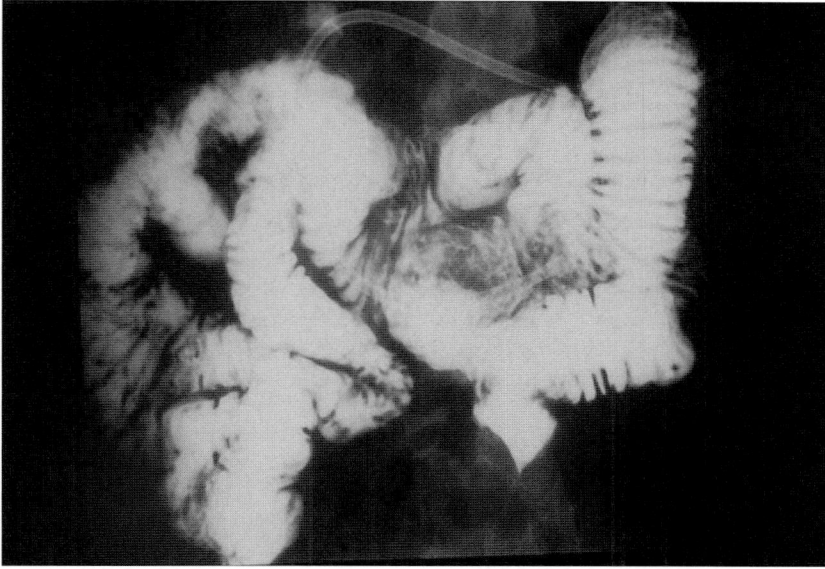

**Figure 2**   Upper gastrointestinal series showing the duodenal segment of the pancreaticoduodenal graft anastomosed side-to-side to the proximal jejunum.

Before the abdomen was closed, an abdominal drain was usually placed in the fossa of Douglas to drain the peripancreatic fluid collections. In all our cases, the renal transplant has been placed extraperitoneally in the left fossa in a standard fashion with a separate incision (Figs. 1 and 2).

## IMMUNOSUPPRESSION AND ANTICOAGULATION

When segmental pancreatic grafts were used, systemic anticoagulation was achieved by heparin and warfarin sodium. However, with whole organ pancreatic-duodenal grafts, no heparin or warfarin was given. The patient only received 500 mL of dextrane daily for five days. As prophylaxis against infections, ampicillin 1 g q. 6 h. and cephotaxin 1 g q. 6 h. are given for two days. A standard quadruple immunosuppressive protocol including cyclosporine or tacrolimus, azathioprine or CellCept, prednisolone, and a one-week course of antithymocyte globulin has been used in the vast majority of cases.

## MONITORING FOR REJECTION

To monitor the pancreatic graft, pancreas-specific serum amylase and fasting and postprandial blood glucose levels were routinely assessed. However, when rejection occurs in recipients of combined renal and pancreatic graft, signs of impaired functions, i.e., a rise in serum creatinine, usually precede signs of impaired pancreatic function by a few days, and consequently monitoring for rejection is mainly based on monitoring of renal function. When a pancreatic duct catheter was used, a decline in amylase activity and the appearance of activated lymphocytes in the pancreatic juice were indicative of rejection (5). The treatment for rejection has consisted of methylprednisolone at a total dose of 1.25 g and, in case of a steroid-resistant rejection, OKT3.

## PATIENTS

All recipients suffered from type I diabetes of long duration. Most of the transplantations were performed on uremic diabetic patients; in 134 instances a combined renal and pancreatic transplantation was performed and in six instances the pancreatic transplantation was performed in a patient who already had a renal graft. A further eight combined renal and pancreatic

**Table 1**  Combined Renal and Pancreatic Transplantation: Results by Era

|           |                                                      | 1 Yr patient survival (%) | 1 Yr graft survival (%) |
|-----------|------------------------------------------------------|---------------------------|--------------------------|
| 1974–1983 | Before ciclosporin                                   | 80                        | 27                       |
| 1983–1987 | Segmental grafts                                     | 90                        | 67                       |
| 1988–1990 | Pacreaticoduodenal grafts, roux loop                 | 82                        | 73                       |
| 1991–2000 | Pancreaticoduodenal grafts, simple duodenojejunostomy | 100                      | 87                       |

transplantations were performed in eight pre-uremic recipients (mean creatinine 192 μmol/L, range 164–250 μmol/L). Twenty-nine non- or pre-uremic diabetic patients received pancreatic transplants alone (6). The indications included hyperlabile diabetes with or without defective hormonal counter-regulation (five patients), severe progressive angiopathy (one patient), rapidly progressing retinopathy (two patients), severe neuropathy (four patients), and pre-uremic nephropathy (17 patients). Of the 169 diabetic patients, 11 underwent a second transplantation after the first had failed.

## RESULTS

Considerable improvements in the overall results have occurred with time. When the series is divided into different patient categories, it is obvious that the best results were obtained in uremic diabetic recipients of combined renal and pancreatic grafts from the same donor. In the latest series of combined transplantations, the one-year patient and pancreatic survival rates have been 100% and 87%, respectively (Table 1). Refinements in technique and improvements in immunosuppressive protocols, harvesting, and preservation have all contributed to the improvement in results. In the first part of the segmental graft series, graft losses because of technical complications, mainly pancreatic fistulas, were approximately 13%. This figure has been reduced to 1% in the most recent part of the series. When the graft losses in the segmental graft series are analyzed carefully, it seems that many of the pancreatic fistulas were secondary to severe graft pancreatitis. When graft pancreatitis occurs in a pancreaticoduodenal graft, the risk for enteric leakage is much reduced. In fact, with the use of pancreaticoduodenal grafts, there has been only one case of enteric leakage, not from the anastomosis but from the stapled end of the duodenal segment. After that case, the staple line has always been reinforced by a running 4.0 maxon suture. The incidence of graft pancreatitis has been reduced by using organs from heart-beating rather than controlled non-heart-beating donors and by the adoption of the University of Wisconsin solution. However, ischemic graft pancreatitis still constitutes a major problem and has been the sole reason for graft losses in recent years. Most of these cases of ischemic pancreatitis are the result of donor factors and donor events beyond our control.

## CONCLUSION

When a pancreatic transplant program was started in Stockholm in 1974, we chose to explore the enteric drainage technique from the very start. Initially, this technique had a bad reputation because of enteric leakages and ensuing abdominal infections. However, when the pancreatic transplantations performed during these years are analyzed retrospectively, it seems that many of the problems encountered are not caused by the enteric drainage technique per se, but rather by suboptimal donor handling, procurement procedures, and preservation solutions. Thus, the majority of the complications were a consequence of graft pancreatitis rather than enteric leakage. Today, the technique for whole organ pancreaticoduodenal transplantation with enteric exocrine diversion has evolved into a safe, routine procedure and has been adopted worldwide as the standard procedure for pancreatic transplantation. As the technical complication rate has thus been drastically reduced, attention has been focused more on the benefits of the procedure than on the hazards. In the early days, much effort was undertaken to show that combined pancreas–kidney transplantation was no more dangerous than kidney transplantation alone in a diabetic patient. Today, it has been shown (7) that long-term patient survival after combined renal and pancreatic transplantation is very much superior to that after kidney transplantation alone. Thus, with a safe technique at hand, the question is no longer whether it is acceptable or ethical to subject a diabetic patient with end-stage nephropathy to a combined pancreas and kidney transplantation but rather whether it is ethical to withhold this procedure from the patient.

## REFERENCES

1. Tydén G, Brattström C, Lundgren G, Östman J, Gunnarsson R, Groth CG. Improved results in pancreatic transplantation by avoiding non-immunological graft failures. Transplantation 1987; 43:674–676.
2. Tydén G, Brattström C, Häggmark A, Groth CG. Studies on the exocrine secretion of human segmental pancreatic grafts. Surg Gynecol Obstet 1987; 164:404–408.
3. Tydén G, Tibell A, Groth CG. Pancreatico-duodenal transplantation with enteric exocrine drainage: Technical aspects. Clin Transplant 1991; 5:36–39.
4. Tydén G, Tibell A, Sandberg J, Brattström C, Groth CG. Improved results with a simplified technique for pancreatico-duodenal transplantation with enteric exocrine drainage. Clin Transplant 1996; 10:306–309.
5. Reinholt FP, Tydén G, Bohman S-O, Brattström C, Groth CG. Pancreatic juice cytology in the diagnosis of pancreatic graft rejection. Clin Transplant 1988; 2:127–133.
6. Tydén G, Bolinder J, Tibell A, Reinholt F, Östman J, Groth CG. Experience with single pancreatic transplantation in pre-uremic diabetic recipients in Stockholm. Transplant Proc 1992; 24:852–853.
7. Tydén G, Bolinder J, Solders G, Brattström C, Tibell A, Groth CG. Improved survival in IDDM patients with end-stage diabetic nephropathy ten years after combined pancreas and kidney transplantation. Transplantation 1999; 67:645–648.

# 34 Pancreas Transplantation at the University of Louvain Saint Luc Hospital in Brussels (Belgium) and the EUROSPK Trial

**Jean-Paul Squifflet**

*Department of Abdominal Surgery and Transplantation, University of Liege, Liege, Belgium*

## INTRODUCTION

Clinical pancreas transplantation started in 1982 at the University of Louvain (UCL) Saint Luc Hospital in Brussels, Belgium, with the concomitant introduction of cyclosporin A in the immunosuppressive (IS) therapy regimen. The program was largely sponsored by D.E.R. Sutherland, following the University of Minnesota experience in that field (1). It slowly grew during the late 1980s. Nevertheless, the proportion of pancreas transplant and/or diabetic recipients remained low compared to the number of cadaver and live donor kidney recipients who were transplanted during the same period (Fig. 1). Since 1990, the number of pancreas cases stabilized for several reasons. The main one was the opening of pancreas programs in all seven Belgian kidney transplant centers. Despite an increasing number of deceased donors, the number of pancreas transplants remained stable in the country (Fig. 2). Other reasons could be the decreasing number of patients with type 1 diabetes on dialysis and the increasing number of type 2 diabetes patients (Fig. 3), better pretransplant medical care, the implementation of intensive insulin therapy, and other confounding factors such as the general incidence of diabetes in the country.

## POPULATION

From November 1982 until June 20, 2005, 87 pancreas transplants were performed at UCL in 82 kidney recipients and one liver recipient (three kidney recipients and the liver recipient received two pancreases). During the same period, two pancreas transplantations alone were performed in two nonuremic diabetic recipients. The first 64 primary simultaneous pancreas kidney (SPK) procedures (November 1982 to June 2001) will be the basis of the current analysis (Fig. 4). Two SPK recipients had previously received a pancreas transplantation alone and a kidney transplant alone each: the first pancreas failed for technical reasons, while the first kidney failed because of chronic rejection. Eight other SPK recipients eventually received a second kidney graft after failure of the first kidney, one a second pancreas graft after thrombosis of the first transplant, and one a second SPK.

Finally, one simultaneous pancreas and liver (SPL) recipient received eventually a second pancreas graft; both pancreases failed from recurrent diabetes 17 and three months after transplantation.

## SURGICAL TECHNIQUE

Surgical technique varied according to the era of transplantation (Fig. 5). From November 10, 1982 to July 28, 1986, 10 pancreases (group 1) were implanted along with a kidney graft according to the Swedish technique (2): the segmental pancreatic graft was drained into a Roux-en-Y loop by performing a pancreaticojejunostomy with systemic venous drainage.

From January 5, 1987 to August 18, 1997, 44 SPK recipients (group 2) underwent whole pancreas transplantation with a duodenal segment. The exocrine secretions were drained into the bladder with systemic venous drainage (3,4). Because of metabolic acidosis, chemical cystitis, and chronic urethritis, five of 44 duodenocystostomies were converted to side-to-side pancreaticoduodenoileostomies.

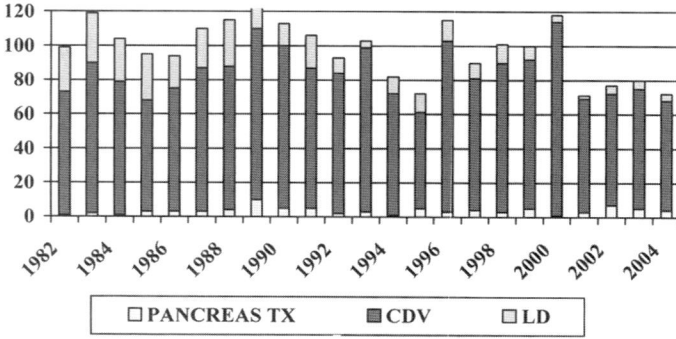

Figure 1 University of Louvain kidney and pancreas transplantation population.

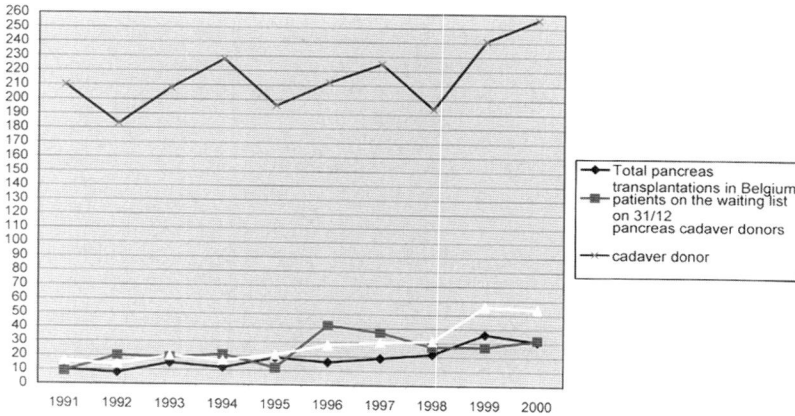

Figure 2 Number of pancreas transplants compared to number of pancreas cadaver donors in Belgium during the last decade (Eurotransplant data).

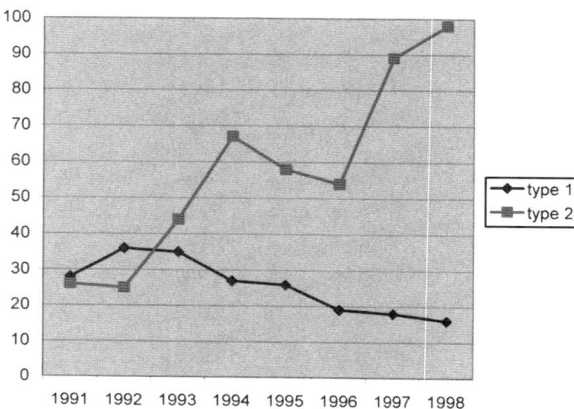

Figure 3 Number of patients on dialysis with type 1 and type 2 diabetes in the southern part of Belgium (French-speaking dialysis registry).

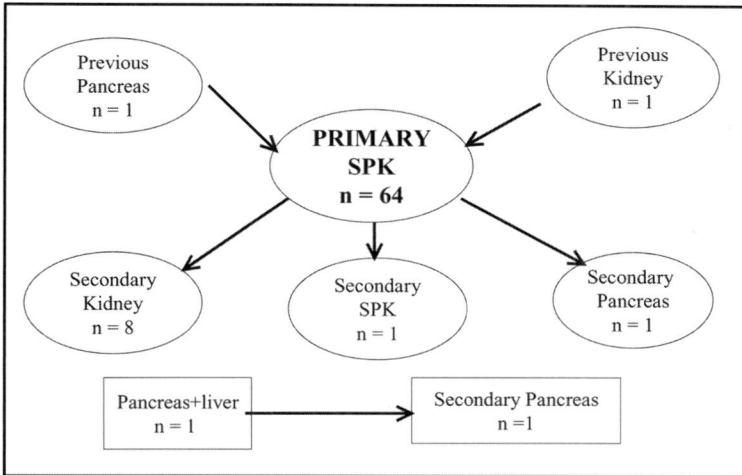

**Figure 4** University of Louvain pancreas transplantation population: 69 pancreas grafts in 65 patients.

Finally, since December 16, 1997, 10 SPK recipients (group 3) have undergone whole pancreas transplantation with a side-to-side duodenoileostomy (5,6). The venous drainage was systemic in four (a) and portal in six (b).

## IS THERAPY

All SPK recipients except one (Table 1) received induction therapy that consisted of a 10- to 14-day course of either antilymphocyte globulin (Pressimum®, Behringwerke, Germany) or antithymocyte globulin (R-ATG®, Fresenius, Germany). For the patients included in the EUROSPK protocol, the ATG course was shortened (see below).

The calcineurin inhibitor in groups 1 and 2 was cyclosporine (cyclo) in combination with azathioprine (Aza-Imuran®—Glaxo Wellcome) ($n = 52$) and prednisone ($n = 54$).

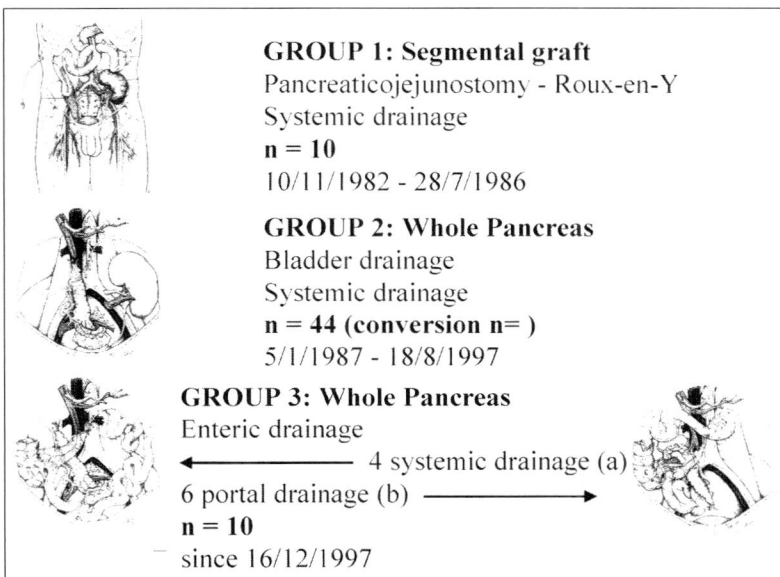

**GROUP 1: Segmental graft**
Pancreaticojejunostomy - Roux-en-Y
Systemic drainage
**n = 10**
10/11/1982 - 28/7/1986

**GROUP 2: Whole Pancreas**
Bladder drainage
Systemic drainage
**n = 44 (conversion n= )**
5/1/1987 - 18/8/1997

**GROUP 3: Whole Pancreas**
Enteric drainage
← ——————— 4 systemic drainage (a)
6 portal drainage (b) ——————→
**n = 10**
since 16/12/1997

**Figure 5** University of Louvain pancreas transplantation: the surgical technique in the three groups.

**Table 1**  University of Louvain Pancreas Transplantation: Immunosuppressive Therapy

| Induction | Group 1 (*n* = 10) | Group 2 (*n* = 44) | Group 3 (*n* = 10) | Total (*n* = 64) |
|---|---|---|---|---|
| NI | 1 | 0 | 0 | 1 |
| ALS | 4 | 10 | 0 | 14 |
| ATG | 5 | 34 | 10 | 49 |
| Immunosuppression: | | | | |
| Cyclo–Pred | 2 | 0 | 0 | 2 |
| Cyclo–Aza–Pred | 8 | 44 | 1 | 53 |
| Cyclo–MMF–Pred | 0 | 0 | 3 | 3 |
| Tacro–MMF–Pred | 0 | 0 | 6 | 6 |

*Abbreviations*: ALS, antilymphocyte serum; ATG, antithymocyte globulin; Cyclo, cyclosporine; Pred, prednisone; Aza, azathioprine; MMF, mycophenolate mofetil; Tacro, tacrolimus; NI, no induction.

When mycophenolate mofetil (MMF) (Cellcept[R]—Roche) became available, all recipients in group 3 received it along with either microemulsion of cyclosporine (Neoral[R]—Novartis) or tacrolimus [Tacro-Prograf[R]—Fujisawa (now Astellas)].

## RESULTS

The mean donor age increased with the era of transplantation, and was only 28.7 years and 28.9 years in groups 1 and 2, respectively, and 39.5 years in group 3. The mean recipient age increased also from 36.7 years in group 1 to 38.2 and 40.5 years in groups 2 and 3, respectively.

One-, two-, and five-year actual patient (Table 2), pancreas (Table 3), and kidney (Table 4) survival improved over time. The causes of patient deaths, and pancreas and kidney graft losses in groups 1 and 2 are illustrated in Table 5.

Noteworthy is the course of the pancreas liver recipient (SPL). That 34-old-year gentleman received an SPL cadaver transplant on September 22, 1988 for sclerosing cholangitis and type 1 diabetes. The IS therapy consisted of a quadruple drug regimen with R-ATG induction, cyclo, Aza, and steroids. A first acute liver rejection was treated with methyprednisolone boluses and OKT3 on day 6. The gentleman did well without insulin therapy for one year. On March 1990, after a two-month period without any laboratory studies, the person came in with a high blood glucose level, a fall in the urinary amylase, and normal serum lipase and amylase levels. The liver biopsy was not contributory, while the transcystoscopic biopsy failed to give enough tissue. The duodenal segment was macroscopically normal. The patient refused an open biopsy and any rejection treatment, and resumed insulin therapy. Eight years later, the patient asked for a second pancreas transplant; the patient's hepatic function was normal under cyclo monotherapy.

On April 4, 1998, the patient received a second cadaver pancreas transplant, which was placed in the right iliac fossa in the same position where the first transplant had been placed (and which was removed during the same operation). Surprisingly, the first pancreas transplant was macroscopically atrophic but microscopically demonstrated normal appearing islets (Fig. 6). Immunological staining confirmed the absence of insulin cells in the islet. The patient did well without insulin therapy under cyclo, MMF, and low-dose steroids. On July 7, 1998, the patient was again hospitalized for hyperglycemic events and a 50% fall in the urinary amylase. Despite rapid treatment for rejection, including boluses of methylprednisolone and R-ATG, the urine amylase content continued to fall, and the patient resumed insulin therapy. The angiogram confirmed an excellent perfusion of the pancreas graft but the biopsy did not have enough material. The anti-IAC512/IA2 antibody ratio was 0.8 (normal <1.0) while anti-GAD65 antibodies were positive (90.4 U.; normal range <3.4). This suggested the recurrence of diabetes in the transplanted pancreas.

**Table 2**  University of Louvain Pancreas Transplantation: Actual Patient Survival According to the Period of Transplantation

| Years | Group 1 (%) (*n* = 10) | Group 2 (%) (*n* = 44) | Group 3 (%) (*n* = 10) | Total (%) (*n* = 64) |
|---|---|---|---|---|
| 1 | 60 | 86.3 | 100 | 84.1 |
| 2 | 60 | 81.8 | 100 | 79.3 |
| 5 | 60 | 74.3 | — | 71.4 |

**Table 3** University of Louvain Pancreas Transplantation: Actual Pancreas Graft Survival According to the Period of Transplantation

| Years | Group 1 (%) (n = 10) | Group 2 (%) (n = 44) | Group 3 (%) (n = 10) | Total (%) (n = 64) |
|---|---|---|---|---|
| 1 | 50 | 72.7 | 100 | 73 |
| 2 | 40 | 68.2 | 100 | 65.5 |
| 5 | 40 | 61.5 | — | 57.1 |

## ISLET RESEARCH

In parallel with the clinical pancreas program, an islet research program was developed at UCL, using a pig to baboon xenotransplant model (7,8). Using the same basic quadruple IS therapy as in the clinic, pig islets were prepared in Geneva (by Prof. P. H. Morel at Islet Laboratory, Department of Transplantation and Abdominal Surgery, Geneva, Switzerland) and implanted into totally pancreatectomized baboons. Despite the heavy IS therapy, they failed to demonstrate long-term function (9).

Following the animal research collaboration with the University of Geneva, a clinical islet research laboratory opened on 9/2000 at UCL: it is functioning jointly with the Swiss–French Gragil Consortium (10). The bone and tissue bank sterile structure houses the Ricordi chamber where human pancreases are currently processed.

## THE EUROSPK PROTOCOL

In January 1997, during the Kühtai Pancreas Transplantation Workshop, Prof. W. Land took the initiative to propose collaboration among 11 pancreas transplantation centers (10 in Europe and one in Israel). They designed the EUROSPK 001 protocol, which aimed to compared the microemulsion formulation of cyclosporine (Neoral—Novartis) with tacrolimus (Prograf—Fujisawa)-based IS therapy regimen, along with a short course (four days) of R-ATG (Fresenius—Germany) induction therapy. MMF (Cellcept—Roche, Switzerland) bid was added, and steroids were to be discontinued by month six. This prospective randomized study included over100 patients in each arm. Data at three years were analyzed at UCL and recently published in a special issue of *Nephrology, Dialysis, and Transplantation* (11).

One hundred and three patients were randomized to receive tacrolimus (initial dose: 0.2 mg/kg/day po) and 102 to cyclosporine-ME (7 mg/kg/day po). The R-ATG dosage was 4 mg/kg/day. Fewer patients receiving tacrolimus (36.9%) than cyclosporine-ME (57.8%) were discontinued from treatment ($p = 0.003$). The initial episodes of biopsy-proven rejection were moderate or severe in just one out of 31 (3%) tacrolimus-treated patients, compared with 11 out of 39 (28%) patients receiving cyclosporine-ME ($p = 0.009$). While three-year patient and kidney survival rates were similar in the two treatment groups, pancreas survival was superior with tacrolimus (89.2% vs. 72.4%; $p = 0.002$). Thrombosis resulted in pancreas graft loss in 10 patients receiving cyclosporine-ME and in only two receiving tacrolimus ($p = 0.02$). The overall adverse event frequency was similar in both groups, but MMF intolerance was more frequent with tacrolimus while hyperlipidemia was more frequent with cyclosporine-ME.

In this three-year study, tacrolimus was more effective than cyclosporine-ME in preventing moderate or severe kidney or pancreas rejection after SPK transplantation. It also provided superior pancreas survival and reduced the risk of pancreatic thrombosis.

**Table 4** University of Louvain Pancreas Transplantation: Actual Kidney Graft Survival According to the Period of Transplantation

| Years | Group 1 (%) (n = 10) | Group 2 (%) (n = 44) | Group 3 (%) (n = 10) | Total (%) (n = 64) |
|---|---|---|---|---|
| 1 | 60 | 79.5 | 100 | 79.3 |
| 2 | 60 | 72.7 | 100 | 72.5 |
| 5 | 60 | 58.9 | — | 59.2 |

**Table 5** University of Louvain Pancreas Transplantation: Causes of Patient Death, Pancreas and Kidney Graft Losses in Groups 1 and 2

| | Group 1 (n = 10) | Group 2 (n = 44) | Total (n = 64) |
|---|---|---|---|
| Causes of death | 6 | 17 | 23 |
| Cardiovascular | 2 | 4 | 6 |
| Infection | 4 | 3 | 7 |
| LPD | 0 | 1 | 1 |
| Various | 0 | 9 | 9 |
| Causes of pancreas loss[a] | 8 (1) | 15 (6) | 23 (7) |
| Technical failure[b] | 3 | 2 | 5 |
| Thrombosis | 0 | 4 | 4 |
| Acute rejection | 0 | 0 | 0 |
| Chronic rejection | 1 | 7 | 8 |
| Infection | 1 | 0 | 1 |
| Various[c] | 3 | 2 | 5 |
| Causes of kidney loss[d] | 6 (1) | 21 (6) | 27 (7) |
| Technical failure[e] | 2 | 2 | 4 |
| Acute rejection | 0 | 2 | 2 |
| Chronic rejection | 4 | 15 | 19 |
| Various | 0 | 2 | 2 |
| Group 3: no deaths, no pancreas and kidney losses | | | |

[a]Values in parentheses represent death with functioning pancreas.
[b]Hemorrhage, leakage, pancreatitis.
[c]Type 2, poor function, multisystemic.
[d]Values in parentheses represent death with functioning kidney.
[e]PNF, leakage, hemorrhage.
*Abbreviations*: LPD, lymphoproliferative disorder; PNF, primary nonfunction.

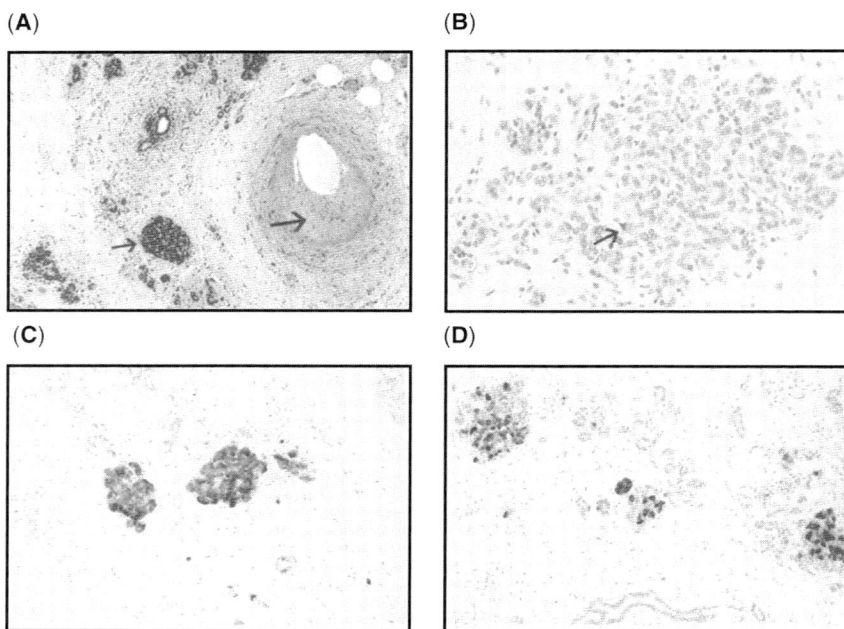

**Figure 6** Histology of the pancreas graft in a simultaneous pancreas–liver recipient. (**A**) The pancreas is atrophic and fibroinflammatory tissue replaces the exocrine glands in many areas. The islets persist (*arrow*) but the endocrine cell cytoplasms are poorly developed. Obliterative endothelitis is observed in several vessels (*arrow*). H&E. staining; 10×. (**B–D**) Immunoperoxydase staining with antibodies directed against insulin (**B**; 20×), glucagon and somatostatin cells (**C**) and (10×). Insulin cells are still present in few islets (**B**, *arrow*); glucagon and somatostatin cells are still very numerous in these islets.

Other analyses demonstrated that, except for lipid profiles, no major differences in metabolic effects or blood pressure control were observed over the three years in SPK transplant patients receiving immunosuppression based on tacrolimus or cyclosporine-ME. In view of the potential risk of hypertension, antihypertensive strategies should be implemented for all patients.

The incidence of CMV infection was also the same in both groups. Ganciclovir prophylaxis effectively prevented CMV infection, especially in higher-risk groups, and was associated with a reduced incidence of rejection compared with aciclovir prophylaxis. Short-term induction therapy with R-ATG was effective and well tolerated in patients undergoing SPK transplantation. Tacrolimus was the preferred IS agent, resulting in fewer cases of pancreas graft loss and drug discontinuation compared with cyclosporine-ME. A long-term analysis of corticosteroid withdrawal in SPK transplantation is necessary to confirm these early results and to evaluate the positive effects on glucose metabolism and hypertension. There was also no evidence that human leukocyte antigen matching was associated with improved kidney or pancreas survival. However, a higher rate of acute rejection was observed with worse human leukocyte antigen matching, and this might impact long-term survival.

## CONCLUSIONS

The data and results of pancreas transplantation at UCL compare favorably with pancreas transplant outcomes for U.S. cases reported to the United Network for Organ Sharing and non-U.S. cases reported to the International Pancreas Transplant Registry (12).

Unfortunately, the number of SPK transplants is not increasing in Belgium in spite of a large deceased donor pool. The low rate of solitary pancreas transplantation, mostly PAK, may be explained by the strict selection of SPK candidates so that the high-risk recipients are offered kidney transplant alone without the secondary possibility of PAK.

Despite a decreasing rate of type 1 diabetic nephropathy in Belgium, uncontrolled diabetes has other secondary complications, which impairs quality of life. The decreasing incidence of rejection encountered in the EUROSPK protocol with the R-ATG induction therapy and a Tacro–MMF-based IS therapy may allow diabetologists to screen more candidates for SPK or solitary pancreas transplantation.

## ACKNOWLEDGMENTS

Mr. Piet Vanormelingen who collected the Eurotransplant data, Mrs. Madeleine Putmans for secretarial assistance, and Prof. B. Lengele, M.D., Ph.D. (Department of Anatomy) who realized with utmost talent the figures and anatomic reproductions. The UCL Pancreas Transplantation Program comprises: Department of Kidney and Pancreas Transplantation: Prof. J. P. Squifflet, M.D., Ph.D., Mr. J. Malaise, M.D., D. Chaib-Eddour, M.D. Department of Nephrology: Prof. Y. Pirson, M.D., Mr. E. Goffin, M.D. Department of Diabetology: Mr. B. Vandeleene, M.D. Department of Immunohematology: Prof. D. Latinne, M.D., Ph.D. Department of Pathology: Prof. J. Rahier, M.D., Ph.D., Prof. J. P. Cosijns, M.D., Ph.D. Islet Research: Mr. D. Dufrane, M.D., Ph.D. and Prof. J. P. Squifflet, M.D., Ph.D The EUROSPK comprises: The EUROSPK Advisory Board: Prof. W. Land (Chairman—Munchen, Germany), Prof. J. M. Dubernard (Lyon, France), Prof. C.G. Groth (Huddinge, Sweden), Prof. R. Landgraf (Munchen, Germany), Prof. R. Margreiter (Innsbruck, Austria), and Prof. Y. Vanrenterghem (Leuven, Belgium) The EUROSPK members: Prof Neuhaus, Dr. A. Kahl, Mrs. Uhl, Mrs. Engelking (Berlin, Germany) Dr. W.O. Bechstein (Bochum, Germany) Prof. W. Land, Prof. R. Landgraf, Dr. W. D. Illner, Dr. C. Dieterle, Dr. A. Tarabichi, Dr. Schneeberger, Dr. Arbogast (Munchen, Germany) Dr. M. Stangl (Munchen, Germany) Dr. F. Saudek, Dr. P. Boucek, Dr. T. Jedinakovà, Dr. R. Koznarova, Mrs. V. Nemcova, Mrs. J. Cerna (Prague, Tchekia) Prof. R. Margreiter, Prof. A. Königsrainer, Dr. W. Steurer (Innsbruck, Germany) Prof. L. Fernandez-Cruz, Dr. M.J. Ricart (Barcelona, Spain) Dr. R. Nakache (Tel-Aviv, Israël) Prof A. Secchi, Dr R. Caldara (Milano, Italy) Prof. Y. Vanrenterghem, Prof. J. Pirenne, Prof. B. Maes, Dr. D. Kuypers, Dr. W. Coosemans, Dr. P. Evenepoel, Dr. Th. Messian (Leuven, Belgium) Prof. G. Tyden, Dr. J. Sandberg (Huddinge, Sweden) Prof J. P. Squifflet, Dr. J. Malaise, Mrs. D. Van Ophem (Brussels, Belgium) Prof. P. Morel, Dr. T. Berney, Dr. J. Oberholzer, Dr. P. Majno, Dr. C. Toso, Mrs. F. Roch (Geneva, Switzerland) The EUROSPK speakers: Prof. J.P. Squifflet, Dr. J. Malaise, Mrs. D. Van Ophem (Brussels, Belgium) The UCL Pancreas program is supported by a grant from "La fondation Louvain." Xeno islet research was supported by FRSM Grant No 3.4591.92 and 3.4584.93 from "Fonds de la recherche Scientifique Médicale" (Brussels, Belgium). The EUROSPK trial is an investigator-driven study supported in part by Fujisawa GmbH and Hoffman-La Roche AG. J.P. Squifflet is recipient of the Nessim Habif Prize (University of Geneva—Switzerland).

## REFERENCES

1. Squifflet J-P. Pancreas Transplantation: Experimental and Clinical Studies. Basel, Switzerland: Karger, 1990.
2. Groth CG, Collste H, Lundgren G. Successful outcome of segmental human pancreatic transplantation with enteric exocrine diversion after modifications in technique. Lancet 1982; 2:522–524.
3. Nghiem DD, Corry RJ. Technique of simultaneous pancreaticoduodenal transplantation with urinary drainage of pancreatic secretion. Am J Surg 1987; 153:405–406.
4. Sollinger HW, Cook K, Kamps D. Clinical and experimental experience with pancreaticocystostomy for exocrine pancreatic drainage in pancreas transplantation. Transplant Proc 1984; 16:749–751.
5. Kelly WD, Lillehei RC, Merkel FK. Allotransplantation of the pancreas and duodenum along with the kidney in diabetic nephropathy. Surgery 1967; 61:827–835.
6. Starzl TE, Iwatsuki S, Shaw BW Jr., et al. Pancreaticoduodenal transplantation in humans. Surg Gynecol Obstet 1984; 159:265–272.
7. Alexancre GPJ, Latinne D, Carlier M, et al. ABO-incompatibility and organ transplantation. Transplant Rev 1991; 5(4):230–241.
8. Besse T, Duck L, Latine D, et al. Effect of plasmapheresis and splenectomy on parameters involved in vascular rejection of discordant xenografts in the swine to baboon model. Transplant Proc 1994; 26:1042–1044.
9. Bühler LH, Deng S, O'neil J, et al. Adult porcine islet transplantation in baboons treated with conventional immunosuppression or a non-myeloablative regimen and CD 154 blockade. Xenotransplantation 2002; 9: 3–13.
10. Oberholzer J, Benhamou PY, Toso C, et al. Human Islet Transplantation Network for the treatment of type 1 diabetes: first (1999–2000) data from the Swiss–French Gragil consortium. Am J Transplant 2001; 1(suppl 1):182.
11. Saudek F, Malaise J, Margreiter R. EUROSPK Study Group. Tacrolimus versus cyclosporine in primary simultaneous pancreas–kidney (SPK) transplantation. Preliminary results of a multicentre trial. Am J Transplant 2001; 1(suppl 1):159.
12. Gruessner C, Sutherland DER. Pancreas transplant outcomes for United States (US) cases reported to the United Network for Organ Sharing (UNOS) and Non-US cases reported to the International Pancreas Transplant Registry (IPTR) as of October 2000. In: Cecka, Terasaki, eds. Clinical Transplants 2000. Chapter 4. Los Angeles, CA: UCL Immunogenetics Center, 2001:44–71.

# 35 | Retroperitoneal Pancreas Transplantation with Portal-Enteric Drainage

**Ugo Boggi, Fabio Vistoli, and Marco Del Chiaro**
*U.O. di Chirurgia nell'Uremico e nel Diabetico, University of Pisa, Pisa, Italy*

**Stefano Signori and Franco Mosca**
*U.O. di Chirurgia Generale e Trapianti, University of Pisa, Pisa, Italy*

Forty years after the first clinical pancreas transplant was performed by Kelly et al. (1), the ideal technique for pancreas transplantation has yet to be defined. Although currently whole pancreaticoduodenal grafts are preferred to segmental ones (2), controversy continues regarding the site of both the venous and exocrine drainage. On a priori grounds, the results of pancreas transplantation should be the best when endocrine activity is delivered through the portal system and exocrine secretions are drained into the gut. The first attempts to comply with these principles date back to the mid-1980s and involved either segmental (3) or whole pancreas grafts (4). A number of different techniques were described, including venous drainage directly into the portal vein (5) or into the splenic vein (6,7), the inferior mesenteric vein (8), and the superior mesenteric vein (9). Similarly, different sites were selected for exocrine drainage including the stomach (10), the duodenum (11), the small bowel (7,8,10,11), and the urinary tract (4,5). Unfortunately, most of these early series meet with high complication rates, both from enteric leaks and vascular complications. Accordingly, portal drainage of pancreas grafts did not gain widespread popularity until the 1990s, following the experimental work by Shokouh-Amiri et al. in a porcine model (12,13) and the encouraging results of the ensuing clinical experience by the Memphis group (9,14,15). In subsequent series and studies portal-enteric drainage of pancreas grafts neither increased the surgical risk nor jeopardized patient and graft survival when compared to either systemic-bladder drainage (14,16–18) or systemic-enteric drainage (19). The main incentives to the use of portal-enteric drainage for pancreas transplantation are achievement of physiologic peripheral insulin levels (20), improvement of lipoprotein composition (21–24), and a possible immunologic advantage, resulting in fewer rejection episodes (25), although there is no final evidence that either patient survival or graft survival is improved long term with portal drainage compared to systemic drainage. Currently, a growing number of centers in the United States and in Europe electively employ portal-enteric drainage for pancreas transplantation. Data from the International Pancreas Transplant Registry show that 25% ($n = 1091$) of U.S. primary pancreas transplants performed during 1996–2002 were drained into the portal vein (26).

The technique of pancreas transplantation with portal-enteric drainage that is currently adopted by most centers is the one described by Gaber et al. (9) or a modification thereof (17,18,27). All these techniques, however, draw inspiration from the same basic principles. Firstly, the graft is located intraperitoneally. Secondly, the donor portal vein is anastomosed into the recipient's superior mesenteric vein, or into one of its main tributary branches, which are approached by direct dissection through the mesenteric root. Thirdly, the arterial supply requires a rather long Y iliac donor graft brought down to the recipient's common iliac artery through a window made in the distal ileal mesentery. Fourthly, the tail of the pancreas is anchored to the anterior abdominal wall to permit subsequent percutaneous allograft biopsies (19,28,29). Alleged surgical advantages of Gaber's technique include intraperitoneal graft placement, which is generally thought to be important to reduce the incidence of peripancreatic fluid collections and consequently the risk of intra-abdominal infection (30,31), and to increase ease of access to and improved exposure of the superior mesenteric vein (19), especially in nonobese patients, making venous anastomosis easier as compared to pelvic graft placement with anastomosis to the iliac vein (19). This technique, however, is not without criticism. The dissection of the superior mesenteric vein can be technically demanding, or overtly impracticable in obese recipients with a thickened mesentery and a deep superior mesenteric vein (16). Arterial reconstruction can be difficult, and requires a rather long donor Y iliac graft (16,19), or even an additional extension donor graft (17,27). Percutaneous allograft biopsy, although possible in most patients, may be complicated by the presence of bowel loops between the graft and the abdominal wall.

We herein describe a new technique for retroperitoneal pancreas transplantation with portal-enteric drainage (32). Placement of the pancreas in the right paracolic, retroperitoneal space facilitates the construction of arterial anastomosis using a short donor graft and improves graft accessibility for postoperative ultrasound surveillance and percutaneous biopsy.

## PANCREAS RECOVERY AND PREPARATION

Deceased donors aged less than 55 years, without a history of diabetes, pancreatic trauma, or chronic pancreatic disease, can be considered for pancreas donation. Hyperglycemia or hyperamylasemia, hemodynamic instability (including short-lived episodes of cardiac arrest) requiring either low or high doses of vasopressors, and long periods in the intensive care unit are not considered absolute contraindications. The final decision to accept a pancreas is mainly based on the gross appearance of the graft and the vessels, and on the quality of visceral perfusion (33).

The pancreas is usually recovered from heart-beating multiorgan deceased donors. Indeed, en bloc recovery of the liver and the pancreas is currently standard practice both in the United States and in Europe, since it has been clearly shown that both the liver and the pancreas can function well after combined liver–pancreas recovery (33,34). Concurrent recovery of the pancreas and the small bowel for transplantation into different recipients is also possible, but it is technically demanding and can be difficult to organize (33,35).

Different recovery techniques may be employed for the pancreas (36,37). The authors prefer the quick en bloc method that they have described (33). Potential advantages of this method include ease and a safe donor operation regardless of operative conditions, and standardization of both in vivo maneuvers and ex vivo maneuvers (33).

Back-table preparation of the pancreas graft is performed according to standard methods, but attention should be paid to cut the peripheral branches of the donor iliac Y-graft as short as possible. Indeed, placement of the pancreas graft in the right paracolic region usually requires the use of a short arterial graft (Fig. 1) in order to avoid the kinking of the peripheral branches, which is more likely to occur with the splenic artery. No venous extension graft is necessary.

Before packing the pancreas graft for cold storage, as shown in Figure 2, a large bore Foley catheter is inserted to the level of the second portion of the duodenum. The catheter is used to create a closed drainage system that is utilized, after graft reperfusion, to empty the duodenum; this prevents duodenal swelling or contamination of the surgical field following duodenal venting.

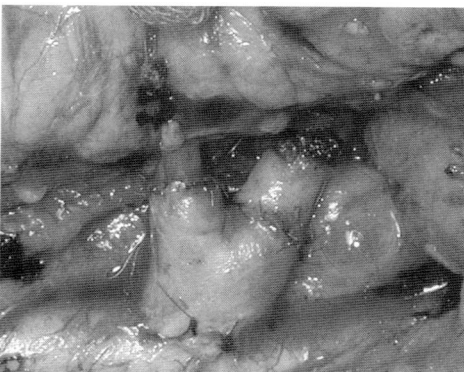

**Figure 1** Intraoperative picture showing the short arterial Y-graft.

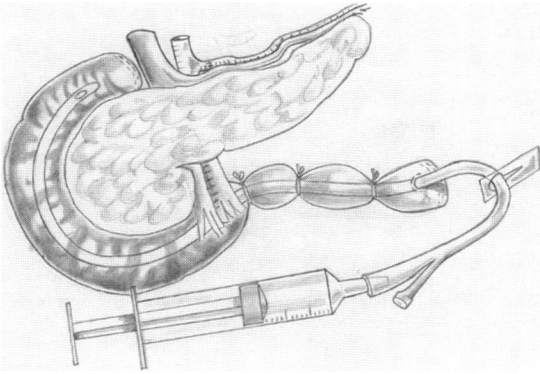

**Figure 2** A Foley catheter is inserted into the first jejunal loop and threaded back to the second duodenal portion.

## TRANSPLANT PROCEDURE

The recipient is anesthetized in the supine position and the entire abdomen is prepped and draped. A midline incision is made from the xiphoid process and carried down to near the pubis. The right colon is fully mobilized and the superior mesenteric vein and its main tributary branches are approached from the right posterolateral side (Fig. 3) according to the same steps commonly followed for proximal venous control in pancreatoduodenectomy (38). A Kocher maneuver, however, is not performed, and dissection is carried out exclusively along the anterior surface of the head of the pancreas and the third duodenal portion until the superior mesenteric vein is encountered and dissected off. The superior mesenteric vein is mobilized from just below the neck of the pancreas down to the mesenteric root, at the point where two large veins merge to give rise to the main trunk of the superior mesenteric vein itself (Fig. 4). The ileocolic vein and the first jejunal vein are also mobilized in preparation for cross-clamping. Additional venous tributaries, such as the middle colic vein, the right gastroepiploic vein, and the anterior superior pancreaticoduodenal vein, may be ligated and divided to achieve complete mobilization of the superior mesenteric vein. The ileocolic artery may course medially to the superior mesenteric vein (Fig. 5A), although in most patients it is found in a lateral position (Fig. 5B). Whether a lateral ileocolic artery complicates the

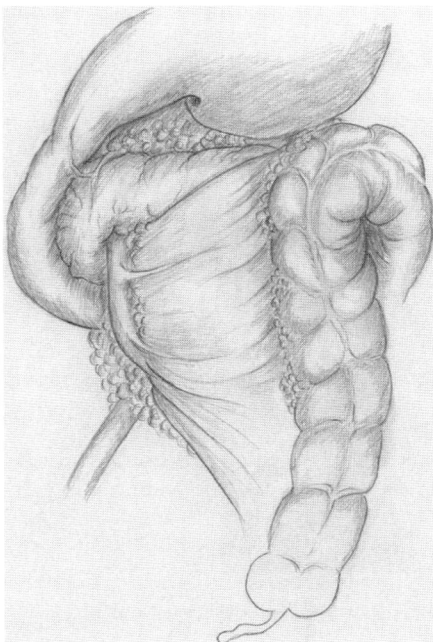

**Figure 3** Mobilization of the right colon allows simultaneous access to the superior mesenteric vein and the common iliac artery.

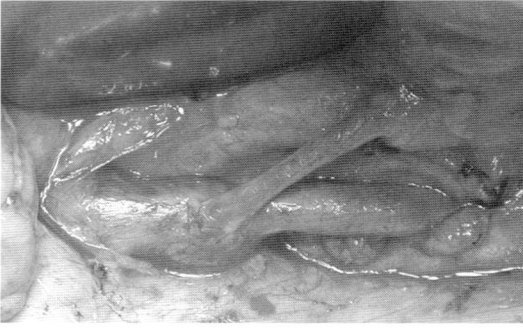

**Figure 4** Superior mesenteric vein mobilized and ready for anastomosis.

construction of the venous anastomosis depends on the vascular anatomy of each recipient. Usually, after wide mobilization, the ileocolic artery can be displaced caudally, thus clearing the lateral aspect of the superior mesenteric vein. However, in a minority of patients, division of the ileocolic artery may be necessary to improve exposure of the anastomotic site.

The common iliac artery is approached next and is encircled as close to its origin as possible, while sparing the parasympathetic plexus. All lymphatics are carefully ligated both in the retroperitoneum and in the mesenteric root.

The pancreas graft is then unpacked and examined to determine if the portal vein needs to be trimmed and to decide the length of the venotomy in the recipient. Following systematic heparinization with 5000 units of heparin, the superior mesenteric vein and its tributary branches are clamped individually. A longitudinal venotomy, matching the diameter of donor portal vein, is then made on the right lateral aspect of the superior mesenteric vein without "unroofing" the vessel. The venous anastomosis is created end-to-side between donor portal vein and recipient superior mesenteric vein using 6-0 polypropylene and employing a fine suture technique with multiple small suture bites. Construction of venous anastomosis begins with placement of stay sutures at the two corners of the anastomosis. Each half of the suture in the proximal corner of the anastomosis is run around half of the circumference of the anastomosis. The posterior half is first brought inside the lumen of the donor's portal vein and then the continuous suture is performed from within the lumen. After removing the stay suture placed at the right corner, the second half of the suture is run over and over on the anterior wall, thus completing the anastomosis. The two half running sutures are then tied with a growth factor, the donor portal vein is clamped, the blood flow through the superior mesenteric vein is restored, and the anastomosis is checked for bleeding sites. The arterial anastomosis is then created end-to-side between donor's Y iliac graft and recipient's common iliac artery using two half-running sutures of 5-0 polypropylene (Fig. 6). The arterial anastomosis is usually created according to the same technique described for the venous anastomosis. However, in obese patients with deep artery, the "parachute" suture technique

**(A)**                                   **(B)**

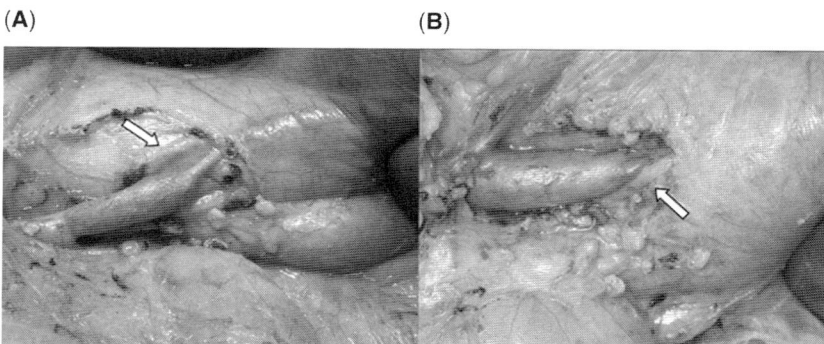

**Figure 5** (**A**) Ileocolic artery (*arrow*) running medially to the superior mesenteric vein. (**B**) Ileocolic artery (*arrow*) running laterally to the superior mesenteric vein.

(A)                                              (B)

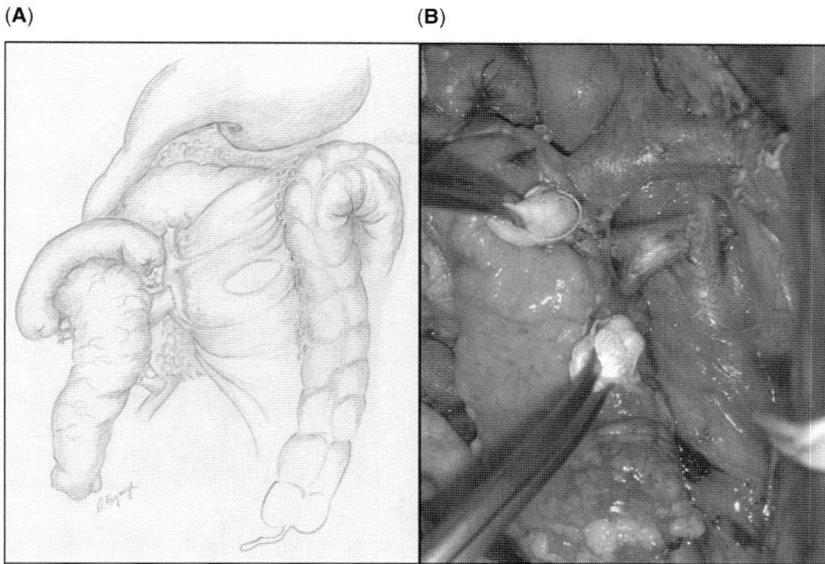

**Figure 6** (**A**) Retroperitoneal pancreas transplantation with portal-enteric drainage. Pancreas graft shown after reperfusion. (**B**) Intraoperative picture of a pancreas graft after reperfusion. Note how short the arterial graft was trimmed.

may be more convenient: several bites are placed around the proximal corner of the anastomosis with a double-armed polypropylene suture, before the donor Y arterial graft is lowered in place; the anastomosis is then completed and only one knot is required.

Following graft reperfusion, hemostasis is carefully achieved by selective ligature and fine polypropylene sutures. As a part of prophylaxis for graft thrombosis, heparin is not reversed. When hemostasis is judged to be adequate, a Roux-en-Y jejunal limb is prepared for drainage of exocrine secretions. The distal end-to-side jejuno-jejunostomy is performed first, and hemostasis is further verified before constructing the duodeno-jejunostomy. The Roux-en-Y limb is then brought to the right flank region through a window made in an avascular portion of the right colon mesentery. As the jejunal limb crosses the superior mesenteric vein proximal to the venous anastomosis, care is taken to avoid any tension on the mesentery. The Foley catheter placed in the duodenum during back-table preparation of the pancreas graft and used to drain pancreatic secretions after reperfusion is now removed. A side-to-side duodeno-jejunostomy is then performed with an outer layer of interrupted nonadsorbable sutures and an inner running layer of 3-0 adsorbable sutures (Fig. 7A). Closed suction drains are then placed around the pancreas and the colon is brought back to its native position, thus completely covering the pancreas and making it a retroperitoneal organ (Fig. 7B).

As the appendix comes to lie close to the tail of the pancreas graft at the end of the procedure, an elective appendectomy is routinely performed. This facilitates the differential diagnosis in patients who develop abdominal pain in the right flank/iliac fossa region after the transplant. Before closure, the abdomen is copiously irrigated with warm saline solution containing amphotericin (10 mg/1000 mL).

## POSTOPERATIVE MANAGEMENT/GRAFT SURVEILLANCE

All patients are managed with a central line and receive a continuous insulin infusion during the procedure. The infusion pump is stopped when blood glucose levels are less than 150 mg/dL. Prophylactic infusions of somatostatin (6 mg/day) and gabexate mesilate (1 g/day) are started before graft reperfusion and maintained during the early posttransplant period until complete normalization of pancreatic enzymes.

All patients receive antibiotic prophylaxis for one week, consisting of cefuroxime 1 g two times a day, and single-strength sulfamethoxazole–trimethoprim for six months. Antifungal

(A)                                                    (B)

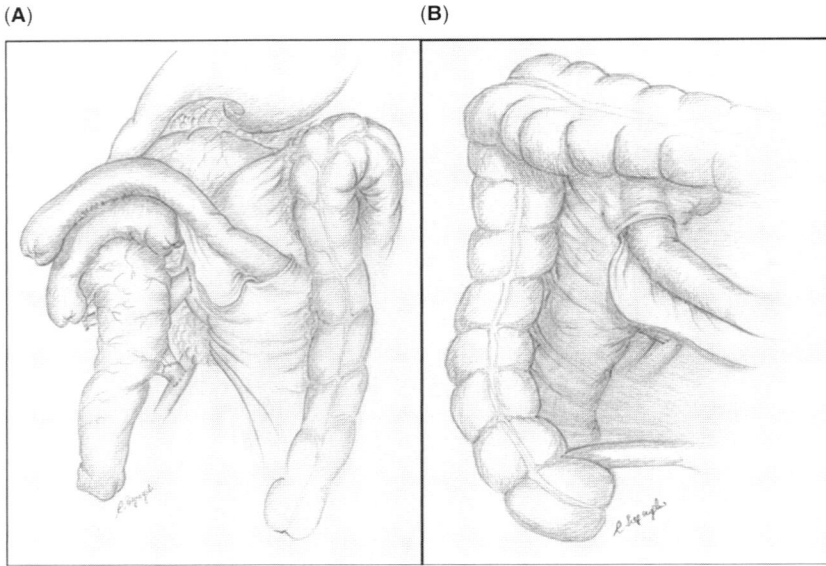

**Figure 7** (**A**) Side-to-side duodeno-jejunostomy. Note that the Roux-en Y loop is constructed intentionally long in order to avoid compression of the superior mesenteric vein distally to the venous anastomosis. (**B**) Right colon brought back to its native position. The pancreas graft is barely visible behind the tight colon mesentery and lies in a retroperitoneal position.

prophylaxis includes oral fluconazole 400 mg/day for two weeks. Antiviral prophylaxis with ganciclovir is employed in all recipients, but dosages and length of administration are individualized based on the donor and recipient antibody status.

Pancreas–kidney patients receive antithrombotic prophylaxis with subcutaneous calcium heparin (0.2 cm³ three times a day) during the first posttransplant week and from posttransplant day three with oral aspirin (100 mg/day) for six months. Recipients of solitary pancreas grafts receive heparin infusion, either an immediate full dose (15 U/kg/hr) or a progressively increasing dose (300 U/hr on transplantation day up to 500 U/hr on posttransplantation day five), followed by oral warfarin sodium for six months.

Intra-abdominal drains are removed as early as possible in accordance with daily measured output and amylase concentration. Duplex ultrasonography is performed daily during the first posttransplant week, regardless of endocrine pancreas graft function, and whenever clinically indicated thereafter.

## RESULTS

Retroperitoneal pancreas transplantation with portal-enteric drainage was successfully accomplished in all but three patients (110/113; 97.3%), including three recipients (2.7%) whose body mass index exceeded 30 kg/m². Systemic venous drainage was utilized in three recipients due to morbid obesity (body mass index >35 kg/m²) ($n = 2$) and the incidental intraoperative diagnosis of chronic liver disease ($n = 1$). Indeed, despite normal liver enzymes and function, one patient was diagnosed with liver cirrhosis at the time of initial surgical exploration. Since the patient was already committed to immunosuppression, because of a previous kidney transplant, we decided to proceed with the pancreas transplant, but opted against venous drainage of the graft into the portal system.

The approach to the superior mesenteric vein from the right retroperitoneal aspect was not associated with any specific difficulty or complication, even in overweight (body mass index 25–30 kg/m²) or obese (body mass index 30–35 kg/m²) patients with a thickened mesentery. In addition, the arterial anastomosis was not found to be more technically demanding compared to pancreas transplantation with systemic venous drainage. More specifically, the length of the donor Y-graft was always sufficient to reach the recipient's common iliac artery easily, despite keeping both the common limb and the peripheral branches intentionally as short as possible (Figs. 1 and 6B).

Three recipients underwent pancreas transplantation with portal enteric drainage despite previous islet cell infusions into the portal vein. In these recipients, before attempting any dissection, portal pressure was measured through cannulation of a small mesenteric vein. Interestingly enough, portal pressure was within the normal range in all patients despite previous multiple infusions of islets in all cases (range: 2–3). No primary pancreas nonfunction occurred; one patient (0.9%) developed delayed endocrine graft function (39).

After a minimum follow-up period of four months (mean $21.2 \pm 11.9$ months) 15 recipients (13.6%) required a relaparotomy. Indications for relaparotomy were bleeding ($n=5$), need for allograft pancreatectomy because of either hyperacute/accelerated rejection ($n=3$) or vein thrombosis ($n=2$), leak from the duodeno-jejunal anastomosis ($n=2$), bleeding and vein thrombectomy ($n=1$), and small bowel occlusion from a bezoar ($n=1$). One patient had a negative relaparotomy. No patient underwent multiple relaparotomies, and the mean number of relaparotomies per patient was 0.14. The relaparotomy rate was 7.1% for simultaneous pancreas–kidney transplant (SPK) (0.07 relaparotomies per patient) and 17.6% (0.18 relaparotomies per patient) for solitary pancreas transplant recipients (SPTx). Excluding the patients diagnosed with either irreversible early acute rejection or complete vein thrombosis, no recipient lost the graft following relaparotomy. The mean interval between pancreas transplantation and relaparotomy was $5.7 \pm 2.3$ days for SPK and $13.4 \pm 20.5$ days for SPTx. The leading cause for relaparotomy was bleeding. Most patients with hemorrhage (5/6; 83.3%) were recipients of SPTx treated with heparin infusions. At relaparotomy, no specific bleeding site was identified, but we felt that evacuation of peripancreatic hematoma was useful to prevent subsequent infection. Finally, it is important to underscore that aggressive prophylaxis for thrombosis, despite necessitating six relaparotomies, reduced the incidence of graft loss due to thrombosis to 1.8% (2/110).

Nonocclusive thrombi were identified in the splenic vein by duplex ultrasonography and confirmed at CT scan in six patients (5.4%). All of these recipients were anticoagulated at therapeutic dosages with heparin and then were treated with warfarin sodium for six months. Two recipients were also treated with urokinase infusion into the Y-iliac graft; one of them bled and underwent concurrent evacuation of peripancreatic hematoma and venous thrombectomy. None of these patients lost graft function.

Ten patients (9.1%) developed peripancreatic fluid collections, all successfully treated by observation ($n=7$) or percutaneous drainage ($n=3$). Enteric bleeding occurred in eight recipients (7.3%). None of them died, none lost graft function, and all but two were treated nonoperatively.

Overall, hospital stay averaged 25.9 days ($\pm 14.0$ days) and the 30-day readmission rate was 10.9%. The mean number of readmissions per patient was 0.11 ($\pm 0.03$). The corresponding

(A)                                                (B)

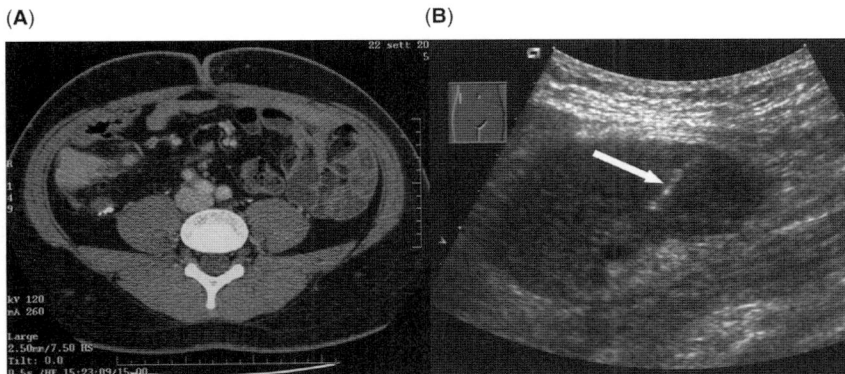

Figure 8   (A) Computed tomography scan demonstrating a pancreas graft relegated in the retroperitoneum. Lack of interposing bowel loops improves graft accessibility for percutaneous biopsy. (B) Ultrasound-guided percutaneous biopsy of a pancreas graft. Arrow points at needle.

**Table 1**  Results of Pancreas Transplantation with Portal-Enteric Drainage and Intraperitoneal Graft Placement

| First author | Gaber | Newell | Stratta | Reddy | Cattral | Stratta | Stratta | Stratta |
|---|---|---|---|---|---|---|---|---|
| Reference | 14 | 18 | 29 | 28 | 17 | 40 | 19 | 15 |
| Year | 1995 | 1996 | 1999 | 1999 | 2000 | 2001 | 2001 | 2003 |
| Number of transplants | 19 | 12 | 28 | 83 | 20 | 126 | 27 | 67 |
| Type of transplant | SPK | SPK | SPK | 65 SPK  18 SPT | SPK | 90 SPK  36 SPT | SPK | SPK |
| Mean cold ischemia (hr) | NA | NA | 12.9 | NA | 10.5 | 13 | 15.3 | 15.4 |
| 1-year patient survival (%) | 88% | 83% | 86% | 84%[a] and 94%[b] | 100% | 89% | 96% | 97% |
| 1-year pancreas survival (%) | 71% | 75% | 82% | 48%[a] and 89%[b] | 100% | 76% | 85% | 82% |
| Relaparotomy (%) | NA | NA | 25% | 38% | 20% | 37% | 26% | 28% |
| Multiple relaparotomies (%) | NA | NA | 11% | 14% | 0 | NA | 0 | NA |
| Relaparotomy per patient ($n$) | NA | NA | 0.4 | 0.7 | 0.2 | 0.4 | 0.2 | 0.3 |
| Mean length of hospital stay (days) | NA | 11.9 | 12.5 | NA | 13 | NA | 12.8 | 12.5 |
| Mean number of readmissions per patient ($n$) | NA | NA | 2.9 | NA | 1.2 | NA | 2.2 | 2.5 |
| Acute rejection (%) | NA | 67% | 21% | NA | 15% | 44% | 33% | 28% |
| Graft loss due to thrombosis (%) | 10.5% | 0 | 3.5% | 14% | 10% | 11% | 4% | 7.5% |
| Enteric bleeding (requiring transfusion) (%) | 5.2% | NA | NA | 1.5% | 10% | NA | NA | NA |

[a]With surgical complications.
[b]Without surgical complications.
*Abbreviation:* NA, not available.

figures for SPK and SPTx were 27.8 (±15.0 days), 9.5%, 0.09 (±0.03) and 24.6 (±13.3 days), 11.8%, 0.12 (±0.03), respectively.

Overall, the acute pancreas rejection rate was 6.3% (7/110); all rejections occurred in SPTx (7/68; 10.3%) recipients. Percutaneous pancreas biopsy was planned and successfully performed in three recipients under ultrasound guidance. The direct apposition of the body-tail of the graft to the lateral abdominal wall along the right retroperitoneal space greatly facilitated performance of percutaneous biopsy (Fig. 8A, B). No biopsy-related complication was observed.

Two patients died with functioning grafts, one from sudden cardiac death and the other from bone marrow aplasia, respectively. Eight pancreases were lost to acute rejection ($n = 3$), early thrombosis ($n = 2$), chronic rejection ($n = 2$), and late (six months) arterial thrombosis ($n = 1$), respectively. Overall one-year patient and pancreas survival rates were 98.1% and 90.7%, respectively; for SPK, they were 97.6% and 97.6%, and for SPTx, they were 98.4% and 86.0%.

## CONCLUSIONS

Our results compare favorably with other series of pancreas transplantation with portal-enteric drainage (Table 1) (14,15,17–19,28,29,40). Overall, three grafts were lost due to thrombosis (2.7%), and the relaparotomy rate was 13.6%. Interestingly, no patient required more than one relaparotomy, and none died after repeat surgery. Moreover, excluding the three cases of allograft pancreatectomy for irreversible rejection, no patient lost pancreas graft or kidney graft after repeat surgery. In our view, the good patient and graft survival after relaparotomy can be explained by meticulous postoperative care and early surgical re-exploration in all patients suspected to have surgical complications. Although this policy is not new to pancreas transplantation, as recently underscored by Humar et al. (41), it is noteworthy that this approach did not result in a high relaparotomy rate. Early reintervention may have avoided multiple relaparotomies, which have been reported to occur between 6% and 14% following pancreas transplantation with portal-enteric drainage (14,15,17–19,28,29,40). In our experience, most relaparotomies were for bleeding from vigorous anticoagulation, while only a minority was required because of actual surgical complications. Although we acknowledge that surgical complications can result from any of the multiple technical pitfalls associated with graft recovery, preservation, and transplantation, and that they may also be related to the multiple biological factors of the donor or the recipient, we also believe that retroperitoneal pancreas transplantation with portal-enteric drainage does not increase the surgical risk associated with pancreas transplantation.

We conclude that retroperitoneal pancreas transplantation with portal-enteric drainage has distinct technical advantages over the classic methods that have been based on intraperitoneal graft placement, and does not seem to incur any additional risks. We suggest that this technique should be included in the repertoire of pancreas transplant surgeons.

## REFERENCES

1. Kelly WD, Lillehei RC, Merkel FK, Iezuki Y, Goetz FC. Allotransplantation of the pancreas and duodenum along with the kidney in diabetic nephropathy. Surgery 1967; 61:827–837.
2. Stratta RJ, Taylor RJ, Gill IS. Pancreas transplantation: a managed cure approach to diabetes. Curr Probl Surg 1996; 33:709–808.
3. Calne RY. Paratopic segmental pancreas grafting: a technique with portal venous drainage. Lancet 1984; 1:595–597.
4. Gil Vernet JM, Fernandez-Cruz L, Caralps A, Andreu J, Figuerola D. Whole organ and pancreaticoureterostomy in clinical pancreas transplantation. Transplant Proc 1985; 17:2019–2022.
5. Muhlbacher F, Gnant MF, Auinger M, et al. Pancreatic venous drainage to the portal vein: a new method in human pancreas transplantation. Transplant Proc 1990; 22:636–637.
6. Ishitani MB, Rosenlof LK, Hanks JB, Pruett TL. Successful paratopic pancreas transplantation: a report of three cases with venous portal drainage and enteric exocrine drainage. Clin Transplant 1993; 7:28–32.
7. Rosenlof LK, Earnhardt RC, Pruett TL, et al. Pancreas transplantation. An initial experience with systemic and portal drainage of pancreatic allografts. Ann Surg 1992; 215:586–597.

8.  Sutherland DE, Goetz FC, Moudry KC, Abouna GM, Najarian JS. Use of recipient mesenteric vessels for revascularization of segmental pancreas grafts: technical and metabolic considerations. Transplant Proc 1987; 19:2300–2304.
9.  Gaber AO, Shokouh-Amiri H, Grewal HP, Britt LG. A technique for portal pancreatic transplantation with enteric drainage. Surg Gyncol Obstet 1993; 177:417–419.
10. Tyden G, Wilczek H, Lundgren G, et al. Experience with 21 intraperitoneal segmental pancreatic transplants with enteric and gastric exocrine diversion in humans. Transplant Proc 1985; 17:331–335.
11. Shokouh-Amiri MH, Gaber AO, Gaber LW, et al. Pancreas transplantation with portal venous drainage and enteric exocrine diversion. Transplant Proc 1992; 24:776–777.
12. Shokouh-Amiri MH, Rahimi-Saber S, Andersen HO, Jensen SL. Pancreas autotransplantation in pig with systemic or portal venous drainage. Effect on the endocrine pancreatic function after transplantation. Transplantation 1996; 61:1004–1009.
13. Shokouh-Amiri MH, Falholt K, Holst JJ, Rahimi-Saber S, Orbaek Andersen H, Jensen SL. Pancreas endocrine function in pigs after segmental pancreas autotransplantation with either systemic or portal venous drainage. Transplant Proc 1992; 24:799–800.
14. Gaber AO, Shokouh-Amiri MH, Hathaway DK, et al. Results of pancreas transplantation with portal venous and enteric drainage. Ann Surg 1995; 221:613–624.
15. Stratta RJ, Shokouh-Amiri MH, Egidi MF, et al. Long-term experience with simultaneous kidney–pancreas transplantation with portal-enteric drainage and tacrolimus/mycophenolate mofetil-based immunosuppression. Clin Transplant 2003; 17:69–77.
16. Stratta RJ, Gaber AO, Shokouh-Amiri MH, et al. A prospective comparison of systemic-bladder versus portal-enteric drainage in vascularized pancreas transplantation. Surgery 2000; 127:217–226.
17. Cattral MS, Bigam DL, Hemming AW, et al. Portal venous and enteric exocrine drainage versus systemic venous and bladder exocrine drainage of pancreas grafts: clinical outcome of 40 consecutive transplant recipients. Ann Surg 2000; 232:688–695.
18. Newell KA, Bruce DS, Cronin DC, et al. Comparison of pancreas transplantation with portal venous and enteric exocrine drainage to the standard technique utilizing bladder drainage of exocrine secretions. Transplantation 1996; 62:1353–1356.
19. Stratta RJ, Shokouh-Amiri MH, Egidi MF, et al. A prospective comparison of simultaneous kidney–pancreas transplantation with systemic-enteric versus portal-enteric drainage. Ann Surg 2001; 233:740–751.
20. Gaber AO, Shokouh-Amiri H, Hathaway DK, et al. Pancreas transplantation with portal venous and enteric drainage eliminates hyperinsulinemia and reduces postoperative complications. Transplant Proc 1993; 25:1176–1178.
21. Coppelli A, Giannarelli R, Mariotti R, et al. Pancreas transplant alone determines early improvement of cardiovascular risk factors and cardiac function in type 1 diabetic patients. Transplantation 2003; 76:974–976.
22. Carpentier A, Patterson BW, Uffelman KD, et al. The effect of systemic versus portal insulin delivery in pancreas transplantation on insulin action and VLDL metabolism. Diabetes 2001; 50:1402–1413.
23. Bagdade JD, Ritter MC, Kitabchi AE, et al. Differing effects of pancreas-kidney transplantation with systemic versus portal venous drainage on cholesteryl ester transfer in IDDM subjects. Diabet Care 1996; 19:1108–1112.
24. Philosophe B, Farney AC, Schweitzer EJ, et al. Superiority of portal venous drainage over systemic venous drainage in pancreas transplantation: a retrospective study. Ann Surg 2001; 234:689–696.
25. Nymann T, Hathaway DK, Shokouh-Amiri MH, et al. Patterns of acute rejection in portal-enteric versus systemic-bladder pancreas–kidney transplantation. Clin Transplant 1998; 12:175–183.
26. International Pancreas Transplant registry: annual report 2002. Newsletter 2003: 15(1): 5–20.
27. Bigam DL, Hemming AW, Sanabria JR, Cattral MS. Innominate artery interposition graft simplifies the portal venous drainage method of pancreas transplantation. Transplantation 1999; 68:314–315.
28. Reddy KS, Stratta RJ, Shokouh-Amiri MH, Alloway R, Egidi MF, Gaber AO. Surgical complications after pancreas transplantation with portal-enteric drainage. J Am Coll Surg 1999; 189:305–313.
29. Stratta RJ, Gaber AO, Shokouh-Amiri MH, et al. Evolution in pancreas transplantation techniques: simultaneous kidney–pancreas transplantation using portal-enteric drainage without antilymphocyte induction. Ann Surg 1999; 229:701–712.
30. Ozaki CF, Stratta RJ, Taylor RJ, Langnas AN, Bynon JS, Shaw BW Jr. Surgical complications in solitary pancreas and combined pancreas–kidney transplantations. Am J Surg 1992; 164:546–551.
31. Brayman KL, Weber M, Sutherland DER. In: Trede M, Carter DC, eds. Pancreatic and Islet Cell Transplantation. New York: Churchill Livingstone, 1997:637–665.
32. Boggi U, Vistoli F, Del Chiaro M, et al. Retroperitoneal pancreas transplantation with portal-enteric drainage. Transplant Proc 2004; 36:571–574.
33. Boggi U, Vistoli F, Del Chiaro M, et al. A simplified technique for the en-bloc procurement of abdominal organs that is suitable for pancreas and small bowel transplantation. Surgery 2004; 135:629–641.
34. Dunn DL, Morel P, Schlumpf R, et al. Evidence that combined procurement of pancreas and liver grafts does not affect transplant outcome. Transplantation 1991; 51:150–157.
35. Abu-Elmagd K, Fung J, Bueno J, et al. Logistics and technique for procurement of intestinal, pancreatic and hepatic grafts from the same donor. Ann Surg 2000; 232:680–687.

36. Nghiem DD. A technique for concomitant whole duodenopancreatectomy and hepatectomy for transplantation in the multiple organ donor. Surg Gynecol Obstet 1989; 169:257–258.
37. Bandlien KO, Mittal VK, Toledo-Pereyra LH. Procurement and workbench procedures in preparation of pancreatic allografts. Factors essential for a successful pancreas transplant. Am Surg 1988; 54:578–581.
38. Jones L, Russel C, Mosca F, et al. Standard Kausch–Whipple pancreatoduodenectomy. Dig Surg 1999; 16:297–304.
39. Troppmann C, Gruessner AC, Papalois BE, et al. Delayed endocrine pancreas graft function after simultaneous pancreas–kidney transplantation. Incidence, risk factors and impact on long-term outcome. Transplantation 1996; 61:1323–1330.
40. Stratta RJ, Gaber AO, Shokouh-Amiri MH, et al. A 9-year experience with 126 pancreas transplants with portal-enteric drainage. Transplant Proc 2001; 33:1687–1688.
41. Humar A, Kandaswamy R, Granger D, Gruessner RW, Gruessner AC, Sutherland DE. Decreased surgical risks of pancreas transplantation in the modern era. Ann Surg 2000; 231:269–275.

# Index